Golden Notes in
Surgery

Golden Notes in
Surgery

As per Competency Based Medical Education Curriculum (NMC)

K Jayarama Shenoy MBBS MS (Surgery)
Professor and *Former* Head of Surgery
Kasturba Medical College, Mangaluru
Karnataka, India

Forewords
Lt Gen Dr M D Venkatesh
Dr M Vijayakumar
Dr K Ramesh Reddy

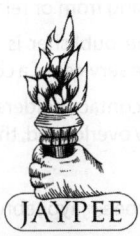

JAYPEE BROTHERS MEDICAL PUBLISHERS
The Health Sciences Publisher
New Delhi | London

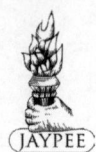 **Jaypee Brothers Medical Publishers (P) Ltd**

Headquarters
Jaypee Brothers Medical Publishers (P) Ltd
EMCA House, 23/23-B
Ansari Road, Daryaganj
New Delhi 110 002, India
Landline: +91-11-23272143, +91-11-23272703
+91-11-23282021, +91-11-23245672
Email: jaypee@jaypeebrothers.com

Corporate Office
Jaypee Brothers Medical Publishers (P) Ltd
4838/24, Ansari Road, Daryaganj
New Delhi 110 002, India
Phone: +91-11-43574357
Fax: +91-11-43574314
Email: jaypee@jaypeebrothers.com

Overseas Office
J.P. Medical Ltd
83 Victoria Street, London
SW1H 0HW (UK)
Phone: +44 20 3170 8910
Fax: +44 (0)20 3008 6180
Email: info@jpmedpub.com

Website: www.jaypeebrothers.com
Website: www.jaypeedigital.com

© 2023, Jaypee Brothers Medical Publishers

The views and opinions expressed in this book are solely those of the original contributor(s)/author(s) and do not necessarily represent those of editor(s) and publisher of the book.

All rights reserved. No part of this publication may be reproduced, stored or transmitted in any form or by any means, electronic, mechanical, photocopying, recording or otherwise, without the prior permission in writing of the publishers.

All brand names and product names used in this book are trade names, service marks, trademarks or registered trademarks of their respective owners. The publisher is not associated with any product or vendor mentioned in this book.

Medical knowledge and practice change constantly. This book is designed to provide accurate, authoritative information about the subject matter in question. However, readers are advised to check the most current information available on the current treatment and procedures included and check information from the manufacturer of each product to be administered, to verify the recommended dose, formula, method and duration of administration, adverse effects and contraindications. It is the responsibility of the practitioner to take all appropriate safety precautions. Neither the publisher nor the author(s)/editor(s) assume any liability for any injury and/or damage to persons or property arising from or related to use of material in this book.

This book is sold on the understanding that the publisher is not engaged in providing professional medical services. If such advice or services are required, the services of a competent medical professional should be sought.

Every effort has been made where necessary to contact holders of copyright to obtain permission to reproduce copyright material. If any have been inadvertently overlooked, the publisher will be pleased to make the necessary arrangements at the first opportunity.

Inquiries for bulk sales may be solicited at: jaypee@jaypeebrothers.com

Golden Notes in Surgery

First Edition: **2023**

ISBN: 978-93-5465-140-3

Printed at India at Rajkamal Electric Press, Kundli, Haryana.

Dedicated to

My Mother
Late **Lakshmidevi Shenoy**
and
My Father
Late **Kudige Umanath Shenoy**

Foreword

It gives me great pleasure to be writing the Foreword for the book titled *Golden Notes in Surgery* authored by my dear friend Dr K Jayarama Shenoy, Professor of Surgery, Kasturba Medical College, Mangaluru, Karnataka, India. This handbook is primarily authored keeping in mind the Competency-based medical education (CBME) for undergraduate education. This book is intended to benefit final MBBS students and those preparing for the proposed National Exit Test (NExT). Dr Shenoy has used his over four decades of teaching and professional experience in Surgery to the fullest in authoring this remarkable work. The book has been written in a lucid and simple language structured in 7 sections and 30 chapters covering 30 essential competencies in Surgery as mandated by NMC for MBBS program. Tables, illustrations, handwritten diagrams and photographs have been very judiciously used to emphasize important points for easy understanding and retention. The contents of this handbook are current, well-researched and up-to-date. I am sure that, this easy to read book will be very helpful students of surgery in their preparation for their examinations. This book can also help Junior Residents/PG Students in Surgery as a quick reference book. I congratulate my friend Dr K Jayarama Shenoy for his committed efforts towards authoring a quality handbook for the benefit of undergraduate and postgraduate medical students. I congratulate the author and the publishers for this remarkable effort and I am sure that this book will be a welcome addition as study material for students of Surgery and should find a place in the undergraduate medical libraries of all medical colleges.

Lt Gen Dr M D Venkatesh
VSM (Rtd)
Vice Chancellor
Manipal Academy of Higher Education
Manipal, Karnataka, India

Foreword

Everyday a new technology is introduced in the field of Medicine and every month a new technique is getting described in the field of surgery. This necessitates an update in every sphere of medical education. The National Medical Council has proposed a new syllabus CBME (Competency-Based Medical Education).

In this background, it is necessary someone with experience of decades of teaching write a book to help the surgical students to understand the subject better. Dr K Jayarama Shenoy has done that job through this book. For a few experienced teachers, it may look redundant. But, as a teacher, I feel a readily readable and easily retainable book is a welcome change, from the routine ones.

With the volumes of the subject increasing day by day, students preparing for the examination may find it difficult to interact and answer the way, it is required in the concerned examination.

The newly appointed young teachers on the other hand, may find this book handy for preparing for taking classes, as per the new CBME syllabus.

In a nutshell, Dr K Jayarama Shenoy has done a wonderful venture and I sincerely hope the student community will benefit from the same.

Dr M Vijayakumar
MBBS DNB MCh FRCS FACS FICS
Vice Chancellor
Yenepoya (Deemed to be University)
Deralakatte, Mangaluru, Karnataka, India

Foreword

"Golden Notes in Surgery"—a book by Dr K Jayaram Shenoy, covering various aspects of surgical topics is a welcome move. My association with Professor Jayaram Shenoy dates back to 1987 when I joined as a postgraduate student of general surgery in Kasturba Medical College, Mangaluru, Karnataka, India. He was as energetic young assistant professor and was always accessible to postgraduate student. He was the first contact to clarify our doubts and discuss various aspects of general surgery. He taught us the basic techniques of surgery. He is a good teacher and I am sure, from his vast experience over last few decades, compiling the various aspects of general surgery as a book, will be of immense help to the MBBS students pursing the CBME syllabus of NMC and also for postgraduate students.

He has included chapters like ethics which every surgeon should read. While taking us through the various chapters of the book, we come across topics in general surgery sharing his experiences. I strongly feel that, general surgery is a subject which can be only learnt from senior surgeons from their experience and complicated situations they faced and how they managed them. Dr K Jayaram Shenoy did exactly that and I congratulate him for this initiative and I am sure this book will be one of the popular referral book of general surgery.

Dr K Ramesh Reddy
MS MCh (Pediatric Surgery)
Director of Medical Education
Government of Telangana
Hyderabad, Telangana, India

Preface

Golden Notes in Surgery is not a substitute for textbooks. It only guides the medical students in learning the concepts of Surgery, as a boost to their preparation for National Exit Examination (NEXT)/final examination in Surgery. It consists of the 30 broad competencies as mandated by the NMC in the CBME syllabus. Briefly outlined are the topics under surgical specialties and subjects like surgical ethics, audit, legal aspects of surgery and hospital waste management, the book contains 191 tables for easy reference and about 125 figures which include my handwritten descriptive diagrams, clinical and operative photographs, all from my personal collection. I have also given 620 typical questions (long and short answer type) against respective topics for benefit of students.

The book is also expected to help the Junior Residents in surgery (MS/DNB) to learn the basic concepts, which they can apply in their academics and clinical practice of surgery.

The junior faculty of surgery in various colleges are expected to find this book useful in preparing their lessons for any class—theory, clinical or short group teaching.

This book presents the lecture notes, I have compiled during my teaching career in surgery since 1984, reasonably updated to contemporary levels, with the help of literature available in public domain, including, but not limited to, the textbooks and manuals enlisted in the bibliography, WHO monograms, various journals and online resources like the Medscape and drjosephtm.blogspot.com.

I have avoided any plagiarism and violation of copyright to the best of my belief.

I hope the book serves its purpose of strengthening the knowledge-based professional learning.

K Jayarama Shenoy

Acknowledgments

I bow to Almighty for blessing me with the strength, courage and vision in conceptualizing, writing and working for the successful launching of this book. I owe my teaching career to Kasturba Medical College, Mangaluru, Karnataka, India and my surgical and clinical skills to my work at Government Wenlock Hospital, Mangaluru.

I am grateful to Dr Ramdas M Pai, Chancellor of Manipal Academy of Higher Education for my appointment as a teacher in surgery under Manipal, Dr HS Ballal, Pro-Chancellor for his unstinted support and help, and Lt Gen Dr MD Venkatesh, Vice-Chancellor for inspiring and boosting my morale.

I am indebted to Dr M Vijayakumar, Vice-Chancellor, Yenepoya (Deemed to be University), Deralakatte, Mangalore and Dr K Ramesh Reddy, Director of Medical Education, Government of Telangana State, for encouraging and supporting this academic work.

I thank, Dr Dilip Nayak, Pro-Vice Chancellor, MAHE; Dr M Venkatraya Prabhu, *Former* Pro-Vice-Chancellor, MAHE, Manipal; Dr Unnikrishnan, Dean and Dr Ashfaque Mohammed, Head of Surgery, KMC, Mangaluru for their constant support.

My friend, Dr Ramdas Naik, Professor of Pathology, Yenepoya Medical College was instrumental in inspiring me to write this book during the gloom of the COVID pandemic.

The kind inputs from Dr GG Lakshman Prabhu, Head of Urology, KMC, Mangaluru, for great help in writing chapters on urology.

I cherish with gratitude the skills, knowledge and blessings I got from my mentor Dr TM Joseph (Cardiothoracic Surgeon at Medical Trust Hospital, Kochi—1983-84) and from all my teachers, in particular, Professor SR Kaulgud (Mysore Medical College), Professor CR Ballal and *Late* Professor K Prakash Rao (KMC, Mangaluru).

I shall always be grateful to all my colleagues, students and fraternity at large for their help, cooperation and encouragement.

I am pleased to thank Shri Jitendar P Vij (Group Chairman), Mr Ankit Vij (Managing Director), Mr MS Mani (Group President) and Ms Pooja Bhandari [Director–Production (Books and Journals)] M/s Jaypee Brothers Medical Publishers (P) Ltd, Delhi, for the successful completion and publication of this book. I am obliged to Dr Madhu Choudhury (Director-Educational Publishing) and the team of Jaypee Brothers for their help in ensuring the success of this book.

K Jayarama Shenoy

Contents

Section 1: Basics in Surgery

1. **Metabolic Response to Injury** 3
   - Neuroendocrine Reflex Response: Modulates the Immune Response *4*
   - Homeostatic Response to Injury *5*
   - Diagnosis of SIRS *7*

2. **Shock** 10
   - Shock *10*
   - Septic Shock *15*
   - Other Forms of Shock *15*

3. **Blood and Blood Components** 17
   - Blood Transfusion *17*
   - Indications for Blood Transfusion *19*
   - Massive Blood Transfusion *19*
   - Complications of Blood Transfusion *19*
   - Blood Substitutes *20*
   - Plasma Substitutes *20*

4. **Burns** 21
   - Mechanism of Burns *21*
   - Depth of Burns *21*
   - Types of Burns *22*
   - Classification of Burns Based on Body Surface Area (BSA) *22*
   - Pathophysiology of Burns *22*
   - Assessment of Burns Patient and Management *23*
   - Surgery in Acute Burns *26*
   - Nutrition in Burns *26*
   - Inhalation Burns Injuries *27*
   - Electrical Burns *27*
   - Cold Injuries *28*
   - Frostbite *28*
   - Radiation Burns (Good to Know) *28*
   - Medico-Legal Aspects in Burn Injuries *28*
   - Legalities of the Award of Disability by Various Competent Authorities *30*
   - Impairment and Disability *30*
   - Legal Rights of Burns Survivors for Compensation *30*

5. **Wound Healing and Wound Care** 32
   - Wounds *32*
   - Chronic Wound Healing (Abnormal Healing) *34*

- Assessment and Treatment of Acute Wound 35
- Burst Abdomen 36
- Diabetic Ulcers 37
- Negative Pressure Wound Closure Therapy (NPWT) 38
- Pressure Sores 38
- Hypertrophic Scar 39
- Keloid 39
- Contracture 40
- Skin Grafts 40
- Flaps 40

6. **Surgical Infections and Hand Infections** 45
    - Surgical Infections 45
    - The Decisive Period—The 4 Hours Interval 46
    - Surgical Site Infection 47
    - Microbiology of Surgical Infections 47
    - Antimicrobial Treatment of Surgical Infection 48
    - Short Notes Questions 49
    - Acute Cellulitis and Lymphangitis 51
    - Tetanus 53
    - Gas Gangrene 55

    ### Hand Infections 56
    - Paronychia 56
    - Felon (Terminal Pulp Space Abscess) 56
    - Webspace Abscess (Collar-Button Abscess) 57
    - Acute Suppurative Flexor Tenosynovitis 57
    - Midpalmar Abscess 58
    - Thenar Space 59

Section 2: Essential Topics in General Surgery

7. **Surgical Audit and Research** 63
    - Audit and Service Evaluation 63
    - Audit Cycle 64
    - Steps of Conducting Clinical Research (Must Know) 65
    - Details of Research Study Designs (Good to Know) 66

8. **Ethics in Surgery** 68
    - Informed Consent 69
    - Confidentiality 70
    - Medico-Legal Issues in Surgical Practice 71
    - "On Table Death" and Post-operative Death 72

9. Investigation of the Surgical Patient and Basis of Cancer Therapy 74
- Biopsy 76
- Imaging: In a Surgical Patient 76

10. Pre, Intra and Post-operative Management 82
Perioperative Management 82

11. Anesthesia and Pain Relief, Day Care Surgery and Safe General Surgery 88
Anesthesia and Pain Relief 88

Management of Chronic Pain 94

Day Care Surgery 96

Safe General Surgery 99

12. Nutrition and Fluid Therapy 101
- Physiology of Body Nutrition 101
- Parenteral Nutrition 103
- Types of Fluids Used 105

13. Transplantation 107
- Immunosuppressive Therapy 108
- Transplantation and Immunosuppression 109
- Mechanism of Graft Rejection 109
- Donor Recipient Matching 110
- The Tissue: Typing Laboratory 110
- Organ Transplantation in Practice 111
- Liver Transplantation (Orthotopic) 111
- Graft Dysfunction 112
- Legal, Social and Ethical Issues 113

14. Basic Surgical Skills 115
- Beginning of Antisepsis and Disinfection 115
- Methods of Sterilization and Disinfection 115
- Surgical Approaches 116
- Abdominal Incisions 117
- Drains 118
- Suturing 119

15. Hospital Waste Disposal 120
Disposal of Hospital Waste 121

16. Minimally Invasive Surgery and Bariatric Surgery 124
- Minimally Invasive Surgery 124
- Conversion to Open Surgery 127

***Bariatric Surgery* 129**
- Surgery for Obesity and Diabetes *129*
- Obesity Surgery *130*
- Types of Bariatric Surgery *130*

17. Trauma **133**
- Mass Casualties *135*
- War Surgery: Mass Injuries due to War (Conflicts) *136*
- Damage Control Surgery *136*

***Neurotrauma* 138**
- Pathophysiology of Head Injury *138*
- Types of Hematomas in Head Trauma *139*
- Chronic Subdural Hematoma *139*
- Clinical Assessment of Head Injury *140*
- Principles of Treatment of Head Injury *141*
- Soft Tissue Injuries *144*

***Chest Trauma* 145**
- Pathophysiology of Chest Injuries *145*

Section 3: Skin, Face, Mouth, Oropharynx, Salivary Glands and Jaws

18. Infections and Tumors of Skin **155**
- Anatomy and Function of Skin and Adnexa *155*
- Infections of Skin *156*
- Lipoma *156*
- Neurofibroma *157*
- Hemangioma *157*
- Arteriovenous Fistula (AV Fistula) *159*
- Branham's Bradycardiac Sign *159*
- Benign Lesions of Skin and Subcutaneous Tissue *160*
- Malignant Melanoma of Skin *162*
- Systemic Therapy *165*
- Basal Cell Carcinoma *165*
- Squamous Cell Carcinoma *166*
- Microscopy *166*
- Malignant Soft Tissue Tumors *167*

19. Developmental Anomalies of Face, Tumors and Swellings of Gums and Jaws **170**
- Craniofacial Anomalies: The "Omens" *170*
- Cleft Lip and Palate *170*
- Epulis ("Epulides" Pleural) *172*
- Swellings of Jaw *172*

- Dentigerous Cyst (Follicular Odontome) *173*
- Dental Cyst *173*
- Adamantinoma *174*

20. Oropharyngeal Cancer 175
- Premalignant Lesions of Oral Cavity *175*
- Oral and Oropharyngeal Cancers *176*
- Oral Cancers *179*
- Management of Secondaries in Neck Nodes *182*

21. Salivary Glands 186
- Surgical Anatomy of Salivary Glands *186*
- Disorders of Salivary Glands *187*
- Xerostomia *188*
- Cysts: Ranula *188*
- Submandibular Salivary Gland and Parotid Disorders *188*
- Salivary Calculi *189*
- Acute Sialadenitis and Parotid Abscess *190*
- Acute Bacterial (Suppurative) Parotitis and Parotid Abscess *190*
- Frey's Syndrome (Auriculotemporal Syndrome) *191*
- Sialadenosis (Sialosis) *192*
- Classification of Salivary Gland Tumors *192*
- Primary Malignancies of Salivary Glands *195*
- Treatment of Salivary Malignancies (General) *195*
- Adenoid Cystic Carcinoma (Cylidromatous Carcinoma) *196*
- Acinic Cell Tumor *196*
- Malignancy in a Mixed Tumor *196*
- Minor Salivary Gland Tumors *197*

Section 4: Endocrines and the Breast

22. Thyroid and Parathyroid 201
- Embryology *201*
- Ectopic Thyroid and Thyroglossal Cyst *201*
- Congenital Thyroid Disorders *203*
- Thyroglossal Cyst *204*
- Goiter (Goitre) any Enlargement of Thyroid Gland *205*
- Diffuse Hyperplastic Goiter and Nodular Goiter *206*
- Investigations for Thyroid Disorders *206*
- Toxic Goitre (Toxic Goiter) *207*
- Toxic Multinodular Goiter (Plummer's Disease) *208*
- Treatment of Thyrotoxicosis (Very Important Topic) *211*
- Treatment of Toxic (Multi) Nodular Goiter *211*

- Thyroiditis *212*
- Hashimoto's Thyroiditis *213*
- Thyroidectomy: Definitions *213*
- Thyroid Malignancies *214*
- Differentiated Thyroid Carcinoma *214*
- Medullary Thyroid Carcinoma *215*
- Treatment of Thyroid Cancers *217*
- Management of Discrete (Solitary) Thyroid Nodules *218*

Parathyroids

- Hypoparathyroidism *220*
- Pseudohypoparathyroidism *221*
- Hyperparathyroidism *221*
- Primary Hyperparathyroidism *221*
- Secondary Hyperparathyroidism *223*

23. The Adrenal Glands 225

- Applied Anatomy of Adrenal Glands *225*
- Disorders of Adrenal Glands *226*
- Incidentaloma *226*
- Investigations in any Adrenal Mass *227*
- Primary Hyperaldosteronism *227*
- Cushing's Syndrome *228*
- Adrenogenital Syndrome *228*
- Tumors of Adrenal *229*
- Tumors of Adrenal Medulla *230*
- Neuroblastoma *231*
- Pheochromocytoma *231*

24. The Pancreas - Exocrine and Endocrine 233

- Anatomy of the Pancreas *233*
- Functions of the Pancreas *234*
- Serum Amylase *234*
- Lipase *235*
- Annular Pancreas *236*
- Mucoviscidosis (Cystic Fibrosis—CF) *236*
- Pancreatic Fistula *237*
- Pancreatitis *238*
- Acute Pancreatitis *238*
- Clinical Features of Acute Pancreatitis *239*
- Complications of Acute Pancreatitis *240*
- Management of Acute Pancreatitis *241*
- Local Complications and Management *242*
- Acute Peripancreatic Fluid Collection *242*
- Sterile and Infected Pancreatic Necrosis *242*

- Pseudocyst of Pancreas 243
- Chronic Pancreatitis 244
- Surgery in Chronic Pancreatitis 245
- Pancreatic Tumors: Exocrine and Endocrine 246
- Tumors of the Pancreas 246
- Exocrine Pancreatic Tumors 247
- Pathology 248
- Staging of Pancreatic Cancer 249
- Tumor Node Metastasis Stage 249
- Treatment of Carcinoma of Pancreas 251
- Palliative Surgery 251
- Palliation in Pancreatic Cancer 251
- Endocrine Tumors or Pancreas Neuroectodermal Tumors (PNET) 252
- Diagnosis and Treatment of PNETS 253
- Glucagonoma 253
- Somatostatinoma 253

25. The Breast 255
- Diseases of Breast 255
- Evaluation of Breast Diseases 257
- Mammography 258
- Benign Breast Diseases 259
- Acute Mastitis and Breast Abscess 260
- Aberrations of Normal Differentiation and Involution 262
- Mastalgia 263
- Benign Tumors of the Breast 264
- Treatment Algorithm for Breast Lumps 264
- Galactocele 266
- Carcinoma Breast 267
- Management of Carcinoma Breast 271
- Treatment of Carcinoma Breast 272
- Surgical Operations 272
- Surgery for Axillary Node Metastases 273
- Hormone Therapy 275
- Chemotherapy 275
- Biological Therapy 276
- Treatment of Non-invasive Breast Cancer 277
- Treatment of Invasive Carcinoma of Breast 277
- Treatment of Locally Advanced Breast Cancer 278
- Inflammatory Carcinoma of Breast 279
- Treatment of Metastatic Carcinoma Breast 279
- Recurrent Carcinoma of Breast 279
- Palliation 280
- Rehabilitation in Breast Cancer 280

Section 5: Cardiothoracic and Vascular System

26. Cardiothoracic Surgery 283
- Principles of Cardiopulmonary Bypass 283
- Surgery for Coronary Artery Disease 285
- Echocardiography 285
- Surgery for Valvular Heart Disease 286
- Role of Surgery for Congenital Heart Diseases 288
- Cyanotic Heart Diseases 289
- Acyanotic Heart Diseases 289
- Pleural Effusion 291
- Empyema Thoracis 292
- Empyema Necessitans 292
- Surgery for Medical Conditions 293
- Lung Cysts 293
- Mesothelioma of Pleura 293
- Tumors of the Chest Wall 293
- Lung Tumors 295
- Lung Cancers 296
- Small Cell Lung Cancer (SCLC) (Oat Cell Cancer) 296
- Non-Small Cell Lung Cancer (NSCLC) 297
- Metastatic Lung Cancers 299
- Mediastinal Diseases and Principles of Management 300
- Treatment of Mediastinal Mass Lesions 301
- Thymoma 301

27. Arteries, Veins and Lymphatics 304

Arterial Diseases 304
- Occlusive Arterial Disease of the Extremities 304
- Gangrene 306
- Signs Elicited on Examination of Ischemic Limb 306
- Diagnosis and Management 307
- Treatment of Acute Limb Ischemia (ALI)—Must be Started Immediately 309
- Treatment of Chronic Limb Ischemia 310
- Surgical Treatment 310
- Vasospastic Conditions and Arteritis 311
- Raynaud's Disease and Syndrome 312

Veins 317
- Applied Anatomy of Venous System of Lower Limbs 317
- Venous Pathophysiology 317
- Venous Hypertension and Chronic Venous Insufficiency 318
- Chronic Venous Insufficiency 318
- Deep Venous Thrombosis 322

Lymphatic System 324
- Lymphedema 324
- Classification of Lymphedema 324
- Treatment of Lymphedema 326
- Acute Lymphangitis 327

Lymphomas 328
- Burkitt's Lymphoma 329
- Hodgkin's Lymphoma 329
- Clinical Features of Lymphomas 329
- Investigations and Diagnosis 331
- Treatment of Lymphoma 331
- Tips for Examination of Lymphatic System 332

Section 6: Hernia, Peritoneum and the Digestive Tract

28. Abdominal Cavity, Hernia and Digestive Tract 337

28.1: Hernia, Peritoneum and Retroperitoneum 337

Herniology 337
- Hernia 337
- Etiology and Pathogenesis of Hernia 337
- Principles of Treatment of Hernia 339
- Groin Hernias (Herniae) 339
- Surgical Anatomy of Femoral Hernia 340
- Classification of Groin Hernias 340
- Nyhus' Classification of Groin Hernia 340
- Fruchaud's Myopectineal Orifice 341
- Inguinal Hernia 342
- Sliding Hernia 342
- Tension Repairs 344
- Surgery for Femoral Hernia 345
- Ventral Hernias 346
- Epigastric Hernia 346
- Incisional Hernia 347
- Rare Hernias 348
- Parastomal Hernia 348

The Peritoneum 349
- Peritoneal Cavity 349
- Peritonitis 349
- Acute Peritonitis 349
- Factors Spreading/Deciding Severity 350
- Peritonitis: Clinical Features 351

- Treatment of Acute Peritonitis 352
- Special Types of Peritonitis 352
- Bile Peritonitis 353
- Meconium Peritonitis 353
- Abdominal Tuberculosis 354
- Tuberculous Peritonitis 354
- Complications of Acute Peritonitis and Intraperitoneal Abscess 355
- Localised Intra-abdominal Abscess 355
- Pelvic Abscess 356
- Subphrenic Spaces and Abscess 356
- Subdiaphragmatic Abscess 357
- Mesenteric Cysts 358
- Carcinomatosis Peritonei 359
- Pseudomyxoma Peritonei 360

Retroperitoneum 361

- Retroperitoneal Pathology 361
- Retroperitoneal Tumors 361
- Retroperitoneal Lipoma 361
- Retroperitoneal Sarcoma 361

28.2: Esophagus and Stomach 363

Esophagus 363

- Applied Anatomy of Esophagus 363
- Lower Esophageal Sphincter 364
- Evaluation of Dysphagia 366
- Esophageal Perforations 366
- Esophageal Diverticula 368
- Classification of Esophageal Motility Disorders 368
- Achalasia Cardia 369
- Esophageal Atresia and Tracheoesophageal Fistula 370
- Gastroesophageal Reflux Disease (GERD/GORD) 371
- Esophageal Hiatus Hernia 372
- Carcinoma of Esophagus 375
- Staging Esophageal Carcinoma 376
- Treatment of Esophageal Carcinoma 377
- Surgery for Esophageal Carcinoma 378
- Radiotherapy and Chemotherapy (Combination) 379
- Palliation in Carcinoma Esophagus 379

Stomach 380

- Applied Anatomy and Physiology of Stomach 380
- Nerve Supply to the Stomach 381
- Microscopy of Gastroduodenal Mucosa 381

- Surgical Physiology of Stomach and Duodenum 383
- Investigation of Stomach and Duodenum: Gastric Function Study 384
- Gastrin 385
- Hypergastrinemia 385
- Helicobacter Pylori 385
- Congenital Hypertrophic Pyloric Stenosis 386
- Gastritis 387
- Peptic Ulcer 388
- Pathology of Peptic Ulcers 388
- Complications of Peptic Ulcer 392
- Hematemesis and Melena 393
- Bleeding Peptic Ulcer: Massive Bleed 394
- Pyloric Stenosis in Duodenal Ulcer 395
- Gastric Volvulus 396
- Acute Dilatation of Stomach 397
- Gastric Cancer 397
- Pathology of Gastric Cancer 398
- Treatment of Carcinoma Stomach 401
- Summary of Treatment of Gastric Carcinoma 402
- Palliation in Gastric Cancer 403
- Other Tumors of Stomach 403
- Gastric Lymphoma 404
- Zollinger-Ellison Syndrome 404

28.3: Spleen, Liver, and Biliary Tract 406

Spleen 406

- Spleen 406
- Splenunculi 407
- Splenic Rupture 408
- Splenic Trauma 409

Liver 411

- Anatomy of Liver 411
- Alfa-fetoprotein 412
- Acute Liver Failure 413
- Liver Injuries 413
- Infectious Conditions of the Liver 415
- Amebic Liver Abscess 415
- Pyogenic Abscess 417
- Portal Pyemia 418
- Hydatid Cyst of Liver 418
- Tumors of the Liver 420
- Palliative Therapy for HCC 423

- Metastatic Tumors *423*
- Portal Hypertension (PHT) *424*
- Etiopathogenesis *425*
- Exclude Non-variceal Bleed *427*

Biliary Tract 431
- Applied Anatomy of Biliary System *431*
- Percutaneous Transhepatic Cholangiography *434*
- Intraoperative Imaging Techniques *434*
- Extrahepatic Biliary Atresia *435*
- Choledochal Cyst *436*
- Gallstones (Cholelithiasis) *436*
- Gallstones *436*
- Pathogenesis of Gallstone Formation *437*
- Pathology and Complications of Gallstones *438*
- Chronic Cholecystitis *439*
- Acute Cholecystitis *439*
- Emergency Cholecystectomy *441*
- Choledocholithiasis (Stone in the Bile Duct) *442*
- T-tube Cholangiography *444*
- Biliary Strictures *444*
- Cholangiocarcinoma of Bile Ducts *444*
- Carcinoma of Gallbladder *445*
- Obstructive Jaundice *445*
- Extrahepatic Biliary Obstruction (Surgical Jaundice) *445*
- Courvoisier's Law *447*
- Surgery in Obstructive Jaundice *448*
- Management Algorithm for Surgical Jaundice *449*

28.4: The Intestines *451*
- Anatomy of Small Intestine *451*
- Anatomy of the Large Intestine *452*
- Lymphatic Drainage of the Colon *453*
- Intestinal Diverticulae *454*
- Meckel's Diverticulum *454*
- Crohn's Disease *455*
- Imaging in Crohn's Disease *457*
- Tuberculosis of the Intestines *459*
- Surgical Complications of Typhoid *460*
- Surgical Complications of Roundworm (Ascaris Lumbricoides) *461*
- Pneumatosis Cystoides Intestinalis (PCI) *462*
- Ileal Strictures *462*
- Blind Loop Syndrome *463*
- Enterocutaneous Fistula *463*

- Small Intestinal Tumors 464
- Peutz–Jeghers Syndrome 464
- Malignant Tumors of Small Bowel 464
- Short Gut Syndrome (SGS) 466
- Intestinal Obstruction 468
- Pathophysiology of Intestinal Obstruction (Dynamic) 468
- Strangulated Obstruction 469
- Paralytic Ileus 469
- Clinical Features of Acute Intestinal Obstruction 470
- Simple v/s Strangulated Obstruction 470
- Chronology of Symptoms Related to Level of Obstruction 470
- Paralytic Ileus 472
- Pseudo-obstruction 472
- Colonic Pseudo-obstruction 472
- Volvulus of Intestines 472
- Ileosigmoid Knotting (Compound Volvulus) 474
- Cecal Volvulus 474
- Intussusception 475
- Acute Intussusception 475
- Intestinal Obstruction due to Internal Hernias 478
- Neonatal Intestinal Obstruction 478
- Duodenal Atresia 478
- Midgut Malrotation 479
- Associated Anomalies 20–25% 479
- Meconium Ileus 480
- Chronic Large Bowel Obstruction 481
- Mesenteric Vascular Insufficiency (with/without Occlusion) 481
- Chronic Mesenteric Ischemia (Mesenteric Angina) 482

28.5: The Vermiform Appendix 483
- Diseases of the Vermiform Appendix 483
- Acute Appendicitis 484
- Clinical Signs in Acute Appendicitis 486
- Differential Diagnosis of Acute Appendicitis 486
- Appendix Mass (Appendicular Phlegmon) 488
- Appendix Abscess 488
- Mucocele of Appendix 489
- Pseudomyxoma Peritonei (PMP) 490
- Carcinoid of the Appendix—Syn: Argentaffinoma 490
- Mass in the Right Iliac Fossa 491

The Large Intestine 492
- Chronic Large Bowel Obstruction 492
- Hirschsprung's Disease (Congenital Megacolon) 492

- Diverticulosis Coli 493
- Ulcerative Colitis (UC) 495
- Surgical Manifestations of Intestinal Amebiasis 497
- Ischemic Colitis 498
- Chronic Constipation 499
- Treatment of Chronic Constipation and Coloparesis 500
- Colostomy 500
- Lower Gastrointestinal Bleeding 501
- Surgery in Acute GI Bleed: General Principles 503

Anorectal Surgery 505
- Surgical Anatomy of Rectum 505
- Emryology of Rectum and Anal Canal 505
- Lymphatic Drainage of Rectum and Anal Canal 508
- Puborectalis Sling of Levator Ani is the Key to Continence 510
- Invertogram 513
- Rectal Injuries 514

28.6: Tumors of Colon, Rectum and Anal Canal 515

Tumors of Large Intestine 515
- Tumors of Large Intestine 515
- Hereditary Polyposis Syndromes 516
- Colorectal Cancers 516
- Etiological Factors for Colorectal Carcinoma 517
- Spread of Colorectal Carcinoma 518
- Surgery for Colonic Carcinoma 522
- Carcinoma Rectum 524
- Rectal Lymphatics 524
- Anal Carcinoma 528

Anal Canal 529
- Etiology and Pathogenesis of Anorectal Abscesses 529
- Etiology of Anorectal Abscesses 529
- Pathogenesis: Anorectal Abscess 529
- Anorectal Fistula 530
- Goodsall's Rule 531
- Pelvirectal (Supralevator) Fistula (Extrasphincteric) 533
- Pilonidal Sinus 533
- Sacrococcygeal Pilonidal Sinus 533
- Hemorrhoids 536
- Anal Cushions " Corpus Cavernosum Recti" of Stelzner 537
- Principles of Stapled Hemorrhoidopexy (Syn: MIPH) 539
- Thrombosed External Piles (Short Notes) 539
- Fissure in Ano 540
- Prolapse of the Rectum 542

Section 7: Urogenital Surgery

29. Kidney, Ureters and the Bladder 547

Hematuria, Congenital Disorders, Infections and Obstructive Pathology 548

- Hematuria 548
- Embryology of Urogenital System 550
- Congenital Abnormalities 550
- Ectopic Kidney/Crossed Renal Ectopia 551
- Horseshoe Kidney 551
- Cystic Diseases of the Kidney 551
- Autosomal Dominant Polycystic Kidney Disease 551
- Urinary Tract Infections 553
- Acute Pyelonephritis 553
- Chronic Pyelonephritis 554
- Emphysematous Pyelonephritis 555
- Genitourinary Tuberculosis 556
- Thimble Bladder 558
- Vesico-ureteric Reflux 558
- Lower Urinary Tract Infection and Cystitis 559
- Schistosomiasis (Bilharziasis) of the Bladder 561
- Hydronephrosis 562

Renal Calculi and Renal Tumors 567

- Urolithiasis 567
- Pain, Hematuria and Fever 569
- Extracorporeal Shockwave Lithotripsy 570
- Percutaneous Nephrolithotomy (PCNL) 570
- Staghorn Calculus 571
- Lower Urinary Tract Stones 572
- Upper Tract Transitional Cell Carcinoma 577
- Wilms' Tumor (Nephroblastoma) 578
- Additional Reading - Good to Know 579
- Investigations in Surgery of Urinary Tract 579
- CT Scan—Renal Cysts 579
- Renal Trauma 581

Lower Urinary Tract: Bladder, Prostate and Urethra 582

- Surgical Anatomy of the Bladder 582
- Congenital Defects of the Bladder 583
- Rupture of Bladder: Trauma 583
- Bladder Diverticula 586
- Neoplasms of the Bladder 587
- Carcinoma of the Bladder 587
- Disorders of Prostate 590

- Benign Prostatic Hyperplasia 591
- Acute Prostatitis 594
- Chronic Prostatitis 594
- Prostatic Abscess 594
- Carcinoma Prostate 595
- Anatomy of Urethra 599
- Posterior Urethral Valves 599
- Hypospadias 599
- Injuries to the Male Urethra 600
- Urethral Stricture 601

30. Scrotum, Testis and the Penis 604
- Balanoposthitis 605
- Carcinoma of Penis 606
- Premalignant Conditions 606
- Pathology of Carcinoma of Penis 606
- Staging 607
- Undescended Testis 609
- Vanishing Testis 610
- Acute Epididymo-orchitis 610
- Chronic Epididymitis 611
- Torsion of the Testis 613
- Epididymal Cysts 618
- Pyocele 619
- Staging of Testicular Tumors 621
- Treatment of Testicular Tumor 622
- Tumors of Scrotum 623

Bibliography 625

Index 627

Competency Table

Competency number	Competency: The student should be able to	Suggested teaching/learning method	Suggested assessment method	Section/ Chapter No.	Page No.
	Metabolic Response to Injury				
SU1.1	Describe basic concepts of homeostasis, enumerate the metabolic changes in injury and their mediators	Lecture, bedside clinic, small group discussion	Written/viva voce	1/1	3–5
SU1.2	Describe the factors that affect the metabolic response to injury	Lecture, bedside clinic, small group discussion	Written/viva voce	1/1	5–7
SU1.3	Describe basic concepts of perioperative care	Lecture, bedside clinic, small group discussion	Written/viva voce	1/1	8
	Shock				
SU2.1	Describe pathophysiology of shock, types of shock and principles of resuscitation including fluid replacement and monitoring	Lecture, small group discussion	Written/viva voce	1/2	9-13
SU2.2	Describe the clinical features of shock and its appropriate treatment	Lecture, small group discussion	Written/viva voce	1/2	13-15
SU2.3	Communicate and counsel patients and families about the treatment and prognosis of shock demonstrating empathy and care	DOAP session	Skill assessment	1/2	16
	Blood and Blood Components				
SU3.1	Describe the indications and appropriate use of blood and blood products and complications of blood transfusion	Lecture, small group discussion	Written/viva voce	1/3	17-19
SU3.2	Observe blood transfusions	Small group discussion, DOAP session	Skills assessment/ logbook	1/3	19-20
SU3.3	Counsel patients and family/friends for blood transfusion and blood donation	DOAP session	Skills assessment	1/3	
	Burns				
SU4.1	Elicit document and present history in a case of burns and perform physical examination. Describe pathophysiology of burns	Lecture, small group discussion	Written/ Viva voce	1/4	21-23
SU4.2	Describe clinical features, diagnose, type and extent of burns and plan appropriate treatment	Lecture, small group discussion	Written/ Viva voce	1/4	24-27

Competency number	Competency: The student should be able to	Suggested teaching/learning method	Suggested assessment method	Section/ Chapter No.	Page No.
SU4.3	Discuss the medicolegal aspects in burn injuries	Lecture, small group discussion	Written/ Viva voce	1/4	28-31
SU4.4	Communicate and counsel patients and families on the outcome and rehabilitation demonstrating empathy and care	Small group discussion, role play, skills assessment	Viva voce	1/4	31
Wound Healing and Wound Care					
SU5.1	Describe normal wound healing and factors affecting healing	Lecture, small group discussion	Written/viva voce	1/5	32–34
SU5.2	Elicit, document and present a history in a patient presenting with wounds	Lecture, small group discussion	Written/viva voce	1/5	32–34
SU5.3	Differentiate the various types of wounds, plan and observe management of wounds	Lecture, small group discussion	Written/viva voce	1/5	35-41
SU5.4	Discuss medico legal aspects of wounds	Lecture, small group discussion	Written/viva voce	1/5	42-44
Surgical Infections					
SU6.1	Define and describe the aetiology and pathogenesis of surgical Infections	Lecture, small group discussion	Written/viva voce	1/6	45-56
SU6.2	Enumerate prophylactic and therapeutic antibiotics plan appropriate management	Lecture, small group discussion	Written/viva voce	1/6	56-60
Surgical Audit and Research					
SU7.1	Describe the planning and conduct of surgical audit	Lecture, small group discussion	Written/viva voce	2/7	63-64
SU7.2	Describe the principles and steps of clinical research in general surgery	Lecture, small group discussion	Written/viva voce	2/7	64-67
Ethics					
SU8.1	Describe the principles of ethics as it pertains to general surgery	Lecture, small group discussion	Written/viva voce/skill assessment	2/8	68-71
SU8.2	Demonstrate professionalism and empathy to the patient undergoing general surgery	Lecture, small group discussion, DOAP session	Written/viva voce/skill assessment	2/8	
SU8.3	Discuss medicolegal issues in surgical practice	Lecture, small group discussion	Written/viva voce/skill assessment	2/8	71-73
Investigation of Surgical Patient					
SU9.1	Choose appropriate biochemical, microbiological, pathological, imaging investigations and interpret the investigative data in a surgical patient	Lecture, small group discussion	Written/viva voce	2/9	74-77

Competency number	Competency: The student should be able to	Suggested teaching/learning method	Suggested assessment method	Section/Chapter No.	Page No.
SU9.2	Biological basis for early detection of cancer and multidisciplinary approach in management of cancer	Lecture, small group discussion	Written/viva voce	2/9	77-80
SU9.3	Communicate the results of surgical investigations and counsel the patient appropriately	DOAP session	Skill assessment	2/9	81
Pre, Intra and Postoperative Management					
SU10.1	Describe the principles of perioperative management of common surgical procedures	Lecture, small group discussion	Written/viva voce	2/10	82-87
SU10.2	Describe the steps and obtain informed consent in a simulated environment	DOAP session	Skill assessment/logbook	2/10	
SU10.3	Observe common surgical procedures and assist in minor surgical procedures; Observe emergency lifesaving surgical procedures	DOAP sessions	Logbook	2/10	
SU10.4	Perform basic surgical skills such as First aid including suturing and minor surgical procedures in simulated environment	DOAP session	Skill assessment	2/10	
Anesthesia and Pain Management					
SU11.1	Describe principles of preoperative assessment	Lecture, small group discussion	Written/viva voce	2/11	88
SU11.2	Enumerate the principles of general, regional, and local anaesthesia	Lecture, small group discussion	Written/viva voce	2/11	88-93
SU11.3	Demonstrate maintenance of an airway in a mannequin or equivalent	DOAP session	Skill assessment	2/11	88-93
SU11.4	Enumerate the indications and principles of day care general surgery	Lecture, small group discussion	Written/viva voce	2/11	93-95
SU11.5	Describe principles of providing post-operative pain relief and management of chronic pain	Lecture, small group discussion	Written/viva voce	2/11	96-98
SU11.6	Describe principles of safe general surgery	Lecture, small group discussion	Written/viva voce	2/11	100
Nutrition and Fluid Therapy					
SU12.1	Enumerate the causes and consequences of malnutrition in the surgical patient	Lecture, small group discussion, bedside clinic	Written/viva voce	2/12	101-104
SU12.2	Describe and discuss the methods of estimation and replacement of the fluid and electrolyte requirements in the surgical patient	Lecture, small group discussion, bedside clinic	Written/viva voce	2/12	104-106

Competency number	Competency: The student should be able to	Suggested teaching/learning method	Suggested assessment method	Section/ Chapter No.	Page No.
SU12.3	Discuss the nutritional requirements of surgical patients, the methods of providing nutritional support and their complications	Lecture, small group discussion, bedside clinic	Written/viva voce	2/12	104–106
Transplantation					
SU13.1	Describe the immunological basis of organ transplantation	Lecture, small group discussion	Written/viva voce	2/13	107-108
SU13.2	Discuss the principles of immunosuppressive therapy. Enumerate indications, describe surgical principles, management of organ transplantation	Lecture, small group discussion	Written/viva voce	2/13	108-112
SU13.3	Discuss the legal and ethical issues concerning organ donation	Lecture, small group discussion	Written/viva voce	2/13	113
SU13.4	Counsel patients and relatives on organ donation in a simulated environment	DOAP session	Skill assessment	2/13	
Basic Surgical Skills					
SU14.1	Describe aseptic techniques, sterilization and disinfection	Lecture, small group discussion	Written/viva voce	2/14	115-116
SU14.2	Describe surgical approaches, incisions and the use of appropriate instruments in surgery in general	Lecture, small group discussion	Written/viva voce	2/14	116-118
SU14.3	Describe the materials and methods used for surgical wound closure and anastomosis (sutures, knots and needles)	Lecture, small group discussion	Written/viva voce	2/14	119
SU14.4	Demonstrate the techniques of asepsis and suturing in a simulated environment	DOAP session	Skill assessment/ logbook	2/14	
Biohazard Disposal					
SU15.1	Describe classification of hospital waste and appropriate methods of disposal	Lecture, small group discussion	Written/viva voce	2/15	120-123
Minimally Invasive General Surgery					
SU16.1	Minimally invasive general surgery: Describe indications advantages and disadvantages of minimally invasive general surgery	Lecture, demonstration bedside clinic, discussion	Theory/ practical / orals/written/ viva voce	2/16	124-132
Trauma					
SU17.1	Describe the principles of first aid	Lecture, small group discussion	Written/viva voce	2/17	133-135
SU17.2	Demonstrate the steps in basic life support; transport of injured patient in a simulated environment	DOAP session	Skill assessment	2/17	

Competency number	Competency: The student should be able to	Suggested teaching/learning method	Suggested assessment method	Section/Chapter No.	Page No.
SU17.3	Describe the principles in management of mass casualties	Lecture, small group discussion	Written/viva voce	2/17	135-137
SU17.4	Describe pathophysiology, mechanism of head injuries	Lecture, small group discussion	Written/viva voce	2/17	138-140
SU17.5	Describe clinical features for neurological assessment and GCS in head injuries	Lecture, small group discussion	Written/viva voce	2/17	140-143
SU17.6	Chose appropriate investigations and discuss the principles of management of head injuries	Lecture, small group discussion	Written/viva voce	2/17	140-143
SU17.7	Describe the clinical features of soft tissue injuries. Chose appropriate investigations and discuss the principles of management	Lecture, small group discussion	Written/viva voce	2/17	143-144
SU17.8	Describe the pathophysiology of chest injuries	Lecture, small group discussion	Written/viva voce	2/17	145-148
SU17.9	Describe the clinical features and principles of management of chest injuries	Lecture, small group discussion	Written/viva voce	2/17	148-152
SU17.10	Demonstrate airway maintenance. Recognize and manage tension pneumothorax, hemothorax and flail chest in simulated environment	DOAP session	Skill assessment/ logbook	2/17	
Skin and Subcutaneous Tissue					
SU18.1	Describe the pathogenesis, clinical features and management of various cutaneous and subcutaneous infections	Lecture, small group discussion	Written/viva voce	3/18	153-156
SU18.2	Classify skin tumors. Differentiate different skin tumors and discuss their management	Lecture, small group discussion	Written/viva voce/skill assessment	3/18	157-169
SU18.3	Describe and demonstrate the clinical examination of surgical patient including swelling and order relevant investigation for diagnosis. Describe and discuss appropriate treatment plan	Bedside clinic, small group discussion, DOAP session	Skill assessment	3/18	
Developmental Anomalies of Face, Mouth and Jaws					
SU19.1	Describe the etiology and classification of cleft lip and palate	Lecture, small group discussion	Written/viva voce	3/19	170-172
SU19.2	Describe the principles of reconstruction of cleft lip and palate	Lecture, small group discussion	Written/viva voce	3/19	172-174
Oropharyngeal Cancer					
SU20.1	Describe etiopathogenesis of oral cancer symptoms and signs of oropharyngeal cancer	Lecture, small group discussion	Written/viva voce	3/20	175-178

Competency number	Competency: The student should be able to	Suggested teaching/learning method	Suggested assessment method	Section/ Chapter No.	Page No.
SU20.2	Enumerate the appropriate investigations and discuss the Principles of treatment	Lecture, small group discussion	Written/viva voce	3/20	179-185
Disorders of Salivary Glands					
SU21.1	Describe surgical anatomy of the salivary glands, pathology, and clinical presentation of disorders of salivary glands	Lecture, small group discussion	Written/viva voce	3/21	186-197
SU21.2	Enumerate the appropriate investigations and describe the principles of treatment of disorders of salivary glands	Lecture, small group discussion	Written/viva voce	3/21	186-197
Endocrine General Surgery: Thyroid and Parathyroid					
SU22.1	Describe the applied anatomy and physiology of thyroid	Lecture, small group discussion	Written/viva voce	4/22	201-203
SU22.2	Describe the etiopathogenesis of thyroidal swellings	Lecture, small group discussion	Written/viva voce	4/22	203-213
SU22.3	Demonstrate and document the correct clinical examination of thyroid swellings and discus the differential diagnosis andtheir management	Bedside clinic	Skill assessment	4/22	
SU22.4	Describe the clinical features, classification and principles of management of thyroid cancer	Lecture, small group discussion	Written/viva voce	4/22	214-219
SU22.5	Describe the applied anatomy of parathyroid	Lecture, small group discussion	Written/viva voce	4/22	220
SU22.6	Describe and discuss the clinical features of hypo-and hyperparathyroidism and the principles of their management	Lecture, small group discussion	Written/viva voce	4/22	220-224
Adrenal Glands					
SU23.1	Describe the applied anatomy of adrenal glands	Lecture, small group discussion	Written/viva voce	4/23	225-226
SU23.2	Describe the etiology, clinical features and principles of management of disorders of adrenal gland	Lecture, small group discussion	Written/viva voce	4/23	226-229
SU23.3	Describe the clinical features, principles of investigation and management of adrenal tumors	Lecture, small group discussion, demonstration	Written/viva voce	4/23	229-232
Pancreas					
SU24.1	Describe the clinical features, principles of investigation, prognosis and management of pancreatitis	Lecture, small group discussion	Written/viva voce	4/24	233-245

Competency Table   xxxix

Competency number	Competency: The student should be able to	Suggested teaching/learning method	Suggested assessment method	Section/Chapter No.	Page No.
SU24.2	Describe the clinical features, principles of investigation, prognosis and management of pancreatic endocrine tumors	Lecture, small group discussion, demonstration	Written/viva voce	4/24	246-254
SU24.3	Describe the principles of investigation and management of pancreatic disorders including pancreatitis and endocrine tumors	Lecture, small group discussion, demonstration	Written/viva voce/skill assessment	4/24	246-254
Breast					
SU25.1	Describe applied anatomy and appropriate investigations for breast disease	Lecture, small group discussion	Written/viva voce/skill assessment	4/25	255-259
SU25.2	Describe the etiopathogenesis, clinical features and principles of management of benign breast disease including infections of the breast	Lecture, small group discussion	Written/viva voce/skill assessment	4/25	259-267
SU25.3	Describe the etiopathogenesis, clinical features, Investigations and principles of treatment of benign and malignant tumors of breast	Lecture, small group discussion, demonstration	Written/viva voce/skill assessment	4/25	267-280
SU25.4	Counsel the patient and obtain informed consent for treatment of malignant conditions of the breast	DOAP session	Skill assessment	4/25	
SU25.5	Demonstrate the correct technique to palpate the breast for breast swelling in a mannequin or equivalent	DOAP session	Skill assessment	4/25	
Cardiothoracic General Surgery—Chest-Heart and Lungs					
SU26.1	Outline the role of surgery in the management of coronary heart disease, valvular heart diseases and congenital heart diseases	Lecture, small group discussion	Written/viva voce	5/26	283-290
SU26.2	Chest wall and pleural diseases—surgical aspects of lung abscess, pleural effusions, empyema thoracis. mesothelioma pleura: Hemothorax, pneumothorax, tumors of chest wall	Lecture, small group discussion	Written/viva voce	5/26	291-294
SU26.3	Describe the clinical features of mediastinal diseases and the principles of management	Lecture, small group discussion	Written/viva voce	5/26	300-303
SU26.4	Describe the etiology, pathogenesis, clinical features of tumors of lung and the principles of management	Lecture, small group discussion	Written/viva voce	5/26	300-303

Competency Table

Competency number	Competency: The student should be able to	Suggested teaching/learning method	Suggested assessment method	Section/Chapter No.	Page No.
Vascular Diseases					
SU27.1	Describe the etiopathogenesis, clinical features, investigations and principles of treatment of occlusive arterial disease	Lecture, small group discussion	Written/viva voce/skill assessment	5/27	304-310
SU27.2	Demonstrate the correct examination of the vascular system and enumerate and describe the investigation of vascular disease	DOAP session	Skill assessment	5/27	
SU27.3	Describe clinical features, investigations and principles of management of vasospastic disorders	Lecture, small group discussion	Written/viva voce	5/27	315
SU27.4	Describe the types of gangrene and principles of amputation	Lecture, small group discussion	Written/viva voce/skill assessment	5/27	311-314
SU27.5	Describe the applied anatomy of venous system of lower limb	Lecture, small group discussion	Written/viva voce	5/27	316-319
SU27.6	Describe pathophysiology, clinical features, Investigations and principles of management of DVT and Varicose veins	Lecture, small group discussion, demonstration	Written/viva voce/skill assessment	5/27	319-323
SU27.7	Describe pathophysiology, clinical features, investigations and principles of management of Lymph edema, lymphangitis and Lymphomas	Lecture, small group discussion	Written/viva voce/skill assessment	5/27	324-327
SU27.8	Demonstrate the correct examination of the lymphatic system	DOAP session, bedside clinic	Skill assessment	5/27	328-333
Abdominal Cavity, Hernia and Digestive Tract					
SU28.1	Describe pathophysiology, clinical features, Investigations and principles of management of hernias	Lecture, small group discussion	Written/viva voce/skill assessment	6/28 -1	337-348
SU28.2	Demonstrate the correct technique to examine the patient with hernia and identify different types of hernias	DOAP session, bedside clinic	Skill assessment	6/28-1	
SU28.3	Describe causes, clinical features, complications and principles of management of peritonitis	Lecture, small group discussion, bedside clinic	Written/viva voce	6/28 -1	349-355
SU28.4	Describe pathophysiology, clinical features, investigations and principles of management of intra-abdominal abscess, mesenteric cyst, and retroperitoneal tumors	Lecture, small group discussion, demonstration	Written/viva voce	6/28-1	355-380
SU28.5	Describe the applied anatomy and physiology of esophagus	Lecture, small group discussion, demonstration	Written/viva voce	6/28 -2	363-365

Competency number	Competency: The student should be able to	Suggested teaching/learning method	Suggested assessment method	Section/Chapter No.	Page No.
SU28.6	Describe the clinical features, investigations and principles of management of benign and malignant disorders of esophagus	Lecture, small group discussion, demonstration	Written/viva voce	6/28 -2	365-379
SU28.7	Describe the applied anatomy and physiology of stomach	Lecture, small group discussion	Written/viva voce	6/28 -2	380-386
SU28.8	Describe and discuss the etiology, the clinical features, investigations and principles of management of congenital hypertrophic pyloric stenosis, peptic ulcer disease, carcinoma stomach	Lecture, small group discussion	Written/viva voce	6/28 -2	386-405
SU28.9	Demonstrate the correct technique of examination of a patient with disorders of the stomach	Lecture, small group discussion	Written/viva voce/skill assessment	6/28 -2	
SU28.10	Describe the applied anatomy of liver. Describe the clinical features, Investigations and principles of management of liver abscess, hydatid disease, injuries and tumors of the liver	DOAP session, bedside clinic	Skill assessment	6/28--3	411-430
SU28.11	Describe the applied anatomy of spleen. Describe the clinical features, investigations and principles of management of splenic injuries. Describe the post-splenectomy sepsis prophylaxis	Lecture, small group discussion, demonstration	Written/viva voce	6/28- 3	406-410
SU28.12	Describe the applied anatomy of biliary system. Describe the clinical features, investigations and principles of management of diseases of biliary system	Lecture, small group discussion, demonstration	Written/viva voce	6/28- 3	431-450
SU28.13	Describe the applied anatomy of small and large intestine	Lecture, small group discussion, demonstration	Written/viva voce	6/28- 4	451-467
SU28.14	Describe the clinical features, investigations and principles of management of disorders of small and large intestine including neonatal obstruction and short gut syndrome	Lecture, small group discussion, demonstration	Written/viva voce	6/28-4	468-482
SU28.15	Describe the clinical features, investigations and principles of management of diseases of appendix including appendicitis and its complications	Lecture, small group discussion, demonstration	Written/viva voce/skill assessment	6/28-5	483-491
SU28.16	Describe applied anatomy including congenital anomalies of the rectum and anal canal	Lecture, small group discussion, demonstration	Written/viva voce/skill assessment	6/28-6	492-504

Competency number	Competency: The student should be able to	Suggested teaching/learning method	Suggested assessment method	Section/Chapter No.	Page No.
SU28.17	Describe the clinical features, investigations and principles of management of common anorectal diseases	Lecture, small group discussion, demonstration	Written/viva voce/skill assessment	6/28-6	505-538
SU28.18	Describe and demonstrate clinical examination of abdomen. Order relevant investigations. Describe and discuss appropriate treatment plan	Bedside clinic, DOAP session, small group discussion	Skill assessment	6/28-6	
	Urinary System				
SU29.1	Describe the causes, investigations and principles of management of hematuria	Lecture, small group discussion	Written/viva voce	7/29	547-550
SU29.2	Describe the clinical features, investigations and principles of management of congenital anomalies of genitourinary system	Lecture, small group discussion	Written/viva voce	7/29	550-559
SU29.3	Describe the clinical features, Investigations and principles of management of urinary tract infections	Lecture, small group discussion	Written/viva voce	7/29	553-562
SU29.4	Describe the clinical features, investigations and principles of management of hydronephrosis	Lecture, small group discussion	Written/viva voce	7/29	562-566
SU29.5	Describe the clinical features, investigations and principles of management of renal calculi	Lecture, small group discussion	Written/viva voce	7/29	567-573
SU29.6	Describe the clinical features, investigations and principles of management of renal tumors	Lecture, small group discussion	Written/viva voce	7/29	573-581
SU29.7	Describe the principles of management of acute and chronic retention of urine	Lecture, small group discussion	Written/viva voce	7/29	582-587
SU29.8	Describe the clinical features, investigations and principles of management of bladder cancer	Lecture, small group discussion	Written/viva voce	7/29	587-589
SU29.9	Describe the clinical features, investigations and principles of management of disorders of prostate	Lecture, small group discussion	Written/viva voce/skill assessment	7/29	590-597
SU29.10	Demonstrate a digital rectal examination of the prostate in a mannequin or equivalent	DOAP session	Skill assessment	7/29	598
SU29.11	Describe clinical features, investigations and management of urethral strictures	Lecture, small group discussion, demonstration	Written/viva voce/skill assessment	7/29	599-603

Competency number	Competency: The student should be able to	Suggested teaching/learning method	Suggested assessment method	Section/Chapter No.	Page No.
	Penis, Testis and Scrotum				
SU30.1	Describe the clinical features, investigations and principles of management of phimosis, paraphimosis and carcinoma penis	Lecture, small group discussion, demonstration	Written/viva voce/skill assessment	7/30	604-609
SU30.2	Describe the applied anatomy clinical features, investigations and principles of management of undescended testis	Lecture, small group discussion, demonstration	Written/viva voce/skill assessment	7/30	609-610
SU30.3	Describe the applied anatomy clinical features, investigations and principles of management of epidydimo-orchitis	Lecture, small group discussion, demonstration	Written/viva voce/skill assessment	7/30	609-610
SU30.4	Describe the applied anatomy clinical features, investigations and principles of management of varicocele	Lecture, small group discussion, demonstration	Written/viva voce/skill assessment	7/30	611-615
SU30.5	Describe the applied anatomy, clinical features, investigations and principles of management of hydrocele	Lecture, small group discussion, demonstration	Written/viva voce/skill assessment	7/30	616-619
SU30.6	Describe classification, clinical features, investigations and principles of management of tumors of testis	Lecture, small group discussion, demonstration	Written/viva voce/skill assessment	7/30	619-624

Plate 1

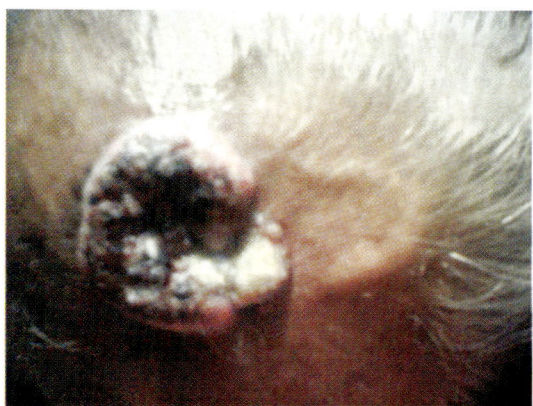

Squamous cell carcinoma scalp
(*Refer* Chapter 18, Page 166)

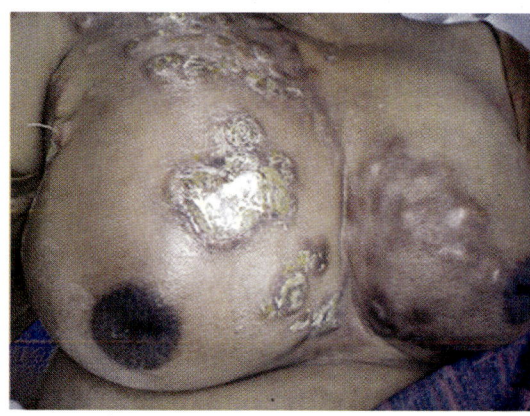

Fig. 25.5: Cancer en cuirasse

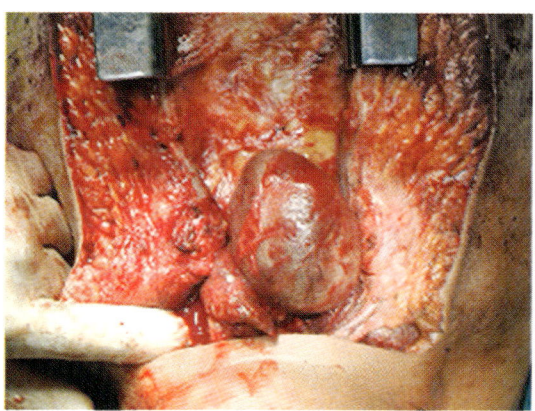

Fig. 22.4: Intra thoracic goitre

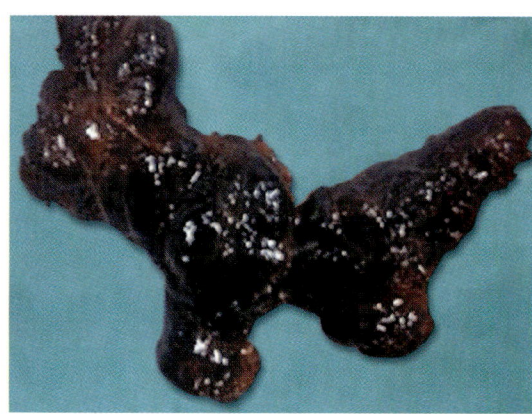

Fig. 22.3: Multinodular goiter with retrosternal nodule

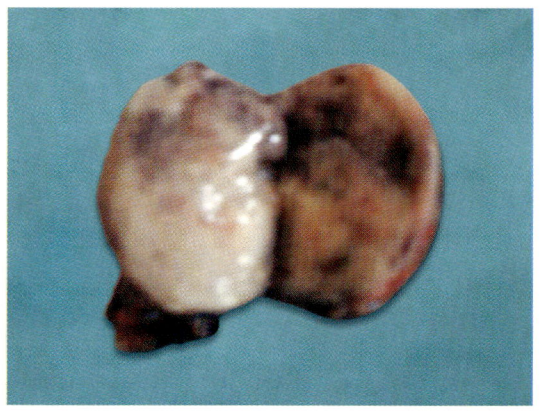

Fig 23.1: Adrenal pheochromocytoma

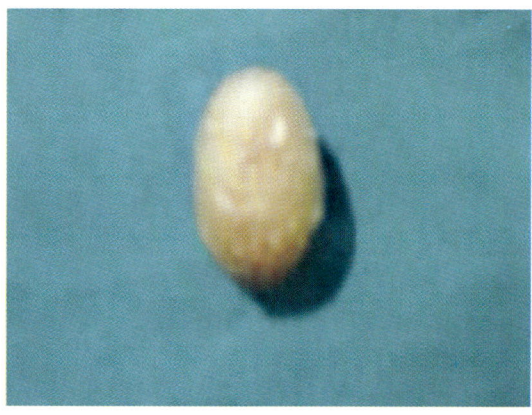

Fig. 28B-2: Pure cholesterol stone

Plate 2

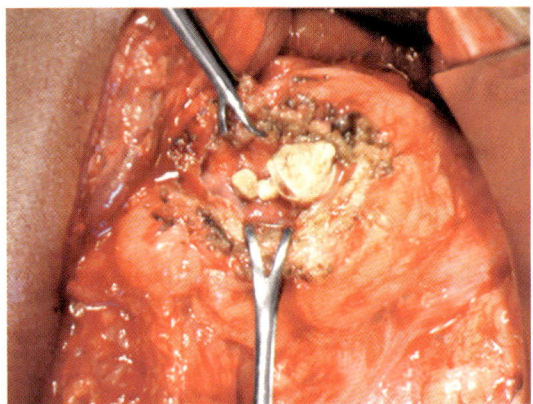

Fig. 24.3: Pancreatic stone retrieval

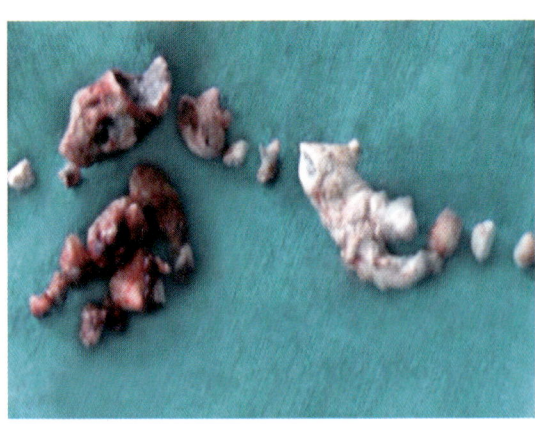

Fig. 24.4: Pancreatic stones removed from head to tail

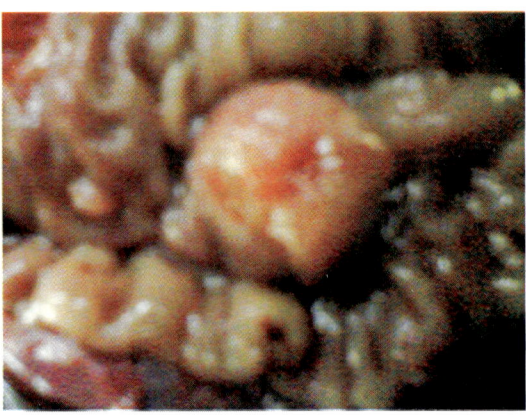

Fig. 24.5: Ampullary tumor

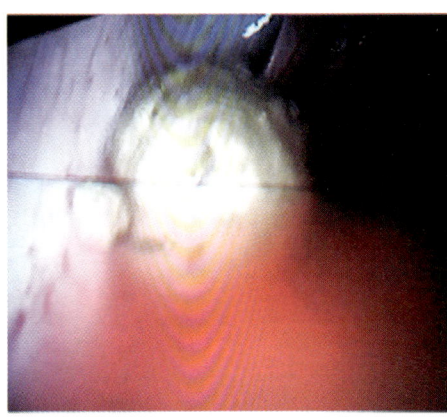

Fig. 28A-3: Fecolith in peritoneum from perforated appendix

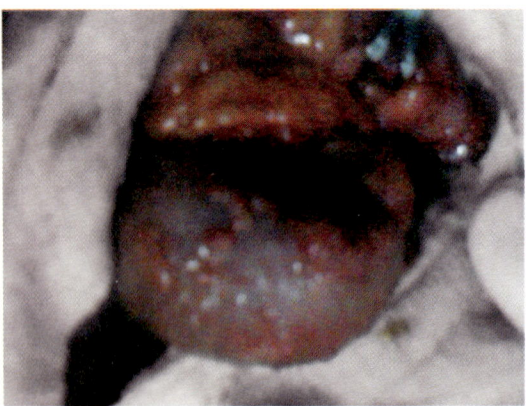

Fig 28A-4: TB ileum and appendicitis

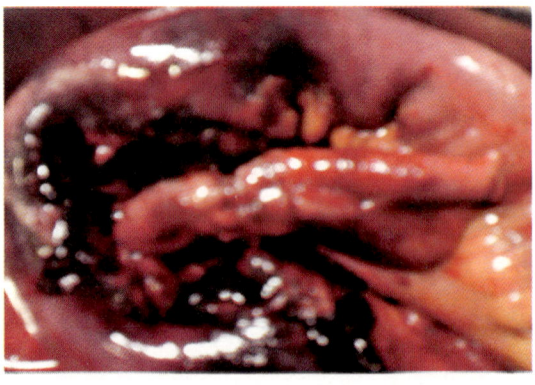

Fig. 28A-5: Ileal gangrene due to thormbosis of mesentery in post-ileal appendicitis

Plate 3

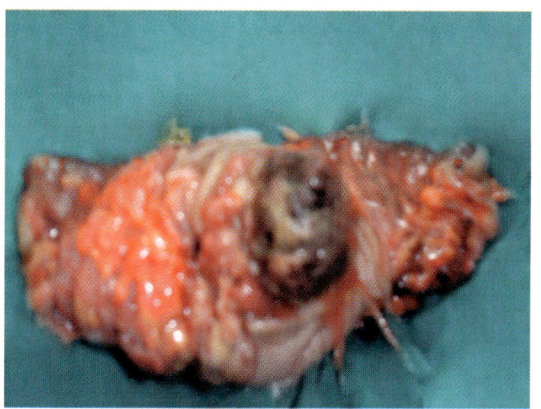

Fig. 28C-5A: Polypoid colonic carcinoma

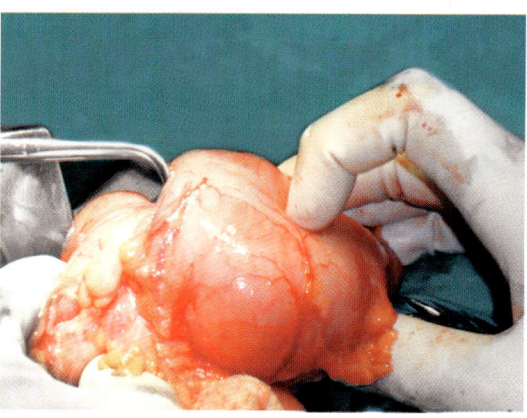

Fig. 28C-5B: Intussusception

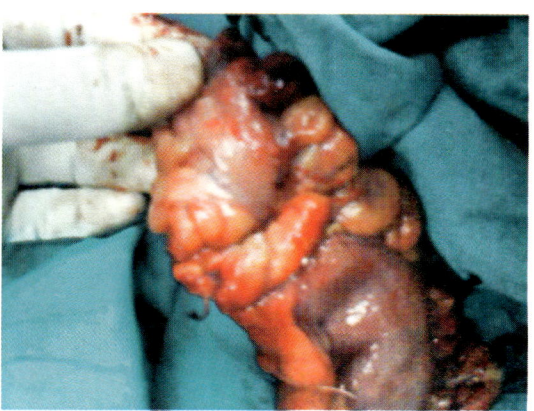

Fig. 28C-5C: Annular sigmoid carcinoma

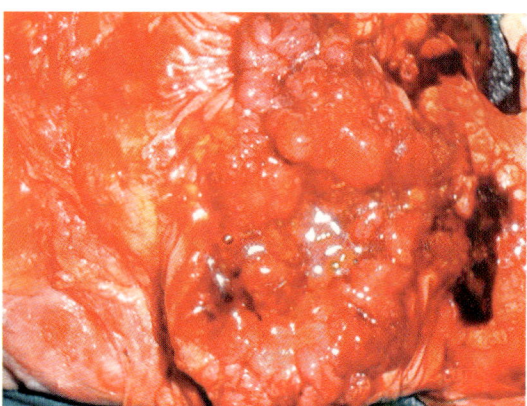

Fig. 28C-5D: Ulcerative carcinoma cecum

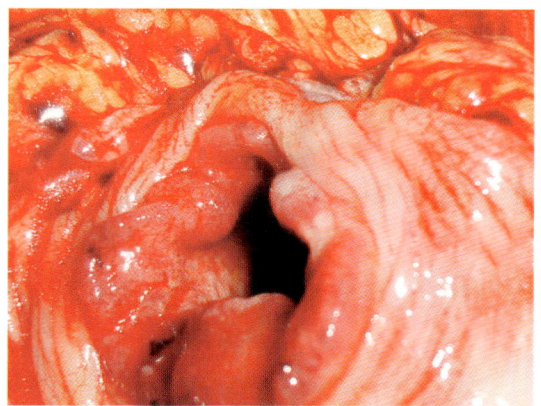

Fig. 28C-5E: Annular carcinoma descending colon

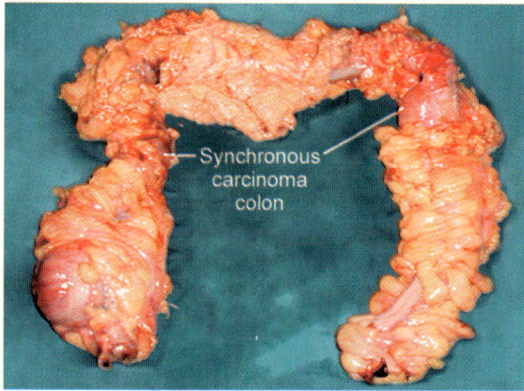

Fig. 28C-5F: Synchronous carcinoma ascending and descending colon

Plate 4

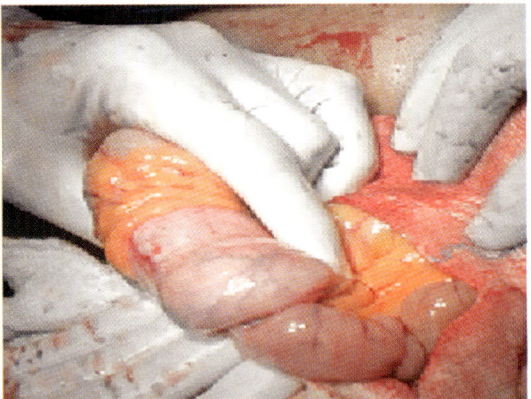

Fig. 28O-9: Acute ileo-ileo colic intussusception

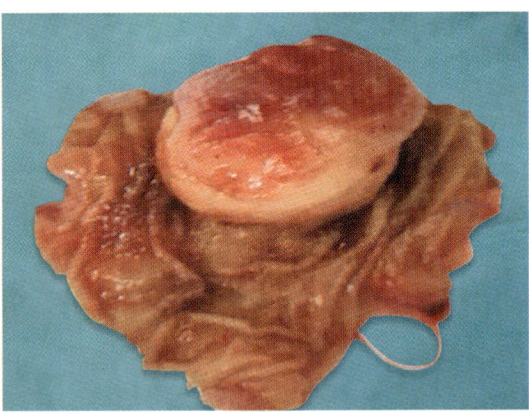

Fig. 28O-10: Submucous lipoma in intussusception

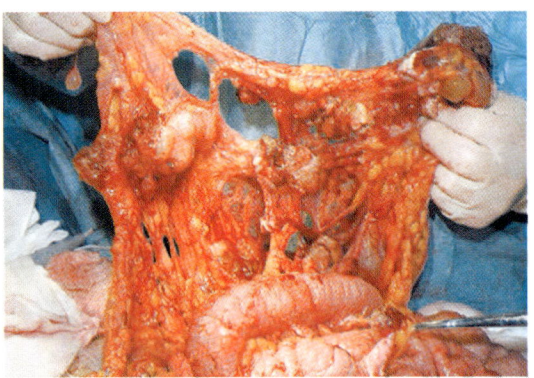

Fig. 28A-6: Pseudomyxoma peritonei

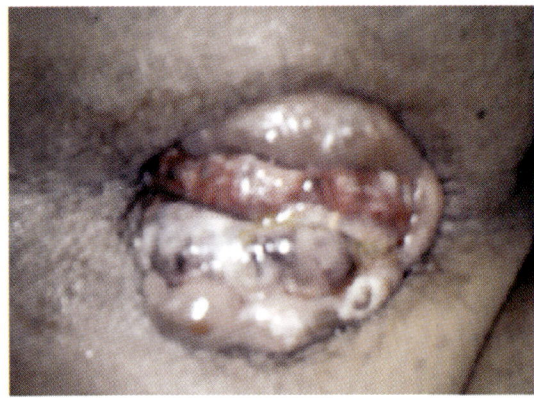

Fig. 28P-3: Acute prolapsed hemorrhoids with gangrene

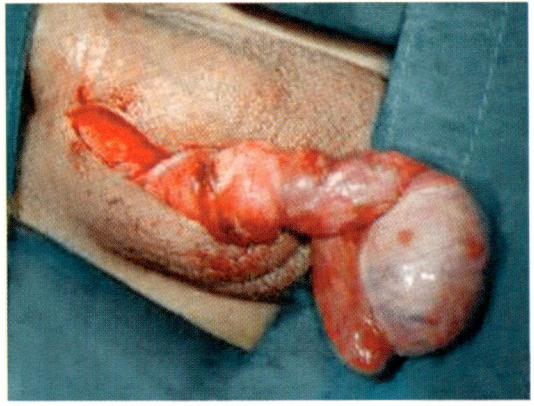

Fig. 30.3: Early torsion—detorsion done

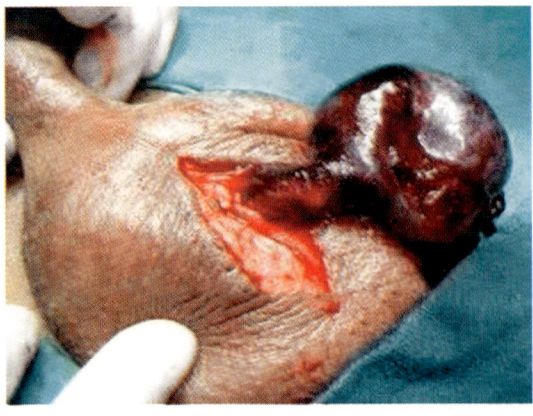

Fig. 30.4: Gangrenous torsion

Section 1

Basics in Surgery

1. Metabolic Response to Injury
2. Shock
3. Blood and Blood Components
4. Burns
5. Wound Healing and Wound Care
6. Surgical Infections and Hand Infections

Metabolic Response to Injury

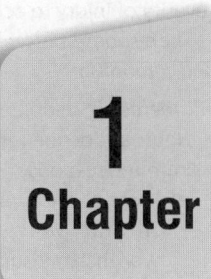
Chapter 1

SU1.1	Describe basic concepts of homeostasis, enumerate the metabolic changes in injury and their mediators.
SU1.2	Describe the factors that affect the metabolic response to injury.
SU1.3	Describe basic concepts of perioperative care.
Also read along with chapter SU 10.1–2 perioperative care	

SU1.1: Describe basic concepts of homeostasis, enumerate the metabolic changes in injury and their mediators.

SU1.2: Describe the factors that affect the metabolic response to injury.

Q. Define homeostasis. Add a brief note on homeostatic control system.

Homeostasis is a dynamic process to maintain the body constancy (internal milieu) against the challenges through the complex homeostatic responses from the body systems involving the brain, nerves, heart, lungs, kidneys, liver and spleen.

The responses to injury effect healing and survival in mild /moderate trauma, but the severely injured patient needs artificial support for survival and restoration milieu—called the 'open loop' system.

Basic Concepts of Homeostasis

Homeostatic Control System

Closed loop: This is a loop of body responses that help healing, which stop upon restoration of homeostasis. viz., the loop "injury-signals- to effect healing and negative feedback loop stops the response" regulated by a negative feedback loop".

Open loop: In severe injury—external intervention, medical or surgical is a must for return to normalcy to resolve the etiological factor that triggered the injury.

No alternatives to interventions, no feedback mechanism. Hence called "Open loop".

Homeostatic Response to Injury

- The response to injury is graded and directly proportional to the severity of injury.
- The responses are—physiological, metabolic, and immunological.

Factors influencing the response:
- Genetic make up
- Severity of injury
- Time lapsed after the insult.

Example: An injury or surgery of average gravity causes transient systemic signs and calorie loss while a severe one leads to systemic inflammatory response and may cause multi organ failure.

Q. Describe the metabolic stress response to surgery and trauma.

Summary of Homeostatic Metabolic Response to Trauma

Homeostasis maintains internal milieu against challenges through the complex responses.

Section 1: Basics in Surgery

The response to injury is proportional to the severity of injury to achieve survival and healing.

The response is essentially - immobilization anorexia and catabolism.

The metabolic response to surgery and trauma:
- Neuroendocrine reflex response - modulates the immune response
  - Acute phase aiming at short term survival
  - Chronic phase—muscle wasting due to hypothalamic suppression led endocrine failure.
- Mediators of the metabolic response to injury:
  - Formation of endogenous damage-associated molecular patterns (DAMPs) and their interaction with pattern recognition receptors—the PRRs on cell surfaces of immune and non-immune cells to initiate an aseptic systemic inflammatory response to injury.
- Cellular stress responses: Cytokines—on hypothalamus, liver and skeletal muscle.

The inflammatory signals—activate the main stress responses and evoke the cell defenses.
- The immunological response—involves both innate and adaptive immune system responses. A proinflammatory response syndrome (immunostimulant response) followed by a compensatory anti-inflammatory response syndrome (CARS)—immunosuppressive
- Adaptive changes:
  - Endogenous cytokine antagonists act at systemic level (anti-inflammatory)
  - The endogenous resolution agonists act locally at injury site level.
- The acute phase protein response (APPR) (protein metabolism) in the liver
  - Stimulation of positive acute phase proteins (fibrinogen and CRP)
  - Suppression of acute negative phase reactors (albumin)
- Insulin resistance: Cortisol induced
- Starvation: Protein loss and loss of adipose tissue

Closed loop: The response and resolution happen in a sequential way and therapy is watching and supporting this.

Open loop: The resolution and repair fail due to the lurking pathogenic factors and intervention becomes inevitable - the close loop fails and calls for open loop of intervention to relieve the cause of injury, (example—a hematoma may resolve and without intervention but needs intervention of evacuation for avoiding infection or effect on tissues.

FOR DETAILED READING

NEUROENDOCRINE REFLEX RESPONSE: MODULATES THE IMMUNE RESPONSE

The central nervous system is sensitized by the:
- Neural afferent input (afferent nociceptive neurons, the spinal cord, thalamus, hypothalamus and pituitary) to the regulatory areas of brain.
- Soluble mediators of the SIRS, providing information on inflammatory response to injury.

Biphasic Neuroendocrine Response to Injury

- **Acute phase** response aims at short-term survival.
  - Stimulation of hypothalamus and pituitary to release CRH and ACTH respectively leading to
  - Hypersecretion of counter-regulatory hormones—cortisol, glucagon, adrenaline.
  - Hypersecretion of prolactin.
  - Growth hormone (GH)—lipolytic and anti-insulin and proinflammatory.
  - Lowered sensitivity to insulin and low circulatory levels of insulin like growth factor-1 (IGF-1) and inactivation of peripheral thyroid hormones.
- **Chronic phase:** Causes muscle wasting due to hypothalamic suppression and hyposecretion of the respective hormones.

Mediators of the Metabolic Response to Injury

Formation of endogenous damage-associated molecular patterns (DAMPs) after cell injury. pattern recognition receptors (PPRs) are on the cells-their function is to sense the invading pathogens. The DAMPs are sensed by the PRRs on cell surface.

The DAMPs interact with the receptors on immune and non-immune cells to *initiate an aseptic (sterile) systemic inflammatory response to injury*.

The clinical picture of SIRS after injury is often the same as the one of septic conditions, because **DAMP** molecules and septic pathogens are sensed by the same PRRs.

Chapter 1: Metabolic Response to Injury

Cellular Stress Responses

- **Cytokines—act on**
  - The hypothalamus to cause: Pyrexia and increased hypothalamic response to stress.
  - The skeletal muscles to induce proteolysis.
  - In the liver-to promote acute phase protein production.
- **The inflammatory signals**—activate the main stress responses and evoke the cell defenses and products to restore homeostasis.
- **The responses**
  - The oxidative stress response; the heat shock protein response.
  - The unfolded protein response; autophagy; pyroptosis.

HOMEOSTATIC RESPONSE TO INJURY

See **Table 1.1**.

Systemic Inflammatory Response Syndrome (SIRS): Injury Induced

Regulation of SIRS

- By transcriptional events and microRNA synthesis.
- By close networking of the cells, mediators, signaling mechanisms and pathways.

> **Q. Short answer on pathogenesis of SIRS after trauma.**
>
> **Pathogenesis of SIRS after Trauma**
> *The Immunological Consequence of Major Injury*
> The innate primary immune system response neutrophils, dendritic cells and macrophages) along with the adaptive immune system (T cells, B cells) induces the metabolic response to trauma.
> - First 24 hours: Proinflammatory phase—release of proinflammatory cytokines (e.g. IL-1, IL-6 and TNFα).
> - After 24 hours: Anti-inflammatory phase—rapidly increased release of anti inflammatory—cytokine antagonists and soluble receptors (e.g. IL-1Ra, TNF-sR).

Table 1.1: Homeostastic response to injury.

Injury— evokes afferent nociceptive pathways to stimulate the following: ↓	In turn the following are stimulated	Resultant plasma levels	Changes in body metabolism
1. **CNS** – Spinal cord – Hypothalamus—CRF stimulates pituitary	ACTH Growth hormone (GH)	**Increased levels** Cortisol	Lipolysis in fat cells
2. The sympathetic nervous system	Adrenal →	Adrenaline	Liver—glycogen breakdown
3. Pancreas	Pancreas →	Glucagon	Gluconeogenesis Skeletal muscle Protein degradation
			Hepatic acute phase Protein synthesis
4. The immune system	Interaction between— Adaptive immune ↕ system and Innate immune system	**Increased** IL-1 TNF IL-6 IL-8 **Decreased** Insulin IGF-1 Testosterone T3, T4	 Pyrexia Hypermetabolism

The *compensatory anti-inflammatory response syndrome (CARS)*—caused by a prolonged or excessive anti-inflammatory, cytokine antagonistic response leading to counter inflammatory response syndrome—where the immunity is suppressed and risk of infection is raised.

- **Proinflammatory mediators:** Cytokines
  The proinflammatory cytokines cause the following:
  - Peripheral insulin resistance.
  - Nitric oxide [NO] and prostanoids (act via COX-2 receptors).
  - Changes in organ function— excessive vasoconstriction via endogenous factors such as endothelin-1, e.g. renal underperfusion.
- **Release of Endogenous cytokine antagonists into the circulation**—act to control the proinflammatory response.
- **Adaptive changes:**
  - **Counter-inflammatory response:** Due to release of by IL-4, -5, -9 and -13 and transforming growth factor beta [TGFβ]. They can lead to **compensatory anti-inflammatory response syndrome (CARS) and results in immunosuppression** and increased susceptibility to opportunistic (nosocomial) infection.
  - **Specialized pro-resolving mediators (SPM):** Fatty acid derived local mediators limit the acute inflammation and help return to homeostasis.
  - **Hyperglycemia:** Can worsen the inflammatory response, formation of excess oxygen free radicals in the mitochondria and enhance cytokine production.

Summary of Adaptive Changes

The body attempts to resolve or minimize the homeostatic disorder induced by inflammation:
- *Endogenous cytokine antagonists*—act at systemic level (anti-inflammatory agents)
- *The endogenous resolution agonists*—act local tissue level:
  - Induce clearance of apoptotic polymorphs and microbial components.
  - Reduce proinflammatory cytokines and lipid mediators
  - Help clearing of debris in inflammatory atmosphere.

Genetic response: Endotoxemia is associated with changes in mRNA expression in leukocytes. This postulates the role of genetic expression in SIRS.

Q. What are the acute phase proteins and their role in trauma? (short notes)

The acute phase protein response (APPR) (protein metabolism) in the liver.

- The daily protein turnover of the body is about 150–200 g. Over 50% this occurs in the liver and skeletal muscle mass (approx 4 kilograms).
- The liver synthesizes proteins—for renewal of structural proteins (50%) and for renewal of export proteins (50%), e.g., albumin.
- The normal transcapillary escape rate (TER) of albumin exceeds the synthesis by ten times.
- Increased capillary permeability (high TER) after trauma/sepsis leads to three times increase in extravascular loss of albumin.
- *The body's response to insult is through the circulating peripheral blood mononuclear cells which release the proinflammatory cytokines (including IL-1, IL-6 and TNF - alfa).*

Action of the proinflammatory cytokines:
- *Increase the hepatic synthesis of positive acute phase proteins,* e.g., fibrinogen and C-reactive protein (CRP) by mobilizing valuable protein reserves in muscles, to help healing.
- Suppression of negative acute phase reactants and fall in the export proteins like albumin (mainly due to transcapillary leak).

This leads to high plasma levels of positive reactants (e.g., CRP) and low levels of negative reactants (e.g., albumin).

Insulin resistance: Proportional to the severity of injury.

This causes post trauma hyperglycemia—due to increase in glucose production; decreased glucose uptake in peripheral tissues and the decreased responsiveness of insulin-regulated glucose transporter proteins due to proinflammatory cytokines.

Treatment: Insulin infusions under monitoring (to avoid hypoglycemia).

Starvation

Adaptive changes lead to reduction in the pace of weight loss and urinary loss of nitrogen helping a starving person survive upto 2 months.

The adaptive responses fail after major injuries and body reserves deplete rapidly. Daily urinary nitrogen loss of 10-20 g (amounting to loss of upto 500 g of muscle mass).

Changes in body composition following injury

Composition of body mass: In a 60 kg person, 60% (35-36 kg) is water, 12 kg of fat, 10 kg is protein (skeletal 3.5-4 kg visceral 7 kg and 3 kg mineral).

Proteolysis: By stress response

- The skeletal muscles—limbs—causing asthenia and exhaustion, chest wall and intercostals and diaphragm, leading to hypoventilation, respiratory insufficiency and infection.
- Smooth muscle—gut—motility and digestive imbalance
- Myocardium—usually spared.

Impact of trauma

- Loss of adipose tissue
- Loss of proteins.

Sepsis is SIRS with a Documented Infection

Severe sepsis or sepsis syndrome is sepsis with evidence of failure of one or more organs: Respiratory (acute respiratory distress syndrome), cardiovascular (septic shock follows compromise of cardiac function and fall in peripheral vascular resistance), renal (usually acute tubular necrosis), hepatic, blood coagulation systems or central nervous system.

Q. What are the diagnostic criteria for SIRS? (Short notes).

DIAGNOSIS OF SIRS

Criteria for Systemic Inflammatory Response Syndrome (SIRS)

SIRS is diagnosed by presence of any two of the following:
- Body temperature above 38°C or below 36°C
- Heart rate over 90 per minute.
- Respiration rate over 20 per minute.
- Total WBC count above 12000 per cu mm or below 4000 per cu mm.

Criteria for SIRS (Detailed)

- *General criteria:*
  - Fever—high temperature >38.3°C or hypothermia core temp <36°C.
  - Heart rate >90 bpm
- *Hemodynamic criteria:*
  - Arterial hypotension (Sys. BP <90 mm Hg, mean AP <70, or fall of over 40 mm Hg)
  - Tachypnea
  - Altered mental status
  - Significant edema or positive fluid balance (>20 mL/kg over 24 hours)
  - Hyperglycemia in the absence of diabetes
- *Inflammatory parameters:*
  - Leukocytosis (WBC >12,000 or leukopenia-WBC <4,000)
  - Plasma C-reactive protein >2 s.d. above normal value
  - Plasma procalcitonin >2 s.d. above normal value
- *Organ dysfunction criteria:*
  - Arterial blood: Hypoxemia
  - Acute oliguria, rising creatinine, high bilirubin levels, paralytic Ileus
  - Coagulation abnormalities, thrombocytopenia
- *Tissue perfusion criteria:*
  - Hyperlactatemia
  - Decreased capillary filling

Q. Write a note on the Ebb and Flow model of metabolic response to trauma.

The metabolic stress response to surgery and trauma—divided into ebb and flow phases.

The 'Ebb and flow' (David Cuthbertson's) model **(Table 1.2).**

Q. Enumerate steps to avoid or reduce systemic damage due to response to trauma.

The measures to control and limit the metabolic response benefit the postoperative patient.
This is to control the factors contributing to the metabolic response to trauma:
- Initiators and regulators of the response: The immune system, cardiovascular system, sympathetic nervous system, ascending reticular formation and limbic system—initiate and regulate the metabolic response.
- Aggravators of the response: Pre and postoperative fasting, dehydration, anesthesia and sepsis, acute medical illness or severe mental stress.

Section 1: Basics in Surgery

Table 1.2: The 'Ebb and flow' (David Cuthbertson's) model.

Injury	Ebb phase	Flow phase: Two subphases	
		Catabolic phase	Anabolic (recovery phase)
Duration	24–48 hours	3–10 days	Weeks
Response of body systems	Shock	Catabolism—SIRS	Anabolism
Aim of the phase	To conserve circulating volume and energy stores for recovery and repair	Mobilize energy from stores for recovery and repair—protein and fat loss weight loss, nitrogen loss, insulin resistance	Restoration of normal phase
Regulators	Neuroendocrine: Catecholamines aldosterone	Hormones and pro-Inflammatory cytokines—plus continued neuroendocrine phase	Anti-inflammatory cytokines and adoptive mechanisms
Treatment	Resuscitation	Monitoring and intervention, nutritional maintenance and not hyperalimentation	Supportive

- Avoidable factors that worsen the response to injury:
  - Hemorrhage
  - Hypothermia
  - Edema of tissue
  - Organ underperfusion
  - Starvation
  - Immobility

Measures to maintain body weight and nitrogen equilibrium after major elective surgery.
- Blocking the neuroendocrine stress response—epidural analgesia or similar techniques.
- Providing early oral/enteral feeding.
- Avoidance of excessive intravenous fluids—mainly saline (the early postoperative fluid can be avoided by regulating fluid balance during operation.
- Early mobilization.

SU1.3: Describe basic concepts of perioperative care.

Q. Describe concept of "open loop approach" in perioperative care.

Goal
Early recovery with minimum residual sequelae; 'Stress-free' peri operative care is the theme of modern surgery.

Goal of Elective Surgical Approach
Faster restoration of normal milieu by minimizing the homeostatic response of the body.

Key factor: Minimising the stress of injury (operative injury) by modifying homeostatic responses which evoke release of mediators and mobilize the body reserves through catabolism.

Example of minimizing the primary insult of surgery are minimal access surgery and 'stress-free' perioperative care of enhanced recovery after surgery (ERAS).

Basis of Intervention in Emergency Surgery
The "open loop" approach of homeostatic response forms the basis of perioperative care, (refer previous section SU1.1) wherein restoration of homeostasis is possible *only with medical/surgical intervention to ensure resolution* of the primary etiology that deranges the homeostasis.

In emergency surgery, the tissue trauma, hypovolemia and/or sepsis often worsens the primary problem. The tissue trauma, hypovolemia and sepsis often worsen the primary problem and a combined intervention helps early restoration of homeostasis. This involves:

1. Active resuscitation
2. Surgical intervention against the primary pathology (e.g., gangrene)
3. Critical care to provide organ support.

Q. Write short note on enhanced recovery after surgery (ERAS).

Rationale

Avoidance of the exposure to the surgical stress, prolonged fasting and excessive fluid load (saline) to minimize the postoperative metabolic response to the injury and stress.

Thereby reduce the long-term sequelae of stress inflammatory response to surgical trauma, e.g., minimal access surgical techniques to reduce severity of operative trauma and enhance the recovery and restoration of homeostasis.

Useful Measures under ERAS

- Minimal access techniques
- Minimal periods of starvation
- Blockade of afferent painful stimuli (e.g. epidural analgesia, spinal analgesia)
- Early mobilization.

Measures for Early Recovery

- Suppression of triggers of neuroendocrine response and inflammatory response:
- Suppression of innate immunity at the time of surgery by blocking the neuroendocrine response.

Epidural anesthesia in open surgery—

1. Achieves analgesia
2. Blocks the cortisol release
3. Reduces postoperative insulin resistance and
4. Reduces protein catabolism.

- Patient controlled analgesia in laparoscopic surgery (small wound and minimal tissue trauma).
- Opioid-sparing analgesia to improve gut function and enhance overall recovery.
- Beta-blockers and statins—improve long-term survival after major surgery.

Please also refer Chapter 10 on page 82.

Chapter 2: Shock

SU2.1	Describe pathophysiology of shock, types of shock and principles of resuscitation including fluid replacement and monitoring.
SU2.2	Describe the clinical features of shock and its appropriate treatment.
SU2.3	Communicate and counsel patients and families about the treatment and prognosis of shock demonstrating empathy and care.

SU.2.1: Describe pathophysiology of shock, types of shock and principles of resuscitation including fluid replacement and monitoring.

SU2.2: Describe the clinical features of shock and its appropriate treatment.

Q. Define shock. Classify shock and describe pathophysiology of shock.

SHOCK

Refer **Table 2.1** for pathophysiology of shock.

Table 2.1: Hemodynamic changes and their causes in shock.

Type of shock	Cause	Venous pressure	Cardiac output	Peripheral resistance
Cardiogenic shock	Primary failure of the heart to pump blood to the tissues	High	Low	High
Obstructive shock	Mechanical obstruction of cardiac filling	High	Low	High
Hypovolemic shock	Low circulating volume	Low	Low	High
Distributive shock	Vasodilatation	Low	Very high	Low
• Anaphylaxis	Histamine release			
• Neurogenic shock—trauma/spinal cord injury	Loss of vasomotor tone and sympathetic outflow			
• Septic shock: Microvascular A-V shunting, failure of cellular O_2 take up	Bacterial products (endotoxin), immune factors (humoral/cellular)			
Late septic shock: Fluid loss into interstitial spaces + myocardial depression	hypovolemia—added to vasodilatation	Normal/ low	Low	Low
Endocrine shock: Adrenal insufficiency hypothyroidism	Combination: Hypovolemic, cardiogenic or distributive shock	Low	Low	Low
Hyperthyroidism		High	High	High/ normal

Definition: A systemic state of failure to meet the metabolic demands of cells due to inadequate perfusion and delivery of glucose and oxygen or failure of cells to utilize the same.

Classification of Shock

Based on the primary mechanism causing the shock syndrome.

(*Note:* All types of shock states are characterised by systemic tissue hypoperfusion, often with combination of the different mechanisms).
- Cardiogenic shock
- Obstructive shock
- Distributive shock—septic (vasogenic), neurogenic, traumatic, anaphylactic
- Endocrine shock
- Hypovolemic shock.

Cardiogenic Shock

Due to **primary failure of the heart to pump** blood to the tissues.

Causes of cardiogenic shock:
- Myocardial infarction, blunt myocardial injury
- Valvular heart disease, cardiac dysrhythmias, and cardiomyopathy
- Myocardial depression secondary to sepsis, or medications (drugs or medicines)
- Venous hypertension with pulmonary or systemic edema.

Obstructive Shock

Due to mechanical obstruction of cardiac filling causing a reduction in preload and a fall in cardiac output.

Causes: Massive pulmonary embolus, cardiac tamponade, tension pneumothorax, air embolus.

Distributive Shock

Septic shock, anaphylaxis and spinal cord injury.

> **Q. What is distributive shock? Enumerate the factors in its etiology. (Short note)**
>
> Distributive shock has a combination of inadequate organ perfusion, vascular dilatation with hypotension, low systemic vascular resistance, low after load and a *very high cardiac output.*

Cause of vasodilatation

Anaphylaxis—histamine release
Spinal cord injury—failure of sympathetic outflow and vascular tone (neurogenic shock)
In sepsis it may be due to:
- Release of bacterial products (endotoxin)
- The activation of immune system(cellular and humoral components
- There is maldistribution of blood flow at a microvascular level with arteriovenous shunting and dysfunction of cellular utilization of oxygen
- Hypovolemia added in late septic shock—due to fluid loss into interstitial spaces
- Myocardial depression—often added in late septic shock.

Endocrine Shock

Combination of **hypovolemic, cardiogenic or distributive shock**.

Causes: Acute adrenal insufficiency; hypo- and hyperthyroidism.
- **Acute adrenal insufficiency:** Causes hypovolemia and a poor response to catecholamines.
- **Hypothyroidism:** Low vascular and cardiac responsiveness to circulating catecholamines causing neurogenic shock like picture—low cardiac output, (bradycardia, negative inotropic effect and associated cardiomyopathy).
- **Thyrotoxicosis:** Causes a high-output cardiac failure.

Hypovolemic Shock

It is due to reduced circulating volume. It is the most common form of shock and also is a component of other forms.
- **Hemorrhagic shock:** Revealed, external visible hemorrhage, stabs, vascular injuries.
  - Or concealed hemorrhage: Intrathoracic, intra-abdominal, major fractures.
- **Non-hemorrhagic causes:** Poor fluid intake (dehydration), excessive fluid loss due to vomiting, diarrhea, evaporation(heat), third space losses—ileus, gastric dilatation, pancreatitis, interstitial space loss (sepsis, anaphylaxis) urinary loss (e.g. diabetes insipidus, diuresis).

Pathophysiology of Shock

The main feature of any type of shock is **decreased tissue perfusion and cellular metabolism resulting in** neuroendocrine and inflammatory responses, proportional to the degree and duration of shock.

The responses are caused by the etiology of shock itself (e.g., hypovolemia or neurogenic or cellular mediators).

- **Cellular changes:**
  - Hypoxic cells turn to anaerobic metabolism, producing lactic acid, causing systemic metabolic acidosis and depletion of intracellular glucose.
  - Release of enzymes from intracellular lysosomes causing cell lysis. Failure of sodium potassium pump and escape of intracellular molecules (mainly potassium) into bloodstream.
- **Microvascular changes: a-v shunting**
- **Hypoxia and acidosis—leads to**
  - Activation of the immune and coagulation systems
  - Activation of complement and prime neutrophils to produce oxygen free radicals and cytokines causing endothelial damage in capillary bed and resultant leak of fluid, tissue edema worsening the hypoxia.
- **Changes in cardiovascular system:** Systemic vasoconstriction (cold extremity) and tachycardia—caused by catecholamines released to counter the drop in cardiac preload and afterload (except in septic shock).
- **Respiratory system:** Tachypnea and high minute volume to flush carbon dioxide to counter metabolic acidosis causing respiratory alkalosis.
- **Renal system:** Low urine output, increased renal reabsorption of sodium and water—due to decreased perfusion pressure which leads to low GFR, and stimulation of renin-angiotensin-aldosterone axis and further vasoconstriction.
- **Endocrine system:** Vasoconstriction and renal resorption of water and sodium, stimulation of renin-angiotensin axis; release of adrenal cortisol and ADH from posterior pituitary.

> **Q. What is ischemia-reperfusion syndrome? (Short notes)**
>
> **Ischemia–reperfusion Syndrome**
> - Shock causes tissue hypoperfusion and tissue hypoxia with organ damage and compensatory activation of inflammation. After restoration of normal circulation, further injury is inflicted.
> - Potassium and lactic acid causes myocardial depression, vasodilatation and hypotension.
> - The cellular and humoral factors released by hypoxic damage circulate and cause endothelial damage in lungs and kidneys leading to acute lung injury and acute renal injury, multiple organ failure and death.
>
> Reperfusion injury can't be avoided, *but its severity can be reduced by reducing duration and severity of tissue hypoperfusion.*

> **Q. Write briefly on role of cytokines in shock. (Short notes)**
>
> **Inflammatory Mediators of Shock - The Cytokines**
> - **Pro-inflammatory:** The tumor necrosis factor (TNF) - alfa, interferon TGF, platelet activating factor (PAF) and interleukins (IL-1, IL-2, IL-6 and IL-8)
> - **Anti-inflammatory:** (IL-4, IL-10 and IL-13, prostaglandin E2)—all suppressing immunity and increasing susceptibility to sepsis.
> - **Chemokines:** A specific set of cytokines, which bind sites on leukocyte to induce chemotaxis of leukocytes. Their role is still not fully understood.

Severity of Shock

Stage of Compensation

Aims to sustain blood flow to lungs and brain by reducing the flow to less essential organ systems.

- **Compensated stage:** Renal, pulmonary and cerebral flow is adequately maintained. Reduced perfusion to the skin, muscle and gastrointestinal tract. But there is systemic metabolic acidosis and activation of humoral and cellular elements.
- Tachycardia, cold peripheries and may be the only signs with normal blood pressure and urine output.
- If prolonged beyond 12 hours, the compensatory state can lead to multiple organ failure and death due to the ischemia, reperfusion syndrome.

Stage of Decompensation
- Loss of over 30% of circulating blood volume causes failure of compensatory mechanisms leads to renal, respiratory and cardiovascular decompensation causing hypotension.

> Q. Classify severity of shock with clinical parameters. (Short notes).

Clinical classification of severity of shock is described in **Table 2.2**.

Distributive shock: Warm peripheries (capillaries with good filling), hypotension.

End Results of Shock
- Recovery—good response to resuscitation and appropriate treatment
- Unsustainable shock—failing systems are not responsive to resuscitative measures
- Multiple organ failure (over 60% mortality)—two or more systems fail
    - Clotting
    - Coagulopathy
    - Acute respiratory distress syndrome
    - Acute renal failure
    - Cardiovascular failure
- Death.

> Q. Describe management of shock in general and special notes on each type. (Long Answer).

Management of Shock

The general management of shock is common to all types as given below:

Goal of treatment is to restore cellular and organ perfusion.

Main points: Resuscitation, investigations, monitoring, fluid therapy, therapy specific to the type of shock.

Resuscitation
- **Resuscitation** is the mainstay of treatment of any shock.
- Assessment of degree and type of shock and planning respective treatment follows resuscitation.

Resuscitation of Airway, Breathing and Cardiovascular System
- Patent airway and ventilation to ensure oxygenation is ensured.
- Cardiovascular resuscitation.
- Diagnosis—clinical diagnosis of cause and type of shock
    - Rapid clinical examination
    - Empirical fluid resuscitation - to treat as hypovolemia—(as the common feature)
    - Further diagnosis—go all out next
    - Hemorrhagic shock—internal bleeds—trauma, GI bleeds, aortic aneurysmal rupture.

Investigations

Carried out concurrently with fluid resuscitation.
- Blood
    - Hematocrit, electrolytes, renal and hepatic functions
    - Culture for bacteremia.
    - Parameters of inflammation and cell damage—CRP, LDH, IL6
    - Coagulopathy—coagulation profile, fibrin degradation product levels, d-Dimer.
- Urine culture and routine analysis
- Imaging
    - Ultrasonography and Doppler—abdominal organ, aorta and veins
    - Focused assessment with sonography in trauma (FAST)
    - X-ray chest
    - CT scan to chest and abdomen.

Table 2.2: Classification of severity of shock.

Severity	Tachycardia	Blood pressure	Tachypnea	Urine output	Mental state	Skin
Mild	+/++	Normal	Present	Low, high color	Anxious	Moist cool
Moderate	+++	Starts falling	More	0.5 mL/kg/h	Drowsy	Cold, dry
Severe	+++, thready pulse	Very low	Acidotic breathing	Zero	Unconscious	Cold, dry

Monitoring in Shock

- Urine output—measures renal perfusion
- Blood pressure—pulse oximetry
- ECG
- Central venous pressure
- Base deficit and serum lactate—measure of perfusion of bowel and muscle
- Intra-arterial catheter for drawing blood samples for arterial blood gas analysis
- Measurement of intra-arterial blood pressure

Cardiac output
- **Non-invasive monitoring:** For example, Doppler ultrasound.
- **Invasive monitoring:** Pulmonary artery catheterization (Swan-Ganz catheter) that also measures the pulmonary artery wedge pressure.

The measurement of cardiac output, end diastolic volume (preload) and systemic vascular resistance and blood volume is done to differentiate between hypovolemia, distributive, cardiogenic shock (they may coexist). This helps plan the fluid and vasopressor therapy.

Fluid Resuscitation Therapy in Shock

- First-line therapy is fluid resuscitation by infusing intravenous fluids, along with ascertaining the cause of shock.
- Correction of hypovolemia and restoration of preload must be done before starting of inotropes and definitive therapy for the type of shock.

In Hemorrhagic Shock

- Bleeding is controlled at the earliest—to avoid hypothermia and dilution of coagulation factors.
- Resuscitation is done concurrently with surgery to control bleeding.

In Others Types

- Example, obstructive shock.
- *Hypovolemia is corrected* before surgical intervention, to reduce risk of end organ failure induced by additional surgical trauma.
- Danger of using inotropic or chronotropic agents—deplete the myocardium of oxygen stores, reduce diastolic filling and coronary perfusion, and dramatically reduce diastolic filling and therefore coronary perfusion. This leads to unresuscitatable shock.
- Central venous catheters—appropriate for monitoring than fluid replacement therapy.

End Points of Resuscitation

Ensuring adequate tissue perfusion and avoidance of occult hypoperfusion.

Occult Hypoperfusion

It is detected by markers of organ perfusion/tissue oxygenation are abnormal—lactic acid, pH, blood gases, acid base status.

Pulse oximetry, urine output, blood pressure show normal values.

Specific Management in Different Types of Shock

> **Q. Classify hemorrhage. Describe clinical features and management of hemorrhagic shock. (Long Answer)**

Hemorrhage

- **Types:** Overt (revealed) or occult (concealed), external or internal.
- **Pathophysiology (discussed in previous sections)**
- **Clinical features (Table 2.3)**

Important Points in Management of Hemorrhagic Shock

Prevention of hypothermia, coagulopathy and lactic acidemia/acidosis (lethal triad). Control of hemorrhage and restoration of lost volume.

- Fluid resuscitation should be started and be concurrently done with controlling hemorrhage at the earliest - to prevent hypothermia and coagulopathy.
- Blood and fluid should be adequately warmed.
- **Damage control resuscitation (DCR):**
  - Promote hemostasis—early administration of plasma and platelets to achieve a balanced resuscitation; minimizing the use of crystalloid and artificial colloid like dextrans
  - Permissive hypotension—keeping low blood pressure helps reducing bleeding along with hemostatic measures.

Table 2.3: Classification of hemorrhage.

Class	I	II	III	IV
Blood loss—volume in mL	Less than 750	750–1500	1500–2000	>2000
Percentage of blood volume	Less than 15%	15–30%	30–40%	>40
Heart rate (beats per min)	Below 100	Above 100	Above 120	Above 140
Hypotension	None	Orthostatic	Present	Severe
Neurological state	Normal	Anxious	Confused and drowsy	Severely drowsy

Emergency interventions: Surgical and non-surgical:
- **Surgical:** Thoracotomy/laparotomy and splenectomy or exploration of vessel injuries of limbs or neck.
- **Non-surgical control:**
  - Endoscopic hemostasis for bleeding varices, angiodysplasia
  - Radiological intervention—transarterial embolisation of bleeding vessels.

Note: All measures under general management of shock are undertaken as described in previous section.

> **Q. Principles of treatment of septic shock. (Short notes).**

SEPTIC SHOCK
- It is a vasodilatory shock/distributive shock.
- *Unlike in other types,* the peripheral capillary dilatation causes warm peripheries and not cold.
- Circulatory catecholamine levels and cardiac output are high but there is hypotension. (Details discussed under pathophysiology, resuscitation and monitoring).

Treatment of Septic Shock
Principles of Therapy
- Fluid resuscitation (refer general steps of management)
- Administration of appropriate antibiotic therapy
- Control of the source of infection
- Surgery—to remove source of sepsis (organ or pus).

Antibiotic Therapy
Best guess antibiotic based on the likely source of sepsis and on the lab reports after the availability. Generally this consists of an anti beta-lactam cephalosporin or meropenem (against gram-negative gut bacteria), anti-anaerobic agent like metronidazole and an anti-MRSA agent like linezolid. Aztreonam is preferred in patients with renal compromise.

Control of Source of Infection
- Drainage of infected fluid collections.
- Removal of infected foreign bodies or a necrotic tissue or gangrenous organ (bowel) or debridement of devitalized tissues and amputation of a septic limb.

Monitoring Involves Measurement
Of physiologic parameters and markers of organ perfusion and tissue oxygenation to determine and follow the efficacy of resuscitation.

OTHER FORMS OF SHOCK
Obstructive Shock
Preload of heart should be restored by action like correcting congestive failure, release of pericardial tamponade or venous obstruction.

Systemic Inflammatory Response Syndrome (SIRS) in Shock
This is explained in Chapter 1 (SU1.1) on metabolic response to injury.

Multiple Organ Dysfunction Syndrome (MODS)
- Irreversible cellular injury of all tissues leading to failure of two or more organ systems, viz., heart, kidney, lung, liver, gut.
- Any cause of shock can lead to SIRS and MODS.
- Hemodynamic instability due to distributive shock and coagulopathy are seen.

> **SU2.3: Communicate and counsel patients and families about the treatment and prognosis of shock demonstrating empathy and care—DOAP**
>
> *(Only salient principles are given here as it is a DOAP practical session)*

Counseling the Patient

To seek and get his cooperation in treatment; to relieve the patient of his apprehension and to boost the patient's morale.

Counseling the Family of the Patient

This is equally important. The doctor should first sit with his co members of the health care team (like other specialties) who are involved in the treatment and decide about what has to be conveyed to the family members.

The family is taken into confidence about the patient's condition, the nature/gravity of the complications and the chances of survival. It is pertinent to discuss the pros and cons of each part of treatment and the need for of the same, clearly convincing them of the limitation. The costs of the treatment especially the resuscitative part in the intensive care and the specific measures like the surgical or non surgical interventions are explained in detail.

Being empathetic during the discussion will have a positive impact on the patient's psyche. The family of the patients will also expect and appreciate empathy from the doctors. If possible two doctors of the team can join together in the discussion with patient and family.

Blood and Blood Components

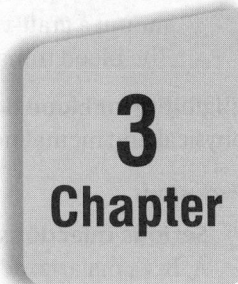
Chapter 3

SU3.1	Describe the indications and appropriate use of blood and blood products and complications of blood transfusion.
	SU3.2 and SU3.3 are included in SU3.1
SU3.2	Observe blood transfusions.
SU3.3	Counsel patients and family/friends for blood transfusion and blood donation.

SU3.1: Describe the indications and appropriate use of blood and blood products and complications of blood transfusion.
The competencies SU3.2 and SU3.3 are incorporated in SU3.1.

BLOOD TRANSFUSION
- First recorded successful transfusion in 1818.
- Use of blood and blood products must always be judicious
- Currently whole blood is rarely transfused; instead, its fractions are transfused according to the specific needs of the situation.

Blood Groups
- **ABO system:** Consists of three allelic genes—A, B and O—highly antigenic proteins with naturally occurring antibodies in the serum. It can be four phenotypes.
  - ABO phenotypes: A, B, AB and O
- Rhesus D group—Rh positive (+ve) and Rh negative (–ve).

Compatibility
Donor's group should be the same as that of recipient.
- In situations of grave emergency, O group is used as a universal donor to transfuse any other group patients. (O cells don't have any surface antigens and can match any group).
- AB can receive AB, A, B or O group (universal recipient)
- Rh negative blood can be transfused to a Rh positive person (converse is incompatible).

Matching
ABO group and Rh type of the recipient and donor are tested and recorded.
- Red blood cells of donors are matched against sera of recipients for compatibility as well as the presence of irregular red cell antibodies.

Transfusion reactions—result from antibodies from in the recipient's serum, which are incompatible with donor's cells.

Types
- Acute hemolytic reaction
  - Severe immune-related transfusion reactions due to ABO incompatibility
  - Potentially fatal intravascular hemolysis and multiple organ failure.
- Antigen reactions are usually milder and self-limiting
- Non-hemolytic: Due to
  - Febrile transfusion reactions—fever, chills or rigors

- Caused by leukocytes in transfused blood mount a graft-versus-host response
- The blood transfusion must be stopped

Eligibility for blood donation: Any one in good physical and mental health can donate blood.

Exclusions

- **Serious infectious diseases:** HIV, hepatitis A, B, C, malaria, active tuberculosis.
- Persons in extremes of age children below 16 and elderly above 60 years (generally).
- Known malignancy or post-treatment state.
- Advanced systemic disorders—heart failure, pulmonary liver and renal failure.
- Active immunological disorders.
- **Temporary exclusions:** Anemia (hemoglobin level below 10 g%).
- Underweight (below 45 kg) and malnutrition.

> Q. Enumerate indications for blood transfusions, write briefly on the blood components and fractions available and enlist complications of transfusions.

Collection of Blood and Storage

- Blood is collected in bags with 75 mL of citrate phosphate dextrose (CPD) solution; stored at 4°C. Shelf life: For 3 weeks.
- **CPDA solution:** CPD and adenosine—shelf life prolonged to 5 weeks
- SAG-M (Saline, Adenine, Glucose-Mannitol)—shelf life - 5 weeks
  - Used to store packed cells at 2–4°C
  - Contains no protein and hence albumin supplementation needed after every 4 units.

Shelf Life of Blood Components in Stored Blood

- Red cells—3 weeks but lose capacity to release oxygen after 7 days.
- WBC—2 days
- Platelets—1 day
- Clotting factors—1–2 days.

About 450 mL of blood is drawn from the donor. The donated blood is leukodepleted to reduce the immunogenicity of the transfusion. The blood is then processed into **subcomponents**.

Individual components are stored:
- **Whole blood:** Rarely used.
  - Advantages over packed cells, if fresh, metabolically active and rich in coagulation factors.
  - Disadvantage: Rich in leukocytes—immunogenicity high.
- **Autologous blood:** Patient's own blood is collected 2 to 3 weeks before surgery for retransfusion during the operation. Similarly, during surgery blood can be collected in a cell-saver which washes and collects red blood cells which can then be returned to the patient.
- **Packed red cells:** Obtained by centrifuging whole blood to separate plasma.
- **Obtained:** Each unit—330 mL, with a hematocrit of 60–70%, stored in a SAG-M solution (Refer above).
- **Fresh-frozen plasma (FFP)** extracted from fresh blood and is rich in coagulation factors; stored at –40 to –50°C, with a 2-year shelf life.
  - Use: In the treatment of hemorrhage due to coagulopathy.
  - Note: Rh positive can be given to Rh negative women in emergency.
- **Cryoprecipitate:** Rich in factor VIII and fibrinogen
  - It is the supernatant precipitate of FFP; has a shelf life of 2 years when stored at –30°C.
  - Uses: In hemophiliacs, von Willebrand's disease and low fibrinogen states.
- **Human albumin 4.5%—prepared by** repeated fractionations
  - Stored in liquid form at 4°C
  - Shelf life: For several months
- **Platelets:**
  - *Pooled platelet concentrate:* Contain about 250 trillion cells per 100 mL.
  - *A shelf life:* 5 days when stored at 20–24°C.
  - **Use:**
    - Thrombocytopenia or
    - Bleeding or to reduce bleeding in surgeries in those with platelet dysfunction due to aspirin or clopidogrel therapy.

Factor VIII and IX concentrate—hemophilia and factor IX deficiency.

- **Prothrombin complex concentrate**
  - Contains factors II, IX and X and VII may be included.
  - VII can be separated) or produced separately.
  - Purified concentrates prepared from pooled plasma.
  - **Use:** Emergency reversal of anticoagulant (warfarin) therapy in uncontrolled hemorrhage.
- **Fibrinogen:** Obtained by organic liquid fractionation of plasma.
  - Stored in dried form.
  - **Use:** DIC and afibrinogenemia.

> Q. What are indications for blood transfusions? (Short notes)

INDICATIONS FOR BLOOD TRANSFUSION

Blood transfusions should be generally avoided and considered only if it is a must.
- Acute blood loss—for restoring circulating volume and ensuring tissue oxygenation.
  - Major trauma—blood loss exceeding 15% of total body volume to replace
  - Major surgeries—operative loss
- Perioperative—deficiency of blood to ensure oxygenation
  - For hemoglobin level—if below 6 g with no active bleed or below 8 g and there is operative bleeding.
- For correction of deficiency of coagulation factors or platelets (blood fractions transfused)
- Adjunct to cancer treatment to correct anemia.
- **Treatment of anemia:** Chronic anemia—if there is no over bleeding or the patient has to undergo a major surgery.

> Q. Define massive transfusion and enlist complications of massive transfusion. (Short notes)

MASSIVE BLOOD TRANSFUSION

- Transfusion of blood equivalent to blood volume of the person in less than 24 hours (5-6 liters in adults and , 85 mL/kg body weight in infants).
- Replacement of 50% of blood volume in 3 hours
- Single transfusion of blood more than 2,500 mL or 4 units in one hour.

Indication

- Major polytrauma.
- Primary surgical bleeding.

COMPLICATIONS OF BLOOD TRANSFUSION

Complications from a Single Transfusion

- **Non-hemolytic:** Allergic reaction, febrile transfusion reaction
- **Hemolytic:** Incompatibility related reaction
- **Infection:** Bacterial, viral (hepatitis, HIV), malaria
- Acute renal failure
- Thrombophlebitis
- Air embolism
- Congestive cardiac failure
- FFP- induced acute lung injury (ALI)—acute respiratory distress syndrome (ARDS).

Complications from Massive Transfusion

- Hypothermia
- Hyperkalemia; hypokalemia
- Hypocalcemia
- Disseminated intravascular coagulation (DIC)/other type of coagulopathy—dilutional thrombocytopenia
- Iron overload.

Management of Coagulopathy

Indication for Correction of Coagulopathy

- During or after massive transfusion—both before or after manifestation of coagulopathy.
- Coagulopathy due to surgery.
- Prevention of dilutional coagulopathy in resuscitation of patients in active hemorrhage.

Section 1: Basics in Surgery

What should be done?
- Transfuse units of FFP, platelets and red cells in a ratio of 1: 1:1 to reduce chances of dilutional coagulopathy.
- Correction of existing coagulopathy—coagulation factors, platelet concentrates.
- Routine monitoring, laboratory tests—fibrinogen, clotting time, activated partial thromboplastin time (APTT), prothrombin time (PT), fibrinogen degradation products (FDP), d-Dimer (DD)
- Empirical tranexamic acid (anti-fibrinolytic).

Acute Lung Injury: After Blood Transfusion

Mechanism
- Donor plasma antibody against HLA and leukocyte specific antigens of recipient.
- Or it is due to recipient's antibody against donor leukocytes.
- *Clinical features*: Breathlessness, hypoxia, hypotension, fever
- Chest X-ray or CT scan—show bilateral diffuse parenchymal infiltrate.
- Treatment—need ventilator support.
- Recovery—good with prompt treatment.

Transfusion-related Graft-versus-host Disease (TGVHD)
- Post transfusion—pancytopenia, toxic epidermal necrosis, liver dysfunction
- Common in immunosuppressed, lymphoma, leukemic patients
- Due to immune response of the donor lymphocytes against host tissues
- Any type of blood products including leukocyte reduced blood can cause the condition
- Rare but mortality—over 90%.

Q. Write a short notes on blood substitutes.

BLOOD SUBSTITUTES
- Alternative to human blood.
- Avoids potential immunogenic and infectious complications associated with transfusion.
- Oxygen-carrying blood substitutes under biomimetic or abiotic.

Biomimetic substitutes—haemoglobin-based oxygen-carrier. Stroma-free hemoglobin

Abiotic substitutes are synthetic oxygen carriers - perfluorocarbon-based perfluorodecalin.

PLASMA SUBSTITUTES

Human Albumin 4.5%
- Plasma fractionation is done using organic liquids and heat to extract albumin which is stored at 4°C for—1 g of albumin binds with 14 mL of water
- **Indications:** Cirrhosis, burns, nephrotic syndrome.

Dextrans: Plasma Volume Expanders
- Polysaccharides—molecular weights 40,000.
- After adding yeast—one gram of dextran binds with 20 mL of water to raise the plasma volume.
  - Low molecular weight dextran (40,000 mol wt)
  - High molecular weight dextran mol wt 70000 or 110,000.

Gelatin—mol wt 30,000 - up to 1000 mL of 3.4–4% solution.
- But it is less effective than dextran.
- **Hydroxyethyl starch:** It contains starch, sodium hydroxide, ethylene oxide. It is a good plasma volume expander but lasts only for 6 hours.

Burns

SU4.1	Elicit document and present history in a case of burns and perform physical examination. Describe pathophysiology of burns.
SU4.2	Describe clinical features, diagnose type and extent of burns and plan appropriate treatment.
SU4.3	Discuss the medicolegal aspects in burn injuries.
SU4.4	Communicate and counsel patients and families on the outcome and rehabilitation demonstrating empathy and care. Demonstration

SU4.1: Elicit document and present history in a case of burns and perform physical examination. Describe pathophysiology of burns.
Refer under history taking and clinical evaluation

SU4.2: Describe clinical features, diagnose type and extent of burns and plan appropriate treatment.

Q. Classify burns - according to mechanism, based on depth, thickness, surface area.

MECHANISM OF BURNS

- Thermal injury
  - Dry heat: Contact with hot subjects, heat of combustion, hot gases
  - Wet heat: Hot liquids—water, oil
- Chemical burns: Acid, alkali
- Electrical burns
- Radiation burns: Ionizing radiation, non-ionizing—ultraviolet rays
- Special: Inhalation burns—steam, chemical fumes, smoke.

Classification of burns based on depth of burns (as given in **Table 4.1**).

DEPTH OF BURNS (TABLE 4.1)

Table 4.1: Depth of burns.

Degree	Depth of burns	Clinical picture	Signs
Superficial burns Degree 1	Epidermis only	Erythema	Sensation intact, hyperemia
Superficial burns Degree 2	Papillary dermis (superficial partial thickness)	Vesicles, red, painful	Capillary circulation intact Sign of blanching, hyperesthesia
	Reticular dermis (deep partial thickness)	Depigmentation	No capillary blanching Pin prick sensation intact
Deep burns Degree 3	Full thickness of skin Subcutaneous tissue	Necrotic skin	Leathery surface, charred No pain Sensation lost
Degree 4	Deeper muscles and or bone	Full thickness necrosis	

TYPES OF BURNS

- **Partial thickness burns:** Erythematous, painful, vesicles—**first or second** degree burn.
- **Full thickness burns:** Affects all layers of the skin—charred, insensitive—**third degree** burns

CLASSIFICATION OF BURNS BASED ON BODY SURFACE AREA (BSA)

- **Mild:**
  - Less than 15% of BSA (10% in children)—partial thickness.
  - Or < 2% full thickness.
- **Moderate:**
  - 15-25% BSA—partial thickness burns (10-20% in children).
  - 2-10% BSA of full thickness burns.
- **Severe:**
  - Above 25% BSA in adults and 20% in children—partial thickness.
  - All full thickness burns of over 10%.
  - All inhalation and electrical burns.
  - Burns associated with major fractures and systemic trauma.
  - Burns involving eyes, ears, feet, hands, perineum.

Surface Area of Burns as a Percentage of the Body Surface Area

- Minor burns are calculated with palm as a guide. (The area of palm is taken as 1% of TBSA).
- **Wallace's rule of "9":** Used for the first assessment of the burns **(Table 4.2)**.

Table 4.2: Wallace's rule of nine.

Parts of body	Adults surface area	Children
Head and neck	9%	18%
Upper limb	9 × 2 = 18%	18%
Lower limb	18 × 2 = 36%	14 × 2 = 28%
Front of chest and abdominal wall	9 × 2 = 18%	18%
Back of chest and abdominal wall	9 × 2 = 18%	18% together
Perineum	1%	

> **Q. Describe pathophysiology of burns** (Please refer box below for brief answer).

PATHOPHYSIOLOGY OF BURNS

Pathophysiology of burns
Coagulation necrosis of skin and subcutaneous tissues, cell damage and release of intracellular molecules into circulation, evoking an inflammatory response and complex circulatory changes.

Inflammation and circulatory changes—happen first 36 hours after the injury.
- Burns produce an inflammatory reaction causing increased vascular permeability.
- Heat causes alteration of proteins, releases neuropeptides and activate complement, degranulation of mast cells and leukocytes, releasing free radicals, further damage to the tissue.
- Mast cells release cytokines such as tumor necrosis factor alpha (TNF-α). and in turn, the inflammatory cells and secondary cytokines (IL-6).

This results in increased permeability of blood vessels causing:
- A net flow of water, solutes and proteins from the intravascular to the extravascular space.
- This causes—hypovolemia, hypoproteinemia and hypoxemia.
- Burns of over 15% of TBSA and results in shock.
- Circulatory failure—hypovolemia, myocardial depression (burns toxins).
- Renal failure, pulmonary edema due to exudation.
- Shock—hypovolemic and distributive shock.

Immunological changes: Due to inflammatory changes:
- Suppression of cell-mediated immunity. Increased susceptibility to infections.
- Acute lung injury—due to cytokines and added infections.

Changes in the intestines and abdomen: Microvascular damage and ischemia of the gut mucosa - stress (curling) ulcers of stomach. Abdominal compartment syndrome—ileus, and translocation of gut bacteria leading to life threatening septicemia.

Metabolic changes: Hypermetabolism, negative nitrogen balance and metabolic acidosis electrolyte imbalance (hyperkalemia, hyponatremia), SIADH.

Sepsis: In burn patient—from burn site, bowel, lungs, bladder, catheters, venous lines and worsened by comorbidities like diabetes, steroids, and HIV.

> **Q. Short notes: Inhalation burns, circumferential burns and eschar.**

Inhalation burns: They pose grave threat to life due to burns and edema of airway tract often with loss of respiratory epithelium - involving face, oronasal apertures, supraglottic and subglottic airway. This leads to respiratory failure and carbon monoxide poisoning.
- Full-thickness burns to the chest can restrict respiratory movements.

Circumferential burns: Cause constricting effect on limb circulation or on chest movement.

Electrical burns: They cause local damage and additional myocardial injury leading to bradyarrhythmias and arrest.

Chemical burns: Acid burns—cause coagulation necrosis and long-term fibrosis.
Alkaline burns—liquefaction necrosis and deeper burns with worse consequences.

Eschar
Formed by the coagulation necrosis of proteins and charring with resultant shrinkage of dermis. It forms a tough protective cover over the burn wound. Infection can occur under the eschar in circumferential burns. The eschar may cause constricting effect on limb circulation or respiratory movements of chest wall.

> **Q. How do you assess and manage a burns patient?**

ASSESSMENT OF BURNS PATIENT AND MANAGEMENT

At the Site of Injury

Pre-hospitalization Care
- Remove from burn source
- Cooling (around 15°C)—15 min upto 1 hour
- Elevation of head in airway burn; elevation of limb in limb burns
- Oxygen
- Fluids started
- Cover wound with sterile (or clean) cloth
- Ensure safety to the rescuer.

Management at First Point of Care

Emergency—primary survey carried out simultaneously with assessment.

History—most important in assessing nature and severity and hence planning treatment.
- Mechanism of burns, nature of burns, identify burn source, duration of exposure and area of contact with heat source, temperature of the source, part of the body exposed.
- Is there an inhalation burn? fumes inhaled?
- Chemical—swallowed or fumes.
- Explosions can cause barotraumas to the eardrums and lungs and may also cause blunt trauma.

Primary Survey

Primary survey—conducted following ATLS principles of ACS.

Burn patient is evaluated and treated like one of multi trauma. Associated injuries are missed in burns due to blasts, fall, industrial accidents.
- **Airway**—assessment and secure.
    - Inhalation injury anticipated.
    - Physical signs—include hoarseness, stridor, facial burns, singed facial hair, expectoration of carbonaceous sputum, and presence of carbon in the oropharynx.
    - Early tracheal intubation in case of facial and neck swelling. Inhalation burns suspected.
- **Breathing**—is evaluated for effort, depth of respiration, and auscultation of breath sounds.
    - Wheezing or rales—(inhalation injury or aspiration of gastric contents).
    - Beware of: Early pulmonary insufficiency and respiratory failure.
    - Oxygen delivered at lower tidal volumes to maintain " permissive hypercapnia".
- **Circulation: Most important step in early burns management.**
    - Aggressive and prompt fluid resuscitation.
    - Full-thickness circumferential burns of extremity or neck burns requires escharotomy (to maintain circulation in the limb).
- **Disability:** Neurological condition—assessed.
- **Exposure- and control of environment:**
    - All clothes removed (to avoid further burns and chemical damage.

- Irrigation of injuries with water or saline to remove harmful residues.
- Removal of all constricting gadgets and jewellery.

Secondary Survey

Burn-specific secondary survey
- Depth of burn—classified and managed based on depth.
- Percentage of total body surface area (TBSA) estimated. Small areas calculated by hand (as - 1% each) and large areas by "rule of nines"
- To plan fluid resuscitation and decide on transferring the patient a specialized burn center.

Transfer to a Burn Center

Age and TBSA of burn percentage are two most important prognostic factors.

Criteria for Shifting to a Specialized Center

- Partial-thickness burns greater than 10% BSA.
- Any full-thickness burn.
- Burns that involve the face, hands, feet, genitalia, perineum, or major joints.
- Any inhalation, chemical, or electrical injury (including lightning).
- Burn injury in patients medical comorbidities.
- Burns in combination with significant associated polytrauma.
- Burns in patients with psychiatric illness.
- Burns with suspected suicide or homicidal actions.

Fluids—most important to start fluid resuscitation at the earliest.

Management at the Burns Unit

- **Oxygen—humidified oxygen—face mask or after intubation.**
- **Intravenous access—for patients with >15% burns.**
  - Large peripheral venous line (14 g or 16 g)
  - Avoiding lower limb.

- **Fluid resuscitation:**
  - Most important in improving survival—reducing the impact of burns shock.
  - Early and aggressive volume resuscitation must be undertaken in all cases of with burns of over 20% total body surface area (TBSA).
  - Fluid resuscitation is done as per various formulae available.
  - Administered fluids—include crystalloids and colloids.

Parkland Formula

- Exclusive crystalloid based resuscitation.
- Lactated Ringer solution is the preferred crystalloid
- Volume of fluid to be replaced in the first 24 hours—4 mL per kilogram of body weight per percentage burns.
- Total percentage body surface area × weight (kg) × 4 = volume (mL).
- Half this volume is given in the first 8 hours and the second half in the next 16 hours—infused with adjustments being made as clinical conditions, size and depth of burns evolve.
- Over-resuscitation is avoided to prevent congestive complications such as abdominal compartment syndrome. For children weighing 30 kg or less, 5% dextrose in one-quarter normal saline helps restoration of fluid and glucose reserves.

Colloid-containing Solutions

- Their role is debated.
- Avoided until after the first 24 hours postburn (capillary leak diminishes).
- Some use albumin later in the first 24 hours and in patients with large burns.

Muir and Barclay Colloid-based Formula

- Calculated rations to be given over specified periods.
- 0.5 × percentage body surface area burnt × weight = one ration.
- First 12 hours 3 rations over 12 hrs. One ration of crystalloid per each 4 hour period.

- Next 12 hours— 2 intervals over next 12 hrs. One ration of crystalloid per each 6 hour period along with colloid (albumin) supplementation.
- Subsequent 12 hours—one ration of crystalloid and albumin.
- Blood transfusions are given, if needed, only after 48 hours.

Monitoring of Resuscitation

Measurement of:
- **Urine output:** Best guide of perfusion (normal urine output is 0.5 to 0.1 mL/kg weight per hour)
  The rate of fluid infusion is increased if the output falls below 0.5 mL/kg/hr.
- Hematocrit—to assess hydration state.
- Acid-base balance—to assess tissue perfusion
- CVP monitoring
- Transesophageal ultrasound—to assess cardiac input.

Relief of Pain

Acute Pain
- Analgesia very important,
- Superficial burns—non-narcotic analgsics—paracetamol and NSAIDs; topical cooling is often soothing.
- Large burns and deep dermal burns: Opiates—intravenous opiates.

Post Acute Phase: In Large Burns
- **Continuous analgesia:** For patients with larger area of burns. Infusions followed by oral tablets—slow-release morphine.
- **For dressing or esharotomy:** General anesthesia or intravenous midazolam and ketamine.

Additional Measures
- **Indwelling Foley catheter**—monitor hourly urine output (index of perfusion)
- **Nasogastric tube**—to tackle paralytic adynamic ileus.
- **Continuous pulse oximetry**—to measure oxygen saturation
- *Note:* Carbon monoxide poisoning can show falsely elevated levels.

Laboratory Evaluation
- Urinalysis—routine, proteinuria, myoglobinuria.
- Complete blood cell count, electrolytes, arterial blood-gas evaluation and renal parameters.
- Arterial carboxyhemoglobin—in inhalation/suspected CO poisoning.
- β-human chorionic gonadotropin—to detect pregnancy.

Electrocardiogram—electrical burns - and in assessing the arrhythmias during fluid replacement.

Tetanus Prophylaxis
- 0.5 mL of tetanus toxoid is given intramuscularly.
- Human tetanus immunoglobulin 250 to 500 units intramuscularly if not immunized previously.

Burns Wound Care
- **Early irrigation and debridement**—using normal saline and sterile instruments to remove all loose epidermal skin layers.
- **Blisters:** They permit healing in a sterile milieu and protect the underlying dermis too. Blisters are left alone in small superficial burns but are debrided in large and deep partial thickness burns to relieve tension, to remove inflammatory mediators and to prevent infection.
- **Topical antimicrobial agents—mainstay of wound care**
  Burn wound sepsis:
  - Gram-negative organisms: *Pseudomonas aeruginosa* and fungi.
  - Gram-positive organisms: *Staphylococcus aureus* and group A streptococci.

Diagnosis: Biopsy Eschar—shows organism load of 1 million per gram of tissue.

Treatment: Excision of infected eschar and topical/systemic antibiotic therapy.

Topical applications: Silver sulfadiazine cream 1%. 0.5% silver nitrate solution, Mafenide acetate cream.

- **Dressings**
  - **Biologic dressings**—allograft (cadaver skin) and xenograft (pig skin). These dressings provide the advantages of ease of acquisition and application while providing barrier protection and a biologic bed under which dermis can granulate.
  - **Synthetic dressings** have become an attractive alternative for early wound coverage. Collagen-coated silicone membrane—prevents moisture loss.

> Q. Enlist principles of surgical procedures in burns.

SURGERY IN ACUTE BURNS

- **Escharotomy—to divide constricting eschar.** In full-thickness circumferential burns of the neck, extremities to restore tissue ischemia due to constricting effect and edema. Or to release restriction of respiratory movements in the chest.
- **Early tangential excision of burn eschar—for deep dermal burns (deep 2nd degree)** to the level of bleeding capillaries done after the resuscitation phase.
- **Early excision and grafting—for all full thickness burns**
  - **All necrotic tissue excised and wound cover given: Temporary or permanent** benefits survival, blood loss, incidence of sepsis, and length of stay
  - **Split-thickness skin grafts (autografts):** For very large wounds, split-thickness skin grafts can be meshed up to 4:1.
  Temporary: Synthetic grafts or heterologous grafts (xenograft).
- **Delayed reconstruction—for full thickness burns.**
- **Scar management: Reconstruction after division or excision**
  Early intervention against contractures:
  - Eyes—grafting to prevent exposure keratitis.
  - Contracture over joints
  - Burn alopecia—unburnt skin expansion done.

Techniques
- Z-plasty
- A transposition flap—for wider scars
- A full-thickness graft or vascularized tissue as in a free flap—for large scars
- Split skin graft.

Keloids
- Pressure dressings—worn for a period of 6–18 months.
- Silicone patches—to speed up the scar maturation.

> Q. How do you manage the nutritional requirement in burns patient.

NUTRITION IN BURNS

It is a hypermetabolic state (upto 200% of normal) proportionate to the size of the burn. The daily estimated metabolic requirement (EMR)—is calculated from the *Curreri formula*:

EMR = 25 kcal × body weight (kg) + (40 kcal × %BSA).

Protein losses in burn patients replaced by administering 1.5 to 2 g/kg of protein per day.
- **Enteral feeding**—the preferred route when tolerated
  - It is administered through an enteral feeding tube, started within first 24 hours. It shortens the hospital stay by reducing the risk of infection and catabolic response.
- **Total parenteral nutrition**—only if the patient is unable to tolerate enteral feeding. Initiated after fluid resuscitation
  - **Daily vitamin supplementation:** Vitamin C, thiamine, Riboflavin, nicotinamide 500 mg and zinc.

Prophylaxis Against Complications
- **Gastroduodenal stress ulcers:** Proton-pump inhibitors (pantoprazole or esomeprazole) or H-2 blockers—ranitidine/famotidine).
- **Venous thromboembolism (VTE):** Heparin or low molecular weight heparin (dalteparin or enoxaparin).

Sepsis

- **Prophylactic antibiotics**—(piperacillin tazobactam) against infection in wound, respiratory tract and urine.
- Fluid resuscitation with crystalloids.
- Vasopressors for hemodynamic support.
- Transfusion - for hemoglobin levels below.
- Ventilatory support - as needed
- Maintenance of blood glucose less than 180 mg/dL.
- Psychological and psychiatric consultation—counseling.

Physiotherapy: Limbs, chest.

Management of Special Circumstances

Age

- Infants and elderly individuals—highest risk patient
- Age is a major determinant on outcome.
- Infants—common form of child abuse.
- Elderly patients usually have comorbid medical problems and decreased physiologic reserve.

INHALATION BURNS INJURIES

Q. Describe inhalation burns injuries.

Also refer Pathophysiology of burns along with this section.

Management

- **Minor inhalation injury**—humidified oxygen is delivered.
- **Major injuries**
  - Endotracheal intubation for airway protection.
  - Pulmonary toilet of viscous secretions.
  - Bronchodilators can be given to treat bronchospasm whereas nebulized heparin and N-acetylcysteine can limit cast formation.
  - Extubation at the earliest possible.

Carbon Monoxide Poisoning

- Suspected by a history of exposure in a confined space,
- Nausea, vomiting, headache, mental status changes, and cherry-red lips.
- Carbon monoxide binds to hemoglobin with an affinity 240 times greater than that of oxygen, resulting in extremely slow dissociation
- Arterial carboxyhemoglobin level >5% in nonsmokers >10% in smokers is taken as high. The patient is started on oxygen—100% oxygen via non-rebreathing mask, continued until normal levels are achieved. Hyperbaric oxygen treatment is used as adjunct to oxygen in CO poisonings and burns.

Q. Write a short notes on electrical burns.

ELECTRICAL BURNS

They cause local tissue damage and myocardial damage in addition.

Complications

- Cardiopulmonary arrest (more common with alternating current)
- Thrombosis, sudden fall and fractures
- Rhabdomyolysis—release of myoglobin from injured cells of deep tissues to cause acute renal failure. Dark urine is seen first.

Treatment

- Intravenous lactated Ringer solution is used to maintain a urine output of at least 2 mL/kg/hr.
- Monitoring for bradycardia and arrest which may happen days after the injury.
- May need administration of atropine round the clock.

Chemical Injury

Alkali or acid or organic (petroleum) compounds.

Treatment

Immediate removal of the offending agent.

- Irrigation with abundant water for 30 minutes or more.
- Alkali burns penetrate more deeply than acid burns and require longer periods of irrigation.
- Neutralizing the chemicals is not preferred as the reaction generates heat.

Q. Write a short note on cold injuries.

COLD INJURIES

Hypothermia

- A core body temperature less than 35°C.
- Mild 32° to 35°C; moderate is 32°C - 30°C; and severe is less than 30°C.

Signs of Hypothermia

- Skin—cold, pale or cyanotic.
- Lower level of consciousness, dysrhythmias (asystole happens below 28°C).

Management

- Cardiac monitoring, resuscitation, rewarming
- Cardiopulmonary resuscitation maintained until rewarming the patient to 36°C.

Rewarming Methods

- Passive rewarming—blankets to cover the body and head (warming rate-0.5° and 2°C hourly).
- Active external warming includes the use of heating blankets or a heated forced-air system, which can increase rewarming rates by 1 °C per hour
- Active internal rewarming—fluids and oxygen, (warming rate of 1° to 2°C per hour).
- Active invasive rewarming methods warm -faster at a rate 1° to 4°C per hour, e.g., warmed peritoneal lavage, thoracostomy lavage, and bladder lavage.
- Extracorporeal rewarming of blood—rapid rewarming—1-2 degree every 5 minutes.
  - Heated hemodialysis or via a continuous venovenous bypass circuit.

Q. What is frostbite? How do you manage the same? Short notes.

FROSTBITE

- Formation of intracellular ice crystals and microvascular occlusion.
- Factors affecting severity: Temperature, duration of exposure, conditions promoting rapid heat loss such as wind velocity, moisture, open wounds
- The fingers, toes, nose and ears are most vulnerable.

Classification

- **First degree:** Hyperemia and edema, without skin necrosis.
- **Second degree:** Superficial vesicle formation.
- **Third degree:** Hemorrhagic bullae and full-thickness necrosis.
- **Fourth degree:** Gangrene with full-thickness involvement of skin, muscle, and bone.

Treatment

- Rapid rewarming in a warm water bath between 40° and 42°C until the tissue perfusion returns.
- Elevation of part—to reduce edema.
- Escharotomy for severe injury.
- Amputation—only for gangrene; late recoveries often happen and hence early amputation has no role.

RADIATION BURNS (GOOD TO KNOW)

- Localised radiation damage
- Lethal dose—desquamation of skin—slow death.
- Non-lethal radiation—observe for effects.
  - Local effect—may be ulcer.
  - Systemic effects—GI tract—ulcers, diarrhea, hematochezia.
  - Immuno suppression.

Local treatment—for ulcers (ulcer excision and a vasculrized graft).

Systemic—supportive treatment—fluids, calories, symptomatic therapy against vomiting, diarrhea.
Management of infection.

SU4.3: Discuss the medico-legal aspects in burn injuries.

MEDICO-LEGAL ASPECTS IN BURN INJURIES

Burn injuries inflict severe systemic trauma, mortality, short and long-term morbidity among survivors, along with the economic, social, psychological and emotional impact on the victim.

The burns trauma often raises suspicion of a background of crime or unnatural act as the cause.

The health care provider is obliged to inform the legal authority of all the information on these accidents.
- A large percentage of accidental burn injuries are preventable.
- Burns in domestic and industrial environments are often due to negligence.
- Burns injuries also happen among psychiatric patients, intoxication (alcohol or drug addicts)
- Suicidal burns are most common, especially women and children.
- Child abuse and domestic violence are frequently the cause of burns.
- Social crimes (sexual abuse, riots and violence) frequently involve homicidal burns.

Q. What are the responsibilities of a doctor in management of burns? (Short notes)

Summary of Medico-legal Issues in Burns Management (the Doctor's Responsibilities):
- Informing the police
- Issuing death certificates—cause of death after getting a medicolegal post mortem.
- Dealing with a burns injury in a female—married or unmarried (dowry problem and death); suicide or homicide.
- Disability and disfigurement—for award of compensation by authorities.
- Quantifying the permanent physical Impairment and issuing authenticated certificate
  - Assessing and quantifying impairment (not disability).
  - Obligation to testify; in a court of law on the degree of physical impairment.
- Plight and rights of burns survivor—physical, economic, emotional and vocational loss entitles them to compensation.
- Also spouses are entitled to compensation for loss of consortium.
- Workmen's compensation for industrial and insurance claims.

Details

Information to the Police

Legal and civic duty (as per IPC): Code of Criminal Procedures in section 39—mandates every citizen (includes the doctor) to inform the police of any incidence harmful to human beings.
- The police must be informed at the time of first visit of the patient for treatment or got admitted.
- Inform and notify police of all burns injuries with suspicion of unnatural cause:
  - All major burns when received
  - Unexplained severity, not matching with the history or circumstances
  - Patients received after several days of burns or patients received without proper treatment
  - Patients in moribund state—likely to die of burns.
  - Patients received dead
  - Mass casualties.(industrial accidents, natural disasters)
- Death certificate in burns injuries
  - Cause of death—is ensured by—hence a medico-legal postmortem is a must.
  - Police Officer in charge of the case, writes down a report on the dead body—panchnama. Fills an inquest for a medico-legal post mortem. Later, the body is taken to nearby health establishment equipped with postmortem facilities. Or the body is shifted to a morgue for later postmortem, the next day morning.

Burn Injuries in a Married Female

Domestic Violence
- **Dowry problem:** Police suspect—a dowry related issue in all burns with circumstantial evidences and investigations are done under a senior officer of the rank of DCP.
- **Death:** Governed by section 304B of IPC (specifies dowry deaths and punishment).

Disability and Disfigurement

Burn survivors suffer from disfigurement, emotional stress, loss of self-esteem, long-term injury due to burn injury or repeated corrective surgical procedures like skin grafting or correction of deformities.

> **Q. Enumerate the guidelines in deciding compensation for disability in a burns victim.**

LEGALITIES OF THE AWARD OF DISABILITY BY VARIOUS COMPETENT AUTHORITIES

Workmen's Compensation Act of 1923 and the Motor Vehicle Insurance Act—applied. Physical impairment may cause limitations of functional capacity of the patient—limitations may be termed as "disability to sustain" or "disability to earn livelihood".

The following terms are from the definitions adopted by the World Health Organization (WHO).

IMPAIRMENT AND DISABILITY

Physical impairment and functional limitations lead to disability.

Physical Impairment
- Permanent or temporary, reversible
- Psychological or anatomical loss—paralysis amputation, diabetic retinopathy
- Burn disfigurement or contracture.

Functional Limitations
- Partial or total inability to perform motor, sensory or mental functions.
- The doctor has to quantify and classify them as regressive or progressive.

Disability
- Deficiency in performing any activity. "Activities" in accordance with the age, gender and essential parts of daily living such as self-care, social and economic activity.
- Disability may be permanent, long-term or short-term.

Permanent Physical Impairment (PPI) and Permanent Disability
- There are physical, social, psychological and vocational effects to disability as well.
- A medical person thus needs to evaluate permanent physical impairment and to testify in a court of law, if called as an expert witness.
- Physical impairment certificates—issued by registered doctors (MCI Act 1956 or NMC 2020)
- Medical doctors must restrict to evaluating and certifying physical impairment and not certify disability, which is not purely a medical condition.
- If burn injury occurs as a workplace accident, the Workmen's Compensation Act is applicable.

Disability
Disability divided into three periods:
1. **Permanent disability:** Certified only after quantifying permanent physical disability.
2. **Temporary total disability:** Certified during the period of treating the individual who is totally physically impaired.
3. **Temporary partial disability:** The period after recovering from total physical impairment.

Ultimate legal compensation may be awarded usually for the permanent physical impairment, leading to permanent disability.

Plight and Rights of Burns Survivor
Suffering of the earning member affects economic strength and morale of the entire family. The management of burns is long, painful and costly.

The challenges for the burn survivor:
- Physical and emotional trauma
- An injury that leaves one in pain
- Disfigurement
- Organ damage
- Metabolic and biochemical damage
- Sensitivity to temperature change.

> **Q. What are the legal rights of burns survivors.**

LEGAL RIGHTS OF BURNS SURVIVORS FOR COMPENSATION

Compensation can be claimed by the burn victim depending on the cause of the burn injury.

Compensatory Damages
- For current medical expenses—hospitalization, surgeries emergency, reconstructive and cosmetic counseling, physical therapy, occupational therapy.

- Lost wages—actual and anticipated future loss
- Anticipated future medical expenses.
- Mental or emotional pain and suffering (past and anticipated in the future).
- Disfigurement, any physical or mental impairment or disability.
- Loss of consortium—compensation payable to spouse of a burns victim due to the injury destroying the spousal relations.

Indian Legal Enforcements

- Persons with Disabilities Act 1995 for compensation from the state.
- Mental retardation and Multiple Disabilities Act, 1999.
- Disability means "a person suffering from not less than forty percent of any disability as certified by a medical authority—include blindness, low vision, hearing impairment, locomotor disability or cerebral palsy, mental retardation, mental illness and persons cured of leprosy.

The Rehabilitation Council of India Act, 1992

The Rehabilitation Council of India (RCI) was set up by the Government of India in 1986 to regulate and standardise.
- To standardize training courses and prescribe standards of education for professionals dealing with people with disabilities.
- To regulate these standards in all training institutions uniformly throughout the country
- To promote research in rehabilitation and special education
- To maintain Central Rehabilitation Register for registration of professionals.

> **SU4.4: Communicate and counsel patients and families on the outcome and rehabilitation demonstrating empathy and care. DOAP session.**
> *Only key principles given.*

After evaluation and emergency measures, the treating doctor shares the details with responsible family members. The patient's morale should be boosted by talking to him about the positive progress made during treatment and encouraging him to communicate freely.

It is not an easy job to share a gloomy picture with the patient of family.

To the patient in presence of his family. He is explained that he is ill for a short period and he is improving. If there is a significant impairment of function, he may be told that he would be entitled to compensation and his job is secure, he is assured of relief from pain and symptoms. Show him pictures and recorded success stories. He is also assured that he is not alone and he would get his life back and his cooperation is sought for.

To the family only: One's concerns are shared fully with them including the worst possible scenario, explaining all the existing and anticipated complications. But the same should be done with empathy. They are reassured of one's cooperation in settling the financial entitlements, legal issues and rehabilitation of the patient.

Wound Healing and Wound Care

Chapter 5

SU5.1	Describe normal wound healing and factors affecting healing.
SU5.2	Elicit, document and present a history in a patient presenting with wounds.
SU5.3	Differentiate the various types of wounds, plan and observe management of wounds.
SU5.4	Discuss medico-legal aspects of wounds.

SU5.1: Describe normal wound healing and factors affecting healing.

SU5.2: Elicit, document and present a history in a patient presenting with wounds.

SU5.3: Differentiate the various types of wounds, plan and observe management of wounds.

WOUNDS

Introduction

Healing follows all injuries. Acute wound healing follows normal orderly process of healing, but chronic wound healing does not and often hence requires intervention to facilitate healing.

Q. Describe normal wound healing and factors affecting healing.

Acute Wound Healing (Normal Healing) (Table 5.1)

Physiology: A sequence of events lead to healing of an injured tissue.

Healing process is a balance of repair and regeneration of tissue.

- **The inflammatory phase**—early wound healing
- **The proliferative phase**—intermediate healing
- **The remodeling phase (maturing phase)**—late phase of wound healing.

Table 5.1: Summary—phases of wound healing.

1.	**The inflammatory phase** Early wound healing Day 0 to day 3	Hemostasis (pre-inflammatory)
		Inflammatory phase
		Post-inflammatory destructive phase
2.	**The proliferative phase** Intermediate healing 3 days to 3 weeks	Fibroblast migration and proliferation
		Angiogenesis
		Epithelialization
3.	**The remodeling phase (maturing phase)** Late phase of wound healing Day 21 to 6 months	Deposition of collagen and other matrix proteins lasts for 2–4 weeks
		Wound contraction—4 to 15 days
		Scar formation and remodeling—21 day to 6 months

Inflammatory Phase (Early Wound Healing) (0 to 3 days)

Hemostasis (pre-inflammatory), inflammatory phase and post-inflammatory destructive phase.

Hemostasis

Tissue trauma—bleeding—vasoconstriction—initiation of coagulation—stimulation of fibrin—activation of platelets, formation of fibrin matrix covering the wound—by cell attachment and cytokine reservoir.

Inflammatory Phase (0 to 3 days)

Three plasma-based systems are activated by injury:
1. The coagulation cascade
2. The complement cascade
3. The kinin cascade.

Leukocytes are attracted by the pro-inflammatory response and migrate to the extravascular space in the wound. The migrated polymorphs release cytokines such as TNF-alpha and interleukin-1 that enhance the inflammatory response and local vasodilation.

Post-inflammatory Destructive Phase

- Cytokines induce migration of monocytes into the wound and differentiation into macrophages. Monocytes—phagocytize bacteria and damaged tissue and release cytokines for inflammatory cell recruitment and fibroblast proliferation.
- The inflammatory phase, continues beyond 4th day indefinitely in case of wound that heal by secondary or tertiary intention.
- **Clinical features of this phase:** Rubor (redness), tumor (swelling), calor (heat) and dolor (pain).

Proliferative Phase (Intermediate Wound Healing) 2–3 days to 3 Weeks

Events

1. Fibroblast migration and proliferation, 2. Angiogenesis, and 3. Epithelialization.
- **Fibroblast migration (mesenchymal cells) from normal tissue to wound** - induced by chemotactic cytokines—after days 2–4.
- Angiogenesis—to restore the vasculature disrupted by trauma.
- **Epithelialization—by migration of epithelial cells happens from the edges of the wound and from remaining epidermal skin appendages. Speed is about 1 mm per day.**

This **covers the wound to** restore the barrier against the external atmosphere.

Primarily closed wounds get epithelial cover by 24 to 48 hours.

Remodeling Phase (Maturing Phase) (Late Wound Healing)

Events

- Deposition of collagen and other matrix proteins (glycosaminoglycans and proteoglycans): Fibroblasts synthesise the proteins.
- Wound contraction.
- Scar formation and remodeling—21 days to 6 months.

Collagen Deposition

- Secreted by fibroblasts at a high pace for 2–4 weeks,
- Provides tensile strength to the wound.
- Cross-linkage of collagen fibers facilitated by—oxygen, vitamin C, alpha-ketoglutarate and iron

Wound Contraction

- Starts by day 4–5 and lasts for 12 to 15 days.
- Decrease in wound size.
- The contraction of myofibroblasts causes the movement of the wound edge toward the center of the wound.
- The wound remains open but smaller.

Scar Formation and Remodeling—from 21 days to 6 months

- The final wound-healing event to gain 80% of normal tensile strength (TS) at 6 months and thereafter reaching a plateau at 12 months—below the normal TS.
- Remodeling: Breaking down and replacement of new collagen, which is denser and organized along the lines of stress.

> **Q. Short notes: What is healing by primary intention?**

Classification of wound healing
- Healing by primary intention:
  - Wound edges well apposed
  - Clean and linear scar, minimal scar
- Healing with secondary intention
  - An open wound heals by granulation, contraction followed by epithelialization
  - Here the inflammatory and proliferative responses are exaggerated
  - Poor scar
- Healing by tertiary intention (Syn: Delayed primary intention)
  - Wound left open initially, e.g., contaminated wound
  - Edges brought together later when condition suits

Wound Healing in Specific Tissues
Nerve
- Wallerian degeneration of axon—distal to the wound.
- Proximal degeneration upto the last node of ranvier.
- Regeneration of nerve fibers, which sprout from the cut proximal end, by neurotrophism— mediated by growth factors, hormones and other extracellular matrix trophins.

Neuroma Formation
Happens in nerve regeneration—due to overgrowth of nerve fibers coupled with poor approximation.

Bone
- Periosteal and endosteal proliferation forms the callus (immature bone).
- Consists of osteoid (osteoblasts lay down hydroxyapatite and mineralize the osteoid).
- Cortex and the medullary cavity are restored in the remodeling phase.

Primary healing occurs with minimal callus formation: If fracture ends are accurately apposed and rigidly fixed, callus formation is minimal

Secondary healing due to inappropriate apposition and a gap: Causes delayed union, non-union or malunion.

> **Q. What are the factors affecting wound healing and describe the specific role of these.**

CHRONIC WOUND HEALING (ABNORMAL HEALING)
Pathophysiology
The delayed healing process caused by disruption of the normal healing process, (generally— slowing or arrest of the inflammatory or proliferative phases).

The chronic wounds have increased levels of matrix metalloproteinases, which bind and inhibit the growth factors and cytokines in the wound.

Delayed healing may result in loss of function or poor cosmetic outcome.

Local Factors
Prolonging the Inflammatory Phase
- Foreign bodies
- Repetitive trauma
- Venous insufficiency—distention and capillary damage triggering an inflammatory response
- Active infection
- Biofilms: Made of groups of cells held by extracellular matrix and bacteria with low virulence and antibiotic resistance, adherent to a surface like a catheter implant or chronic wound.

Prolonging Proliferative Phase
- Necrotic tissue prevents new tissue growth (crush injuries, devitalization).
- Hypoxia/ischemia—deficient nutrients and oxygen—failure of collagen deposition.
- Growth factor deficiency—impairs signaling pathways of inflammation, migration, and maturation and causes stagnation of wound healing.
- Excessive matrix protein degradation—inhibits cell function.

Radiation—inhibits local response in general.

Systemic Factors
- Smoking
- Chronic renal insufficiency
- Chronic liver disease
- Diabetes mellitus
- Steroids
- Antimetabolites (anti-cancer therapy)
- Collagen vascular disease.

> **SU5.3:** Differentiate the various types of wounds, plan and observe management of wounds.

Q. Describe management of the acute wound.

Aim
- To secure healing of the wound by primary intention.
- Thereby to reduce the inflammatory and proliferative responses of the body.

Types of Wounds
Based on severity of wound or mechanics of:

Severity of Damage
- Abrasions—(only upto dermis)
- Contusions (skin cover intact)
- Incised wounds—through full thickness
- Laceration—element of tissue avulsion in full thickness wound
- Indeterminate wound—shape, depth, devitalization, damage cannot be defined.

Mechanism of injury: Penetrating or blunt.

Management of Wounds Based upon their Type

Types of Wounds—Tidy and Untidy
- **Tidy wounds:** Clean, incise, tissues are healthy, little or no loss of tissue.
- **Untidy wounds:** Contaminated, irregular wounds, tissues are often crushed and devitalized with tissue loss.

Aim
To convert untidy to tidy by removing devitalized and all contaminated tissue.

- **Tidy wound:** Primary repair.
- **Untidy wound with contaminated wound with dead tissue:** Debridement (one or more sittings).

Q. What is second look surgery? (Short notes)

Second look surgery
In major injuries related to bullets, missiles, explosions or natural disasters (e.g., earthquake) the initial assessments on vitality of structures are often inconclusive. Sometimes late devitalization may also follow. This is managed by repeated surgical explorations to evaluate and remove devitalized tissues before a definitive repair can be done.

Q. Describe the evaluation of a wound and principles of management.

- Complete clinical examination of the patient and the wound in particular.
- Initial management along acute trauma life support (ATLS) principles
- Wound toilet and exploration for a proper assessment and diagnosis.
- Removal of contaminants and devitalized tissues (debridement)
- Repair of tissues and replacement of lost tissues if any.
- Wound closure—skin suturing without tensions.

ASSESSMENT AND TREATMENT OF ACUTE WOUND
- **History:** Time and mechanism of injury, administration of tetanus immunoglobulin and toxoid, analgesia or anesthesia, tourniquet for visualizing wound, assessment of pain, movement and sensation.
- Washing of all wounds, thorough debridement until fresh bleeding is seen. Vitality of structure is the factor to decide on immediate or delayed repair.

Primary Wound Repair
In a tidy wound including repair of nerve, arteries and tendons.
- Splinting of limb wounds
- Active mobilization of limbs
- Skin cover.

Special Situations
Compartment Syndrome: See Below

Q. Write a short notes on acute compartment syndrome.

- Raised intracompartmental pressure in closed fascial compartment can endanger vascularity of the limb and need emergent action.
- Severe pain, pain on passive movement of the affected compartment muscles.
- Distal sensory deficit and late sign of impalpable distal pulsation.

Measurement of compartment pressure is done by placing a catheter in the compartment. A pressure exceeding 30 mm Hg is diagnostic of the syndrome.

Treatment

(1) Emergency fasciotomy—long multiple fasciotomies if needed.

Complications of fasciotomy

Release of muscle protein and myoglobinuria with glomerular blockage and renal failure.

(2) Amputation of the limb—is required if tissue is already necrotic with demarcation of non viable tissues.

Q. Describe etiology, pathology, clinical features and management of necrotising soft-tissue infections.

These are polymicrobial infections affecting soft tissues, mainly subcutaneous, fascial and muscular planes, they are often life threatening.

Common Organisms

- *Gram-positive aerobes: Staphylococcus aureus, Streptococcus pyogenes*, beta-hemolytic *Streptococcus* (*S. viridans*)
- Gram-negative (*Escherichia coli, Pseudomonas*)
- **Anaerobes:** *Clostridium*, Bacteroides.

Types of Necrotizing Infections

- **Clostridial:** Gas gangrene
- **Non-clostridial:** Streptococcal gangrene and necrotizing fasciitis.

The infection commonly follows an injury or surgery with wound contamination.

Patients with poor immunity are susceptible. Sudden presentation and rapid progression.

Clinical Features

Typical necrotizing fasciitis.
- Severe pain, fever—(absent in those with compromised immunity, e.g., diabetics).
- Erythema and severe edema beyond area of erythema.
- Skin blistering, serous and greyish drainage.
- Crepitus (gas forming organisms—*Pseudomonas, Proteus*).

Complications

- Focal cutaneous gangrene—after 2–3 days.
- Septic shock, coagulopathy and multiorgan failure (especially *Strepto. pyogenes*).

Treatment of Necrotizing Fasciitis

Aggressive antibiotic therapy—piperacillin with tazobactam, clindamycin and metronidazole.

Surgery

Liberal surgical excision of necrotic tissue.
- Tissue biopsies are taken for histological study and bacterial sensitivity too.
- Secondary skin grafting for the raw areas.

Q. Burst abdomen. (Generally a short question but may be a long answer question).

BURST ABDOMEN

Syn: Abdominal wound dehiscence, acute wound failure.

A condition characterized by disruption of a wound laparotomy. It has a high mortality.

An innocuous looking seemingly healing wound of laparotomy is seen giving way between the postoperative days 5 and 8 leading to evisceration of the bowel loops.

Pathogenesis

It is due to the failure of acute wound healing involving the rectus sheath or the linea alba.

Contributing Factors

- Underlying abdominal pathology and sepsis—local or systemic.

- Patient
  - *Preoperative:* Nutritional deficiency, hypoproteinemia, anemia, ascites, systemic disease like tuberculosis, renal failure or chronic liver disease, chronic cough, diabetes, chemotherapy, irradiation, steroid and immunosuppressive therapy.
  - *Postoperative:*
    - Cough, deep wound infection
    - Distension—paralytic ileus.
- Technical factors
  - **Suturing techniques:** Mainly of the musculoaponeurotic layer by tight suturing, causing necrosis.
  - **Type of incision:** Vertical incisions are more prone for dehiscence than transverse incisions.
    - This is due to the tension across the vertically sutured fascial layer.
  - **Type of suture material:** Absorbable suture material like catgut and use of short length of suture contributes to dehiscence.

Treatment

Note:
Immediate action to correct:
- Hypovolemia, electrolyte imbalance, anemia and sepsis, intravenous fluids and electrolytes.
- Broad spectrum antibiotic like piperacillin—tazobactam
- Blood and plasma transfusion as needed
- Monitoring of urine output
- Nasogastric tube aspiration to decompress the bowel.

Immediate surgery—under general anesthesia once the patient is stabilized. Bowel returned to abdomen—saline wash to the bowel.
Closure is difficult due to distended abdomen.

Wound closure: Options.
1. Immediate closure with tension sutures with interrupted nonabsorbable sutures (e.g., polypropylene or polyamide.
2. Temporary lax approximation of edges leaving the dehisced gap open but fitted with a bogota bag to cover the bowel.

This is followed by a delayed definitive closure of the wound after the ileus and sepsis settle.
3. A temporary dressing or mesh covered by dressing (to prevent adhesions) and delayed closure of the wound.

Postoperative problems to be anticipated:
- Ileus
- Sepsis
- Abdominal compartment syndrome
- Thromboembolism.

Chronic Wounds and Ulcers

Management

Aim: Achieve wound healing by external assistance to compensate for the defective stages of wound healing:
- Determination of causes of failure of early wound healing
- Identify the specific defective stage of healing.
- Plan specific measures.

Diabetic ulcer is a typical chronic wound and hence described as an index cause hereunder:

Q. Describe pathology and management of diabetic ulcers of limbs.

DIABETIC ULCERS

Evaluation

- The extent of the wound
- The peripheral circulation
- The degree of sensory loss are recorded
- Web spaces and nails should be examined for evidence of mycotic infection.

Ulcers: Due to vasculopathy, neuropathy and arthropathy.

Site of ulceration: Plantar surface of the metatarsals and the metatarsal head.

Investigation

- Plain X-ray of the foot or CT scan for osteomyelitis and air in tissue
- Nerve conduction test for neuropathy
- Doppler study of arteries—ankle-brachial index measurements for vascular insufficiency.

Treatment

- Diabetic shoe or orthotic device—offloading of the ulcer.
- Clean wounds are treated with minimal debridement and damp gauze
- Hydrogel-based dressings, alginate, hydrocolloid
- Negative-pressure wound closure therapy (NPWT) that removes excess wound exudate, which inhibits wound healing.
- Recombinant human basic fibroblast growth factor (rhbFGF) improves healing.
- Bioengineered living tissues: Composites of a structural mesh and cultured keratinocytes. (Cells are taken from neonatal sources).
- Metallic silver-impregnated dressings. Silver has broad antimicrobial properties.
- Hyperbaric oxygen treatment (HBOT) acts against local hypoxia and hastens healing.

Infected Diabetic Foot Ulcer

- Inpatient wound care
- Broad-spectrum antibiotic therapy
- Wound exploration and drainage of infected and necrotic tissue.

Prevention

Most important management of the diabetic foot—hygiene and daily inspection for tissue trauma prevent injury. Custom-made shoes to relieve pressure.

> **Q. Negative pressure wound closure therapy. (Short notes)**

NEGATIVE PRESSURE WOUND CLOSURE THERAPY (NPWT)

Syn: Vacuum-assisted closure

Mechanism of Action of Negative Pressure

- Removes interstitial fluid and increases blood flow.
- This causes reduction in edema, which in turn, causes reduction in bacterial counts and promotes cell proliferation leading to granulation formation suitable for graft or a flap.
- Intermittent negative pressure (at approx –125 mm Hg) applied over the wound.
- It hastens debridement and the granulation in chronic wounds and ulcers.
- A foam dressing cut to the shape and size of the wound is placed; a drain is placed over the same and wound sealed with adhesive film. Vacuum is applied to the drain.

> **Q. Write short note on decubitus ulcers.**

PRESSURE SORES

Syn: Decubitus ulcers, bed sores.

Pathophysiology

- Prolonged pressure on to soft tissue over bony prominences, causes ischemic ulceration.
- Usually seen in immobility and paralysis.
- **Sites:** Sacrum greater trochanter, heels and occiput.

Pressure Sore Stages

- **Stage I:** Non blanchable erythema of intact skin (generally reversible with intervention)
- **Stage II:** Partial-thickness skin loss involving epidermis or dermis (abrasion, blister, shallow crater)
- **Stage III:**
  - Full-thickness skin loss—with necrosis of subcutaneous tissue.
  - Underlying tissue and fascia not involved.
- **Stage IV:** Full-thickness skin loss with damage to underlying fascia, tendon, or joint capsule.

Unstageable

Full-thickness tissue loss—depth of ulcer unknown due to slough and/or eschar in wound bed, e.g., ischium or greater tuberosity.

Prevention

Skin Care

Moisturizing the skin and protection from dampness of fluids.
Frequent change of position every 2–3 hours.

Support surfaces to take off pressure points.

- Static support surfaces. Water bed or air, gel or foam—for low risk patients.
- Dynamic support surfaces. They redistribute pressure actively, e.g., alternating and low air-loss mattresses—for high-risk patients.

Nutrition: To meet caloric and protein requirements.

Treatment of Pressure Sores

Pressure relief is the most important factor in healing.

Surgical Treatment

- Most pressure ulcers heal spontaneously when pressure is relieved.
- **Surgery:**
  Options include - simple closure, split-thickness skin grafting, creation of a musculocutaneous flap, debridement, necrosectomy and escharotomy.

Wound cleansing: Saline irrigation

Dressing:
- Should ensure a moist wound base
- Enzymatic debridement with topical agents such as collagenase.
- Hydrocolloid dressings.
- Negative pressure wound therapy (NPWT).
- Recombinant human basic fibroblast growth factor (rhbFGF) improves healing in pressure ulcers.

Control of Infection and Bacterial Colonization

- Topical wound cleansing.
- Re-exploration of the wound and debridement - for active infection purulence, surrounding cellulitis, or foul odor.

Nutrition: 30 to 35 kcal/kg body weight and 1.25 to 1.5 g protein/kg body weight.

Treatment of Necrotising Fasciitis

Aggressive antibiotic therapy—piperacillin with tazobactam, clindamycin and metronidazole.

Surgery

- Liberal surgical excision of necrotic tissue.
- Tissue biopsies are taken for histological study and bacterial sensitivity too.
- Secondary skin grafting for the raw areas.

Scars

- Maturation phase may take upto 1 year or even more.
- **Immature scar** is hard, pink, raised and itchy—reorganization of collagen fibers to align with the lines of stress with interweaving to derive strength. Plenty of fibroblasts and blood vessels.
- **Mature scar** (after about 3 months): Pale, softer and flat, rarely itchy and it contains mature collagen denser with fewer fibroblasts and blood vessels finally acellular.
- **Aberrations:** Scars may be atrophic, hypertrophic and keloid.
- **Atrophic scar** is pale, flat and stretched in areas of tension—thin dermis hence traumatized easily excision and resuturing may help.

> **Q. Short notes: Describe hypertrophic scars and keloid.**

HYPERTROPHIC SCAR

Excessive scar tissue, not extending beyond the limits of the original incision or wound.

Cause

A prolonged inflammatory phase of wound healing and wrong scar siting (e.g., across the lines of skin tension).

KELOID

Excessive scarring extending beyond the boundaries of the original incision or wound.
It has excessive collagen (of type III collagen) with hypervascularity.

Etiology is not clear but it is associated with following factors:
- Deeply pigmented skin
- Elevated levels of growth factor
- Tendency if inheritance
- Certain areas of the body are more prone for keloids (e.g., a triangle between the points—the xiphisternum and both shoulder tips).

The treatment of both hypertrophic and keloid scars is difficult.
- Pressure—elasticated garments and local moulds
- Silicone gel sheeting (mechanism unknown)
- Intralesional steroid injection (triamcinolone)

- **Surgical excision:** All surgeries have a high rate of recurrence.
  - Excision and steroid injection.
  - Intralesional excision (keloids only)
  - Excision and postoperative radiation (external beam or brachytherapy)
  - Laser—to reduce redness (which may resolve in any event)
  - Vitamin E or palm oil massage (unproven).

CONTRACTURE

A deformity flowing shortening of a scar over a joint or an area joining two body.
A tight web may cause:
- Restriction of movement of joints—hyperextension or hyperflexion.
- Neck: Restriction of neck extension—difficulty in breathing and swallowing.

Treatment
- Scar excision or/and revision.
- Single or multiple sittings.
- Multiple Z- plasties, skin grafting, rotation flap preconstruction.
- Physiotherapy before and after surgery with splintage is vital to the success of treatment.

SKIN GRAFTS

> **Q. Describe different ways of covering skin defects.**

Classification

Free Grafts
Take up nutrition from the recipient area for survival.
1. Partial thickness graft
2. Dermal grafts
3. Full thickness graft.

Partial Thickness Skin Graft
Epithelium and superficial dermal layer included.

Advantage
Most commonly used, most defects can be closed—technically easier, graft take up rates are high.

Disadvantage
- Poor cosmetic appearance.
- Graft won't take up on bare bone and tendon without paratenon.
- Graft contraction and shrinkage leads to disfigurement.
- Easily breaks and hence cannot be used on weight bearing or friction prone areas.

Contraindication
Pre graft culture from the wound grows *Pseudomonas* or streptococci.

Dermal Grafts
- Epithelium and appendages are removed and only dermal layer is used.
- Epidermis is shaved off and only a partial thickness of dermis is used.
- Used in facial defects, intra-oral or intra-vaginal defects.

Disadvantage
Technical expertise required.

Full Thickness Grafts
- Cosmetically better as it will not shrink
- Recipient area should be vascularized to take up the graft.

FLAPS
A flap is a unit of tissue that is transferred from the donor site to recipient site, with an intact blood supply.

Classification of Flaps
Based on:

Type of Blood Supply
- Random flap—example, local cutaneous flaps
- Axial flap—example, muscle flaps.

Type of Tissue to be Transferred

Type of Tissue Transfer
- Skin—full-thickness cutaneous flaps
- Fascia
- Muscle
- Bone

- Visceral—example, colon; small intestine omentum
- Composite
  - Fasciocutaneous—example, radial forearm flap, deltopectoral flap.
  - Myocutaneous—example, myocutaneous flaps—example, pectoralis major myocutaneous flaps, latissimus dorsi myocutaneous flap.
    Transverse rectus abdominis myocutaneous (TRAM) flap.
  - Osteocutaneous, e.g., fibula flap, pectoralis major along with rib is used for reconstruction of facial defects.
  - Tendocutaneous—example, dorsalis pedis flap.

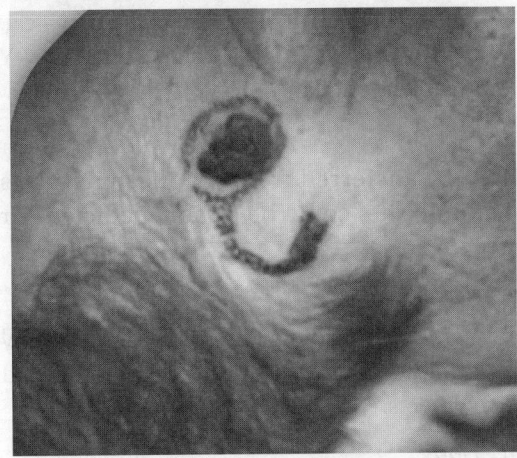

Fig. 5.2: Petal flap for a seborrheic wart

Location of Donor Site

Local or distant (pedicled or free).

Local Flaps

Tissue transferred from an area adjacent to the defect. (**Refer Figures 5.1 to 5.3, Figures 28-R10 and R11**).

Different techniques are used to design the flaps which are named according to the respective
- Design of the flap—e.g. rhomboid flap, Z-plasty (single or multiple), petal flap, butterfly flap
- The person who designed these flaps—e.g. limberg flap

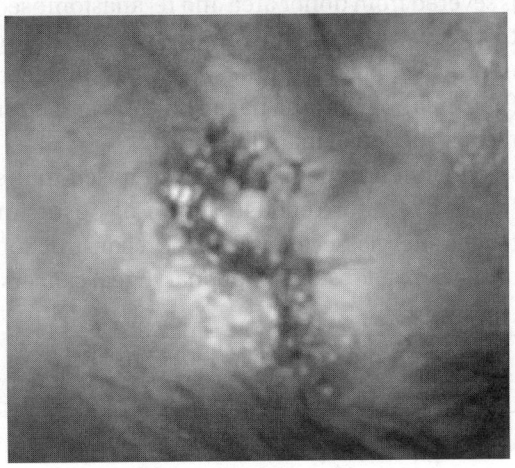

Fig. 5.3: Petal flap completed

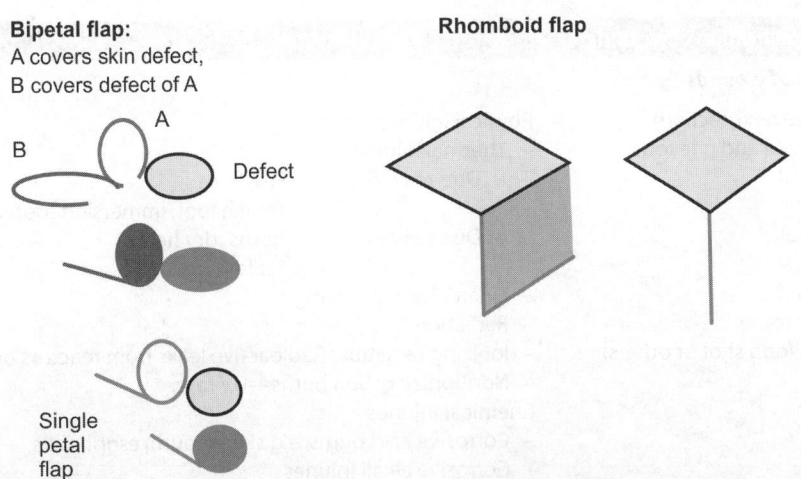

Fig. 5.1: Local flaps—petal flap and rhomboid

- The mechanism deployment of the flap—e.g, local advancement flap, rotation flap or V-Y advancement flap.

Distant Flaps

Tissue transferred from a non-contiguous anatomic site, could be either "pedicled" or "free".

Pedicled Flaps

These are full thickness flaps with blood supply from the donor area useful to cover deep and large defects.

Free Flaps

Microvascular flaps: Here the vascular pedicle is severed from donor area and re-anastomosed to the vessels of the recipient area using microvascular techniques, e.g., vascularized (peroneal perforator based) fibular graft for reconstruction of mandible.

The forearm pedicle is anastomosed to the facial artery for reconstruction of posterior tongue after glossectomy or for the reconstruction of pharynx after surgery for pharyngeal cancers.

> **SU5.4: Discuss medico-legal aspects of wounds.**

Wound or injury is a breach in the natural continuity of any part or tissue of the living body.

Mechanical injuries: As per Indian Penal Code (IPC) Section 44)—injury (44 IPC): Injury is any harm, caused to any person in body, mind, reputation or property.

> **Q. Describe the doctor's legal responsibilities in managing wounds.**

- Wound certification and documentation
- Declaring cause of death
- Testifying in a court of law on wound (to determine homicide or suicide or accidental). The doctors required to document the wounds of a victim in the register and coordinate with the legal authorities.

The doctor' responsibilities' include

- Determine type of wound described in **Table 5.2**.
- Measure the dimensions (length, width, depth) and location of wound in relation to anatomical landmarks.
- Determine height of victim, other contributing factors like heart problems
- Wounds provide evidence of the crime
- Contribute to proof of the severity.

General Principles

The wound is caused by the mechanical force of the movement or static rigidity of the body against a moving object or a combination thereof on most of the cases.

Table 5.2: Classification of wounds.

Classification of wounds

- Medical (see next section)
- Legal—simple and grievous
- Medico-legal
  - Suicidal
  - Homicidal
  - Accidental
  - Fabricated
  - Self inflicted
  - Defence (gun shot or others)
- Physical injuries:
  - Thermal injuries
    » Due to cold: Frostbite
    Trench foot: Immersion foot
    » Due to heat: Burns (dry heat)
    Scalds (wet heat)
  - Electricity: Lightening
  - Radiation
  - Ionizing radiation: Radioactive leaks from reactors or industries
  - Non-ionizing: Sun burns—UV rays.
- Chemical injuries
  - Corrosive acid burns, e.g skin, mouth, esophagus
  - Corrosive alkali injuries
- Explosions

Result of Impact

Impact between force and counter force causes transfer of energy to tissues, which have variable elasticity, density and integrity.

Movement of Body Causes

- Bending, torsion or shearing
- Elongation compression of tissues
- Displacement and deformation

Shear strain is parallel to plane of contact causes rupture of tissue.

Factors Affecting Mechanical Injuries

- Amount of energy discharged by the impact decides the gravity of injury.
- Velocity of impact is more important the mass of the impacting object—higher the velocity, greater is the impact.
- **Time taken to transfer the energy:** Shorter the time period required to transfer the energy, greater the damage.
- **Area of transfer:** Smaller the area, greater the damage.
- **Elasticity of the tissue:** The less elastic the tissue, the greater the damage (e.g., bone)
- Inertia of tissue
- Hydrostatic pressure.

Types of Mechanical Wounds

- Abrasion—damage to superficial layers of skin (epidermis) or mucous membrane.
- **Due to scratches:** Linear—pin, nail
- **Graze:** Sliding, scraping, or grinding abrasions—movement between the skin and some rough surface
- Pressure abrasion, impact abrasion
- Patterned abrasion—very common.

Brush abrasion or gravel rash: It is produced by the violent lateral force against a surface as in dragging over the ground.

Graze

Friction burn (scuff or brush abrasion): It is an extensive, superficial, reddened excoriated area without bleeding and without any linear mark—due to tangential force with the skin covered by clot.

Types of Wounds: Injuries

- The definition of a skin wound or injury as per the pattern of injuries:
- Type of damage to the skin caused by **(Table 5.3)**.
- Measurement of these wounds are essential in medico-legal proceedings.

A Bruise: Escape of Blood from Blood Vessels

- It is generally larger than the object that caused it.
- Bruise is a phenomenon that occurs only in living state (blood circulation needed)
- Documenting bruising and photography.

Bruising in Deep Tissue

- Possibly life-threatening
- Sometimes no external injury
- Revealed in autopsy.

Lacerations

Caused by penetrating, or shearing or blunt force (with or without crushing).

Distinguished from incised wounds by:
- Ragged edge
- Usually have adjacent abrasion/bruise
- Tissue bridges in depth.

Forensic Importance

Lacerations are rarely suicidal and their shape is not related to the object causing it.

Defence wounds are found in cases of assault, as the victim tries to protect oneself—commonly on the ulnar aspect of the forearms and hands.

Suicidal wounds are always in areas accessible to self. And seen in predictable sites like wrist, throat or neck or "pit of abdomen".

Table 5.3: Type of damage to the skin caused.	
Sharp force injuries	*Blunt force injuries*
• Incised wounds • Stab wounds • Chop wounds • Diagnostic/therapeutic wounds • Bullet and missile wounds	• Lacerations • Abrasions • Bruising/contusion

A laceration is often caused by a blunt object stretching and eventually tearing the skin. Underlying structures such as nerves and blood vessels may be torn, at the site of maximum impact, not at ends of the laceration.

Stab Wounds

Forensic Importance

- These wounds reflect the sharp edge of the weapon
- No trace evidence
- Bleeds profusely and prone for hemorrhage and air embolism
- Any penetrable subject can cause these wounds.

Stab Wounds are often the Cause of Death

- Most are homicides.
- Homicidal stab wounds are usually multiple,
- Single homicidal stabbings are always aimed at the heart, or in otherwise partially incapacitated victims, often associated with drugged, drunk, sleeping victims.

Stab v/s Slash Wounds

- Stab wounds are deep and not wide
- Slash wounds are wide and not deep.

Chop Wounds

Chop wounds are caused by heavy instruments with sharp edges, such as axes and machetes.

Diagnostic or Therapeutic Wounds

Often mimic stab wounds are need to be recognized in victims of violence or wounding, e.g., surgical incisions for insertion of intercostal drains, 'cut downs' for deep veins and tracheostomy.

Surgical Infections and Hand Infections

Chapter 6

SU6.1	Define and describe the etiology and pathogenesis of surgical infections.
SU6.2	Enumerate prophylactic and therapeutic antibiotics plan appropriate management.

SURGICAL INFECTIONS

They are infections confronting the surgical patients and include infections seen in the post-operative period—systemic sepsis and localized infection including the local infection of the surgical wound (surgical site wound infection—SSI).

Sepsis is a life threatening state due to infection and the systemic host response to it. It presents with some form of organ dysfunction as a part of variable manifestations.

Definition of Infection of a Wound

The invasion of tissues by organisms due to breach of local and systemic host defenses.

Events following microbial invasion: Invading microbes are confronted by the host defence (local and systemic) which may result in any of the following:
- Eradication
- Containment—may form pus (e.g., a furuncle on surface or abscess within a tissue space or the parenchyma of an organ)
- Loco regional infection (cellulitis, lymphangitis, and aggressive soft tissue infection) with or without distant spread of infection (pyemic abscess) or progression to concurrent systemic infection, e.g., an abscess with bacteremia
- Systemic infection (bacteria or fungus)—due to the failure of host defenses.

Factors weakening the host defence and favoring the spread of infection
- Necrotic wound tissue
- Bacterial toxins—particularly anaerobic endotoxins
- Anaerobic atmosphere in wound
- Bacterial enzymes—to aid spread through the tissues, e.g., gas gangrene—release of hyaluronidase, lecithinase and hemolysin by *Clostridium perfringens*
- Antibiotic resistance—pre-acquired by bacteria through plasmids
- Release of organisms—naturally occurring in human body during perioperative period—into tissue. e.g., microbial contamination—perforation of viscus or operative injury.

Postoperative Infections

Classification of Sources of Infection

Endogenous organisms—on or in the patient at the time of surgery, (e.g. perforated appendix).
Exogenous organisms—from outside the patient.

The cause of hospital acquired infection (HAI)
- Operating theater (inadequate air filtration, poor antisepsis)
- The ward (e.g. poor hand-washing compliance).

The Natural Barriers and Protective Mechanisms against Microbial Invasion
- Mechanical barriers by intact epithelial surfaces: Skin and mucosa—broken down by trauma or surgery.

- **Chemical:** Low gastric pH.
- **Humoral:** antibodies, complement and opsonins.
- **Cellular:** Phagocytic cells, macrophages, polymorphonuclear cells and killer lymphocytes.

Factors Contributing to the Development of Surgical Site Infections (SSI)

- Breach of natural barrier mechanisms—surgical trauma and treatment.
- Virulence and pathogenicity of the organisms present
- Bacterial load (quantum of pathogenic inoculums).

Host Factors: Impaired

- Tissue ischemia, shock
- Immunosuppression
- Caused by radiotherapy, chemotherapy or steroids.

Technical Factors Related to Surgery

- Surgeon factors:
  - Poor technique
  - Devitalization of tissue
  - Large collections or hematoma
  - Excessive dead space.
- Foreign materials, e.g., implants, sutures and drains.
- Type of suture material, e.g, multifilament, silk or cotton suture for skin.
- Antibiotics given during the "decisive period".

> **Q. What is the decisive period in surgical site infections?**

THE DECISIVE PERIOD—THE 4 HOUR INTERVAL

After a tissue trauma (surgery or otherwise), it takes about 4 hours before the bacterial growth establishes sufficiently to cause an infection. All decisions should be taken and enacted during this 4 hour period to be effective in preventing an infection. Hence called the decisive period. All the measures are likely to fail in prevention of infection after this.

Prophylactic antibiotics are given during the decisive period to ensure tissue levels of antibiotics above the minimum inhibitory concentration against the respective organisms.

Weak Host Resistance to Infection

Impaired inflammatory response

- Malnutrition
- Recent rapid weight loss
- The presence of obesity
- Metabolic diseases—diabetes mellitus, uremia and jaundice
- Disseminated malignancy
- Acquired immune deficiency syndrome (AIDS)
- Iatrogenic causes.

Other Factors

- Colonisation of gut by Gram negative bacteria and translocation leads to endotoxemia causing SIRS. Due to failure of gut-associated lymphoid tissue (GALT).
- The excessive release of proinflammatory cytokines and activation of macrophages
- Opportunistic infection—commensals grow virulent due to host resistance, e.g., fungal infection.

> **Q. Classify surgical wounds and give examples. (Short notes)**

The classification of surgical wounds is given in **Table 6.1**.

Table 6.1: Classification of surgical wounds.

	Type of wound	Description	For example, operation
1.	Clean	No contamination of luminal contents	Hernia, thyroid
2.	Clean contaminated	Minimal spillage	Appendix, gallbladder
3.	Contaminated	Luminal contents spilled into operative wound	Colectomy, ileum opened in intestinal obstruction
4.	Dirty	Gross infected material in the operative field	Peritonitis, gangrene of bowel, burst liver abscess

> Q. Define surgical site infections (SSI) and discuss etiopathogenesis and prevention of SSI.

SURGICAL SITE INFECTION (SSI)

Classification of Surgical Site Infection (SSI)

- Superficial surgical site infection (SSSI) the infection of surgical wounds
- Deep SSI (infection in the deeper musculofascial layers)
- Organ space infection (such as an abdominal abscess after an anastomotic leak).

SSI is classified as per severity by various scoring systems:

- **A major SSI** is:
  - As a wound with discharge of large quantities of pus or one requiring drainage.
  - Has systemic symptoms and signs—tachycardia, tachypnea, fever and leukocytosis.
- **Minor SSI**: Wound infection which settles spontaneously without antibiotics.

Southampton Score: 0 to 5

- Based on appearance of wound and presence of major complication (pus and dehiscence).
- Assessment is done over 30 day period of surveillance for a 30-day postoperative period.

Asepsis Score System—Based on

- Additional treatment (antibiotics, drainage of pus, necrosectomy) of wound
- Serous discharges
- Erythema
- Purulent exudate
- Dehiscence of wound—complete separation of deep tissues)
- Isolation of bacteria from wound
- Stay beyond 14 days due to wound infection.

Hospital Acquired Infection (HAI)

Infection acquired from the hospital environment or the staff after surgery or hospitalization.
- SSIs
- Bacteremia due to intravenous and arterial lines)
- Respiratory infections including ICU sepsis (ventilator-pneumonia)
- Urinary tract infections (urinary catheters).

Treatment: Principles

Rapid resuscitation, antibiotics, and source control (refer to next section on treatment).

Preventive Measures Against SSI

- Preoperative preparation: Optimize the patient's condition.
- Clean hand wash by the staff.
- Aseptic techniques.
- Use of triclosan based local disinfectant agents for skin preparation on table.
- Aseptic instrumentation and operation theater practice.
- Preoperative antibiotics—used before surgery in clean contaminated operations
- No antibiotics in clean wounds operation.
- Continuation of antibiotics in contaminated and dirty class operation in cases with significant operative hemorrhage.
- Antibiotic coverage for patients with valvular heart disease or prostheses.
- No use of local antiseptic ointments for the closed operative wound
- Adequate oxygenation during anesthesia.

MICROBIOLOGY OF SURGICAL INFECTIONS

Gram Positive

- Streptococci
- Alfa hemolytic: *Streptococcus viridans*—not usually seen in surgical infections.
- Beta hemolytic: *Streptococcus pyogenes* (resides in the pharynx)
- *Streptococcus faecalis* (*Enterococcus*) in Lancefield group D—synergistic action with other gamma-hemolytic *Streptococcus*
- Anaerobic *Streptococcus*: Peptostreptococcus.

Staphylococci—coagulase positive

- *Staph. aureus*—penicillin sensitive
- Beta-lactamase producing staphylococci (usually hospital strains) are resistant to penicillin.

- But sensitive to flucloxacillin, vancomycin, aminoglycosides and some cephalosporins.
- Methicillin-resistant *Staphylococcus aureus* (MRSA)—sensitive to teicoplanin.

Coagulase negative staphylococci

Staphylococcus epidermidis—skin commensal—endangers prosthetics—ortho and vascular through venous and arterial lines.

Aerobic Gram-negative Bacilli

- Lactose fermenting: *Escherichia coli* and *Klebsiella* spp.
- Non-lactose fermenting: *Proteus*
- Most act synergistically with Bacteroides (cause SSI after bowel surgery)
- *Escherichia coli*—urinary infections and SSI after abdominal surgery.
- Extended-spectrum β-lactamases (ESBLs): Resistant to antibiotics (cephalosporin)

Clostridia: Gram-positive, obligate anaerobes (detalis given in **Table 6.2**).

Table 6.2: Clostridial infections.

Clostridium perfringens	Gas gangrene	Gas forming infection—limbs and perineum
Clostridium tetani	Tetanus	After implantation into tissues or wound
Clostridium difficile - commensal	Pseudomembranous colitis	Destruction of the normal colonic bacterial flora. Following antibiotics and overgrowth of *Cl. diff*.

Q. Pseudomembranous colitis. (Short notes)

Refer above for etiology and pathology.
Colonoscopy: Fibrinous exudate is typical
Laboratory recognition of the toxin

Treatment

Resuscitation—fluid and electrolytes
Antibiotic therapy—metronidazole or vancomycin
Rifaximin 550 mg twice daily—against *Clostridium difficile* for 10 to 14 days

ANTIMICROBIAL TREATMENT OF SURGICAL INFECTION

Role of antibiotics may be—preventive or therapeutic.

- Antibiotics should be used for spreading infections and established infections.
- Antibiotics are an essential supplement and not a substitute to surgical drainage of infected contents like pus and necrosectomy.
- Sensitivity of the organism to antibiotic is determined.

Selection of Antibiotic

- **Monotherapy:** In cases of known sensitivity of the organism, e.g., pus from the wound culture grows MRSA: A specific narrow-spectrum antibiotic, such as vancomycin or teicoplanin is used.
- **Combination therapy: Broad-spectrum antibiotics**
  - When there are several organisms involved (e.g., large bowel surgery).
  - The organism is not known or polymicrobial infection is suspected.

Antimicrobial Therapy in Surgical Infection

- Antimicrobials: Prophylactic or therapeutic
- Antibiotics: Produced by organisms
- Synthetic methods.

Hospitals should have an antibiotic policy and protocol based on the periodic microbiology profiles of antibiotic sensitivity and organisms.

Empirical antibiotics are used in infections pending availability of culture and sensitivity.

Penicillin: Against gram-positive Streptococci and the Clostridia, Actinomyces. As a part of multiple therapy for a mixed infection.

Anti beta lactamase: Flucloxacillin:
- Producing staphylococcal infections
- Soft tissue infections and osteomyelitis.

Beta-lactam penicillins: Ampicillin, amoxicillin and co-amoxiclav:
- Given orally or parenterally.
- Effective against Enterobacteriaceae
- Clavulanic acid—inactivates beta-lactamases

These include resistant strains of *Staphylococcus aureus, E. coli, Haemophilus influenzae, Bacteroides*.
Ineffective against *Klebsiella* or *Pseudomonas*.

Ureidopenicillins: Piperacillin and ticarcillin: A broad spectrum—gram-positive, gram-negative and anaerobic bacteria.

Used in combination with beta lactamase inhibitors (tazobactam or clavulanic acid).
For *Pseudomonas* and *Proteus*.

Cephalosporins

Several beta lactamase-susceptible—cefuroxime, cefotaxime and ceftazidime.
Used in intra-abdominal skin and soft-tissue infections.
Ceftazidime—gram-negative organisms including *Pseudomonas aeruginosa* and *Staphylococcus aureus*.

Aminoglycosides: Gentamicin and tobramycin, amikacin.
Effective against gram-negative Enterobacteriaceae and *Pseudomonas*.
Not effective against anaerobes and streptococci.
Toxicity: Nephrotoxicity ototoxicity.

Imidazole: Metronidazole

Acts against all anaerobic bacteria.
Administered—intravenously, orally or rectally.
- Against bacteroides and clostridia can be treated.

Quinolones: Ciprofloxacin, Ofloxacin

- Activity against both gram-positive and gram-negative bacteria
- Used against *Pseudomonas* infections.

Glycopeptide Antibiotics: Vancomycin and Teicoplanin

- Most active against MRSA and other gram-positive aerobic and anaerobic bacteria, *Clostridium difficile*.
- Nephrotoxic and ototoxic.

Carbapenems: Imipenem meropenem and ertapenem.
- Act against beta lactamases, have a broad-spectrum anaerobic as well as gram-positive organism.

- Extended-spectrum β-lactamase (ESBL) resistant urinary tract infections or serious mixed-spectrum abdominal infections (peritonitis).

SHORT NOTES QUESTIONS

Q. Short notes on abscess.

Localized collection of pus with a containing membranous wall.

Types

Pyogenic (localized), pyemic (metastatic) and cold (no signs of inflammation).

Etiology

- **Acute:** *Staph. aureus* (generally)—localized abscess or metastatic (pyemic) abscess, Gram negative—*E. coli*, Klebsiella.
- **Chronic:** Mycobacterium (cold abscess) and actinomyces.

Pathology

Parts of an abscess:
- **Contents:** Pus—dead and dying white blood cells (neutrophils), toxins.
- **Wall:** Pyogenic membrane—due to an acute inflammatory response.
- A fibrinous exudate, edema and neutrophils.
- **Later:** Granulation tissue (macrophages, fibroblasts and capillary proliferation) leads to collagen deposition—causing fibrous wall.

Complications of an Abscess

- Rupture—sinus, fistula (if communicating with hollow organ)
- Antibioma formation
- Calcification
- Bacteremia and sepsis.

Clinical Features

- **General:** Fever with chills.
- **Local:** Swelling, throbbing pain,
- **Cardinal signs of inflammation:**
  - Calor (heat), rubor (redness), dolor (pain and tenderness) and tumor (swelling).
  - Function laesa (Galen's addition)—affected part will be defunct.

Sign of fluctuation: Diagnostic, but difficult to elicit in tense pus with severe pain.

Differential Diagnosis

- Cellulitis (no fluctuation, no limit, no pus)
- Hematoma
- Aneurysm, e.g., axilla, popliteal fossa
- **Sarcomas:** Rapidly growing tumor may mimic
- Cold abscess.

Q. Describe principles of draining an acute abscess?

Treatment: Of acute pyogenic abscess.

Incision and drainage of pus

- General anesthesia (commonly) aseptic precaution, **under antibiotic coverage**.
- Confirmation of pus by aspiration with a wide bore needle (14G or 16G)—sending it for culture and sensitivity.

Hilton's method of drainage followed:

- Incision at the point of maximum tenderness, along the lines of neurovascular bundle.
- Thrusting the sinus forceps with blades closed and opening them parallel to the bundle.
- Passing the finger tip to break the septa and loculi in the cavity.
- Washing the cavity clear of pus with saline.
- Inserting a drain.
- Dressing the open wound.

Q. Short notes on cold abscess.

Abscess without signs of acute inflammation (warmth and redness) hence the word "cold".

Causes

Tuberculosis, leprosy, actinomycosis.

- Inflammatory response is absent or poor to the chronic infections where pus is formed by liquefied dead tissue with organisms.
- It spreads along the musculofascial planes or along the neurovascular bundles in the deep tissues to point on surface.

Complications

- Secondary bacterial infection (presents like pyogenic abscess)
- Rupture and sinus or fistula formation.

Treatment

Aspiration (not drainage)—no dependent point.
- Non-dependent drainage and primary closure (to prevent fistulation)
- Pus is sent for TB or fungal culture.

Q. Short notes on collar stud abscess.

Collar stud abscess

Typical of tuberculous caseating lymphadenitis where cold abscess in subfascial lymph nodes (e.g., neck or groin) penetrate the fascia and collect in subcutaneous (extra fascial) plane to form two loculi (one deep to fascia and one superficial) connected by a narrow neck giving the appearance of the old fashioned collar studs.

Q. Short notes on boil (furuncle).

- Acute suppurative infection of hair follicle with perifolliculitis due to *Staph. aureus*.
- Pain redness and swelling at the root of hair follicle.
- **Fate of boil:** Resolution (blind boil); suppuration and rupture.

Complications

- Cellulitis
- Axillary boil may lead to hidradenitis suppurativa
- Facial boils progress to cavernous sinus thrombosis
- **Septicemia:** Diabetics and immunocompromised may develop systemic sepsis.

Sites: Any hairy region like thigh back, neck, face, eye lash (stye) and auditory canal.

Treatment

- Antibiotic: Amoxyclav preferred.
- Some cases need an incision and drainage.
- Linezolid for recurrent or multiple boils in diabetics.

Q. Short notes on hidradenitis suppurativa.

- Chronic suppurative infection of apocrine sweat glands.
- **Sites:** Axillae, groin, perineum, scalp.
- **Common groups:** Women, obese, hair men.
- **Predisposing factors:** Fat rich food, smoking, estrogenic medication.

- Poor hygiene, diabetes mellitus, steroid therapy.
- **Bacteriology:** *Staphylococcus aureus* and *Propionibacterium*.

Clinical features
- Young individuals, both sexes involves (more in female) present with multiple sinuses with foul smelling discharge.
- Site: Most common in axilla—more often bilateral.
- Acute exacerbations and remissions are common.

Treatment
- **Mild cases:** Local hygiene application of warmth, trimming of hair.
- Acute exacerbation is treated with cloxacillin and amoxicillin
- Recurrences, diffuse disease and bilateral disease—surgical treatment
  - Radical excision of the apocrine apparatus of the region with, if needed skin grafting or local flap rotation.

Q. Short notes on carbuncle.

Word meaning of carbuncle is charcoal.

Staphylococcal infection of multiple hair follicles with infective gangrene of skin and subcutaneous tissue. The infected units coalesce to form multiple sieve like openings infective gangrene of skin and subcutaneous tissue.

Common sites: Nape of the neck and back, abdominal wall, shoulder.

Clinical features:
Age: After 45
Sex: More in male
Diabetics are more prone to get carbuncle.
Presents with severe pain, fever, multiple vesicles progressing to form sieve like pattern with multiple openings discharging pus and a central necrotic patch with surrounding vesicles with redness, induration and tenderness.

Investigations: 1. Pus for culture, 2. Diabetes mellitus - work up.

Treatment
Carbuncle is a surgical emergency with a high mortality.

Principles of treatment
- Control of diabetes
- Antibiotics: Aggressive; combination—carbapenem or cephalosporin with metronidazole, or depending on culture and sensitivity report.

- **Surgery:** Excision of carbuncle under full anesthesia—cruciate incisions over the ulcerated area and liberal excision of all the infected and necrotic tissue from skin and subcutaneous plane. Considerable bleeding and intraoperative or anesthetic challenges are common. Drainage is done by a cruciate incision and debridement. Thereafter regular dressing of the open wound is done, granulation is formed. Split skin grafting is done after the wound is healthy with coverage of granulation of all dead tissues is done. Excision is done later.

Q. Short notes on: 1. Acute cellulitis and 2. Acute lymphangitis.

ACUTE CELLULITIS AND LYMPHANGITIS

Cellulitis is a non-suppurative **spreading** invasive infection of subcutaneous tissue and fascia/planes, usually following an injury—trivial or deep.

Characterised by signs of inflammation without signs of localization. It can be superficial or deep.

Predisposing factors include diabetes, immunosuppression and old age.

Common sites
The upper and lower limbs or face and neck areas where the subcutaneous tissue is lax.

Organisms
- Streptococcus pyogenes (mostly): Hyaluronidase breaks tissue cement spreading of infection. Streptokinase is the toxin. *Staphylococcus* may be associated.
- **Gram-ve bacteria:** May be associated (more in deep cellulitis) *Klebsiella, E. coli* and *Pseudomonas*.

Complications
- Local suppuration (due to mixed infection)
- infective gangrene of the overlying skin
- Subcutaneous—necrotizing fasciitis
- Bacteremia and septicemia.

Clinical Features
- **General features:** Fever with chills and rigors.

- **Cause**: Triggering of SIRS by the released toxins.
- **Local swelling:** Diffuse with no signs of localization ad no fluctuation.

Differential Diagnosis

- **Lymphangitis:** Similar to cellulitis, but it is in superficial plane and red streaks of inflamed lymphatics seen.
- **Deep vein thrombosis (DVT):** Lower limb.

Investigation

- Blood culture, WBC counts, renal function, liver function tests
- Blood sugar, urine test for ketone bodies, glycosylated hemoglobin estimation
- Venous Doppler and ultrasound of soft tissues to differentiate from DVT and for locating localized collections or abscesses.

Treatment

- **Aggressive antibiotic therapy:** Superficial cellulitis—penicillin and cloxacillin or cephalosporins with amikacin; or piperacillin as a mono therapy for severe cellulitis.
- **Elevation** of limb or part to reduce edema so as to increase the circulation and bandaging.
- **Dressing** (often glycerine dressing is used as it reduces the edema because of its hygroscopic action glycerine magnesium sulphate dressing).
- **Surgery:**
  - *Long fasciotomies for deep cellulitis:* To relieve compartmental pressure, curb anaerobic infection and improve tissue circulation.
  - *Necrosectomy:* For cutaneous gangrene and necrotizing fasciitis.

Q. Short notes on erysipelas.

Erysipelas is an acute streptococcal infection of dermal and superficial lymphatics.

Clinical features

- Sites affected generally: On face, ear lobule, fingers and legs, scrotum, umbilicus
- Raised well demarcated rose pink rash skin rash with cutaneous lymphatic edema

Milian's ear sign: To differentiating from facial cellulitis.
- Rash and redness extends to ear lobule in erysipelas but not in cellulitis, a subcutaneous infection (there is no subcutaneous plane in ear lobule).
- Vesicles and serous discharge.

Differential diagnoses

Angioedema of face, herpes simplex and zoster; contact dermatitis.

Complications

- Early: Septicaemia, pneumonia, meningitis.
- Late: Lymphedema of face or eyelid or limbs.
- Glomerulonephritis.

Treatment

- Antibiotics: Penicillin is the drug of choice
- Macrolides: Azithromycin , erythromycin and clindamycin are also effective
- Long term coverage with Benzathine penicillin monthly injections for 2 year against recurrence.

Q. Short notes on Ludwig's Angina.

Ludwig's angina is a life threatening rapidly spreading cellulitis of sublingual and submandibular spaces affecting the plane between floor of mouth and suprahyoid space.

Etiology

Peritonsillar abscess, dental sepsis (abscess), sialadenitis, injuries—iatrogenic—intubation.

Predisposing Factors

Diabetes mellitus, immunosuppression—post-viral infection, chemotherapy.

Microbiology

Streptococcus viridans, Staphylococcus aureus and anaerobes. Gram-negative: *Klebsiella*.

Complications of Ludwig's Angina

- Laryngeal edema and respiratory distress.
- Mediastinitis
- Aspiration pneumonia.
- Septicaemia.
- Parapharyngeal infection
- Thrombosis of the internal jugular vein and sigmoid sinus
- Death.

Clinical Features

General—h/o infection or dental sepsis, injury retropharynx.
- Fever, diffuse pain in submandibular area
- Tachycardia, halitosis, inability to swallow with salivary drooling, difficulty to speak
- Dyspnea, tachypnea.

Local
- Brawny and diffuse swelling under chin
- Red color, tenderness and induration of floor of mouth.
- Edema tongue, larynx, dysphagia.
- Strider, respiratory distress and cyanosis.

Investigations
- **Blood:** WBC counts, blood sugar
- Ultrasound neck—look for fluid collection and presence of gas
- CT scan or MRI to identify airway obstruction.
- Chest- X-ray and often blood gas analysis (in severe cases) is done.

Differential Diagnosis
- Angioedema of face and neck
- Sublingual
- Hematoma, sialadenitis, lymphadenitis.

Treatment
- Aggressive antibiotic therapy (intravenous)—intravenous penicillin or piperacillin with tazobactam and metronidazole with clindamycin if needed.
- Emergency tracheostomy to relieve a patient in respiratory distress.
- Early surgical release of exudate—whenever distress is severe.

Surgical Decompression
- A curved submental incision and division of mylohyoid to release the closed space pressure and a drain to help escape of the exudates.
- **Steroids:** Hydrocortisone or dexamethasone—against laryngeal edema (emergency).

Q. Discuss etiopathogenesis, clinical features and treatment of tetanus.

TETANUS

A clinical syndrome caused by exotoxins released following infection by *Clostridium tetani*.

Etiology

The spores of *Cl. tetani* enter body through any wound or prick.
Incubation period - about 7-10 days.

Microbiology

Clostridium tetani: A gram positive anaerobic bacterium, bearing terminal spores giving a microscopic picture of drum stick. Spores are in abundance in mud and soil and horse dung.

Pathogenesis

Refer **Table 6.3.**

Predisposing conditions: Road accidents, injuries due to metals and sharp objects, caries teeth, chronic suppurative otitis media with perforation. Inadequate sterilization of instruments in operation and labor theater.

Spores enter wound and germinate in anaerobic conditions into vegetative forms of *Cl. tetani* which grows and releases the exotoxins—tetanolysin and tetanospasmin.

Table 6.3: Pathogenesis of tetanus and clinical effect.

Pathogenesis	Travel through the perineural sheath and lymphatics around the sheath	Clinical effect
Tetanus toxins	Blocks the NMJ (neuromuscular junction)	Hyperexcitability; causes tonic reflex muscle spasm
Tetanospasmin	Enters the central nervous system and gets fixed to nerve tissue (irreversibly) Blocks cholinesterase enzymes at anterior horn cells	Clonic convulsions
Tetanolysin	Through lymphatic and blood circulation	Hemolysis and toxemia

Clinical Features and Complications

> **Q. Define period of onset and period of incubation. (Short notes)**

Incubation Period
- Approx. 7–10 days
- Time interval between the entry of spore and first symptom.

Period of Onset
- Time between appearance of first symptom and first spasm (represents time taken by toxin to get fixed to neuro muscular junction)
- Prognostic value—shorter the period of onset worse is the outcome.

Early Tetanus
- H/o wound, injury operation or procedure
- Fever, tachycardia, anxiety, mild dysphagia, difficulty to breathe, stiff neck and pain in back and neck.

Stage of Tonic Muscle Spasm (Neuromuscular Excitation)

> **Q. Short notes on risus sardonicus.**

- Extremities show stiffness due to tonic spasm
- Spasm of erector spinae causes -hyperextension like a bow, (called "Dhanurvedam" Sanskrit)
- Cranial nerves involvement:
  - V—trigeminal—lock jaw—trismus (masseter and pterygoid spasm)
  - VII—facial—muscle spasm—risus sardonicus
  - VIII—auditory nerve—spasm of stapedius— hyperacusis
  - X—vagus and XII—hypoglossal: dysphagia.

Moderate Tetanus Stage of Clonic Spasm
- Toxin has entered central nervous system and blocked anterior horn cells
- The toxin here cannot be neutralised by immunoglobulin or antitoxin
- Clinical features are hyperstimulation and hence clonic spasm
- Respiratory distress.

Severe Tetanus: Convulsive Stage
- Convulsions, coma
- Toxemia, myocarditis and death are terminal events.

Differential Diagnosis
- Poisoning—strychnine
- Convulsive disorders—status epilepticus
- Stiff jaw and dysphagia—quinsy, dental abscess.

> **Q. Describe the principles of management of tetanus.**

Management of the Tetanus
- **Isolation of patient:** To prevent visual and auditory stimuli from causing spasm or convulsions.
- **Supportive care**
  - Sedation—to avoid excitation—diazepam
  - Ventilation
  - Air
  - Fluid and nutrition
- **Antitoxin (passive immunization)**
  - Neutralizing circulating and unbound tetanus toxin (to prevent it from getting fixed to nerve tissue)
  - Tetanus immuno globulin—3000 to 6000 units intramuscular.
- **Anti-clostridial therapy**—usually for 10 days.
  - Penicillin G (crystalline penicillin) 20 lakh units intravenously every 6 hours with metronidazole 500 mg every 8 hours.
- **Anticonvulsants:**
  - Diazepam intravenous 20 mg 8 hourly (along with oxygen supplementation).
  - Midazolam infusion (short acting)
    * Phenobarbitone
    * Chlorpromazine 25 mg IV Q8H.
- **Mechanical ventilation:** In severe cases:
  - Non-depolarizing muscle relaxants—vecuronium and atracurium
  - Endotracheal intubation and assisted ventilation.
- **Stabilization** of hemodynamics and autonomic nervous system
  - Intravenous fluids
  - Alpha-blockers—phentolamine

- Phenothiazine—chlorpromazine
- Atropine-high doses for cardiovascular stability.

Magnesium sulphate infusion—controls the autonomic dysfunction; intravenous loading dose of 5 g given in 20 minutes followed by infusion for maintenance.

- **Active immunization:** Tetanus toxoid—first dose with immunoglobulin, 2nd after 1 month and 3rd 6 month.
- **Wound management**
  - Wound debridement
  - Local Injection of human tetanus immunoglobulin 500 units into the wound.
- **Management of complications:** Carried out as mentioned below.
  - ARDS, aspiration pneumonia
  - Cardiac—arrhythmias
  - Pulmonary edema
  - Renal—acute renal failure
  - DVT, thromboembolism, sepsis
- **General care:**
  - Symptomatic and supportive—paracetamol, steroids
  - Oral relaxants.

> **Q. Discuss the etiopathogenesis, clinical features and management of gas gangrene.**

GAS GANGRENE

Anaerobic infection caused by group of clostridia led by *Clostridium perfringens, Cl. oedematiens* and *Cl. septicum* along with the saccharolytic clostridia.

These are gram-positive, anaerobic, spore-bearing bacilli. They release collagenase, hyaluronidase, other proteases and alpha toxin to cause toxemia and spread.

High-risk etiological factors: Road accidents, diabetes, immunocompromised states, cancer.

Wounds with necrotic tissue and foreign bodies.

Clinical Features

- Fever, severe pain and crepitus (air crackling).
- Brownish watery exudates sweet odor
- Edema and spreading gangrene.
- Systemic complications with circulatory collapse and organ failure.

Treatment

Aggressive antibiotic therapy: High doses of penicillin—penicillin G—2 million units intravenously 6 hourly.

Metronidazole

Supportive: Fluid, blood transfusion, intensive monitoring, inotropic support if need be.

Early surgery: Liberal necrosectomy—removal of all necrotic material, wound toilet with hydrogen peroxide to release nascent oxygen.

Hyperbaric oxygen chamber therapy.

Hand Infections

Q. Describe the general principles in the diagnosis and treatment of hand infections.

General Considerations

- The key to management of any of disease of the hand is the knowledge of its anatomy.
- The goal of any treatment here is to ensure wound healing, relief of pain, and restoration of function of hand.
- Clinical finding of the most tender spot is diagnostic of pus.
- Early surgical intervention is planned if patient fails to improve after 24 to 48 hours of intravenous antibiotics therapy.
- After any treatment—surgical or otherwise, the hand is always splinted to protect the injured digits and to stretch the collateral ligaments of the injured joints (metacarpophalangeal joints flexed, interphalangeal joints extended).

Causes of Hand Infections

- Trauma is the most common.
- Predisposing factors—diabetes, neuropathies, and immunocompromised states.
- Microbiology:
- *Staphylococcus* and *Streptococcus* are seen in 90% of infections cases.
- Gram negative organisms seen in infections in diabetics, those due to human bites or heavily contaminated injuries.

General Principles of Treatment

- Incision, drainage of pus and debridement.
- Elevation of hand and immobilization—fingers flexed at metacarpophalangeal joints and extension at interphalangeal joints.
- Pus culture and appropriate antibiotic.
- Early mobilization of hand movements.

Q. Write short notes on acute paronychia.

PARONYCHIA

- Paronychia is an infection beneath the nail fold (eponychium). The nail plate invaginates into the dorsal skin of the finger, down to the periosteum of the distal phalanx.
- **Predisposing factors:** Any trauma to the of nail, (at work, or bites or manicures) diabetes is a major risk factor.
- **Microorganism:** Usually *Staphylococcus aureus*.
- The infection may spread around the nail under the eponychium or cause complications due to spread under the nail (subungual plane) causing necrosis of nail and spread to the pulp space resulting in a felon or osteomyelitis of terminal phalanx.
- **Clinical features:** Severe pain and redness of the nail fold and later a yellow area of pus under the fold. Discoloration under the nail indicates complication.
- **Treatment:** Antibiotics—usually cloxacillin or linezolid (in complicated cases).
- Anti diabetic treatment in diabetics.
- **Surgery:** Simple cases—elevation of eponychium and release of pus.
- In case of subungual abscess-excision of nail is required to release the pus and prevent osteomyelitis of phalanx.
- Analgesia and wound dressing.

Chronic paronychia: Commonly seen in those who use hands for washing and cleaning domestic articles, clothes or even work in gardens. Often a fungal infection of the nail supervenes. Diabetics are more prone for the condition. It is a long-standing and a relatively painless condition with sodden nail folds and an unhealthy nail.

Q. Write a short notes on felon.

FELON (TERMINAL PULP SPACE ABSCESS)

- A felon is an abscess of the fingertip involving the terminal pulp space of the finger.
- **Etiology:** Penetrating trauma (most commonly); spread from subungual abscess or paronychia (less common).
- **Microbiology:** Generally *Staphylococcus aureus*.
- **Anatomy:** Terminal pulp space is a closed space between volar skin and distal phalanx

with multiple tough septa fixing the skin to the bone. Any abscess or exudates cause increase in pressure, infective thrombosis of the digital arteries (these are terminal arteries) and cause necrosis, osteomyelitis of the terminal phalanx. The base of the phalanx escapes necrosis as it receives an arterial twig from the digital artery before the artery enters the tough pulp space.
- **Clinical features:** Severe pain and swelling of the finger tip along with fever. Redness and tense pulp space indicate a closed space sepsis. Fluctuation is a late sign.
- **Complications:** Osteomyelitis of terminal phalanx ; spread to the insertion of flexon tendon and tenosynovitis (especially if incision is done too proximally).
- **Treatment:**
  - Antibiotic—generally cloxacillin or linezolid are preferred analgesia.
  - Diabetes, if present, is controlled or excluded.
  - If symptoms do not improve in 24 hours, emergency drainage of the abscess is done under a digital block anesthesia. Incision is done over the point of maximum.

Q. Short notes on whitlow.

Whitlow is any infection of finger tip. But the term is also applied to some non-infective conditions which mimic a finger tip infection and are misdiagnosed.

Generally includes the following:
- Herpetic whitlow—herpes simplex—red painful fingertip with scaling—contagious.
- Staphylococcal whitlow—pulp space infection (felon).
- Fungal whitlow—*Candida albicans*—secondary to a chronic paronychia under nail bed.
- Melanotic whitlow—a subungual melanoma of finger tip—very painful (but not infective).
- Painless whitlow—in syringomyelia—due sensory deficit.

Q. Write short notes on webspace infection.

WEBSPACE ABSCESS (COLLAR-BUTTON ABSCESS)

- Due to subfascial infection of a web space; caused by injury (like pricks). The infection spreads to dorsal web space as the lateral spread is prevented by the skin of the palmar web space, which is adherent to the palmar fascia.
- The web space is swollen and tender on ventral and dorsal sides. The adjacent fingers are held in abduction.
- Incision and drainage is performed with incisions on both volar and dorsal sides separately.
- Other principles of treatment are as given above under general consideration.

Q. Write short notes on suppurative flexor tenosynovitis.

ACUTE SUPPURATIVE FLEXOR TENOSYNOVITIS (FTS)

Flexor tenosynovitis (FTS) is suppurative infection of flexor tendon and sheath of the hand causing disruption of flexor tendon function.

Etiology of FTS
- Penetrating trauma most common.
- Infectious bites (animal, insect or bird).
- Secondary to chronic inflammation as a result of diabetes, sarcoidosis, RA, crystalline deposition, overuse syndromes, psoriatic arthritis, SLE and amyloidosis.

Microbiology: Skin flora (mainly staphylococci and streptococci) are the most common organisms. Infectious bites may cause a different bacterial sepsis (*Pasteurella multocida, Mycobacterium marinum*).

Suppurative FTS is a surgical emergency (as it can cripple a hand very rapidly).

Pathophysiology of Suppurative FTS

The bacteria multiply in the closed space of the flexor tendon sheath causing migration of inflammatory cells and subsequent swelling. There is rapid erosion and necrosis of paratenon causing rupture of tendon, and digital contracture due to adhesions and scarring.

Complications of Suppurative Tenosynovitis
- **Spread to "Parona's space" in forearm:** Directly or by rupture and proximal retraction of flexor tendon into forearm space.
- Early adhesions between tendon and paratenon causes stiffness in flexors.

Clinical Features
Fever, pain and redness.

Signs: Kanavel's "cardinal" signs of flexor tendon sheath infection:
- Fusiform swelling of the affected finger.
- Position of the finger in partial flexion.
- Tenderness along the flexor tendon sheath, over the head of metacarpal—between distal palmar crease and proximal crease of the little finger (main Kanavel sign).
- Severe pain over the flexor sheath upon attempted extension of the finger.

These signs are not present in immunocompromised patients.

Investigation:
- MRI of hand helps delineate the anatomy of the involved tendons and adjoining soft tissues.
- High WBC counts and blood sugar levels.

Treatment
- Empiric intravenous antibiotics—cloxacillin, amikacin and metronidazole.
- Surgical drainage, if improvement is not seen in 24 hours or if imaging shows collection.
- Splint immobilization.
- Elevation until infection is under control.
- **Physiotherapy:** Hand rehabilitation (i.e., range-of-motion exercises and edema control) started at the earliest, once the pain and inflammation are under control.

The treatment of suppurative flexor tenosynovitis is performed as according the stage of presentation as given in **Table 6.4**.

Table 6.4: Michon's stages of suppurative flexor tenosynovitis and appropriate treatment.

Stage	Findings	Treatment
I	Increased fluid in sheath, mainly a serous exudate	Catheter irrigation
II	Purulent fluid, granulomatous synovium	Minimal invasive drainage with or without an indwelling catheter irrigation
III	Necrosis of the tendon, or tendon sheath	Extensive open debridement

Other Measures
- Dressings are continued.
- Splinting of hand in stretched position of flexed metacarpal joint and extended interphalangeal (IP) joint.
- Finger movement are restored at the earliest as soon as the inflammatory signs abate.

Q. Describe midpalmar space and midpalmar abscess.

The **Figure 6.1** depicts a cross-section of midpalm to show the palm spaces.

MIDPALMAR ABSCESS

Anatomy of midpalmar space: This is given in Figure 6.1.

Midpalmar space occupies the hand between the palmar aponeurosis superficially and the 3rd to 5th metacarpals in the depth of the hand. The space is divided into superficial palmar space and deep palmar space by the ulnar bursa, the expanded tendon sheath of the flexor tendons, which are bunched into the superficial flexor sublimis and deeper flexor profundus. The midpalmar space is separated by a tough fibrous septum attached to 3rd metacarpal and tendon sheath of flexor tendons (ulnar bursa) separating it from the thenar space on radial side. Another septum separates from the hypothenar space on the ulnar side.

Proximally the space communicates with Parona's space in forearm through the carpal

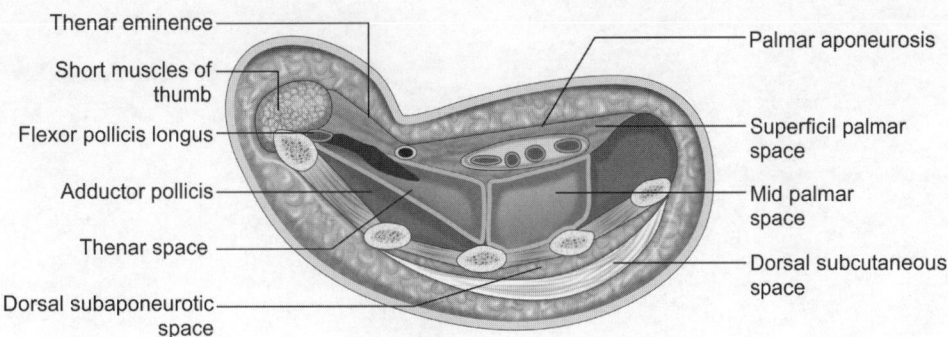

Fig. 6.1: The palmar spaces.

tunnel. The contents of the space include—the superficial and deep flexor tendons, covered by the flexor synovial sheaths (the ulnar bursa), the median nerve and superficial palmar arterial arch.

The space also opens into the medial three web spaces of the fingers distally through narrow lumbrical canals.

Etiology of Infection of Midpalmar Space
- Penetrating direct trauma.
- Spread of infection from web space.
- Suppurative flexor tenosynovitis due to rupture or due to surgical intervention.
- **Predisposing factors:** Diabetes mellitus, HIV, immunocompromised states.
- **Complications:** Suppurative tenosynovitis, spread into Parona's space in forearm.
- Late—contractures and stiff hand.

Clinical Features
- Fever, swelling and redness of hand and pain.
- **Frog hand:** Hand is swollen—on palmar side with loss of concavity of hand and on dorsum (due to inflammatory and lymphatic edema).
- Hand is held with fingers (position of ease).
- However the extension of fingers is not so painful as in a case of tenosynovitis.
- **Differential diagnosis:** Suppurative tenosynovitis (where Kanavel's signs are positive).

Investigation
- MRI of hand for clarity of anatomy of the pathology.
- Ultrasound study to identify and localize pus.

Treatment
- The general principles of management—antibiotics, elevation of hand and analgesia.
- **Surgery:** Performed to drain the abscess—general anesthesia or a proximal block. An arm tourniquet avoids bleeding, helps to identify and avoid damage to the tendons.
- Postoperative wound management, splinting.
- Physiotherapy to restore function of the hand.

> **Q. Short notes on thenar space abscess.**

THENAR SPACE
- It is the fascial compartment in the radial half of hand. A fibrous septum separates the thenar space from midpalmar space on ulnar side tendon of the long flexor of thumb on radial side, short muscles of thumb and flexor tendon of index anteriorly and the short adductor of the thumb posteriorly.
- The synovial sheath of flexor pollicis longus makes the thenar bursa.
- Penetrating trauma is the usual cause of sepsis.

Clinical Features
Fever, swelling and redness of hand and pain over thenar eminence.

Treatment
- Antibiotics and surgical drainage.
- Incision is put over the palmar crease between thenar eminence and palmar hollow.

Section 2

Essential Topics in General Surgery

7. Surgical Audit and Research
8. Ethics in Surgery
9. Investigation of the Surgical Patient and Basis of Cancer Therapy
10. Pre, Intra and Post-operative Management
11. Anesthesia and Pain Relief, Day Care Surgery and Safe General Surgery
12. Nutrition and Fluid Therapy
13. Transplantation
14. Basic Surgical Skills
15. Hospital Waste Disposal
16. Minimally Invasive Surgery and Bariatric Surgery
17. Trauma

Surgical Audit and Research

SU7.1	Describe the planning and conduct of surgical audit.
SU7.2	Describe the principles and steps of clinical research in general surgery.

SU7.1: Describe the planning and conduct of surgical audit.

AUDIT AND SERVICE EVALUATION

Q. What is clinical audit and what is its importance?

Clinical Audit
- It is a process to improve patient care.
- Involves **comparing** the structure, process and outcome of **the given care against predefined** and set criteria and **standards**.
- Personal outcome data contributes to a clinical database that helps continuous monitoring of a surgeon's own performance against the mandated standards.

Service Evaluation
- *It aims to judge the efficacy* of current care of an institution or competence of an individual surgeon/team
- Example, how best can this be? Useful can this be? How adequate is this?
- Does not compare data with set standard (unlike in audit).

In essence, they answer the following questions respectively:

Audit
- Are we at par with the standard of care?
- If not how to do that?

Serviced evaluation
- Are we adequate to meet requirements of the patient?
- Or should we improve?

Features Common to Audit and Service Evaluation
- Surgeon, team and patients are prefixed.
- Interventions (investigations and treatment protocols) are predefined and there is no change in this.
- Both study the existing data plus (if needed) questionnaires and interview with stake-holders.
- No additional interventions or deviation from protocols unlike in a research.
- No randomization involved (unlike a research).
- Help improve the standard of care.

Implications
Audit helps in planning to:
- Improve the standard of care in the institution.
- Improve a surgeon's performance.
- Train the staff to meet the standards.
- It also helps to plan change in antibiotic policy or pre operative protocols, revalidation of licence, and staff recruitments.

Types of Audit
- To improve the quality of care.
- Local—hospital level or district level.
- General—national or state level.

Q. What is an audit cycle? Write a brief note.

AUDIT CYCLE

Audits require certain structured steps to establish an audit cycle:
- A multidisciplinary team to conduct audit on a specified aspect, e.g., (structure, performance of individual or team, protocols etc.).
- Define the audit question.
- Set agreed standards on the audit question.
- *Design* the audit-data against standard—evidence based.
  Involve audit bodies and other institutions for audit if needed.
- Specify time interval of audit (e.g., say over a past 12 months or 6 months)
- Perform the audit and analyse.
- *Gap analysis*
  - *Scenario 1:* Audit shows shortcomings—identify specific steps needed (interventions) to improve and meet the standards (e.g., need for an instrument or training a surgeon or nursing team or improving preop protocols etc.)
  - *Scenario 2:* Audit shows - no shortcomings - meeting all standards - needs are audit after a specified time.
- *Re-audit*—when needed.

Note: Audit may lead sometimes to research.

Research study: Aims to attempt generating new aspects of knowledge or treatment protocols and regimen. Even during an audit project, certain evidence of limited nature may emerge calling for a research study design on further work to confirm a new piece of knowledge or to try a new treatment regimen or a surgery.

SU7.2: Describe the principles and steps of clinical research in general surgery.

Clinical Research

Clinical research involves systematic study of available data and outcomes of exposure to interventions to derive new knowledge and/or to evolve effective newer treatment options to improve outcomes in clinical conditions.

Q. What are the types of clinical study designs? Write briefly about each. (Long notes)

Q. What are the differences between observational and experimental study? (Short notes)

Q. What are the types of observational study and experimental study? (Short notes)

Basic Principles of Clinical Research Studies (Must Know)

Study Designs (Based on Aims of Enquiry) (Must Know)
- Observational study
- Experimental study
- Systematic review and meta analysis.

Observational Study

Patients are not assigned into groups as under control and test (treatment). Inferences are made by surveillance of a given number of participants, to postulate associations between exposure (risk factor) and outcome (result). But the causation cannot be proved.

Types of Designs in Observational Study
- **Case control study:** Analyses—exposure (risk) v/s outcome (disease) in a group of patients with and without disease.
- **Cohort study:** Analyses—exposure (risk) and observe for development of outcome (disease)
  - Prospective cohort study
  - Retrospective cohort study
- **Cross sectional study:** Single time analysis of a cross section of patients.
- **Longitudinal study:** Multiple sampling of similar small cross sections at different intervals.
- **Case series study:** Small set of patients with a specified treatment are studied.

Experimental Studies

Comparison of outcome of two or more treatments (exposures)—involves new intervention.

Types of Designs in Experimental Studies

- **Randomized trials without control:** The researcher or an external person or agency *randomly* allocates the patients to groups undergoing respective treatments.
- **Randomized controlled trials (RCTs):** Patients are assigned to two groups:
  - **Control**—"the non exposure group" (not undergoing the treatment under study)
  - **Treatment group**—or "exposure group" undergoing the treatment under study and **observed for a specified (particular) outcome (effect)**.

  This study design can often establish a causal relationship between a risk factor and outcome.
- **Pragmatic trials:** They attempt to overcome the limitations of RCT—such as strict inclusion and exclusion criteria and the limited generalisability of RCT (due to diversity across populations).

  Claimed to be offering a "real ground" applicability.

Systematic Review and Meta-analysis

Study of all available published literature to evolve consensus from data.
- Qualitatively (systematic review)
- Quantitatively—meta-analysis.

> Q. Describe principles of conducting clinical research.

STEPS OF CONDUCTING CLINICAL RESEARCH (MUST KNOW)

- **Define a topic for research:**
  - Involves identifying a research topic—after discussions, questionnaires, and search.
  - If idea is derived from the above and the that idea then transformed into **a hypothesis.**
  - Next steps revolve around the hypothesis.
- **Study design:** The purpose and direction of research should be clear.
  - The design should define the purpose of study.
  - Be practically feasible in the given specified time, infrastructure sand resources.
  - Be flexible to expand its scope to derive better outcome. There should be clarity on expected outcomes of the study and should address and comply with the **ethical issues** in the study.
  - **The study must possibly foresee the impact of the study.**
- **Type of study**
  - **Observational or experimental?**
  - The study design is drawn accordingly
- **Sample size:** Very important to prove or disprove the hypothesis in the study.
  - Calculating the number of patients required to perform a satisfactory investigation is done on various statistical formulae after considering the parametrers.
  - This helps avoid errors in conclusions—such as:
    - **Type I (false positive):** Wrongly claiming a non-existing benefit or harm when it is not there.
    - **Type II (false negative):** A benefit or harm of significance is missed.
- **Eliminating bias:** Blinding—single or double blinding.
  - **Single blinding:** Blinding the observers—the observers of study are not allowed to know if they are treating the controls or test group.
  - **Double blinding:** Blinding both the observers and patients—here patients also do not know if they are in the test group or control group.
- **Study protocol:** A final summary of research protocol and all details of logistics (work force, place etc.) is given along with the flowchart for convenient reference.
- **Legal and statutory compliance:** Ensure compliance with all Regulatory laws and guidelines.
- **Peer review of protocols:** Institutional or state bodies or institutional scientific committee conducts the same before the study is started.

- **Ethical issues:** Self appraisal, scrutiny by ethics committee and review committee.
- **Research integrity:** Being honest is the most integral part of credibility of research; the research study should ensure—transparency and accountability in its conduct.
- **Statistical analysis:** The most important part of the study with normal distribution of data.
- **Analyzing a scientific article:** Consolidated standards of reporting trials (CONSORT) statement to improve the quality of reporting.
- **Presenting and publishing an article.**

> **Q. What is IMRAD form of a study? (Short notes)**

The study details and results are compiled—in compliance with the IMRAD form—introduction, methods, results and discussion.

And submitted for presentation or publication in the appropriate forum.

The documented and published data from the study contributes to the evolution of consensus on knowledge - viz., **evidence-based surgery**.

> **Q. Write brief note on randomised control study. (Short notes)**

Described under the next section on research study designs.

DETAILS OF RESEARCH STUDY DESIGNS (GOOD TO KNOW)

Observational Study

Case-control Study (Refer Table 7.1)

A given risk factor (exposure) and specific fallout (outcome) are studied to determine the relationship of exposure to outcome. Patients are selected based on presence or absence of the given **outcome of interest**.

The group of patients with disease (sick) are compared to those without disease (control).

Advantages of Case Control Study Design
- Inexpensive and quick assessment to look for association between a risk factor and a disease or between an intervention and outcome of surgery.
- Also useful for investigation of rare diseases.
- Can be used as a sub-study from database of a larger study like randomized trials saving additional cost.

Cohort Study (Table 7.2)

A group of participants, who are free from specified outcome of interest (disease) is selected and followed up over a period of time for development of the specified outcome(disease) in two groups—1) after they are exposed to risk factor or 2) without exposure ot risk factor:

The participants must be free of the specified outcome (e.g., disease or symptoms) before they are recruited for the study. They should be available for follow up over a specified period of time. To evaluate for a development of the outcome.

Types of Cohort Studies
- **Prospective cohort design**
  - Selected participants from the study participants are followed over a long

Table 7.1: Case control study.

Group—with exposure to risk		Group—without exposure to risk	
Have disease	No disease	Have disease	No disease
Number	Number	Number	Number

Table 7.2: Cohort study.

No disease at start—followed over a period **with exposure** to risk factor		No disease at start—followed over a period **without exposure** to risk factor	
Develop disease during period of follow up	No outcome—disease during the period of follow up	Develop disease during period of follow up	No outcome—disease during the period of follow up
Numbers	Numbers	Numbers	Numbers

period for occurence of an outcome or otherwise.
- **Disadvantage:** Long periods of follow up, needs large size of participants.
- **Retrospective cohort design**
  - The selection of participants is from a past database of patients.
  - The outcome of interest is evaluated at the beginning of study and data from a pre-existing population are used to compare exposed and non-exposed members.
  - **Advantage:** This allows quicker completion of studies
  - **Disadvantage:** Based on quality and reliability of data available.

Cross-sectional Studies

Study of a specified population during a single period of observation with reference to exposure and outcomes, which are measured simultaneously.

Advantages
- Low cost, simpler to act, a large amount of information is made available and quickly.
- Can be used to hypothesize causal relation in larger population on risk factors.

Case Series
- This design of study documents the natural course of a disease, the treatment and outcome.
- This is conducted on a small group of patients.
- These reports are useful to document rare disease processes or outcomes.

Experimental Studies

Randomized Controlled Trials (RCTs)

The gold standard design for clinical research: Patients are randomly assigned to **intervention** and **control** groups or "**arms.**"

- **Randomization:** Facilitates unbiased distribution to the study arms of both known and unknown participant **covariates**. Helps minimize the bias in observer's interpretation of the relationship between the under study intervention and the outcome (which is observed for).
- **Blinding:** The allocation of participants to treatment and control groups is **concealed**. It can be utilized with respect to both the investigators and the participants.
  Blinding could be twofold:
  - **Single blinding:** The investigator does not know if he is treating the one from control or treatment group.
  - **Double blinding:** Both investigator and participants also do not know if the respective patients are in the treatment or control group.

  This could raise ethical issues and legal issues as it amounts violation of human rights.

Systematic Review and Meta-analysis

These are **distinct** (though similar) methods for evolving a consensus on data through critical appraisal of existing published literature.

A **systematic review** is a qualitative review of literature.

Principle
- Set a clinical question
- Search of all available published data
- Mark the relevant among the studies
- Analyzing the data—mainly qualitative (may be quantitative too).

A **meta-analysis** is a quantitative statistical analysis of results of searching the literature.

Pooled analysis: In a meta analysis—allows deriving abstraction of individual patient data—to allow homogeneity among the studies.

Ethics in Surgery

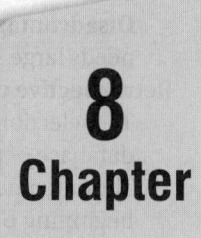
Chapter 8

SU8.1	Describe the principles of ethics as it pertains to general surgery. Studied with help from - forensic medicine AETCOM
SU8.2	Demonstrate professionalism and empathy to the patient undergoing general surgery. DOAP (demonstration - observation - assistance - performance) AETCOM
SU8.3	Discuss medico-legal issues in surgical practice. (With forensic medicine - AETCOM - attitude ethics and communication)

SU8.1: Describe the principles of ethics as it pertains to general surgery.

SU8.2: Demonstrate professionalism and empathy to the patient undergoing general surgery.

The word 'ethics' is derived from Greek word 'ethikos', i.e., arising from custom. Medical and surgical ethics is considered as the principle of proper professional conduct concerning the right and duties of physician himself, his patients and his fellow practitioners. Surgery, ethics and law go hand in hand.

Sushruta Samhita, the oldest literary resource in the field of surgery, describes ethics in detail.

Q. What are the ethical issues in modern medicine and legal issues?

The ethical concepts have evolved since ancient times as given in **Table 8.1**.

The above modules are comparable with difference only in the context of time.

General Ethics on Surgical Training and Practice

- The selection process of student into the discipline surgery, duties and responsibilities of a learning surgeon, their relation to teacher and patient.
- Surgical teachers—their rights and responsibilities.

Table 8.1: Concept of ethical and legal issues in ancient and modern medicine.

The concept of surgical ethics as in *Sushruta Samhita* are grouped as follows:	Surgical ethics in era of modern medicine and their legal extension
• General ethics • Professional and academic ethics • Pre-operative, operative and postoperative ethics • Experimental surgical ethics • Ethics in emergency surgery • Ethics in professional conduct	• Respect for autonomy of patient • Informed consent • Practical application of consent • Matter of life and death • Confidentiality • Maintaining standard of excellence

Chapter 8: Ethics in Surgery

- Learning theoretical knowledge and its practical aspects to get administrative permission.
- Performance of surgery should be only allowed after practical mentoring and surgery should be allowed to be performed only with background of sound theoretical knowledge.
- Surgeon should have a sound knowledge of medicine and related domains (physician who operates when necessary and avoids an unwanted surgery).
- Registration—with regulatory body like the medical council after training.

Professional and Academic Ethics

- Diagnosis of disease with clinical examination before starting any treatment
- Respect autonomy of patients
- Informed consent
- Confidentiality
- Professional conduct
- Empathy.

The autonomy of the patient must be strongly respected by a surgeon.

It should be the right of the patient to choose, accept or to refuse the type of treatment offered by the surgeon, regardless of the surgeon's opinion and advice.

Surgeon has to explain prognosis of the disease, purpose and perceived role of surgery in treating the disease, outcome of surgery, risks involved including the intra and post-operative complications and loss of life. He should also explain alternatives to surgery and fallout of not operating.

Surgeons have a relationship of trust with the patients because they have a duty of care towards the latter, which is for—protecting the life and health of patients and also additionally respecting the autonomy of patients in making choice of treatment.

Preoperative, Operative and Postoperative Ethics

- The importance of clinical examination
- Preparation of patient before any surgical procedure is a must
- Postoperative care.

Ethics in Professional Conduct

A surgeon's actions and conduct during surgery—concern for patient, the team members like the anesthetist, nursing and ancillary staff, his role in encouraging and leading the team are of paramount importance.

Empathy

Also the surgeon's role in empathizing the patient will go a long way in ensuring a better recovery by boosting the morale of patient and that of patient's family. The patient feels that the surgeon is one among "his people". This also helps in boosting the relationship of trust.

Ethics in Emergency Surgery

In emergency cases, the doctor should not apply the routine methods of treatment, instead he should act as if his own house is on fire (*Sushruta*).

Q. Short notes on informed consent.

INFORMED CONSENT

- Patient should be fully informed of the disease, need for treatment with details including the type of surgery, its risks, intended benefits and chances of failure.
- The details of surgery, the need for, complications and hazards also should be explained.
- Any alternative treatments should also be explained.
- The reasons for advising the particular surgery and possible consequences of not operating should be explained.
- This should be done in patient's preferred language, if necessary with help of an interpreter.
- The surgeon should do it himself and not ask his subordinates to do it.
- Patient should be an adult in normal senses, who can understand and take one's decisions.
- Patient should give consent voluntarily only after fully understanding the available options
- Patient should never be coerced into giving consent.

For children, adults in comatose state or those with psychiatric illness: A responsible kin or caretaker can give consent.

It should be recorded on paper, *signed by the surgeon, the patient, patient's family member and testified by witnesses.*

> **Q. Briefly the concept of confidentiality and enumerate the situations to break confidentiality.**

CONFIDENTIALITY

The personal and clinical details of the patient should never be disclosed to any other person or agency including video demonstration in workshops and publicity in media.

Exceptions

- There is a need for another opinion or help in improving the outcome of treatment (inpatient's interest).
- The statutory obligations require disclosure of details to the state authorities (by court orders or in relation to the requirements of public health legislation) in the interests of preventing harm to society, e.g., in situations like epidemics or pandemics and communicable diseases.
- Patients explicitly request for disclosing the details to help them in legal or insurance claims.
- In professional studies and conferences/publications—with the explicit consent of the patient, but without disclosure of identity of the patients.

Deviations from Consent

On table need to perform an extra operation or procedure other than one for which consent is taken may become necessary. An on table decision should be taken only after discussing with patient's attendants and taking their explicit consent.

On Table Death and Postoperative Deaths

- Should be properly documented with reference to the events leading to death and resuscitative measures undertaken.

- All the facts should be properly explained to the responsible family members of the family.
- Empathy and humanitarian approach is always advocated.
- A police complaint should be registered and an autopsy insisted upon.

Situations of Moral Dilemmas

Every surgeon should ask oneself before advising a surgery "Can I treat this patient without this surgery?" If there is a slightest doubt, it is better to avoid surgery.

> **Q. What are the situations of "life and death" and dilemmas on ethical actions in moribund patients.**

Situations of "Life and Death"

- Moribund patient with imminent death or brain dead patients.
- When surgery is a mere surgical exercise with minimal benefits expected.

Dilemmas and Ethical Actions

- To operate or not to? To continue life support or not to?
- Surgeon should ask oneself—what if it is one's kin?
- Will the patient recover by prolonging life support, to live a life with an improved quality?
- Will the patient or the family be harmed economically by offering a surgery just to keep the patient alive?

The patient's family is taken into confidence and a decision taken accordingly.

A patient's explicit wish (if the situation was anticipated by the patient) is followed.

> **Q. Write a note on euthanasia.**

Passive Euthanasia

Discontinuing the life support as may be a difficult and yet pragmatic decision—when it is agreed for and accepted as entirely "in patient's interest".

Active Euthanasia

It is generally unethical, immoral and illegal in most of the countries although some have opened a scope for conditional active euthanasia.

This will raise moral and ethical questions and potentially be a ground for unethical practice.

Research

- To enhance knowledge and to gain higher competence.
- The patient should be taken to confidence and no research should be undertaken which has even slightest risk to patient's interests.
- Any innovation or an entirely new concept of treatment may need ethical regulation and statutory clearance from the local ethics committee and national body respectively.
- The pressure on surgeons from institutions to enhance the performance must be resisted.
- **Ensuring standards of excellence:** Constant updation of knowledge and skills (training) and upgradation of equipments and instruments in diagnostic, operative and postoperative domains.
- **Professional charges:** Should be transparent and clear with no hidden or misleading sections.

> SU8.3: Discuss medico-legal issues in surgical practice.

MEDICO-LEGAL ISSUES IN SURGICAL PRACTICE

- Patient surgeon relationship and surgical services.
- Treating surgical cases where the illness is attributable to criminality or foul play.
  - Burns—suicidal or homicidal.
  - Mob violence involving stab or gun injuries.
- Accident victims of a road mishap, air crash or disasters like land slides or industrial disasters and fall from heights and blunt trauma.

Medico-legal Issues in Patient Surgeon Relationship and Surgical Services

- Patients trust their respective surgeons and the trust is built over the surgeon's qualification, credentials, reputation, communication with the patients and ability to convince the patient of the need for surgery and details of surgery.
- Surgery involves interventions—operative and non-operative to treat the patient.
- A surgery is a planned injury inflicted with the sole intention of treating the illness. Any harm to the patient that may arise or any result that may be short of patient's expectation is unintentional or a necessary step of surgery (e.g., a stab wound to insert a drain or a urinary catheter that may cause cystitis). The unforeseen complications of a surgery may include a disability or death.
- The patient and the family of the patient may feel that the care is short of expected outcome. The complications may be attributable to the surgeon's failure or the shortcomings in the system. Or the same may be fully beyond the surgeon' control. Also there may be a scope for suspecting the breach in ethical norms and violating the patient's right to autonomy and privacy.
- The shortcomings of the treatment may be real or merely perception of the patient's side. The law aims to differentiate a negligence in treatment and a preventable and avoidable deficiency of service from a shortcoming or complication, beyond the control of surgeon or system, despite the adequate following of protocols.
- Any breach of ethical principles provides the ground for litigations and so do the legal non-compliance.

> Q. Enumerate the ethical principles and legal non-compliance leading to litigations against the surgeons.

Criminal Liabilities

- Example, complicity of a surgeon in illegal acts like facilitating a kidney transplant without caring for the legal mandates.
- Operating on a brain dead patient without the knowledge of the patients' relatives.

Unintended Criminal Negligence

- Leaving an instrument of mop in the abdomen.

- Operating—on wrong side, e.g. hernia, knee joint, breast, brain, etc.

Vicarious Responsibility
For any deficiency of services by the nurse or the hospital machinery.

Breach of Confidentiality of the Patient
Divulging details of the patient's illness to third parties without patient's consent, that may harm patient's interests.

Deficiency in Preoperative and Postoperative Care
Deficiency in informed consent and inadequate documentation:
- Informed consent to be taken by the surgeon after an in person explanation to the patient and relatives in the language understood by the patient and relatives.
- The details of surgery, the need for, complications and hazards also should be explained.
- Any alternative treatments should be explained. Also the reasons for advising the particular surgery and possible consequences of not operating should be explained.
- The consent should be voluntary and not out of coercion.
- The same should be documented clearly and signed by the patient, relatives and the surgeon.
- An independent witness should also sign the same.

Deviations from Consent
On table need to perform an extra operation or procedure other than one for which consent is taken may become necessary. An on table decision should be taken only after discussing with patient's attendants and taking their explicit consent.

"ON TABLE DEATH" AND POST-OPERATIVE DEATH
This is an important topic of medico legal and ethical importance related to death of the surgical patient in the operating room.

Q. How do you handle a case of perioperative death?
- Should be properly documented with reference to the events leading to death and resuscitative measures undertaken.
- All the facts should be properly explained to the responsible family members of the family.
- Empathy and humanitarian approach is always advocated.
- A police complaint should be registered and an autopsy insisted upon.

Q. Enlist briefly the doctors' duties in medico-legal issues pertaining to surgical care of accidents, disasters and criminal activities in society.
- First step is recording the facts and informing the police.
- This happens concurrently with resuscitation along the advanced trauma life support (ATLS) principles.
- The legal procedures are adhered to without any let up.
- The accident register should be complete with the facts.
- At each stage of the treatment, the police should be involved and the patient's relatives are kept in loop with the compliance with court orders.
- The discharge of these patients should be documented with full compliance with legal procedures.

Q. Explain the legal provisions to protect rights of patients and Consumer Protection Act (CPA) 1986, amended by new CPA 2019.

Regulation
- The surgical practice is regulated and controlled by the law of the land encompassing the ethical, and moral principles respecting the rights of the patients. The standards are set for providing the treatment.
- The regulatory bodies in India include the Medical Council of India, the statutory body established by the Medical Council Act, largely superseded by the recent

- parliamentary act for the new National Medical Council which provides for the medical education, licensing, credentialing and regulation of practice.
- The patient's rights are also addressed under the criminal law under Indian criminal code and the civil codes.
- Further, the medical care (services of a surgeon) are considered as a service and the patients are considered as consumers paying for the services. The same is regulated by the Consumer Protection Act (CPA) of 1986, amended by the new CPA 2019, enacted and enforced from August 2020.
- The disputes claiming compensations upto 1 crore rupee are filed at the district forum, those up to 10 crore rupee at the state forum and those above 10 crore rupee at the National forum, which is also highest appellate (before the Supreme Court) for disputing the judgments of lower fora. Sadly the patients are often instigated to sue the surgeons and hospitals for compensation and hence the surgeons are under increasing stress of having to face law suits under the consumer protection law.
- Adherence to ethical principles, diligence in enacting the surgical practice and respecting the patient's rights will go a long way in maintaining the professional respect among surgeons and human dignity among the patients.

Investigation of the Surgical Patient and Basis of Cancer Therapy

Chapter 9

SU9.1	Choose appropriate biochemical, microbiological, pathological, imaging investigations and interpret the investigative data in a surgical patient.
SU9.2	Biological basis for early detection of cancer and multidisciplinary approach in management of cancer.
SU9.3	Communicate the results of surgical investigations and counsel the patient appropriately. DOAP session

SU9.1: Choose appropriate biochemical, microbiological, pathological, imaging investigations and interpret the investigative data in a surgical patient.

Note: Specific tests and imaging methods are employed as per the system involved and the same are discussed in respective chapters. This chapter only aims to highlight the "how to go about".

A surgical patient is one under a surgeon's care—for treatment—operative or non-operative.

Goals of Evaluation of the Surgical Patient

- Assessment of patient's functional status.
- Identify the medical ailments and to stratify the medical status, if needed.
- Assessment (and quantification) of the patient's level of risk for the planned procedure.
- Confirmation of state of optimization of the patient's medical condition before surgery.

General Steps

- History and physical examination.
- Routine diagnostic testing is usually not needed minor surgical procedures and young healthy patients (but done only for medico-legal purpose). But the investigatons are done in patients with comorbidities and before major and complex surgeries.

Specific and Special Needs in Preoperative Management

Preoperative laboratory studies and imaging should be decided on an individual basis.

Diagnostic investigations: Clinical diagnosis is confirmed or other diagnoses are established by investigations.

Prior to surgery, a multidisciplinary approach including a cardiologist is employed to determine which noninvasive or invasive measure should be taken to optimize the patient.

- **General:**
  - Blood: Complete blood counts
  - Hemoglobin and hematocrit: To evaluate anemia and blood loss
  - Cell counts: RBC, WBC and platelets
  - ESR and CRP are indications of active inner disease process
  - Renal function
- **Cardiovascular disease:** This is a major cause of post operative mortality in all surgeries and should be detected even in asymptomatic patients.

Risk stratification is done for major adverse cardiac events (MACE), by the operating surgeon, anesthesiologist, and the physician (cardiologist). The details are given in SU10.1 on page 82.

Factors related to the surgical procedure under consideration also convey risk.

Biochemical Investigations in a Surgical Patient

The following are estimated generally:
- Serum electrolyte levels are crucial—sodium, potassium, calcium, chloride and bicarbonate.
- Preoperative hyponatremia needs correction.
- High potassium can be seen in renal dysfunction (diabetic nephropathy) or may result from tissue injury (muscle). It can be arrhythmogenic.
- Low bicarbonate levels indicate acidotic state.
- Coagulation profile is needed when patients with history of bleeding disorders or in patients with is having liver disease or those on antiplatelet/anticoagulants.

Includes—bleeding time, clotting time, activated partial thromboplastin time, prothrombin time with international normalized ratio (INR).

Renal Function
- Blood urea and urea nitrogen levels and serum creatinine
- Elevated in diabetics and obstructive uropathy.

Thyroid function
Parathormone and ionic calcium levels.

Liver Function Tests
- Albumin levels are a function of liver cells.
- Low levels are seen in patients with chronic liver disease and those with renal dysfunction due to protein loss.
- Raised enzyme levels indicate cell damage [alanine transaminase (ALT)/aspartate transaminase (AST)] or obstructive pathology gamma-glutamyl transferase (GGT) or alkaline phosphatase.

- **Pancreatic enzyme levels:** Lipase and amylase are evaluated only in specific patients.
- **Cardiac enzymes:** Creatine kinase MB (CK-MB) and troponins are elevated in patients with acute cardiac damage.

Other Special Biochemical Tests
Example, serum iron levels ferritin levels, iron binding capacity (evaluation of anemia), magnesium levels in patients with sepsis and/or renal dysfunction.

Urine Tests
- Proteins, sugar, pH
- For protein—qualitative and quantitative
- Special tests of urine are done as needed
- Coproporphyrins in abdominal pain due to porphyria (both qualitative and quantitative)
- Urinary vanillylmandelic acid (VMA) or metanephrines—in suspected pheochromocytoma.

Microbiological Investigations in a Surgical Patient

- **Urine analysis**—routine evaluation for proteins, sugar, cells and pH.
- **Urine culture**—when infection is suspected.

Blood examination can be as per diagnosis and system of involvement.

Blood culture for bacteremia.

Immunological study
- RA factor
- ASA titer
- Antinuclear antibody (ANA) in collagen disorders
- Serum immunoglobulins—IgA, IgE, Ig M.

Tumor Markers
- Carcinoembryonic antigen (CEA)—colon and many other GI cancers
- CA 125—ovarian cancers
- CA 19-9—pancreatic cancer.

Pathology
Hematology: To evaluate blood dyscrasias or anemia in a surgical patient.

Q. Explain cytology with examples.

Cytology

Smear Cytology

- Specimen of smear of secretions or excretions—studied for specific malignant cells.
- Brush cytology—at endoscopy or examination.
  Fine needle aspiration cytology (FNAC)—needle aspirates are taken as smears and stained to study the cells in the lesion. However, they can't study the histology of the tissue as in a biopsy.

Q. Explain briefly the types of biopsy.

BIOPSY

A piece of tissue is taken from the lesion for microscopic study and diagnosis. Special stains are used according to the need and diagnosis.

Types of Biopsy

- **Needle biopsy**, e.g., trucut biopsy—a core of tissue is cut and taken into the needle which is subjected to microscopic examination (tissue histology unlike cytology in FNAC). It is an outpatient procedure, avoids general anesthesia.
- **Incision biopsy:** A piece of tissue is taken from a lesion after incising the skin over the same.
- **Excision biopsy:** Small lesions within 3–5 cm size can be entirely removed and examined. The diagnostic biopsy here can also be curative in benign lesions.
- **Edge biopsy** (piece from the edge of the lesion including piece of normal tissue): This allows comparison of the diseased part with the normal structure. The lesions are most actively growing at the edge and hence chances of getting the active cells of the pathology are high, e.g. carcinoma of the foot or oral cavity.
- **Wedge biopsy** (a wedge is taken from middle of a growth or lesion): In lesions like melanoma or fungal granulomas.
- **Punch biopsy:** Punch machine takes a punch and cylindrical specimen from the lesion (as in a wedge biopsy).

IMAGING: IN A SURGICAL PATIENT

The advances in electro medical engineering have revolutionized the diagnostic and therapeutic paradigm in surgical science.

X-Ray

- Oldest and yet the most accessible and affordable.
- X-ray chest for evaluation of lung fields and skeleton, deformity or disease of chest wall and spine, lungs, mediastinum and pericardium, heart and aorta.
- X-ray of the diseased part—as per the need plain or contrast.

Contrast radiography for specific sytems are done as per indication, e.g., ventriculography, intravenous cholangiography, arteriography.

Fistulography and Sinusography

Dye injected into the fistula tract or sinus to delineate before planning the operation.

Ultrasonography (USG)

- It is extensively employed in diagnosis and in monitoring therapeutic response of surgical patients.
- **Advantageous**—accessible, affordable, non invasive and harmless
- **Disadvantage**—heavily interpreter dependent.

Doppler Study

It is an application of ultrasound imaging with addition of a special probe to evaluate the blood flow based on velocity of flow. This helps accurate assessment of arterial and venous obstructions and flow pattern.

Computed Tomography (CT Scanning)

- Clarity in image delineates axial images or further spiral and 3D imaging depending on the type of CT scanner.
- Contrast studies are done as per the system.
- **Disadvantage**—heavy radiation exposure.

Magnetic Resonance Imaging (MRI)

- Allows radiation free imaging of the parts, especially soft parts.

- Often it is complimentary to CT more than a substitute, because each has the limitation and advantages over the other.

Nuclear Medicine in Imaging

These are functional scans where a radio isotope acts as a tracer of diseased cell that take up the isotope. Radioisotopes are chosen as per the system and tissue type (e.g., iodine 123 in thyroid).

Q. Positron emission tomography (PET).

Positron emission tomography (PET) scanning is a functional scan.
- The particular radiotracer is tagged with fluorodeoxyglucose (FDG) and injected, FDG is taken up as food by the active cell of the tumor.
- The radio tracer emits gamma rays which is picked and digital images taken in combination with a CT (or MRI).
- Tumors and lesions usually smaller than 0.5 cm are not seen on CT (structural), but picked by the PET as the radiotracer is taken up by cells that take up glucose (functional).

SU9.2: Biological basis for early detection of cancer and multidisciplinary approach in management of cancer.

"*Cancer*" is a Greek word for "*Crab*".

The malignant transformation of a normal cell to cancer cell has several features:
- The cell foregoes or "forgets" normal rules governing a normal cell
- No contact inhibition as in a normal cell
- No regulation of growth—uncontrolled and unhindered cell division and proliferation.

Failure of apoptosis
Acquires ability to:
- Invade into normal tissue and vessels
- Acquire new blood supply
- Ability to disseminate—by invasion, migration and escape into extravascular space by evoking
- Inflammation in the endothelial cells
- Change in cellular energy metabolism
- Evades detection and elimination—by suppressing or evoking immune responses to camouflage as normal cells.

Q. Short notes on apoptosis.

Apoptosis (Greek word meaning—leaf fall)
- A physiological process (unlike necrosis)
- It is an internal cellular arrangement of programmed cell death and dismantling, with the cellular material is available for recycling. This happens when the cell is old, or when it is defective or defunct or is in wrong place. This is a self regulatory phenomenon in growth, generally controlled by genes like p53 which activates apoptosis to suppress tumor cells (tumor suppressor gene).
- Failure of function of a tumor suppressor gene will cause oncogenesis.

Q. Explain the Gompertzian curve of tumor growth.

Gompertzian curve of tumor growth—generally explains the tumor growth pattern
- The fastest growth happens early and later the same slows down due the cells competing for food and oxygen. The cells grow at an exponential pace until they outpace each other by competing with each other with the result that over 90% of cells die and remaining continue to grow.
- The most rapid growth would be over before the tumor is detected clinically, however early.

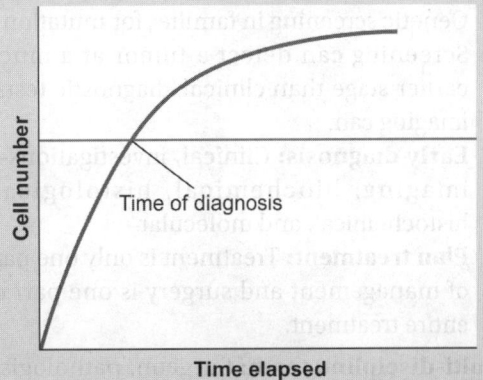

Gompertzian curve of tumor growth

The implications of Gompertzian growth on cancer management
- The tumor is past its rapid growth stage before the physical diagnosis. Tumor is therefore a systemic disease at this stage.
- Tumor cells respond best to chemo and radiotherapy when they grow rapidly.
- The slow growth pattern and multiple mutations in the cells makes it more resistant to therapy—radio or chemo.

The Biological Basis for Early Detection of a Cancer
- Cancer should be killed in early stage and before it spreads.
- The biological investigations aim to detect tumorigenesis at cellular level and some to find changes at molecular level, which helps to detect tumorigenesis and plan cancer prevention.

Inheritance and environment, both are important factors in development of cancer
The role of genes in oncogenesis has made it possible to employ genetic testing and counseling, in the prevention of cancer.

The Management of Cancer
This refers to—prevention, detection, treatment, rehabilitation and palliation.

Prevention
- **Screening:** Easy, inexpensive and harm free tools should be used whenever possible. Genetic screening in families for mutation. Screening can detect a tumor at a much earlier stage than clinical/diagnostic tests/imaging can.
- **Early diagnosis:** Clinical, investigations—imaging, biochemical, histological, histochemical, and molecular.
- **Plan treatment:** Treatment is only one part of management and surgery is one part of entire treatment.

Multi-discipline team: Surgeon, pathologist, diagnostic radiologist, genomic specialist, immunologist, medical oncologist, radiation oncologist, an internist, palliative care specialist and an occupational therapist and can be members of the team to cover all aspects of management and make correct decisions on modality, steps and timing of therapy.

Principles of Cancer Surgery

> Q. Explain the principles and role of surgery in general in management of cancer.

Role of surgery in management of cancer
- **"Ratification of diagnosis":** Diagnosis and staging
  - Staging laparosocopy, e.g., gastric and esophageal cancers, evaluation of malignant ascites
  - Sentinel node biopsy—in cancers of breast and melanoma
  - Orchidectomy—in lymph node tested positive for lymphoma or testicular cancers.
- **Radical surgery:** Curative resection of primary tumour (with area of spread as in a radical gastrectomy)
- **Reductive surgery:** Cytoreductive surgery—debulking of tumor to facilitate non-surgical modalities of cancer therapy by reducing tumor load, e.g., omentectomy and tumor debulking in ovarian cancers before chemotherapy, peritonectomy before hyperthermic intraperitoneal chemotherapy (HIPEC) in pseudomyxoma peritonei)
- **Relief from symptoms:** Palliation of surgical complications of tumor (gastrojejunostomy obstructing gastric cancer or resection of a bleeding intestinal tumor or for pain relief, cholecystoenteric bypass in an inoperable pancreatic cancer).
- **Removal of metastases,** (e.g., resection of metastases in liver or lung in colorectal cancers)
- **Reconstructive surgery,** (e.g., skin graft after wide resection of squamous cell cancers or mandibular reconstruction after wide resection for carcinoma tongue)
- **Restraining against cancer:** Prevention—
  - Resection of premalignant lesions
  - Dysplastic lesions of tongue or colonic polyps
  - Prophylactic mastectomy in patients after testing for BRCA genes.

Chapter 9: Investigation of the Surgical Patient and Basis of Cancer Therapy

Principles of Nonsurgical Treatment of Cancer

- Destroying all the tumor cells is the goal.
- **Dose v/s response:** Optimise the dose of the modality to ensure a response of the patient with least toxicity.
- **Selective toxicity:** Ideally therapy should ensure lethal damage to the tumor, and no damage to normal tissue (not possible fully).
  Optimizing the dose helps in **ensuring selective toxicity** to the tumor with least harm to normal cells.
- **Synergistic effect:** Some modalities or drugs act in a way to enhance the effect of other agents (synergistic effect) - as in a chemoradiation in rectal cancer. Or multidrug regimens in which agents act on different stages of cell cycle.
- **Molecular biology** and pharmacogenomics help understand tumor response better. That opens the scope for designing personalized **(individualised) regimens**.
  - Tumor specific therapy—chemotherapy and biological therapy
  - Patient specific therapy—biological and immunotherapy.
- **Combination therapy:** The combination of different modalities. To enhance effective cancer control, for synergistic benefit and thereby reduce toxicity.

Application of Non-surgical Therapy

- General effects of anti-cancer therapy
- Surgery and radiotherapy—offer loco regional cure or control
- Chemotherapy—systemic and local control.

Intent of Non-surgical Therapy

- Curative radio or chemotherapy.
- Adjuvant to surgery—to prevent local or systemic recurrence—targeting hidden residual or metastatic disease, that is not detected before surgery.
- Neoadjuvant therapy—administered before surgery to facilitate effective surgical clearance; to downstage a tumor and to make a surgical clearance feasible.

Radiotherapy

Q. Explain rationale of radiotherapy in treatment of cancer.

Rationale and principles

- Radiation damages the DNA and kills cells.
- The dose of radiation to inflict lethal damage to a cancer cell is less than that for a normal cell.
- Normal cells tolerate the sublethal damage better than the tumor cells and their DNA can recover from sub lethal damage; tumor DNA can't recover.
- Rapidly dividing cells respond better than slow growing cells or cells at rest.
- Oxygenated cells respond better and hypoxic cells respond poorly.

Ensuring the selective toxicity and evoking best response:

- Define the target for irradiation and planning done for the optimal focused area and minimizing exposure of the normal tissue.
- **Fractional dose of irradiation:**
  - The calculated radiation dose is delivered in multiple smaller fractions that is lethal to cancer and minimal damage to normal cells.
- Remission between the fractions: (Time interval given between fractions)
  - Cell growth cycle is taken into consideration in delivery of radiotherapy.
  - The fractions of radiation dose are withheld to allow the normal cell recovery even as the surviving tumor cells go through cell cycle to the mitotic phase when radiation acts best.

Use of modern digital technology for focused targeting of cancers

Uses

- Delivery of higher radiation doses to cancer tissue
- Delivery of radiation in conformity with any shape and depth of tumor
- Along with avoiding or with minimal damage to normal tissue
- Types of digital techniques in radiotherapy:
  - Intensity-modulated radiation therapy (IMRT)
  - Image-guided radiation therapy (IGRT)
  - Stereotactic ablative radiotherapy (SABR): Small number of fractions in high doses to cure isolated metastases
  - Brachytherapy: Implanting the radioactive source in the tumor.

Combination treatment
Radiotherapy (RT) and chemotherapy (CT) are often given together.

Combination chemotherapy
Helps to reduce probability of development of drug resistance among the tumor cells, (generally acquired by the mutated tumor cells, which lead to expansion of clones of cells resistant to drugs).

Basis of choosing the combination of cytotoxic drugs:
- The drugs should have specific biological actions against different cell functions to get synergistic action to increase their total individual effect on cancer cells.
- All the drugs should be active against the specific tumor.
- The drugs should not have toxicities that are common between them (e.g, two nephrotoxic or cardiotoxic).
- The drugs should be acting at different phases of cell cycle.

Combination CT and RT
- Radiation effect—synergistic with chemotherapy and toxicity too.
- In addition RT can reach areas like brain and testes where drugs may not (e.g., radiation given to brain and meninges—in small cell lung carcinoma, lymphomas.

Q. What is targeted therapy?

Targeted Therapy—Monoclonal Antibodies and PARP Inhibitors

Immunotherapy and Monoclonal Antibodies
- To target the specific tumor antigens and thence kill the cancer cells
- Also in combination with chemotherapy
- As vehicles to deliver the cytotoxic drugs to the specific tumor cells, which are targeted by the monoclonal antibody that is tagged to the chemotherapeutic agent to be delivered to the cancer cell.

Molecular Therapy
Poly (ADP-ribose) polymerase (PARP) inhibitors—a new class of drugs inhibiting the PARP enzyme and promoting tumor cell death. PARP is a a molecular enzyme with a role in cellular growth, regulation and cell DNA repair to allow the cell to recover and hence avoid apoptotic cell death. The same also helps the cancer cells repair themselves and survive. The PARP inhibitor stops the cancer cells being repaired which causes the cells to die and so reduces tumor growth. This is currently used in treatment of carcinoma breast, ovary, prostate pancreas.

Others include:
Tyrosine kinase inhibitors (TKI) that inhibit cancer cell metabolism (e.g., Imatinib and sunitinib against GIST).

CDK 4/6 (cycline dependant kinase) inhibitors—e.g., palbociclib, ribociclib-used against hormone positive breast cancers.

Palliative Therapy: Concept is Changing

The distinction between palliative and curative treatment is blurring due to the development of targeted therapies which control growth of cancer and not eradicate the same.

Palliative treatment, today is not just relief of pain and distressing symptoms, but to make the patient ableto live a near normal life with the cancer, until they die of other reasons, but not of cancer.

So palliation involves symptomatic remedy as well as treating the disease to achieve the same, e.g., palliative radiotherapy for skeletal metastases.

End-of-life Care

- Refers to situations where the death is imminent in a few months.
- Differs from palliative care where patients live for indefinite length of time.
- Involves:
    - Control of troublesome symptoms is one part of end of life care.
    - Counseling the patient and dependents (about bereavement).
    - Help in family bridges and planning of the future of the family with a will or declaration.
    - Spirituality.
    - Passive euthanasia.

Chapter 9: Investigation of the Surgical Patient and Basis of Cancer Therapy

> **SU9.3:** Communicate the results of surgical investigations and counsel the patient appropriately. DOAP session

Principles outlined here:

Steps before Investigations

- Clinical examination followed by discussion with the patient and relatives about the diagnosis, the surgical treatment offered and justification for the same.
- Explain the need for various investigations to confirm the diagnosis, assess the disease state and plan treatment.
- The results of investigations are compiled, in often after discussing with the involved pathologist or radiologist.
- The final treatment plan is drawn after the state of the patient and disease are reassessed, correlating the clinical and investigation reports.

Communication and Counseling of the Patient after Review with Investigation Reports

- Communicate the results to the patient in presence of the relative with whom a preliminary discussion on the reports has been done.
- Disclose the nature of the disease in words that patient can understand sick to words spoken once and don't change them.
- Depending on the knowledge of the patient, the lab reports and imaging reports should be explained with emphasis on the positive aspects of the side the reports to convince the patient of the need for treatment and to boost the latter's morale. For example: Don't say—you have a cancer and it is bad. Say—this report confirms my doubt—there is a "tumor" which could spread if left alone and trouble. Fortunately we have diagnosed it and it can be removed as shown by the reports".

Never demoralize the patient; never give false hopes. Speak the truth.

Pre, Intra and Post-operative Management

10 Chapter

SU10.1	Describe the principles of perioperative management of common surgical procedures.
SU10.2	Describe the steps and obtain informed consent in a simulated environment.
SU10.3	Observe common surgical procedures and assist in minor surgical procedures; observe emergency life-saving surgical procedures.
SU10.4	Perform basic surgical skills such as first aid including suturing and minor surgical procedures in simulated environment.

SU10.2, 10.3 and 10.4 are practical DOAP sessions and are demonstrated in the hospital.

SU10.1: Describe the principles of perioperative management of common surgical procedures.

PERIOPERATIVE MANAGEMENT

- Evaluation
- Care.

Includes: Preoperative, intraoperative and postoperative management.

Goals

- Evaluation of functional status of the patient and identify the medical morbidities.
- Stratification of the risk, for the specified operation.
- Optimisation of the patient's medical condition to minimize the risk and maximize the outcome of surgery.

Preoperative Evaluation

General evaluation of the surgical patient - done for:

- **General and systemic morbidities:** Cardiovascular, pulmonary, renal, metabolic, bleeding disorders, endocrine disorders and others, depending upon patient's history and functional status, urgency and, goal of surgery and its inherent risk.

History and Physical Examination

- Routine diagnostic testing—adds to the clinical diagnosis.
- Complex procedures require detailed lab and imaging tests.
- General risk factors: Advanced age, obesity, diabetes.
- Respiratory system: Chronic obstructive airway disease, asthma, obstructive sleep apnea, smoking, surgical site located near the diaphragm and respiratory functional status.
- Renal disease: Hypertension or diabetes and chronic renal failure—information of the timing and quality of the patient's last dialysis session
- Recording preoperative weight and measuring daily urine output and assess volume status.
- Elevated jugular venous pulsations or lung congestion—hypervolemia.
- Hepatic disorders—history of jaundice, taking hepatotoxic medication, liver diseases.

- Endocrine and metabolic disorders
- Coagulation disorders
- Airway assessment—for anesthesia and post operative management.

Cardiovascular disease: Major cause of death after non-cardiac surgery.

Risk stratification for major adverse cardiac events (MACE) due to major surgery.

> American Heart Association recommended levels: Two risk levels—1. Low-risk (MACE risk <1%) and 2. Elevated risk (MACE risk >1%)

(Includes events - death, Q-wave myocardial infarction and need for revascularization).

Risk factors for perioperative cardiac morbidity and mortality.

Age above 70 years, unstable angina, myocardial infarction within past 6 months, untreated congestive heart failure, valvular heart disease, cardiac arrhythmias, diabetes mellitus, peripheral vascular disease, and functional impairment.

Functional status: Patients with poor functional status have a very high-risk of perioperative cardiac events. It is assessed from a patient's activities of daily living (ADLs)—given in metabolic equivalents (METs). (One MET equals the resting oxygen consumption of an average 40-year-old male). MET grades: excellent (>10 METs), good (7 to 10 METs), moderate (4 to 6 METs), or poor (<4 METs). (Moderate—is classified as the ability to perform usual ADLs.

> **Overall risk** is assessed by cardiac, non-cardiac factors, factors related to the surgical procedure and functional status of the patient.

Risk Factors for Postoperative Acute Renal Failure (ARF)

Major procedures like radical gastrectomy, hepatectomy, AAA repair patient factor:
- High levels of BUN or creatinine
- Intraoperative hypotension, sepsis, CHF, advanced age
- Intravascular volume contraction, and use of nephrotoxic and radionuclide agents.

Preoperative Testing

- **Cardiological tests:** Identification of active cardiac conditions that may require intensive management in emergency and need to delay elective surgeries.
- **Pulmonary disease:**
  - Chest X-ray (CXR) performed for acute symptoms related to pulmonary disease.
  - Arterial blood gas (ABG) a baseline for comparison with postoperative state; cannot predict postoperative pulmonary complications.
  - PFT—pulmonary function testing—if indicated.
- **Renal disease:** Laboratory data. Serum electrolyte and bicarbonate levels.
  - Blood urea nitrogen (BUN) and creatinine.
  - Complete blood cell count (CBC)—anemia or thrombocytopenia.
- Liver function tests
- **Diabetes mellitus:** HbA1c—for glycemic state and control.
  - Blood glucose measured preoperatively and intraoperatively.
  - To prevent unrecognized hyperglycemia or hypoglycemia.

Assessment of risk factors for infectious complications after surgery.

The grading of risk of mortality after surgery are enumerated in **Table 10.1** given below.

Table 10.1: American Society of Anesthesiologists physical status classification system.

ASA grade	Description	30 day mortality (%)
I	Healthy	0.1
II	Mild systemic disease, no functional limitation	0.2–0.4
III	Severe systemic disease, definite functional limitation	1.8–4
IV	Severe systemic disease, constant threat to life	7.8–23
V	Moribund patient unlikely to survive 24 hours with or without operation	9.4–51
E	Emergency operation	

Procedure-specific risk factors:
- **Type of the surgery**—classified as clean, clean-contaminated, contaminated, or dirty, the duration and urgency of the operation (emergency or elective).

Patient-specific risk factors: Age, diabetes, obesity, immunosuppression, malnutrition, pre-existing infection, smoking, and other chronic illness.

Q. Discuss in detail the preoperative prophylaxis and management.

Cardiovascular system—challenges and risks
- Beta blockers—reduce perioperative ischemia and the risk of cardiac death.
- **Patients with recent angioplasty or stenting:** To delay non-cardiac surgery—by at least 6 weeks after coronary angioplasty and placement of bare metal stents
  - They need dual antiplatelet therapy—aspirin 81 mg, and clopidogrel for at least 1 month after stenting for stable ischemic disease and for 12 months after PCI for ACS.
  - The risk of bleeding and thrombosis should be weighed against each other.
- **Patients with pacemakers:** Preoperative—to be on uninhibited mode.
  Intraoperative: Use bipolar diathermy. Internal defibrillators—turned off during surgery.

Pulmonary complications
- Elective operation should be postponed if there is wheezing
- **Pulmonary toilet:** Increasing lung volume by preoperative incentive spirometry.
- **Antibiotics:**
  - Elective operations should be postponed in patients with respiratory infections.
  - Antibiotics—intravenous—used in presence of preoperative infection, emergent surgery in patients, acute pulmonary infections
- **Cessation of smoking:**
- **Bronchodilators:** For obstructive airway disease.

Renal disease

Pre op management
- Timing of dialysis—within 24 hours of the planned operative procedure.
- Intravascular volume status—avoid hypovolemia and volume overload.

- Preventing perioperative renal dysfunction.
- Adequate hydration
- Avoid nephrotoxins—nonsteroidal anti-inflammatory drugs (NSAIDs), aminoglycoside antibiotics, and various anesthetic drugs

Diabetes mellitus
- It is a factor for increased risk of morbidity and mortality.
- Vascular disease is common in diabetics, and silent MI is frequent perioperative death.

Oral hypoglycemic agents should be discontinued the evening before scheduled surgery.

Insulin-dependent diabetics require insulin and glucose preoperatively to prevent ketosis and catabolism. Patients undergoing major surgery should receive one-half of their morning insulin dose and 5% dextrose IV. Subsequent insulin administration—guided by frequent blood glucose.

Infectious complications: At surgical site or in other organ systems.

Q. Write short notes on prophylaxis against surgical site infection.

Prophylaxis of surgical site infection
- **Antimicrobial prophylaxis**—parenteral/non-parenteral
- **Glycemic control**—blood glucose target levels less than 200 mg/dL in all patients.
- **Normothermia**—maintained
- **Oxygenation**
  - Ensure high levels of inspired oxygen (FiO_2) for optimal intra and postoperative tissue oxygenation.
- **Antiseptic prophylaxis**
  - A full bath on the night before the surgery and intraoperative skin preparation using an alcohol based antiseptic.
  - Intraoperative irrigation of deep or subcutaneous tissues with aqueous iodophor solution.
- **Blood transfusion:** Necessary blood products—to prevent/minimize risk of SSI.

Surgery in the elderly

Difference between a patient's chronologic and biologic age is an excellent tool for predicting perioperative morbidity in elderly surgical patients.

Chapter 10: Pre, Intra and Post-operative Management

Assessment
- Screening—as a prognostic tool for early identification of high-risk patients
- Patients aged above 65 years benefit most.
- Shared decision making—multidisciplinary and involving patient's family
- Pre habilitation—preoperative interventions can improve patients' perioperative morbidity and mortality
- Interdisciplinary geriatric co-management

Operative Steps and Postoperative Care

Teamwork (Table 10.2)

Surgery involves a teamwork of anesthesiologists, perioperative nursing team, and surgical technologists, and the support of ancillary services of the hospital.

Preoperative

- Evaluation, discussion with team, review of the condition and optimization as necessary.
- **Surgery:** Identify the patient, examine and mark the site.
- **Anesthesia:** Ensure all requirement for administration of anesthesia, fluids and transfusion.

Positioning

After anesthesia is induced:
- Correcting positioning, make use of gravity in facilitating surgery, strapping the patient to table to avoid falls, padding of all pressure points (elbows, wirsts and heels).
- **Common positions for operations in general surgery**—supine, lithotomy, lateral, and prone jackknife.
- **Supine position:** The positioning of the arms—supinated and abducted facilitates access for the anesthesia team and allows the surgeons to stand closer to the patient.
- **Lithotomy position:** Flexing the hips and knees and abducting the hips—provides exposure of the perineum and abdomen simultaneously.
- Padding the lateral aspect of the knee and legs for preventing injury to the peroneal nerve.
- **Lateral**—is used for operations on the back.
- **Requires**—padding of the hip, shoulder, and axilla.
- **Prone jackknife** position is used for anorectal surgery—but adds difficulty for the anesthesia
- **Extension of the neck**—for facilitating operations on front of neck.
- **Positioning the patient**, is done with provision to change position, e.g., Trendelenburg (head down) or and reverse Trendelenburg positioning and rotation of the bed.
- Diathermy plate—returning electrode—kept away from heart and site of surgery (e.g., thigh for abdominal or neck surgeries).

Preparation

After positioning, the surgical site is prepared.
- Removal hair is done and 10% povidone iodine used for preparing skin.
- Surgical team wears sterile gowns and masks to perform surgeries.
- Each member defines one's role.

Access

Most operations commence by entering or creating a potential space around the target anatomy. Incisions—used as per plan.

Exploration

- "To look down, look around, and then to look Forward".
- Confirm the preoperative diagnosis; to detect unexpected pathology, and look for iatrogenic injury. The decision is taken to proceed with the planned operation and to alter the procedure as per the finding.

Dissection

Sharp dissection or **blunt** dissection—to divide tissue or to separate tissues.

Hemostasis is the control of bleeding. Vessels in capillary beds, arterioles, and venules will retract and stop bleeding on their own.

Table 10.2: Steps of surgical operation.

Preoperative preparation	Preparation
Anesthesia	Access, exploration, dissection and specified procedure
Positioning	Closure

Others need active control:
- Direct pressure—ligation, topical hemostatic agents.
- Energy devices—monopolar or bipolar electrosurgical and ultrasonic devices.

Procedure Proper

Resection or reconstruction or drainage, etc.

Closure

- Hemostasis is obtained.
- Irrigation of site of surgery to confirm hemostasis.
- Reinspect surgical site—for leaks or slipped sutures and staples.
- Surgical drains—if needed.
- Instrument and mop counts taken.

Wound Closure

- Wound dressing.
- Anesthetic recovery and shifting to the postoperative ward.

Postoperative Care

Goal: A good and rapid, safe and least painful recovery from surgery.

The shifting from theater to the postoperative ward is done with details of patient including personal data, details of operation, his preoperative morbidities, allergies, details of fluid, transfusions and along with urine output.

Immediate postoperative observation and treatment:

- Treatment of pain and nausea/vomiting (PONV)
- Monitoring done for level of consciousness and development of complications.

Classification of Postoperative Complications

- Based on time after surgery:
  - Immediate—(within 6 hours of procedure)
  - Early—6-72 hours of surgery
  - Late—after 72 hours of surgery
- Complications specific to system and surgery.

> **Q. Write briefly on how to detect and treat early postoperative respiratory complications.**

Early Detection of Postoperative Respiratory Complications

Assessment of airway patency, respiratory rate and oxygen saturation measurement.

- **Airway obstruction**—treatment: Urgent
  - Upper airway obstruction
  - Caused by laryngospasm, edema, foreign body, vocal cord dysfunction.
  - Action needed: Manual support of the jaw or insertion of an airway.
- **Inadequacy of ventilation**
  - The residual effects of anesthetic gases, opioids and muscle relaxants.
  - Action: Monitoring pulse and respiration and oxygen supplementation.
- **Hypoxemia**
  Causes:
  - Aspiration, bronchospasm, pneumothorax
  - Acute pulmonary edema
  - Acute pulmonary edema.
  Action: Positioning, airway and oxygen, suction of secretions and blood, re-anesthetizing and ventilation.

General Postoperative Complications

- **Hemorrhage:**
  - *Cause:* Coagulation disorder—generalized bleed, arterial or venous source
  - *Aim of treatment:* To stop the bleeding and give supportive treatment—oxygen and fluid; correction of coagulopathy.
- **Wound dehiscence:** Poor healing and dehiscence
- **Drain and wound care** are integral to postoperative care
- **Thrombotic complications**.

> **Q. Write a note on postoperative thrombotic complications.**

- **Thrombophlebitis** - i/v line - local application of heparinoid ointments.
- **Deep venous thrombosis**
  - Anticipated by predisposing high risk factors and nature of surgery.

- Detected by Doppler evaluation and assessed by blood coagulation profiles.

Prophylaxis: Intraoperative or immediate (6 hours) postoperative administration of low molecular weight heparin (enoxaparin or delteparin).

Treatment: Discussed in chapter on venous disorders - heparin - unfracationated or low molecular weight heparin. Thrombolysis, elevation of limb IVC filter.

- **Postoperative pulmonary embolism (PE)**
  - Prophylaxis—early mobilization, intra and postoperative graded muscle pumps.
  - Low molecular weight heparin.

Diagnosis:
  - Suspected in presence of—unexplained dyspnea, hypoxia, tachycardia, or dysrhythmia.
  - ECG, D-dimer, chest radiography and CT scan.
  - Pulmonary angiography.

Treatment:
  - Oxygen, monitoring and support.
  - Thrombolysis—if there is collapse of lung.
  - Anti coagulation and long term, anti coagulation
  - Inferior vena cava filter.

Systemic Complications in Postoperative Period

Pulmonary complications (after recovery)
- Fever, cough, dyspnea, bronchospasm, hypercapnia
- Atelectasis, pneumonia, pleural effusion, pneumothorax and respiratory failure.

Cardiovascular complications
- Hypertension
- Arrhythmias—preventable by proper preoperative and intraoperative care of electrolyte imbalance and hypotension.
- Myocardial ischemia/infarction.

Neurologic complications
Stroke: Will need management with the help of cardiologists and neurologists.
- Surgical stress causes drowsiness, delirium, seizures, stroke.

Urinary and renal complications
- Retention of urine
- Oliguria
- Urinary infection.

Acute renal failure (acute kidney injury)
Diagnosed by
- A low urine output to less than 0.5 mL/kg/h for more than 6 hours
- A rise in serum creatinine of over 26 μmol/L within 48 hours
- Glomerular filtration rate—falls by over 25% in past 7 days (predisposing causes are discussed in the previous section of preoperative care).

Causes
- Intraoperative—hypotension, hypovolemia
- Nephrotoxic drugs—aminoglycosides, NSAIDs, diuretics
- Sepsis
- Myoglobinuria surgery involving renal vessels
- Postrenal—ureteric injury, blocked urethral catheter.

Gastrointestinal complications
- Postoperative nausea and vomiting—drugs, anesthetic agents, metabolic causes like acidosis.
- Postoperative paralytic ileus—surgical trauma, spinal anesthesia, metabolic, sepsis.

Endocrine
- SIADH: Syndrome of inappropriate secretion of ADH from posterior pituitary.
- Hypothyroidism.

Infective complications
Postoperative fever—infection suspected.

Causes: Iatrogenic—IV line, infusion, transfusions, urinary catheters.

Respiratory infections
- Early postoperative—atelectasis
- After 72 hours postoperative—pneumonia, lung abscess, effusion.

Surgical site infection (SSI):
- Needs prophylactic antibiotics in high-risk (refer preoperative care)
- Treated by: Intravenous aggressive antibiotics, draining any collections, opening of the wound and wound dressings.

Intra abdominal and urogenital infections

Fungal infections

Anesthesia and Pain Relief, Day Care Surgery and Safe General Surgery

Chapter 11

SU11.1	Describe principles of preoperative assessment, integrated with anesthesiology.
SU11.2	Enumerate the principles of general, regional, and local anesthesia.
SU11.3	Demonstrate maintenance of an airway in a mannequin or equivalent. DOAP session skill assessment.
SU11.4	Describe principles of providing post-operative pain relief and management of chronic pain.
SU11.5	Enumerate the indications and principles of day care general surgery.
SU11.6	Describe principles of safe general surgery.

Anesthesia and Pain Relief

SU11.1: Describe principles of preoperative assessment.

Q. Describe principles of preoperative assessment. (Long answer question).

Goals of Preoperative Medical Assessment
- To reduce the patient's surgical and anesthetic perioperative morbidity or mortality
- To return him to desirable functioning as quickly as possible.

History and Physical Examination
- With a focus on risk factors for cardiac and pulmonary complications determination of the patient's functional capacity.
- **Laboratory tests and investigations:** When indicated by the patient's medical status, proposed procedure and drug therapy.

Primary Goals of Preoperative Evaluation and Preparation
- Documentation of the indication for surgery, assessment of patient's physical state of health, risk factors for perioperative complications control of comorbidities.
- Discuss the information with the patient about surgery, anesthesia, intraoperative care and postoperative pain (helps reduce the anxiety and facilitates recovery).
- Plans for better patient satisfaction through shorter hospital stay and reduced costs.

Investigations
Complete Blood Counts
- Tests for bleeding diathesis—bleeding and clotting time, APTT, INR and prothrombin time.
- Blood sugar and HbA1c—in diabetics.

Chapter 11: Anesthesia and Pain Relief, Day Care Surgery and Safe General Surgery

- Chest X-ray—patients with pulmonary disease and heart ailments.
- ECG and cardio evaluation—as needed.

Generally, drugs are continued up to and including the morning of operation, with dose adjustments if needed—like insulin or metoprolol.

Some drugs are stopped preoperatively, e,g., the monoamine oxidase inhibitors—2–3 weeks pre-op oral contraceptive pill—6 weeks pre op. (risk of venous thromboembolism).

Aspirin and clopidogrel stopped 7–10 days pre-op and oral anticoagulants—4–5 days pre-op (ensuring INR of level of 1.5).

Perioperative Risk Assessment

Factors Contributing to Perioperative Risk

- Preoperative medical condition of the patient
- The gravity of the proposed surgical procedure
- The type of anesthetic administered.

> **Q. The American Society of Anesthesiologists (ASA) physical status classification.**

The American Society of Anesthesiologists (ASA) physical status classification

ASA 1 - A normal healthy patient
ASA 2 - A patient with mild systemic disease
ASA 3 - A patient with severe systemic disease
ASA 4 - A patient with severe systemic disease that is a constant threat to life
ASA 5 - A moribund patient who is not expected to survive without the operation
ASA 6 - A declared brain dead - organs being removed for donation purpose
E   - An emergency operation.

- Evaluation of cardiovascular, respiratory, neurological and risk, bleeding diathesis
- Pre operative management in patients on anticoagulants (discussed in chapter on preoperative management).

Patients Receiving Oral Anticoagulants (Vitamin K Antagonists)

- Ensure an INR of below 1.5 prior to neuraxial (spinal or epidural) block or surgery.
- For emergency surgery—fresh frozen plasma, vitamin K, or prothrombin complex concentrate

- Elective procedure, anticoagulant therapy must be stopped 4–5 days prior to the surgery and Vit K1 administered 10 mg menadione i/v daily for 3 to 4 doses.

> **SU11.2:** Enumerate the principles of general, regional and local anesthesia.
>
> **SU11.3:** Demonstrate maintenance of an airway in a mannequin or equivalent principles. This is included in Competency SU11.2.
>
> Note: Summary given at the bottom.

Role of Anesthetist—One of a 'Perioperative Physician'

- To optimise the patient for surgery,
- To evaluate and minimize the risk, during surgery
- Post operative care—regarding pain management and restoration of normal function.

Preparation for Anesthesia

Should involve close teamwork between surgeon, anesthetist and other care providers in perioperative care, safety checklists and risk assessments.

Anesthesia may be general, neuraxial, spinal or epidural and loco regional.

General Anesthesia

It has three phases (the triad of general anesthesia)—unconsciousness (loss of awareness), analgesia and muscle relaxation.

Induction of General Anesthesia

> **Q. Enlist the drugs used for induction of anesthesia; note on rapid sequence induction.**

Intravenous Drugs

- Propofol—most frequently, can be used for maintenance of anesthesia (as in TIVA).
- Thiopentone—widely used before propofol.
- Etomidate and ketamine, etomidate derivatives and fospropofol.

Inhalation Agents for Inductions

- Non-pungent sevoflurane
- In children, non-cooperative adults; patients with anticipated difficult airway.

Rapid Sequence Induction (RSI)

- An intravenous anesthetic agent together with rapidly acting muscle relaxant is used
- Suxamethonium (depolarizing) or Rocuronium (non-depolarizing)
- It is a useful technique to secure a rapid access to the airway—(1) when a high risk of aspiration is anticipated and (2) in case of delayed gastric emptying.
- Also used in a patient with delayed gastric emptying.

Q. Write a short notes on total intravenous anesthesia.

Total intravenous anesthesia (TIVA)

- *Induction of anesthesia:* Propofol and the ultra-short acting opioid remifentanil.
- *Maintenance of anesthesia:*
  - Continuous infusion of intravenous agent (propofol)
  - Inhalation agents: Isoflurane, sevoflurane or desflurane
- *Advantages of these drugs:*
  - No cumulative effect
  - Better hemodynamic stability
  - Excellent recovery profile
- *Uses of TIVA*
  - Anesthesia for day-case surgery, neurosurgery
  - During cardiopulmonary bypass and laryngotracheal laser surgery

Management of Airway During Anesthesia

General anesthesia and muscle relaxants cause loss of muscle tone making the patient unable to keep airway open and breath. This mandates mechanical (artificial) ventilation.

Maneuvers

To ensure patency of airway during mask ventilation. These include: Head tilt, chin lift and jaw thrust maneuvers along with oropharyngeal airways, to facilitate bag mask ventilation.

Endotracheal tube—inserted into the trachea to allow breathing (unless muscle relaxants given).

Endotracheal tube with cuff: Allows positive pressure ventilation and prevents aspiration of gastric contents.

Complications of Intubation

- Injury to oral pharyngeal and laryngeal anatomy including vocal cords
- Aspiration of gastric contents
- Accidental esophageal or bronchial intubation
- Inability (failure) to intubate
- Kinking of tube and blockage
- Disconnection and disruption
- Tracheal injuries—immediate (tear) and late (stenosis).

Supraglottic Airways

Laryngeal mask airway (LMA): A supraglottic airway inserted orally to get a snug fit around the larynx. It has an inflatable cuff-fits against the laryngeal aperture and avoids intubation.

- Less traumatic to a patient's airway than endotracheal intubation technique.
- Easy to learn the technique and useful in emergency airway management.

Various Modifications are available

- "I-gel" silicon gel flexible laryngeal mask—has a built in passage for esophageal suction.
- Intubating LMA (ILMA)—allows a blind technique in aiding insertion of a tracheal tube in difficult emergency situations.

Situation of Difficult Intubation

- Difficult or impossible; if compounded by inability to ventilate the patient by bag-mask
- Can lead to catastrophic hypoxia.
  Fiberoptic intubating bronchoscope with topical local anesthetic or under general anesthesia.
- It allows insertion of the endotracheal tube into the trachea under bronchoscopic vision by threading the tube over the bronchoscope.

Double lumen tubes and endobronchial tubes:

- For selective collapse of lung and single lung ventilation, while ventilating the other for ease of surgery
- Used in surgery of the lungs—lobectomy, bronchopleural fistula, thoracoscopic procedures and esophageal surgeries.

Ventilating bronchoscopes and endobronchial catheters: To maintain oxygenation during laryngotracheal surgery.

> Q. Write brief notes on muscle relaxants in general anesthesia. (Short notes)

Muscle Relaxation and Artificial Ventilation
- To facilitate easy surgical access.
- Neuromuscular blocking agents are used for muscle relaxation.

Classification
- **Depolarizing:** It acts by binding to the nicotinic cholinergic receptors, causing opening of the cation channel leading to depolarization and rapid relaxation of muscles, e.g., succinylcholine and suxamethonium.
    - **Advantage:** Quick onset and short duration of action, useful for rapid endotracheal intubation
    - **Adverse effects:** Muscle pain, hyperkalemia, bradycardia, hyperthermia.
- **Non-depolarizing muscle relaxants:** These act by competitive blockade of postsynaptic receptors at the neuromuscular junction with prolonged and predictable duration of action. They need reversal of their action by administration of neostigmine after the procedure.

    Example:
    - Aminosteroid group—pancuronium, vecuronium and rocuronium.
    - Benzylisoquinoline group—atracurium, cisatracurium and mivacurium.

    Rocuronium is an alternative to suxamethonium in a "rapid sequence" induction and its neuromuscular blocking action is selectively reversed by Sugammadex.

Ventilation during Anesthesia
Indication for mechanical ventilation:
- When the patient's spontaneous breathing is inadequate.
- When patient is under muscle relaxants or anesthetic medications.

Types
Pressure Control Ventilation
- The ventilator delivers gas at a particular preset pressure.
- Disadvantage: The actual tidal volume delivered is variable and depends on airway resistance.

Volume Control Ventilation
- The ventilator delivers a preset volume—irrespective of the airway pressure.
- Disadvantage: Can generate high pressure and cause barotrauma to the lungs, pneumothorax.

Positive end expiratory pressure (PEEP): This helps maintaining the functional residual capacity (FRC) and opens collapses alveoli to avoid lung collapse; it also ensures gas exchange and prevents vascular shunting and hence improves lung perfusion.

Intermittent Positive Pressure Ventilation
Combines positive attributes of all the above to negate the disadvantages of the respective modes.

Intra-anesthetic Monitoring
- General—temperature, ventilation parameters and urine output and central venous pressure if needed.
- Cardiovascular—blood pressure, ECG
- Respiratory:
    - Ventilation—pulse oximetry
    - FiO_2—inspired oxygen concentration
    - End tidal carbon dioxide concentration.

Regional Anesthesia
- Central neuraxial
- Peripheral nerve or plexus blocks.

Advantages
Safer in patients unfit for general anesthesia:
- Those with severe cardiopulmonary disease.
- Pelvic surgery and obstetric practice.
- Reduces the need for analgesia.
- Local anesthetic drugs are used:
    - As sole agents for anesthesia or as supplements to general anesthesia.
- Available techniques include:

> **Local and regional anesthesia: Techniques**
> - Topical anesthesia
> - Local infiltration
> - Regional nerve blocks
> - Central neuraxial blocks (spinal and epidural anesthesia

Topical Anesthesia

Application of local anesthetic agents to block nerve endings:
- Lignocaine—2%, 4% gel, 10% solution
- Gel—e.g., for venepuncture
- Spray—for endoscopy and intubation
- Gargle—for oropharyngeal biopsy or drainage of small abscess

Field block - a field is of anesthesia procured by blocking nerve endings by infiltration of an anesthetic drug.

Agents Used
- Lignocaine—maximum dose 3 mg/kg. (7 mg/kg with adrenaline)-short acting.
- Bupivacaine— max. dose 2 mg/kg - long acting, more cardiotoxic, never be used intravenously.
- Levobupivacaine 2 mg/kg—less cardiotoxic.
- Ropivacaine 3-4 mg/kg—less cardiotoxic,
- Prilocaine 6 mg/kg (9 mg/kg with adrenaline) —least systemic toxicity.

Complications of local anesthesia: Anaphylaxis, cardiac arrhythmia, cardiac arrest or convulsions, depressed consciousness.

Nerve blocks—for anesthesia in a defined area:
- Needs perfect knowledge of the sensory nerve supply and local anatomy
- Stimulators are used in localising nerves.
- Sonographic guided regional anesthesia helps to visualize the nerves, e.g., axillary brachial plexus block or wrist blocks for upper limb surgery, interscalene block for shoulder surgery and ankle blocks for surgical procedures of foot.

Complications of nerve blocks:
- General (systemic)—overdose or accidental intravascular injection
- Local—infection or hematoma, thrombophlebitis, nerve damage.

Intravenous Regional Anesthesia (Bier's Block)
- For short surgery of the upper limb (e.g. carpal tunnel release), open reduction of fractures.
- A double tourniquet is applied to the limb to prevent systemic entry of the drug.

A short acting agent is injected intravenously to anesthetize the limb, after exsanguination of the limb using an Esmarch bandage and inflation of proximal cuff of the double tourniquet. It is kept left inflated for 20 minutes to allow binding of the local anesthetic to tissues to prevent systemic entry of the drug.

Agents used: Prilocaine and lignocaine.
Bupivacaine— never used for risk of cardiac toxicity.

Spinal Anesthesia
- Used extensively for lower limb, obstetric and pelvic surgery.
- Spinal anesthesia alone or combined spinal and general anesthesia or sedation
- Injection of a 'single shot' local anesthetic agent intrathecally for a rapid block.
- Addition of an opioid—for postoperative analgesia.
- Drugs used:
  - Bupivacaine 0.5% hyperbaric.
  - Lignocaine 5% (less often used).

Q. What are the complications of spinal anesthesia.

Complications
- Hypotension—due to sympathetic blockade
- "Total spinal"—due to flow of drug to medullary level and respiratory arrest
- Spinal headache—a low pressure headache due to a leak from needle hole in dura
- Cardiac arrest—in hypovolemic patients
- Respiratory depression when used with addition of opioids.

Q. Short note on epidural anesthesia.

Epidural Anesthesia

Injection of anesthetic agent—isobaric bupivacaine 0.5% in epidural space (alone or with—fentanyl)
- For surgery: Repeated "shots: or infusion
- For postoperative analgesia
  - Continuous infusion of diluted dose
  - Patient controlled analgesia (PCA)
- Slower in onset than spinal

Chapter 11: Anesthesia and Pain Relief, Day Care Surgery and Safe General Surgery

- Prolonged analgesia
- Hypotension from sympathetic blockade is amenable for better control.

Used
- For pelvic, abdominal and thoracic procedures
- Postoperative analgesia.

Precautions
- Avoided in bleeding disorders
- Anticoagulants (warfarin) and antiplatelet drugs (aspirin and clopidogrel) must be stopped 5–7 days before the procedure and coagulopathy corrected
- The epidural catheter should be removed only after 12 hours from the last dose of heparin.

Complications
- Accidental spinal injection of large volume of local anesthetics
- Nerve damage, spinal injuries
- Risk of infection and epidural hematoma.

SU11.4: Describe principles of providing postoperative pain relief and management of chronic pain.

- World Health Organization has recognized pain relief as a human right.
- Poorly managed postoperative pain can lead to complications and prolonged rehabilitation
- Traditional postoperative analgesia is opioid based.
- Pain needs to be quantified to be treated effectively. A simple pain scoring with a 10-point pain assessment scale is practiced, (1 is no pain and 10 is the most unbearable pain).

Q. Short note on intravenous patient-controlled analgesia.

Efficacious alternative to conventional systemic analgesia in managing postoperative pain. Patient-controlled analgesia (PCA) allows infusion of the drug through a pump.

Drugs: Morphine, hydromorphone, and fentanyl through the PCA pump.
Requires special equipment and patient gets control over the need for medication used.
But patient and staff require training for proper use and for safety concern.

Management
A multimodal approach to analgesia is given in **Table 11.1**.

Q. Summary: Principles of management postoperative pain. (Long question) (Must know)

The goal for postoperative pain management
- To reduce or eliminate and discomfort and pain with least of side effects.
- Perception of pain varies widely among patients—many combinations in the treatment of pain.
- A multimodal approach helps reduce opioid dose as described in **Table 11.1** given above.

Table 11.1: Multimodality pain management.

A typical illustration of multimodality pain management

Preoperative (pre-emptive)	Postoperative
• Paracetamol 1,000 mg IV in preop • Ketorolac 800 mg IV in preop **Intraoperative** • liposomal bupivacaine—266 mg (long acting—wound infiltration).	• Paracetamol 1,000 mg IV every 6 hours until starting oral paracetamol • NSAID: Diclofenac 75 mg or Ibuprofen 400 to 800 IV—oral later • Patient controlled analgesia (PCA): Morphine for severe pain (scale 6–10)—before starting oral feeds • Tab. Oxycodone 10 mg per oral every 4 hours for moderate pain.

Assessment and preoperative preparation: Involves evaluation and preparation to adjust medications—pain history, physical exam and a pain control plan.

Pre-emptive analgesia: Preoperative initiation of analgesia as part of a multimodal pain management plan. To reduce postoperative pain or analgesic requirements.
Involves—local wound infiltration, epidural or systemic administration prior to surgical incision.

Treatment of postoperative pain
- Agents: Opioid—morphine, oxymorphone, fentanyl. Non-opioid—NSAID, paracetamol.
- Routes: Oral, intravenous, neuraxial, regional
- Modes (patient controlled vs. "as needed").

Modes of postoperative analgesia

Opioid analgesia: Opioids are still the mainstay of postoperative pain.
- Opioids bind to receptors—(peripheral and CNS) and modulate the effect of the nociceptors.
- Administration: Parenteral—IV or IM, neuraxial, oral, transdermal, and rectal routes.
- Agents: Morphine, hydromorphone, and fentanyl.

Intravenous patient-controlled analgesia: Efficacious alternative to conventional systemic analgesia in managing postoperative pain. Patient-controlled analgesia (PCA) allows infusion of the drug through a pump.
Drugs: Morphine, hydromorphone, and fentanyl through the PCA pump.

Epidural and spinal analgesia
- Act as neuraxial regional blocks.
- Used extensively in thoracic, abdominal, and pelvic surgery. Best used in 72 hours post-op.

Epidural analgesia: A catheter inserted into the epidural space in the thoracic or lumbar spine and continuous infusion of local anesthetic agent along with opioids.
Continuous epidural analgesia (CEA): Through a patient controlled epidural pump—lowers the dose requirements for each individual drug.

Nonopioid analgesia: Important component strategy for postoperative pain management.
Nonsteroidal anti-inflammatory agents (NSAIDs)
- Useful in mild to moderate levels of pain.
- Act by evoking anti-inflammatory response by blocking the production of prostaglandins through inhibition of the enzyme cyclooxygenase (COX). They pose a risk of bleeding.

Ketorolac: Injectable NSAID—predominantly COX-1 inhibitor—used as pre-emptive analgesia. Acetaminophen (parcetamol) is a centrally acting analgesic, but lacks peripheral anti-inflammatory effects (Precaution: Maximum daily dose 4000 mg—to avoid hepatotoxicity).

Peripheral nerve blocks: Drug—liposomal bupivacaine 266 mg: Analgesia for up to 72 hours. The transversus abdominis plane (TAP) block for anesthesia of the abdominal wall.

Obese patients: Avoid parenteral opioids due to higher risk of sleep apnea and respiratory depression. Epidural analgesia: Patient-controlled analgesia.

Postoperative pain management in chronic pain patients is challenging.
Their requirement of analgesia is considerably higher.

Management: A multimodal approach to analgesia—regional, local infiltration, and nonopioid systemic analgesia. Opioids—given through transdermal route (fentanyl patch) or PCA pump.

MANAGEMENT OF CHRONIC PAIN

Q. What is chronic pain? Detail the approach and steps in chronic pain management.

Chronic Persistent Pain: Refers to Pain of More than 3 Months' Duration

- **Nociceptive pain:** Activation of pain receptors in skin (cutaneous nociceptors)
  Mechanism: Prolonged ischemia or inflammation causes sensitization of nociceptors and increased transmission in the central nervous system due to exaggerated responses in the dorsal horn of the spinal cord, leading to hypersensitivity and hyperalgesia (allodynia).
- **Neuropathic (or neurogenic) pain**—due to dysfunction in peripheral or central nerves.
  - It may be 'burning', 'shooting' or 'stabbing' type and associated with allodynia, numbness and diminished thermal sensation.
  - It is poorly responsive to opioids.
  Example, trigeminal neuralgia, post-therapeutic and diabetic neuropathy.
  Treatment: Monoaminergic, tricyclic inhibitors and anticonvulsant drugs.

- **Psychogenic pain** is associated with depressive illness; chronic pain and the illness may exacerbate each other.

Surgical patients require treatment of chronic pain from benign or malignant disease.

Acute pain after surgery may progress to chronic pain.

Control of Pain in Benign Disease

Example, postoperative neuropathic pain: Nerve injury and sympathetic dystrophy, chronic inflammatory disease, recurrent infection, degenerative bone or joint disease, phantom limb pain.

- **Local treatment**
  - Local infiltration of local anesthetic and steroids o reduce muscle spasm.
  - Transcutaneous nerve stimulation (TNS)—endorphin mediated analgesia.
  - Nerve decompression.
  - Nerve blocks with alcohol.
- **Drugs (pharmacotherapy)**
  - Paracetamol and NSAIDs. The tricyclic antidepressant drugs.
  - Anticonvulsant agents—for the pain of nerve injury.
  - Pregabalin and gabapentin—reduce spontaneous neuronal activity.
  - Opioid analgesic drugs—oral/transcutaneous patches of fentanyl/morphine, tapentadol
  - Combinations of drugs—can offer minimal side effects.
- **Treatment of pain due to sympathetic hyperactivity:** There is vasoconstriction and abnormal nociception leading to hyperalgesia, allodynia and trophic changes (causalgia).

Management

Multimodal management:
- **Antineuropathic pain drugs:** Pregabalin, gabapentin, amitriptyline.
- Targeted physiotherapy
- Psychological support and counseling.
- **Sympathetic blocks:** Example, stellate ganglion blocks or chemical lumbar sympathectomy by local anesthetic for relief of rest pain in ischemic pain of limbs.

Pain Control in Malignant Disease (Advanced Stages of Cancer)

Principle of Treatment

To encourage the patient to ignore pain and live an active life (with pain)
- **"Step ladder" approach to pain (WHO recommendation)**
  - **Step I: Non-opioids: Analgesics**—Aspirin, paracetamol, NSAIDs, tricyclic antidepressants or anticonvulsants like pregabaline.
  - **Step II: Intermediate strength opioids**—codeine, tramadol
  - **Step III: Strong opioids**—morphine
- **Oral opiate analgesia** is necessary when the non-opioids fail. Fear of addiction to opiates is ignored in cancer.

Oral morphine: Dose should be titrated by giving the drug every 4 hours for a period. Then the daily dose can be divided into two and given through morphine slow release tablets.

- **Infusion of subcutaneous, intravenous, intrathecal or epidural opiate drugs**
  - If a patient is unable to take oral drugs.
  - Usually reserved for acute crises, such as pathological fractures.
- **Ablative (neurolytic) techniques in cancer pain**—used only if the life expectancy is limited.
  - Subcostal phenol injection for a rib metastasis.
  - Coeliac plexus block (alcohol) for pain of pancreatic, gastric or hepatic cancer.
  - Intrathecal neurolytic injection of hyperbaric phenol.
  - Percutaneous anterolateral cordotomy—divides the spinothalamic ascending pain pathway (selective elimination of pain and temperature sensation in a specific area)
  - Antipituitary hormone drugs: Tamoxifen and cyproterone, enables effective pharmacological—therapy for the pain of widespread metastases.
- **Palliative radiotherapy:** Relief of pain in metastatic disease.
- **Adjuvant drugs**
  - Anticonvulsants, tricyclic antidepressants
  - Corticosteroids—against cerebral edema.

Day Care Surgery

> **SU11.5:** Enumerate the indications and principles of day care general surgery.

Conventional surgery involved admission of a patient to a hospital, preparation and performance of operation and postoperative care before discharging the patient.

> **Q. What is day care surgery? What are the contraindications for day care surgery?**

Definition of Day Care Surgery

- **Day surgery**—as the admission and discharge of a patient for a surgical procedure within the 12-hour working day.
- Patient requiring overnight stay—23-hour admission with early morning discharge
- Outpatient surgery—surgery without admission to hospital.
- Short-stay surgery—admission of up to 72 hours
- Procedure room surgery—surgery not requiring full sterile theater facilities.(e.g., drainage of paronychia or small abscess.

Significant Benefits for Both Patient and Healthcare Providers

- Avoiding overnight stay helps—patient's family commitments avoiding disruption of work.
- Saves cost to both patient and hospital. Considerable time, man days, hospital resources.
- Partly sets off the shortage of hospital beds to handle increasing demand for surgical beds.
- Day surgery extends from first patient contact to final discharge.
- Unplanned overnight admissions are minimised:
- This requires ensuring performance of all steps carefully;
  - Surgery should be achievable on day care basis (e.g., rectal resection can't be done)
  - The patient is fit for day care surgery—so as to avoid post operative problems
  - Patient should be fully informed of the concept, and its limitations; The patient should be willing.

Types of Day Care Surgery

> **Q. Describe types of day care surgery. (Short answer)**

- **Office-based care**
  - Example, diagnostic interventions: Biopsy—open or endoscopic biopsy
  - Minor surgeries: Simple excisions of cysts, nails etc.
  - Limitations: Only procedures under local anesthesia. General anesthesia needs additional set up and staff.
- **"Stand alone"—peripheral centers for day surgery**
  - Must be within 30 km of a major parent unit with access to tackle any need for unplanned overnight stay or any complication.
  - Day care surgery performed in isolated or remote centres are usually under local or regional anesthesia or relatively minor cases under general anesthesia.
- **Integrated day surgery centers**
  - Independent unit within a major full fledged hospital facility.
  - A complete unit of reception, ward, theater and recovery areas.
  - But essentially part of a major hospital with flexibility to shift the patient to the major unit in case of emergencies.
  - They can undertake of day surgery of far higher level major cases.
- **Integrated day and short-stay surgery centers**
  - Flexibility in the day and short-stay surgery.
  - Advantages: Can consider more complex cases and patients with lower levels of fitness.
  - Requirements:
    - Dedicated day surgery facilities.
    - Dedicated day ward facility, to focus on the timely recovery and discharge of the patient.

Q. How do you select patients for day care surgery?

Selection of Patients for Day Care Surgery
Surgical Criteria
- **Surgical:** Operations up to 2 hours only are considered, (e.g., appendectomy, hernia repairs, anal fistula surgery, laparoscopic cholecystectomy.
  - Should be able to drink and eat in early post-op period timescale.
  - Should be able to ensure suitable control of pain and be fit for discharge.
- **Medical criteria**
  - Age: No specific age criteria, but functional state of the patient is considered.

  Comorbidities:
  - American Society of Anesthesiologists (ASA) physical status—grade GR II.
  - ASA Gr III—only in "integrated units within a hospital".
  - Diabetes—good control is a must.
  - Epilepsy—should be under control.
  - Obesity—usually those with BMI below 38 are chosen.
  - Bleeding disorders: Avoided (but are not absolutely contraindicated).
  - Patients on anticoagulants: Aspirin and clopidogrel—stopped 5-7 days before surgery Warfarin—stopped 5-6 days before surgery—after evaluation risk of thrombosis (risk of thrombosis v/s bleeding).
- **Patient criteria**
  - Patient should have a well informed and reliable caretaker—for at least 24 hours or more
  - In case of elderly—for longer—to watch for hypotension and risk of internal bleeding.
  - Patient's home should be within an hour's reach of a hospital facility and be accessible for any emergency.
  - Communication with hospital is essential.

Preoperative Assessment and Preparation
- Done by—anesthetist, a specialist nursing team and surgeon, if needed a physician.
- Measurement of blood pressure BMI.
- Past medical history with current medication.
- The comorbidities are optimized after selection of patients.
- An assessment of risk of venous thromboembolism and thromboprophylaxis.

Information and education of the patient and his attendant on day care surgery and consent for admission, operation and discharge and need for shifting to major center if needed.

Perioperative Management
Timing of Surgery
- Major procedures, under general anesthesia are done in early hours of morning to facilitate maximum recovery before evening.
- Operations posted in the afternoon are performed under spinal or regional anesthesia.
- This will reduce the need for overnight admissions.
- Mixed lists have day care cases in morning and inpatient surgeries later.

Anesthesia and Analgesia
Multimodal anesthesia: Optimal dosages of anesthetic agent.
- Preoperative—paracetamol and NSAID.
- Operative: General anesthesia—with sevoflurane or isoflurane.
  - Total intravenous anesthesia (TIVA) techniques using propofol.
  - Opioids—minimal use to reduce PONV.
- Local anesthetic injection into wound—bupivacaine into the wound.

Postoperative Complications
- Same as in inpatient surgery.
- Requires proactive monitoring in the immediate postoperative period.

Surgical Hemorrhage
- **Reactionary:** Occurs 4-6 hours after surgery and is caused by ligature slippage, clot displacement or cessation of vasospasm after mobilisation or coughing.
- **Secondary:** Occurs due to infection eroding a vessel.

These patients require a high index of suspicion and monitoring: Slow recovery, severe abdominal pain.

Elective Day Surgery
- Requires close supervision. Patient should be admitted overnight if there is risk of postoperative hemorrhage after reaching home.
- Postoperative monitoring of vital signs—to alert the recovery team to any underlying bleed.
- Secondary hemorrhage presents several days later, caused by postoperative infection.

Postoperative Nausea and Vomiting (PONV)
IV fluids for hydration antiemetic, e.g. ondansetron, dexamethasone.

Procedures recommended: The procedures mentioned may vary from place to place.
- Varicose vein surgery
- Anal surgery, e.g., hemorrhoidectomy, fistula
- Inguinal/femoral herniae, hydrocoele/varicocoele, circumcision
- Laparoscopic cholecystectomy, appendectomy, fundoplication
- **Breast:** Excision/biopsy breast lesion, sentinel node excision
- Laser prostatectomy, orchidectomy, epididymectomy
- Orthopedics: Dupuytren's fasciectomy, carpal tunnel release
- Arthroscopic surgery—knee or shoulder.

Emergency Day Surgery
Minor cases—drainage of abscesses.

Absolute Contraindications
- Major comorbidities
- Systemic sepsis, unstable diabetes
- If postoperative parenteral analgesia is required.

Discharge-After Assessment of Fitness for Discharge
Advice: Analgesics—paracetamol, NSAIDs (codeine in the western countries).

Discharge Criteria Followed
- Stable vital signs—for at least 1 hour.
- Minimal nausea, vomiting.
- Patient is conscious and well oriented.
- Absence of significant bleeding or wound drainage.
- Adequate pain control with oral analgesia and patient knows how to use the analgesics.
- Able to walk, dress and converse.
- Tolerates oral intake before discharge.
- Has passed urine (if appropriate).
- Has a responsible adult to take them home and to take care.
- Fully instructed (written) about postoperative care and follow up visit.
- Emergency contact number supplied.

Safe General Surgery

SU11.6: Describe principles of safe general surgery.

It is estimated that about 40-45% of medical errors (half of them preventable), occur in the operating theatre.

Safe Surgery concerns—paying the best attention to the problem of patient safety.

The same involves:
- Development of global standards and protocols
- Evolve excellence in patient safety
- Enforcement of evidence-based policies
- Encouragement of research
- Provision of assistance to all countries in necessary areas
- **Medication without harm**
  - Patients and health care professionals, should ensure safety of medication
  - Past errors should guide to prevent future errors by infusing safety into the system.

Definitions
- **Safety:** Freedom from inflicting unintended injury
- **Error: Mistakes**
  - Error of execution—failure to enact a planned action
  - Error of planning—enacting a wrong step to achieve goal of surgery.
  - Error of commission—the wrong step/action.(e.g., cutting the wrong structure)
  - Error of omission—the right step left out (e.g., not keeping a drain after draining an abscess when it should have been).
- **Adverse event:** Harm induced by any intervention—medical or surgical.

Importance of safe surgery: Surgical care is a major part of healthcare. Surgical interventions are increasing in all fields of surgery and calls for the need for safe surgery.

The goal of surgical operation is to save life and alleviate suffering. But, unsafe surgical practice leads to harm, often irreversible.

Half of the complications due to surgery and anesthesia *are preventable.*

How to Achieve Safety
- **Organizational culture**
  - **Systems approach:** Focus on safeguards and barriers to prevent adverse events due to human error.
  - **Avoiding active failures:** Unsafe acts committed by people in direct contact with the patient or system (e.g., mistakes, violations of protocols, etc.)
  - **Correcting latent deficiencies of system:** Example, inexperience, lack of manpower, unavailability of equipment, etc.
  - **Human factors engineering:** Morale boosting of errant staff and correction of mistakes through peer review and audit.
- **Reporting systems:** Collect, review, and learn on safety from adverse events in care.
  - Near misses should also be reported (where an error occurs but escapes causing an adverse event).
- **Patient safety processes**
  - **Root cause analyses (RCAs):** A multi-disciplinary team to develop and implement strategies to prevent future harm through analysis of the actions and events that led to the adverse event.

Quality Improvement
- Goes hand in hand with safety protocols.
- Analysis of results and outcome of implementing the safety and quality steps.

Q. WHO and surgical safety campaign: "Safe surgery saves lives". (Short notes)

Four areas in which dramatic improvements can be achieved in safety of surgical care:
1. Surgical site infection prevention
2. Safe anesthesia
3. Safe surgical teams
4. Measurement of surgical services.

"Five Steps to Safer Surgery" **from National Patient Safety Agency (NPSA)**

1. Briefing
2. Sign-in
3. Timeout—before the start of surgical procedure
4. Sign-out—before any member of team leaves the operating theatre
5. Debriefing.

"**Five Steps to Safer Surgery**" (from National Patient Safety Agency [NPSA]—England and Wales). It is a surgical safety checklist—proved to decrease death rates from 1.5% to 0.8% and serious complications from 11% to 7%.

> **Q. Elucidate the WHO guidelines on safe surgery.**

WHO Surgical Safety Checklist

WHO surgical safety checklist, is a 19-item tool created by WHO in association with the Harvard School of Public Health.

Aims to increase teamwork and communication in surgery and to decrease errors and adverse events.

Checklist Requires

- Items to be checked at three points of the patient journey through theater.
- Use of the checklist for every patient undergoing a surgical procedure.
- Its documentation in the patient's case papers.

Specific checklists are developed for different specialties. Also they are modified according to local needs of the country and area.

The three-point checklist was converted to the Five Steps to Safer Surgery and was introduced in the 'How to Guide' produced by the NPSA.

Significant reduction in both morbidity and mortality has been shown after the Global implementation of the checklist around the world.

Surgical safety checklist (copied from the WHO checklist, published 2009).

Modifications are done to suit the local situations in each part of world given in **Table 11.2**.

Table 11. 2: Surgical safety checklist (copied from the WHO check list, published 2009).

Before induction of anesthesia (with at least nurse and anesthetist)

- Has the patient confirmed his/her identity, site, procedure, and consent? Yes/No
- Is the site marked? Yes/No/Not applicable
- Is the anesthesia machine and medication check complete? Yes/No
- Is the pulse oximeter on the patient and functioning? Yes/No
- Does the patient have a: Known allergy? Yes/No
- Difficult airway or aspiration risk? Yes/No, and equipment/assistance available
- Risk of >500 mL blood loss (7 mL/kg in children)? Yes/No
- Two IVs/central access and fluids

Before skin incision *(with nurse, anesthetist and surgeon)*

- Confirm all team members have introduced themselves by name and role
- Confirm the patient's name, procedure
- Where the incision will be made
- Has antibiotic prophylaxis been given within the last 60 minutes? Yes Not applicable

To the surgeon

- Anticipated critical events to surgeon
- What are the critical or non-routine steps?
- How long will the case take?
- What is the anticipated blood loss?

To anesthetist

- Are there any patient-specific concerns?

To nursing team

- Has sterility (including indicator results) been confirmed?
- Are there equipment issues or any concerns?
- Is essential imaging displayed? Yes Not applicable.

Before patient leaves operating room (with nurse, anesthetist and surgeon)

Nurse verbally confirms

- The name of the procedure
- Completion of instrument, sponge and needle counts
- Specimen labeling (read specimen labels aloud, including patient name)
- Whether there are any equipment problems to be addressed

To surgeon, anesthetist and nurse

- What are the key concerns for recovery and management of this patient?

Nutrition and Fluid Therapy

Chapter 12

SU12.1	Enumerate the causes and consequences of malnutrition in the surgical patient.
SU12.2	Describe and discuss the methods of estimation and replacement of the fluid and electrolyte requirements in the surgical patient.
SU12.3	Discuss the nutritional requirements of surgical patients, the methods of providing nutritional support and their complications.

> **SU12.1: Enumerate the causes and consequences of malnutrition in the surgical patient.**
>
> **SU12.3: Discuss the nutritional requirements of surgical patients, the methods of providing nutritional support and their complications.**

Nutrition is a key player in recovery of surgical patients. Malnourished patients and those with chronic starvation have a higher risk of complications and of death than those with normal state of nutrition. Prolonged protein calorie malnutrition (cachexia or general weakness) and short-term under nutrition (e.g. after trauma, burns or surgery or after with critical illness) affect the recovery after surgery.

PHYSIOLOGY OF BODY NUTRITION

Body mass – made of water 60–70% and ICF 40 + 20 ECF (15% 3/4 interstitial + 5% plasma ¼). The aim of nutritional support is to identify those patients at risk of malnutrition and to ensure that their nutritional requirements are met by the most appropriate route and in a way that minimizes complications.

Daily calorie requirement is linked to body mass index (BMI). Calorie requirement based on BMI:

- Normal and stressed surgical patients: 25 kcal/kg/day. Average 1300–1800 kcal/day.
- Patients with severe stress or burns: 35 to 40 kcal/kg/day, others require in between.

BMI (weight in kg)/(height in meter)^2.
Under weight: <18.5, normal 18.5–24.9
overweight 25–29.9.
Obese: 30–39.9, morbid obesity >40.

Normal metabolism: Involves anabolism (synthesis and storage) and catabolism—mobilization of energy from stored substrates.
- **Anabolic state:** Insulin converts glucose into glycogen and stored in liver and muscles, enough for about 12 hours, as a source of constant glucose for brain and RBCs. It also stores triglycerides in fat cells.
- **Catabolic state:** Beyond 12 hours of fasting, glycogen gets depleted and release of glucagon causes gluconeogenesis from amino acids (alanine and glutamine) and ketones from lipids, for the brain to utilize in lieu of glucose (exclusively after 10 days).

Metabolism during stress: Example: trauma, burns, surgery, extreme mental stress.
Action of counter-regulatory hormones: Adrenal hormones (catecholamines and glucocorticoids —release glucose and lipids from peripheral stores), glucagon and growth hormone.

Result
- Increased energy requirements—10 to 20 times the normal needs (severe sepsis or burns)
- Insulin resistance and glucose intolerance
- Increased gluconeogenesis and protein breakdown. Increased nitrogen requirements, preferential lipolysis and loss of adaptive ketogenesis
- Fluid retention with hypoalbuminemia.

Surgery induces a hypercatabolic state, increasing protein utilization and urinary nitrogen excretion.

Nitrogen balance—important clinical indicator of nutritional status in patient
- Nitrogen balance = (24 hour protein intake/6.25) less (24 hour urinary nitrogen excretion + 4) recovery is shown by shift from catabolic to anabolic parameters (following feeding and wound healing).

Causes of Malnutrition in Surgical Patient
Preoperative State
- Low BMI, (below 18)
- Prolonged starvation, protein calorie deficiency
- Chronic protein loss—renal failure, protein losing enteropathies
- Chronic liver disease due to poor reserves and protein synthesis
- Metabolic disorders.

All the above cause poor wound healing and infections.

Carbohydrate Related
- Diminished uptake of carbohydrates
- Diseases causing intestinal mucosal flattening (Whipple disease celiac sprue).

Fat Related
- Major pancreatic or ileal resection may lead to fat malabsorption due to defective enterohepatic circulation of essential fatty acids (linoleic acid and linolenic acid)
- Deficiencies can cause infection, poor wound healing, thrombocytopenia.

Postoperative State
- Prolonged starvation
- Imbalance in postoperative feeding/nutrition.

- Infections.
- Systemic disorders—renal, endocrine, hepatic.

Surgical Conditions and Surgeries Causing Malnutrition
- Crohn's, pancreatitis, cancer
- Intestinal resection—leaving less than 150 cm of bowel.

Consequences of Malnutrition
- Poor wound healing
- Infection
- Systemic failures
- Poor immunological function
- Specific to individual factors:
  - Protein calorie related problems
  - Trace elements related—neurological, dermatological, integumentary (skin and nails)
  - Emotional and psychological.

Assessment of Malnutrition in Surgical Patients
- Clinical (history)—illness, recent or long-standing
- Starvation due to any cause
- Stress and emotional factors
- Examination—BMI, general systemic examination psychological and psychiatric
- Evaluation for—serum proteins, hepatic dysfunction, renal dysfunction, endocrine disorders.

> **Q. What are ASPEN criteria for diagnosis of malnutrition?**

American Society for Parenteral and Enteral Nutrition (ASPEN) criteria:
Two out of six criteria for a clinical diagnosis of malnutrition:
1. Insufficient energy intake
2. Weight loss
3. Loss of subcutaneous fat
4. Muscle mass loss
5. Localized or general fluid accumulation (may mask weight loss)
6. Diminished functional status (measured by hand grip strength).

Chapter 12: Nutrition and Fluid Therapy

Q. Discuss the nutritional requirements of surgical patients.

Surgery induces a hypercatabolic state, increasing protein utilization and urinary excretion of nitrogen. A knowhow of dietary components, digestive physiology and metabolism helps to plan and administer the nutritional requirements in surgical patients according to individual state.

Glucose

Minimum 200 g/day—increasing demand after surgical stress.

Protein

- Non-stressed patients; 0.8 to 1.2 g/kg body weight/day.
- Critically ill: Upto 1.5 g/kg weight/day.
- In sepsis and burns patients: Upto 1.5 to 2.5 g/kg/day.
- Obese patients require high levels of proteins.

Q. Briefly enlist daily dietary ration of a surgical patient. (Short notes)

Daily dietary ration of a surgical patient should have the following compositions:

Carbohydrates: Provide 50% to 65% of calories. Energy /each gram of glucose—4 kcal.
Fats: Provide 20% to 35% of calories. Energy/gram of fat—9 kcal.
Proteins provide: 10%- 35% of calories. Energy / gram of protein—4 kcal.
Micronutrients: Essential in involved in wound healing and immune function.
This includes vitamins and trace elements—iron, manganese, iodine, zinc, selenium chromium, molybdenum. They serve as cofactors and enzymatic catalysts.

Methods of Providing Nutritional Support and their Complications

Two routes: Enteral and parenteral.

Q. Define and discuss enteral nutrition including the routes, pros and cons.

Enteral nutrition: Mixture of required nutrients given. It is easy, inexpensive, least or non-invasive.

Most physiological— maintains the cytoarchitecture, mucosal integrity (via trophic effects) and absorptive function of GI tract.

Also maintains normal microbial flora. Hence less chance of bacterial translocation into blood stream and endotoxin release.

Complications

- Mechanical—related to tube or feeding (aspiration pneumonia, perforation, slipped tube into respiratory tract), bleeding
- Septic—infections
- GI disturbances, diarrhea, bloating, ileus
- Electrolyte and metabolic imbalances.

Methods—Enteral Nutrition

- Oral—convenient.
  Problems—difficult in unconscious patients, cant be given in major surgeries for fear of inability to take or of aspiration.
- Nasogastric—easy and convenient.
  Disadvantage: Discomfort, infection, misplaced tube entry into respiratory tract, perforation.
- Nasoduodenal/nasojejunal tube—bypasses stomach in feeding, (e.g. in pancreatitis). Needs expertise to introduce.
- Feeding gastrostomy (endoscopic or surgical) or jejunostomy (invasive – surgical).

Timing of Feeding

- Early enteral feeding is generally preferred
- **Contraindications:** Bowel discontinuity, obstruction, acute peritonitis ischemia, high output fistula
- Bolus feeds—20-40 mL/hr gradually increased to meet requirement
- Continuous feeding through tubes—30-40 mL/hr monitor for gastric stasis and aspiration.

Q. Describe types of parenteral nutrition. Discuss its advantages and disadvantages; enumerate the complications.

PARENTERAL NUTRITION

Peripheral parenteral nutrition (PPN)—can cause phlebitis.

- Phlebitis can be avoided by keeping osmolarity of PPN solutions below 900 mOsm (approx. 10% dextrose solution).

Total Parenteral Nutrition (TPN)

Provides complete nutritional requirements.

Route: Central venous access (subclavian or internal jugular vein).

Method of Administration of TPN

- **Continuous TPN** (24 hours)—no need for IV fluid in addition—for prolonged needs
- **Cyclical TPN**—intermittent relief from the infusion pump for stable patients, also for those who need other IV lines and injections.

Complications

- Related to venous catheter—sepsis, phlebitis, extravasation, venous puncture and intrathoracic leaks—hydropneumothorax
- Sepsis—tube, feeding solution, systemic
- Cholestasis—acute and chronic causing biliary cirrhosis.

Overfeeding - Related Complications

- **Excess glucose:** Hyperglycemia, dehydration, hypercapnia, fluid retention
  - Electrolyte abnormalities.
- **Excess fat:** Hypercholesterolemia and hypertriglyceridemia, hypersensitivity
- **Excess amino acids:** Hyperchloremic metabolic acidosis, aminoacidemia, uremia
  - Hypercalcemia, hypophosphatemia, hypokalemia.
- Re-feeding syndrome—hypophosphatemia, hypokalemia, hypomagnesemia.

The nutritional requirements are individualized and accordingly the constitution of nutrient solution, volume of administration, and additives are decided.

Discontinuation of TPN should be gradual and in proportion to the extent of patient's ability to meet over 60% of the daily requirement complete fluid needs orally.

Concern: Rebound hypoglycemia, dehydration, hypophosphatemia.

Q. Short note on refeeding syndrome.

Refeeding Syndrome

- A potentially lethal complication in severely malnourished patients receiving TPN.
- After feeding synthesis begins depleting limited phosphorous store in the body stores, Further, insulin rebound causes induces intracellular shift of potassium and magnesium.
- **Result:** Hypophosphatemia, severe hypokalemia and hypomagnesemia.
- **Immediately lethal:** Arrhythmia and acute heart failure.

Dumping syndrome: Undigested, hyperosmolar food reaches the jejunum, fluid shifts into the intestine to equalize osmotic pressure.

Clinical features: Nausea, tachycardia, bloating, abdominal cramping, diaphoresis and diarrhea.

Enhanced Recovery after Surgery (ERAS)

- Nutritional recommendations and comprehensive set of guidelines for multimodal perioperative management to speed recovery and shorten the duration of hospital stay.
- Includes avoiding fasting prior to surgery, use of carbohydrate-rich beverages up to 2 hours prior to surgery (except in diabetes), to preserve glycogen stores and improve postoperative insulin resistance.

> **SU12.2:** Describe and discuss the methods of estimation and replacement of the fluid and electrolyte requirements in the surgical patient.

Applied Physiology

Body Fluid Compartments 60% of body weight is due to water (36 liter in 60 kg).

Total-body water

- ICF—intracellular fluid compartment (40% of weight)
- ECF—extracellular fluid compartment (20% of weight)
- Intravascular compartment (5%)
- Interstitial compartment (15%)

The ICF and ECF have following distribution of ionic molecules **(Table 12.1)**.

Table 12.1: Distribution of ionic molecules.

	Intracellular compartment	Extracellular compartment
Cation	Potassium—K^+ Magnesium—Mg^{2+}	Sodium (Na^+) is the main cation
Anion	Phosphates (PO_4^-) and negatively charged protein	Chloride—Cl^- Bicarbonate—HCO_3

Water Balance in a Normal Adult Person

Average Intake

2000-2500 mL (oral intake and 500 mL from metabolic oxidative activity in the body).

Daily Water Losses

Urine: 1,000 to 1,500 mL (40-60 mL/hour)—minimum 600-700 mL needed to excrete metabolites.

Stool: 150 mL– 200 mL.

Insensible water loss: About 600–800 mL.
- Skin: 300–400 mL
- Lungs: 400–500 mL

Insensible losses increase with dry atmosphere, hyperventilation fever, and hypermetabolism.

Obligatory losses include: Minimum water loss to maintain normal state—includes minimum losses from kidney, skin and lungs (as given above).

> **Q. Describe the daily fluid requirement in surgical patient.**

Fluid Requirement in Surgical Patient

- Maintenance fluids—based on insensible and obligatory losses to ensure urine out put of 0.5–1 mL/kg/hour.
- Replacement' fluids—to correct pre-existing deficiencies
- Supplemental fluids—to compensate for anticipated additional intestinal and other losses.

Average Daily Requirements: Main Electrolytes

- **Sodium:** 50–70 mM/day
- **Potassium:** 45–50 mM/day
- **Calcium:** 5–6 mM/day
- **Magnesium:** 1 mM/day.

TYPES OF FLUIDS USED

- Crystalloids and colloids
- Osmolality and tonicity of fluid—is considered.

Crystalloids

- **Isotonic crystalloids**
  – Sodium chloride 0.9% saline
  – Lactated Ringer solution (LR)
- **Hypotonic solutions**
  – Dextrose 5%, in water—D5W
  – 0.45% NaCl—half normal saline
- **Hypertonic saline solutions**
  – Alone or combination with colloids (dextran), in patients with shock or burns
  – 10% dextrose, 25% dextrose

Colloid

- **Colloid solutions:** Contain high molecular weight substances—dextran, albumin.
- **Osmolarity:** The penetrability into blood vessels.

Maintenance Fluid Requirements

- This is calculated by various formulas, generally based on a person's body surface area or body weight.
- An average fluid volume of 30–40 mL/kg gives an estimate of daily requirements.

The following are the approximate maintenance fluid requirements (based on body weight):
- 100 mL/kg/day for the first 10 kg
- 50 mL/kg/day for the next 10 kg
- 20 mL/kg/day for every 10 kg thereafter.

(Example, for a 60 kg adult this will be 100 × 10 = 1000; 50 × 10 = 500; 20 × 40 = 800 mL, totalling 2400 mL/day).

Contents of Maintenance Fluid

- Sodium (Na^+)—1 to 2 mmol/kg/day
- Potassium (K^+)—0.5 to 1 mmol/kg/day
- 5% dextrose, 0.45% $NaCl^-$ 30 mmol KCl per liter of fluid is a balanced solution.

The nature and type of replacement fluid is assessed as below:

- If the hematocrit is below 21%, blood transfusion may be required.
- Assessment of the patient:
  - Pulse, BP and central venous pressure
  - Serum electrolytes and hematocrit
  - State of hydration—peripheries, skin turgor, urine output and specific gravity of urine.
- Estimation of losses: Vomiting, ileus, diarrhea, excessive sweating or fluid losses from burns (mainly sodium).

Estimation of Replacement and Supplemental Fluids

Loss from: Fistulae, nasogastric tubes or abnormal urine or fecal losses from drains. Most intestinal fluids are rich in sodium and saline is fluid of choice.

Intraoperative and Postoperative Fluid Management

Preoperative deficit plus ongoing losses including "third space losses".

Intraoperative losses

Include maintenance fluids for the length of the case, hemorrhage and "third-space losses" (peritoneal cavity, pleural cavity, luminal sequestration of intestinal secretions, gastric stasis etc).

Fluids and electrolyte administration

- Lactated Ringer solution is used for replacing intestinal and pancreatic secretions
- Normal saline with potassium chloride (KCl) for replacing gastric secretion.
- Third space loss is carefully tackled with monitoring of electrolyte, urine output.

Albumin replacement only if crystalloids fail to improve the condition.

Blood is used for replacement of severe blood loss.

In conclusion, the surgical patient is given fluids, electrolytes along with the nutrients (macro and micro) as guided by; the preoperative state, nature and gravity of surgical operation and postoperative progress.

Chapter 13

Transplantation

SU13.1	Describe the immunological basis of organ transplantation.
SU13.2	Discuss the principles of immunosuppressive therapy. Enumerate, indications, describe surgical principles, management of organ transplantation.
SU13.3	Discuss the legal and ethical issues concerning organ donation.
SU13.4	Counsel patients and relatives on organ donation in a simulated environment.
	SU13.4 is a practical session and hence clubbed with SU13.2 and SU13.3.

SU13.1: Principles of immunosuppression.

Q. Describe the innate and adaptive arms of human immune system. (Major Question)

The human immune system is made of two arms: The innate and the adaptive (acquired) complementary to each other:
1. **The innate system**—recognizes general challenges and its response is non-specific, direct and without any memory. It enacts these responses through:
   - **The complement cascade**—the activated proteins form formation of the **membrane attack complex (MAC)** and attach to cell membrane and lysis of the pathogen. It also causes opsonization to effect phagocytosis by **antigen-presenting cells (APCs)**.
   - **Natural killer cells**—mainly responsible for body's cancer surveillance. They recognize cells which do not have a self-**major histocompatibility complex (MHC)**
2. **The acquired or adaptive system distinguishes "self" from "non-self":** It recognizes specific foreign antigens in the major histocompatibility complex (MHC), and targets the same.

Q. Describe the human major histocompatibility complexes (MHC). (Short notes)

The human MHCs: A cluster of genes, **human leukocyte antigens (HLA)** located on short arm of chromosome 6.

Types: HLA—2 Classes
- **Class I (A, B, C):** Present on all nucleated cells and made of a heavy chain and β2-microglobulin. They are targets for cytotoxic (CD8) T-cells.
- **Class II (DR, DP, and DQ):** Present on **antigen-presenting cells (APCs)** viz., B cells, dendritic cells and macrophages. They trigger an antibody (humoral) mediated response. They are targets for helper (CD4) T-cells.

Expression of MHC Genes is Codominant

The genes are expressed on both the maternally and the paternally derived chromosomes. Humans have six HLA antigens on each strand of the chromosome 6, having inherited one

MHC complex each from both parents. The are highly polymorphic and widely different in each individual and hence pose difficulty in matching.

An individual may express between 6 and 12 different HLA antigens,

The most important HLA in solid organ transplantation are A, B, and DR.

Type of Adaptive Immune Responses

When confronted with specific challenge.
- **Cell mediated.** Antigens in tissues are exposed to T-cells (in lymph nodes and the spleen). The **T-cell receptor** (TCR) recognizes a specific antigen in the context of the MHC.

  The DNA rearrangement in the thymus, during fetal development enables the T-cells to bind the self MHC without activating response and MHC in those tissues not having exposure to the thymus of the individual evokes the response. This is the cause of immune reactivity after a transplant (allo reactivity).
  - **Helper T-cells (CD4)** recognize exogenous antigens in of MHC class II on the surface of APCs (B-cells, dendrites, and macrophages).
    Activation releases IL-2 and IL_4 (IL-2 transforms B-cell into plasma cells which - produce antibody and IL-4- maturation of cytotoxic T-cells directly kills the cells).
  - **Cytotoxic T-cells (CD8)** recognize the antigens in the context of MHC class I.
- **Antibody mediated (humoral).** B-cells (bone) activate antibody mediated (humoral) immunity aided by IL-4 from helper T-cells which transforms B-cells into plasma cells, to produce antibodies specific to the "non-self".

IMMUNOSUPPRESSIVE THERAPY

The immune apparatus of the recipient treats the grafted organ as "foreign" by recognizing the antigens on the graft cells, mounting an immune response by activating the T cells, which release cytokines and direct T- killer cells and also activate B cells, which produce antibodies against the graft leading to graft rejection.

Immunosuppressive therapy is the cornerstone of successful transplantation by inhibiting the immune cell activation at various stages.

Aim

To maximize graft protection with minimum of side effects.

> **Q. Enlist and write short notes on immunosuppressive agents used in organ transplantation.**

Immunosuppressive agents
- **Non-specific**
  - **Corticosteroids** (prednisone, methylprednisolone) main immunomodulators to suppress inflammatory response, act on lymphocytes to prevent proliferation, neutrophils to prevent migration,
  - Used for induction and maintenance of immunosuppression and for treatment of rejection.
- **Calcineurin inhibitors**: Block IL-2 gene transcription. Ciclosporin, tacrolimus—most important agents for graft survival. Tacrolimus—is more effective in reducing the risk of acute rejection.
- **Antiproliferative agents**
  - Block lymphocyte proliferation
  - Azathioprine, mycophenolic acid
- **ATG** (anti-thymocyte globulin) – blockade of lymphocytes and their depletion
- **mTOR inhibitors**
  - Blockade of IL-2 receptor signal transduction
  - mTOR (Mammalian target of rapamycin) inhibitors: Sirolimus and everolimus
- **Monoclonal antibodies** against lymphocytes—causing their depletion.
  - Anti-CD25   against activated T cells
  - Anti-CD20   B lymphocytes
  - Anti-CD52   all lymphocytes
  - CTLA-4Ig   Blocks T-cell co-stimulation

General principles of immunosuppression in organ transplantation
- Immunosuppression is needed over indefinite period but most needed in the first three months. Immunosuppression increases the risk of infection and malignancy.
- Most regimens—based on calcineurin blockade plus steroids and an antiproliferative agent.

Adverse effects of non-specific immunosuppression

Infection:
- High risk of opportunistic infection, especially by viruses (mainly CMV). Bacterial and fungal infections. Risk of infection is greatest during first six months.
- Chemoprophylaxis is important for high-risk patients.
- Pre-transplant vaccination against community-acquired infection—considered.

Malignancy:
- Post-transplant lymphoproliferative disease (PTLD)—mainly children
- Squamous cancer of the skin—high risk of and recipients should have regular skin review

TRANSPLANTATION AND IMMUNOSUPPRESSION

Definitions "transplantation" means the grafting of any human organ from any living person or deceased person to some other living person for therapeutic purposes, Transplantation of Human Organs Act **(THOA 1994 GOI)**.

Types of Transplantation

- **Based on type of donor**
  - **Allograft:** An organ or tissue transplanted from one individual to another
  - **Isograft:** Transplantation between identical twins
  - **Xenograft:** A graft performed between different species.

  Note:
  - **Alloantigen:** Transplant antigen.
  - **Alloantibody:** Transplant antibodies.
  - **HLA:** Human leukocyte antigen, the main trigger to graft rejection.
- **Site of grafting:**
  - **Orthotopic graft:** A graft placed in its normal anatomical site
    Involves removal of recipient organ: Liver, heart, lungs, intestines, cornea
  - **Heterotopic graft:** A graft placed in a site different from normal location
    No need to remove recipient organ kidney, pancreas.

- **Types of donor**
  - Live donor (LD), e.g., liver, kidney
  - Cadaveric donor: Deceased donor (DD)
    - Donor brain dead (DBD)
    - Donor circulation dead (DCD)
- **Types of grafts**
  - Split organ—part of organ—liver, intestine, pancreas
  - Full organ— kidney, heart, one or both lungs.

Human Leukocyte Antigens (HLA Antigens) (Refer previous section on immunosuppression).

- Are the most common cause of graft rejection
- Their physiological function is to act as antigen recognition units
- Are highly polymorphic (amino acid sequence differs widely between individuals).

HLA-A, -B (class I) and -DR (class II) are most important in organ transplantation.

MECHANISM OF GRAFT REJECTION

> **Q. Describe how a graft is rejected after transplantation.**

T-cell mediated – *activated CD4* through cytokines, *CD8* – mediated target cell death, CD 4 mediated direct cell death and through cytokines, macrophages and *B- cell –antibody* action.

- HLA antigens expressed by graft cells activate T cells and stimulate them to proliferate in response to interleukin-2 (IL- 2) and other T-cell growth factors.
- Activated CD4 T cells, release cytokines and trigger mechanisms for graft rejection.
- Cytotoxic CD8 T cells: The cells that target donor HLA class I antigens expressed by the graft and cause target cell death by releasing lytic molecules such as perforin and granzyme.
- Graft infiltrating CD4 T cells recognise donor HLA class II antigens and mediate direct target cell damage and also by releasing proinflammatory cytokines such as interferon to activate macrophages which act as non-specific effector cells.

- CD4 T cells help: B lymphocytes mature into plasma cells and produce antibodies against the graft cells.

Types of Graft Rejection

Q. Enumerate types of graft rejection and write a note on each.

Hyperacute rejection: Immediate post transplant (1–3 days)
- Immediate graft destruction due to ABO or preformed anti-HLA antibodies
- Characterised by intravascular thrombosis and interstitial hemorrhage.
- Treatment: Removal of graft needed

Accelerated rejection—within a week—reversible
- Is caused by sensitized T-cells that produce a secondary immune response
- Treatment—steroid plus monoclonal antibody—muromonab-CD3

Acute rejection: Acute cellular rejection (ACR)—after one to six weeks—reversible
- It is cell mediated—**T-cell** dependent due to CD8 (T lymphocytes)
  - Cytotoxic and helper T-cell led B-cell-antibody.
- Treatment—methyl prednisolone—antithymocyte globulin.
- Usually reversible.

Chronic rejection—after 6 months—irreversible
- Occurs after first six months, most common cause of graft failure
- Antibodies play an important role
  - Non-immune factors contribute to pathogenesis
  - Characterised by myointimal proliferation in graft arteries—leading to ischemia and fibrosis.

Contributors to chronic rejection
- Acute rejection with vasculitis or recurrent acute rejection
- HLA mismatch
- Immunosuppression—inadequate or inappropriate
- Long cold ischemia time
- Cytomegalovirus (CMV) infection.

Q. What is graft versus host disease?

Graft-versus-host disease (GVHD). (Short notes)
- The reciprocal problem of graft-versus host reaction is occasionally seen following organ transplantation.
- Contrary to the main immunological problem of graft rejection.
- Some donor organs (particularly liver and small bowel) contain large numbers of lymphocytes
- These may react against HLA antigens expressed by recipient tissues, leading to graft-versus-host disease (GVHD)

Features of GVHD
- Frequently involves the skin, causing a characteristic rash on the palms and soles.
- May involve the liver (after small bowel transplantation)
- The gastrointestinal tract (after liver transplantation).
- GVHD is a serious and sometimes fatal complication

DONOR RECIPIENT MATCHING

- HLA matching crucial to organ transplantation (Refer below)
- ABO matching—important.
- O—universal donor, A—donor to A and AB, B- to A and AB, AB donor only to AB recipient.
- Rh typing is not considered in tissue matching.

THE TISSUE: TYPING LABORATORY

Working closely with the transplant team.

Functions

- The HLA typing ('tissue typing') of all potential organ transplant recipients and organ donors —DNA typing techniques for samples of peripheral blood.
- **Cross-match test** - detects preformed circulating antibodies against donor HLA—by incubating recipient sera with donor lymphocytes—either blood or lymphoid tissue. This helps to avert in rapid or hyperacute graft rejection)
- **HLA specificity of circulating anti-HLA antibodies**

- **Determination of the panel reactive antibodies** (PRA): Patient sera are incubated with a panel of latex beads coated with purified HLA molecules (panel of cells of various possible HLA specificities of the donors) and antibody binding detected by flow cytometric analysis.
- **Uses:** To plan the following:
  - Pre-transplant
    » To predict the likelihood of a positive cross-match
    » To plan donor organ allocation.
  - Post-transplant—immunosuppressive therapy.

Graft Dysfunction

> Q. Describe causes of graft dysfunction and rejection.

Causes of allograft dysfunction

Factors determining organ function after transplantation
- Donor characteristics
- Recipient-related factors

Early dysfunction: Ischemia, thrombosis, rejection, drugs, infection, obstructive.
- Primary non-function—irreversible ischemic damage during transplantation
- Delayed function (reversible ischemic injury)
- Thrombosis of the graft vessels arterial or venous
- Hyperacute and acute rejection
- Drug toxicity (e.g., CNI toxicity)
- Infection (e.g., CMV disease in graft
- Mechanical obstruction (ureter/common bile duct).

Late: Chronic rejection, ischemic, recurrent primary disease, obstructive
- Chronic rejection
- Arterial stenosis, recurrence of original disease in graft (glomerulonephritis, hepatitis C)
- Mechanical obstruction (ureter, common bile duct)

Evaluation of Potential Recipients for Organ Transplantation

- Evaluation by multidisciplinary team including surgeon and physician.
- Determine presence of comorbid disease, exclude malignancy and systemic sepsis.
- Evaluate for organ-specific criteria for transplantation—ability to cope psychologically with transplant and comply with immunosuppression.
- Evaluate need for any preparative surgery needed to facilitate transplantation
- Optimise recipient condition prior to transplantation.

Overcoming: Shortage of Organs for Transplantation

- Maximising donation after brain-death (DBD) donation
- Encourage—marginal DBD—deceased donors and circulatory death (DCD) donors
- Increased use of split liver transplantation
- Increased living donor kidney (and liver) transplantation.

ORGAN TRANSPLANTATION IN PRACTICE

- Kidney: Heterotopic
- Pancreatic transplantation: Heterotopic—pancreatic duct anastomosed to urinary bladder
- Liver: Orthotopic
- Cardiac transplantation: Orthotopic—right atrium retained
- Lung transplantation
- Heart-lung
- Renal and heart
- Renal and liver.

LIVER TRANSPLANTATION (ORTHOTOPIC)

> Q. What are the indications for liver transplantation?

Indications for liver transplantation—4 groups
1. **Cirrhosis**
   - Chronic liver failure, non-alcoholic steatohepatitis
   - Primary biliary cirrhosis and sclerosing cholangitis
   - Alcoholic liver disease, viral liver disease
   - Children account for around 10–15% of all liver transplants, biliary atresia is the most common indication
2. **Acute fulminant liver failure**
3. **Metabolic liver disease**
4. **Primary hepatic malignancy.**

Couinaud's liver segments: I–VIII—are depicted in **Figure 13.1**. Segment I is caudate lobe. Each of the segments II to VIII are subdivided into A and B.
- Liver graft is usually made of minimum two and usually three segments of liver.

Types of segmental grafts
- 2 segments—minimum—needed.
- 3 segments usually taken.
- 4 or 5 segments also used sometimes.

One liver may be split into multiple grafts:
A graft may be made of:
- Segment 2, 3 (usually for child); 2, 3, 4
- 4, 5, 8; or 5, 6, 7, 8, or 4, 5, 6, 7, 8.

Steps of Liver Transplantation (Orthotopic transplantation)
- Recipient hepatectomy
- Donor hepatectomy (organ harvest)
- Partial in LD/total in DD and segment wise division
- Transplantation
- Anastomosis: Host vena cava to graft hepatic veins
- Portal vein to portal vein
- Hepatic artery
- Biliary anastomosis.

Kidney Transplantation (Heterotopic Transplantation) (Figure 13.2)
- Kidney transplantation is highly HLA dependent
- Needs complex and prolonged immunosuppression
- Improved results after cyclosporin and tacrolimus
- LD better than DD
- Blood related better than unrelated.

Steps
- Donor nephrectomy: Generally minimal access or open
- Minimum ischemic time
- Transplant in right iliac fossa
- Renal artery to external iliac art or internal iliac trunk
- Renal vein to ext iliac vein
- Ureteric implantation into bladder.

GRAFT DYSFUNCTION

A common problem during the early postoperative phase.

Possible causes are—acute tubular necrosis; arterial/venous thrombosis; urinary leak/obstruction; CNI toxicity; hyperacute/accelerated acute rejection.

Post op Monitoring
- For graft dysfunction
- Rejections
- Immunosuppression—generally tacrolimus and ciclosporin
- Steroids
- Antibiotics
- Antiviral agents (against CMV)—valganciclovir.

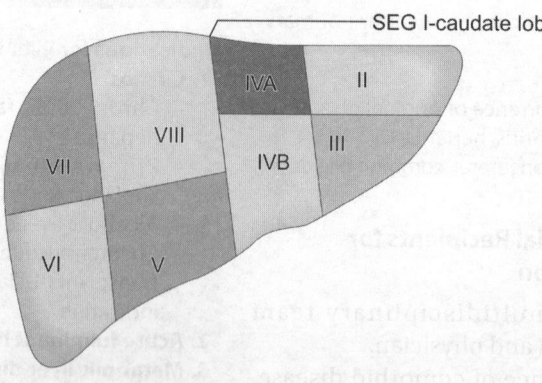

Fig. 13.1: Couinaud's liver segments.

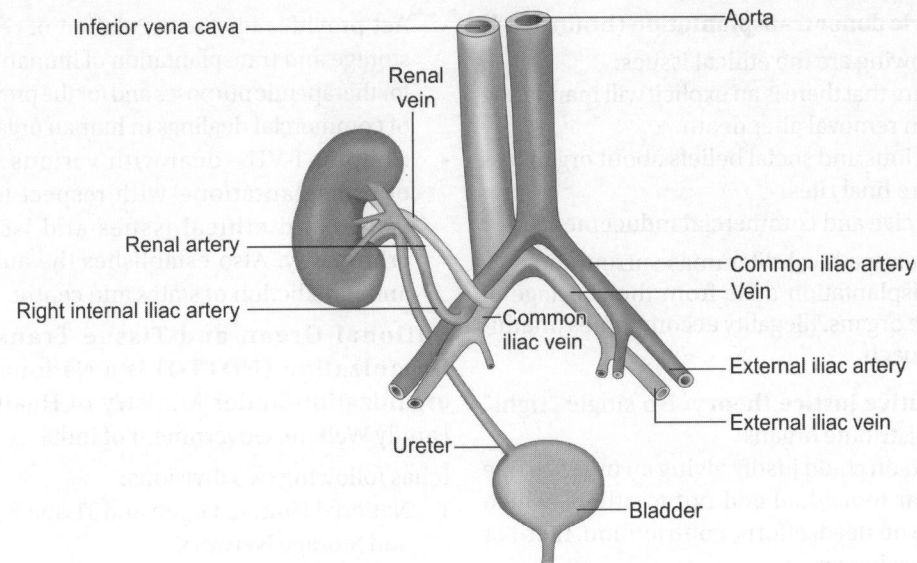

Fig. 13.2: Renal transplantation

> **SU13.3: Discuss the legal and ethical issues concerning organ donation.**

"Transplantation" means the grafting of any human organ from any living person or deceased person to some other living person for therapeutic purposes. THOA 1994 GOI.

LEGAL, SOCIAL AND ETHICAL ISSUES
Ethical and Social Issues

- Preservation and protecting the life has become the concern of medical fraternity. "Organ transplantation" is an issue that needs sensitivity.
- Orienting society to accepting the 'value of life after death' will go a long way in strengthening the acceptance of transplantation as a medical treatment and help build donor pool.
- Ethics mandates enacting "the right" act.

The Ethics of Transplantation: Involves Three Requirements

1. **Medical integrity:** Doctors must command the trust of patients and public, that they do not sacrifice the one anothers' interests.
2. **Scientific validity:** Best use of basic biology and technology to offer a beneficial outcome.
3. **Consent:** Consent of patient and donors based on information adequately presented, weighted and understood, and unforced.

Organs can only be procured wilfully, not forcefully or through inducements.

The abuse, fraud and coercion of paid organ donors are to be curbed.

Payment for organ donation, as incentive or compensation or insurance is msotly denounced but the fraternity is divided in opinion.

Living donor transplantation. It is to be ensured that:

- The organ removal should not impair donor's health or function.
- The benefits to the recipient should outweigh the likely harm to the donor.
- The donation should be altruistic and free from coercion or external pressure.
- The donor and family/relatives including spouse and adult children must be fully informed of the nature of the procedure and the possible (even the rare) complications and possible future health consequences traceable to organ donation.
- This requires the need for follow-up of the donor's health in the future.

Cadaveric donor transplantation (brain dead)

The following are the ethical issues:
- Ensure that there is an explicit will mandating organ removal after death.
- Religious and social beliefs about organ loss before final rites.
- Coercive and commercial inducements.

The primary ethical dilemmas surrounding organ transplantation arise from the shortage of available organs. Illegality accompanies unethical approach.

Distributive justice theory: No single "right" way to distribute organs.

A person could justify giving an organ to one particular individual and not to others, which could be on need, efforts, contribution, merit or market exchanges.

One distributive justice criteria is **equal access**. Organs allocated according to equal access criteria are distributed to patients based on objective factors aimed at limiting bias and ensuring the needy getting the organ.

Arguably, the illegality involving the transplantation involves a nexus between the stake-holders—beneficiary (the recipient), medical enterprise (hospitals, doctors and labs, pharma industry and intermediaries (touts, network) targeting the potential donor.

These factors led the Government of India to enact the central legislation. The Transplantation of Human Organs and Tissues Act, 1994 (THOA 1994) and amend the same in 1994, 1995, 2008 and 2011. The Act as amended upto 2011 regulates organ donation in India.

Transplantation of Human Organs and Tissues Rules, 2014.
- The law allows both deceased and living donors to donate their organs.
- It also identifies brain death as a form of death.
- Act provides for the regulation of removal, storage and transplantation of human organs for therapeutic purposes and for the prevention of commercial dealings in human organs.
- Chapter I-VII—deal with various aspect of transplantation—with respect to legal issues and ethical issues and issues of criminality. Also establishes the authority and jurisdiction of states and centre.

National Organ and Tissue Transplant Organization (NOTTO) is a National level organization under Ministry of Health and Family Welfare, Government of India.

It has following two divisions:
1. National Human Organ and Tissue Removal and Storage Network
2. National Biomaterial Centre.

"National Human Organ and Tissue Removal and Storage Network"(THOA 2011)

Functions:

National Network division of NOTTO would function as apex centre for all India activities of coordination and networking for procurement and distribution of Organs and Tissues and registry of Organs and Tissues Donation and Transplantation in the country.

National Biomaterial Centre (National Tissue Bank)

THOA (Amendment) Act 2011 deals with of tissue donation and registration of Tissue Banks. To establish National level Tissue Bank to fulfill the demands of tissue transplantation—activities for procurement, storage and fulfill distribution of biomaterials. The main thrust and objective of establishing the centre is to **fill up the gap between 'Demand' and 'Supply' as well as 'Quality Assurance' in the availability of various tissues.**

Basic Surgical Skills

Chapter 14

SU14.1	Describe aseptic techniques, sterilization and disinfection.
SU14.2	Describe surgical approaches, incisions and the use of appropriate instruments in surgery in general.
SU14.3	Describe the materials and methods used for surgical wound closure and anastomosis (sutures, knots and needles).
SU14.4	Demonstrate the techniques of asepsis and suturing in a simulated environment.

The reader is advised to refer a detailed chapter on practical aspects of surgical skills and operative surgery.
SU14.1, 14.2 and 14.3 are outlined in brief.
SU14.4 is a practical competency—only principles are mentioned.

> **SU14.1: Describe aseptic techniques antisepsis, disinfection and sterilisation.**

BEGINNING OF ANTISEPSIS AND DISINFECTION

Dr Ignaz Semmelweis of Vienna

The mortality rates of unqualified midwives was around 2% while it was quite high in teaching hospital involving teaching, examining the patient and autopsies. In 1847, Dr Semmelweis instituted a **mandatory hand washing policy for medical students and physicians using a solution of chlorinated lime (calcium hypochlorite)** for washing hands between autopsy work and the examination of patients. This led to fall in the mortality rate fell to about 2%. Later he started washing the medical instruments and the rate decreased to about 1%.

Dr Joseph Lister, 1827-1912, British surgeon and medical scientist introduced the concept of **antiseptic medicine and pioneered preventive medicine**. He started use of phenol for disinfection of instrument and antisepsis.

Definitions

- **Asepsis:** Preventing the microbes from accessing the individual (and hence preventing infection.
- **Antisepsis:** The term refers to inhibition of growth of microorganisms.
- **Disinfection:** Subjecting any surface or object to a process involving is killing of all vegetative bacteria (not spores), fungi and viruses.
- **Sterilization:** A process of removal of all microbes from an object of surface by killing all bactreria including spores, viruses and fungi.

METHODS OF STERILIZATION AND DISINFECTION

Physical Sterilization

Heat—Dry or Wet

Dry Heat

- *Hot-air oven*—induces temperature upto 160–180°C. For at least one hour.

- *Burning and incineration*—for disinfecting articles like hospital dressings.

Wet Heat

- *Boiling:* At temperatures of around 90 to 99°C, it can't kill spores and sme viruses.
- *Autoclave:* It uses steam under pressure.
- At temperature of 120°C for 20 minutes at a pressure of 15 Lb/sq inch or 135°C for 15 minutes.
- A green gelatin strip placed in the tank, it turns black when sterilization is complete.
- All spores and viruses are killed here.
- Most surgical instruments are sterilized by this method including, linen, cotton, dressings.
- However heat sterilization is not suitable for sharp instruments like knife and scissors as the latter get blunted by heat.

Chemical Sterilization

Phenol—the first efficient agent used for disinfection by Lister. It is used as bench mark to test efficacy of other disinfections, taking the efficacy of phenol as 1 (Phenol coefficient).

Other Phenols: Cresol, Lysol

- Chlorhexidine—most polular antiseptic.
- Chloroxylenol (brand dettol).
- Cetrimide is cationic surfactant (cetavlon).
- The popular brand Savlon is made of cetrimide and chlorhexidine.

Halogen Derivatives

- Sodium hypochlorite.
- Bleaching powder.

EUSOL: Edinburg University Solution contains sodium hypochlorite, boric acid and calcium hydroxide.

Alcohols

- Ethyl alcohol 76%
- Isopropyl alcohols are used.

Aldehydes

- *Formaldehyde:* It is used to disinfect indoors like operation room and ICUs, fumigating the rooms with vapors of formaldehyde, obtained by adding potassium permanganate to Formalin solution and keeping the room closed for 12 hours.
- *Glutaraldehyde (Cidex 2%):* This is the most commonly used chemical to sterilize sharp instruments like knife, endoscopes. The instruments should be dipped in glutaraldehyde 10 hours for sterilization.

Ethylene Oxide Gas

This is the most commonly used and cost effective gas to sterilize any instrument including endoscopes.

Radiation

May be ionizing or non-ionizing.
- *Ionizing radiation:* Gamma radiation is used commonly to sterilize suture materials, syringes, needles, disposable tubings like endotracheal tube, urinary catheters etc.
- *Non-ionizing radiation:* Ultraviolet radiation and infrared radiation is used for disinfection of air. Bacteria and many viruses are susceptible to UV rays.

SU14.2 Describe surgical approaches, incisions and the use of appropriate instruments in surgery in general.

SURGICAL APPROACHES

An internal organ can be approached only by breach of anatomical barriers. Accordingly knowledge of anatomy is mandatory for any surgery.
- Abdomen—the approaches are transperitoneal and extraperitoneal
- Thoracic approaches:
  - Transpleural—for lungs, heart and great vessels
  - Extrapleural—for mediastinal and paravertebral pathologies (sternotomy or transcostal approach).

Incisions should be placed along lines of natural development to get better scar.

The reader is advised to refer operative surgery books.

ABDOMINAL INCISIONS

Considerations in choice of incision: The mnemonic "EAS Prasanna," the name of former off-spinner helps
- E: Extensibility—of incision—in case of need for extra access to internal organs.
- A: Accessibility—of organs
- S: Stability—of wound
- P (Prasanna): Precision of technique.

How to Choose an Incision
- Indication—emergency or elective
- Always have a diagnosis for a correct incision to get access to the anatomy and pathology
- If the diagnosis is not precise, use a liberal incision with a provision for modification
- Use an incision you are best at
- Shape and build of patient also modifies incisions.

Upper Abdomen

Upper Midline Incision

From xiphisternum to umbilicus, through to the peritoneum
- Once peritoneum opened just to the right of midline.
- Go to right of falciform ligament.
- Xiphisternum is usually left alone—but may be retracted or cut in need.
- The incision needs to be skirted around the umbilicus in case of extension to the lower abdomen.
- Advantages:
  - Easy to make and easy to close.
  - No major nerves and vessels cut; no muscle damaged.
- Disadvantage: Umbilicus prevents a straight extension downwards.

Lower Midline Incision
- From umbilicus to the symphysis pubis through the linea alba.
- Urinary bladder should be emptied before the incision is made.
- Useful incision for all surgeries on sigmoid and rectum, small bowel, gynecological and urological operation.

Paramedian Incision
- Right or left.
- 2–3 cm from midline, through the skin to open the rectum sheath.
- Starts from below costal margin vertically downwards to a point about 2 cm below the level of umbilicus.
- Avoid too lateral an incision.

(*Note:* Battle's para rectal incision—is away from midline, opening lateral to the rectus muscle it causes damage to the nerves supplying the rectus muscle. And hence the incision is avoided).
- Rectus muscle is separated and retracted off the medial edge of the sheath and here the tendinous intersections—upper, middle and lower are encountered and separated.
- Linea semilunaris: This is the lower edge of posterior rectus sheath, formed by fusion of posterior lamina of internal oblique which ends at this level and the entire muscle joins the external oblique.

Right Subcostal Incision
- About 2 finger below the right costal margin from midline obliquely and parallel to the costal margin upto anterior axillary line.
- It is a muscle cutting incision cutting across the abdominal wall.
- At least 2 cm of upper edge of muscles is kept to get muscle edge for closure of wound.
- Muscles divided along the line of incision—external and internal oblique and the transversus abdominis and also the rectus belly in medial part.
- Vessels—superior epigastric vessels.
- Nerves—intercostal nerves 8, 9 and 10th
- But every effort is made to retract the nerve and avoid cutting the 9th intercostal nerve to avoid complete denervation of the rectus muscle. The incision can be extended to the left side across the midline.

Transverse Incisions
- Transpyloric: Across the epigastrium from one the right to the left costal margin at the level of two costal cartilages. Usually preferred in pediatric surgery for biliary, gastric and pancreatic surgeries.

- **Bucket handle:** An curvilinear incision under the costal margin across the upper epigastrium— preferred for pancreatic surgeries and liver resections.
- **Chevron (inverted Chevron):** Two subcostal incisions joined across the midline.
- **Pfannenstiel:** Suprapubic transverse incision between the two mid inguinal points—rectus sheath incised in the midline and raised as a flap off the recti upto the umbilicus. The two recti are retracted laterally to expose the peritoneum or the bladder. The urological operations are carried out extra peritoneally and abdominal and obstetric or gynaecological surgeries are carried out by opening the peritoneum.
- Flank incisions: For excision of retroperitoneal swellings and drainage of retroperitoneal abscesses, renal and ureteric operations and also lumbar sympathectomy.

Closure

- **Anatomic:** Layered closure—involves closure in layers according to the anatomical structure
  - *Material:* Generally absorbable material like polyglactin is used for peritoneum and non-absorbable material like polypropylene is used for muscle and fascia.
- **Mass closure:** Closure of the abdominal wound as a single layer with approximating sutures through all the layers of the abdomen.
- Peritoneum to be closed or not? Peritoneal mesenchymal cells regenerate in situ in about 72 hours and hence there is no need to close the layer. But presence of fluid, blood and inflammatory exudates—leak through the edges and hence many surgeon prefer to close the perineum to prevent herniation of bowel and adhesion to the raw part of the abdominal wall in the early postoperative phase.

> **Q. What are the indications for use of drains in surgical operations?**

DRAINS

- Generally tube drains are preferred but corrugated drains are also popular.
- **Where to keep:** The drains are kept to the site of collection or expected leak. However in major surgeries, the drains are kept in the most dependent parts of the peritoneal cavity viz., the right and left paracolic gutter, the subhepatic space (Rutherford Morrison's pouch) or in the pelvis through incision in the flanks.
- **How to insert:** Incision is made in the flank and a long bladed Kocher's forceps is introduced avoiding any damage to the bowel inside the abdomen.
- **Fixing the drain:** It is very important to prevent it from slipping and more importantly from getting pulled into the abdomen.
- **Removal**—under aseptic precautions.
- Time of removal—depends on the purpose of the drain.
- Usually after 48 hours when it is to drain a collection, e.g., after cholecystectomy or after a retroperitoneal swelling.
- After 5–7 days when it is kept in anticipation of a leak from a bowel anastomosis.

Other types: Negative suction (vacuum drains) corrugated drains.

Complications

- Infection being carried into abdomen.
- Injury to internal organs while placing.
- Erosion and pressure necrosis of organs or vessels.
- Loss of drain into the internal cavities—due destruction or division while removing.

Thoracic Incisions

Mainly:

- **Median sternotomy:** Vertical split of the sternum for accessing the heart and the great vessels, superior and anterior mediastinal tumors.
- **Antero lateral thoracotomy:** For surgeries on pericardium, heart—mitral valvotomy.
- **Posterolateral thoracotomy:** For most of the lung operations and surgeries on posterior mediastinum.

> SU14.3: Describe the materials and methods used for surgical wound closure and anastomosis (sutures, knots and needles).

SUTURING

Principles

- Asepsis and hemostasis.
- Approximation (coapting) of the wound edges after trimming them.
- Edges must be perpendicular to the surface.
- Ensuring adequate blood supply to the wound.
- Adequate wound support.
- Avoiding tension across the wound edges and in superficial layers; instead shifting the tension to deeper layers of the wound.
- Eversion of the wound edges is preferred to get good healing but wound edges are approximated " at level" in areas like face, neck and scalp.
- Should lead to an acceptably good scar.

Surgical Techniques

The following are the basic instruments used in different designs and modifications thereof:

- Scalpel blade with handle
- Needle holder (driver)
- Needles and suture materials
- Hemostats—curved and straight (popularly called "artery forceps")
- Straight scissors for cutting of the suture
- Tissue forceps toothed and non-toothed
- Gauze—non-woven gauze and mops (non-woven gauze acts like a wick through its capillary suction property and it is preferred to a woven gauze)
- Diathermy or any energy device—for hemostasis.

Hospital Waste Disposal

Chapter 15

| SU15.1 | Describe classification of hospital waste and appropriate methods of disposal. |

Definition of Hospital (Medical) Waste

Any waste which is generated as a by-product of healthcare work and includes any material which could come in contact with the body during diagnosis, drug administration or any type of treatment and medical research.

Q. Classify medical waste.

Classification

Names and categorizations for the different types of medical waste: Each country categorizes differently, but basically depending on the hazardous potential to community and environment.
- UK—2 types: Hazardous and non-hazardous.
- USA—4 types: General, infectious, hazardous and radioactive.

World Health Organisation (WHO) Medical Waste Classifications

- **Infectious waste:** Anything that's infectious or contaminated.
- **Sharps:** Waste like needles, scalpels, broken glass and razors.
- **Pathological waste:** Human or animal tissue, body parts, blood and fluids.
- **Pharmaceutical waste:** Unused and expired drug or medicines, like creams, pills, antibiotics.
- **Genotoxic waste:** Cytotoxic drugs and other hazardous toxic waste, that's carcinogenic, mutagenic or teratogenic.
- **Radioactive waste:** Any waste containing potentially radioactive materials.
- **Chemical waste:** Liquid waste, typically from machines, batteries and disinfectants.
- **General/other waste:** All other, non-hazardous waste.

Medical Waste in the USA: As per US Environment Protection Agency (EPA)

- **General waste**—household and office waste makes the bulk of most medical waste.
- **Infectious waste**—potential to cause an infection in humans, (e.g., blood, waste contaminated with body fluids or human tissue).
- **Hazardous waste**—dangerous, but not infectious, (e.g., needles, blades, discarded surgical equipment, and chemical waste.
- **Radioactive waste**—waste generated from radioactive treatments, (e.g., like cancer therapies) and nuclear medicine (equipment that uses radio isotopes).

Medical Waste in the UK: As per UK Govt Advice

- **Infectious waste**—any waste generated from the treatment of individuals or contaminated with any infectious bodily fluids
- **Cytotoxic/cytostatic waste**—cytotoxic or cytostatic drugs, medicines and items) which come into contact with any toxic or carcinogenic medicine (syringes and tubings used during treatment)

- **Medicinal waste**—non-cytotoxic and non-cytostatic medicine, pills and creams
- **Anatomical waste**—waste from a human or animal, (body parts, blood bags and organs)
- **Offensive waste**—any waste that's non-infectious, including sanitary and nappy waste
- **Domestic or municipal**—all other general, non-clinical waste.

Q. Explain the steps of disposal of hospital waste.

DISPOSAL OF HOSPITAL WASTE

Concept: Waste is an inevitable product of health care and needs disposal. Safe disposal of the waste concerns minimizing its hazardous potential to environment and humanity.

Bio-Medical Waste Management Rules, 2016 along with Bio-Medical Waste Management (Amendment) Rules, 2018 (Ministry of Environment, GOI) regulate the disposal of hospital waste.

Steps of Biomedical Waste (BMW) Management (Refer Table 15.1)

1. Generation, 2. Segregation, 3. Collection, 4. Storage, 5. Treatment, 6. Transport, 7. Disposal.

The respective hospital and health care facility (HCF) are responsible for the steps 1–5 and also treatment of lab and highly infectious waste, which is pre-treated by the HCF.

The service provider is responsible for treatment and disposal at the CBMWTF (Common Biomedical Waste Treatment Facility Center).

Table 15.1: Steps of biomedical waste disposal.

Step 1	Segregation and pre-treatment of waste at the site of generation
Step 2	Collection of segregated waste from all areas of the hospital
Step 3	Transportation of waste from various areas of the hospital to storage site
Step 4	Weighing of bags at storage site
Step 5	Transportation for final disposal

Segregation, Packing, Storage and Transport

As per BMW rules GOI—2016 and 2018.
- Bio-medical waste classified into 4 categories based on treatment options.
- No untreated bio-medical waste shall be mixed with other wastes.
- Untreated human anatomical waste, animal anatomical waste, soiled waste and, biotechnology waste shall not be stored beyond a period of forty-eight hours.
- If required to store beyond 48 hours, the occupier shall ensure that it does not affect human health and inform the SPCC with reason.

Schedules: There are 4 schedules (or parts) in the Bio-medical Waste Management rules, 2016 and Rules 2018:
- **Schedule I (Part-1 and 2):** Categorization and Management of BMW.
- **Schedule II:** Standards for treatment and disposal of BMW.
- **Schedule III:** Prescribed authorities and corresponding duties.
- **Schedule IV:** Label of containers or bags (Part A) and label for transportation of Bio-Medical waste bags or containers (Part B)

Schedule I: Parts 1 and 2: Waste categories and their segregation, collection, treatment, processing and disposal options.

Part 1: BMW: Classified Based on Treatment Options (Described in Table 15.2)

Four categories: Yellow, red, white and blue.

Part 2: Treatment before Storage and Transportation

- **Chemical treatment** - done using at least 10% sodium hypochlorite having 30% residual chlorine for twenty minutes. But as per BMW (amendment) rules, 2018, 1% to 2% sodium hypochlorite should be used.
- There is no need of chemical pre-treatment before incineration, except for microbiological, lab and highly infectious waste.
- **Syringes should be either mutilated or** needles should be cut and or stored in tamper proof, leak proof and puncture proof containers for sharps storage.

Table 15.2: Classification of biomedical waste.

Color code of bag	Type of bag/ container used	Type of waste treatment	Disposal options
Yellow	Non-chlorinated plastic bags	**All anatomical waste** Cytotoxic drugs, expired or discarded medicines with vials/ampoules **Chemical waste**—solid and liquid micro, bio-tech and other clinical lab waste Discarded linen, mattresses, beddings contaminated with blood or body fluids. Also routine mask and gown (2018)	Incineration or plasma pyrolysis or deep burial
Red	Non-chlorinated plastic bags or containers	**Recyclable contaminated waste** Vacutainers, tubing, bottles, intravenous tubes and sets, catheters, urine bags, syringes (without needles) and gloves	Autoclaving/microwaving/ hydroclaving and then sent for recycling, not sent to landfilling
White	Translucent containers: Puncture, leak, and tamper proof	**Waste sharps** Including metal sharps—needles, syringes with fixed needles, needles from needle tip cutter/burner, scalpels, blades	Auto or dry heat sterilization followed by shredding or mutilation or encapsulation
Blue	Cardboard boxes or containers with blue colored marking. (As per BMW rules, 2018) puncture proof and leak proof	Broken/discarded glass medicine vials and ampoules without those contaminated with cytotoxic wastes Metallic implants	Disinfection or autoclaving, microwaving, hydroclaving and **then sent for recycling**

Schedule IV: Part A: Label for Bio-Medical Waste Containers or Bags

Standard symbols are used for – each category of bags, e.g., "cytotoxic hazard " - symbol –"handle with care" or biohazard - symbol –"handle with care.

Note: Schedules II and III are relevant to the service provider and are excluded from this chapter.

Disposal of radioactive medical waste: It is regulated by the radioactive wastes (Atomic Energy Act, 1962).

Summary: Management of Biomedical waste (BMW) hospital waste (given in stepwise detail in Tables 15.3 and 15.4).

Definition and classification—2 categories in UK and 4 categories in USA

WHO classification – 8 categories

BMW disposal is regulated by:

BMW Management Rules- 2016 and 2018 (Ministry of Environment, GOI):

Mainly has 4 schedules regarding steps of BMW management.

Each color category is stored (and pretreated if needed by rules) and transported to the final disposal point—*Common Biomedical Waste Treatment Facility Center (CBMWTFC)*.

Radioactive waste is regulated by the Radioactive wastes (Atomic Energy Act, 1962).

Table 15.3: Schedule I – part – refers – steps of BMW management.

Steps: 1 to 5	1. Segregation and pretreatment 2. Collection from each area 3. Shifting to storage area 4. Weighing the bags 5. Transportation for final disposal

Table 15.4: BMW classified under color codes.

BMW—classified into 4 categories as per respective treatment options and each category is stored and transported in 4 color coded containers.

Yellow	Disposable contaminated waste
Red	Recyclable contaminated waste
White	Sharps, e.g., needles, blades, etc.
Blue–glass	Noncontaminated wastes including implants, medicines

Minimally Invasive Surgery and Bariatric Surgery

16 Chapter

SU16.1	Minimally invasive general surgery.

Q. Describe indications, advantages and disadvantages of minimally invasive general surgery.

MINIMALLY INVASIVE SURGERY

Syn: Minimal access surgery.

Short answer questions
1. What are ports in minimally invasive surgery?
2. Veress' needle.
3. Pneumoperitoneum in minimally invasive surgery. How and why?
4. Enumerate complications of laparoscopic surgery.
5. Hypercarbia in minimally invasive surgery.
6. What are the advantages and disadvantages of minimally invasive surgery?

First laparoscopy in 1901 by Georg Kelling of Dresden with a cystoscope (he termed it 'celioscopy'). Philippe Mouret performed the first video-laparoscopic cholecystectomy in Lyon, France in 1987.

Today—widely applied to all fields and generally renamed as **MIS (MAS)**.
- **MIS:** Minimally invasive surgery
- **MAS:** Minimal access surgery (access wound small).

Principles and Technology

Basic Principles

Laparoscopy is visualization and exploration of abdominal cavity by the use of an endoscope.

The same involves:
- **Entry** into the intraperitoneal cavity.
- Creating **pneumoperitoneum** with CO_2 (less often N_2O); to obtain working space for instruments. The ports have valves that prevent leak of CO_2.
- **Visualization**—through a rigid or semirigid **endoscope** connected to a **light source** and monitors to display operative field.
- **Ports**—are placed at sites suited for the respective procedure.

Laparoscope (telescope)—made of a sheath, eyepiece and tip.

Sheath—rigid or semirigid tube—inserted into the patient through a port.

The telescope has a fiber optic bundle connected to a light source to illuminate surgical field and a CCD chip (charged chip device), to capture the image of the operative field from the laparoscope tip and project the digitized image to a monitor.

Laparoscope size—10 mm is most commonly used, others—7 mm, 5 mm and 3 mm. Larger scopes provide better illumination.

Tip of laparoscopes: Depicted in **Figure 16.1**.

Tip has a rod/lens/prism for view of the field.
- **Flat tips** (0-degree scopes)
- **Angled tips** (commonly 30- or 45-degree) to allow the field of view to be turned around the long axis of the scope.

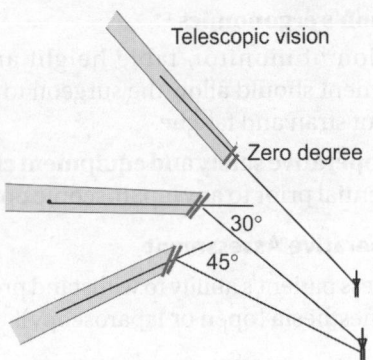

Fig. 16.1: Tip of the telescope

Veress' Needle

A spring loaded needle used to create pneumoperitoneum for laparoscopic surgery. Complications include injuries to bowel and vessels from blind insertion of the needle.

"Open access": It is entry under vision through a small incision and a blunt tip trocar as an alternative to Veress Needle.

Trocar and Sheath

- Outer sheath and inner trocar
- 10 mm is the most commonly used trocar
- 2/3 mm, 5 mm, 7 mm 10, 11, 12 mm, 16 mm are also available
- They are disposable or reusable.

Laparoscopic Instruments

- Long handle to work from a distance
- Involves double fulcrum
- Maximal access—minimal invasion.

Camera

- Basic single chip
- Three chip (splits light into red gree and blue) for better image
- Digital high definition cameras.

Insufflator

To establish pneumoperitoneum.

Gas insufflator: A pressure-limited gas insufflator is used to control the flow of CO_2 into the abdominal cavity.

It has indicators to show (1) the pressure in the abdominal cavity, (2) the flow rate and (3) total volume of gas used to insufflate.

Increase in pressure and fall in pressure (loss of pneumoperitoneum) are warning signs of different problems—technical or of morbid states (physiology).

Light source: Halogen, xenon or LED source.

Anesthesia: General Anesthesia

Operating Laparoscope Set

Equipment: Laparoscopic instrumentation, and instruments for open operation (if conversion to open surgery is required at any point of time), if necessary.

Generally made of the following: More instruments are getting added each day.

- Camera with camera controller—single chip/3-chip or digital HD
- Light source—halogen, xenon or LED
- Telescope
- Monitors for display of operative field
- CO_2 insufflator with gas source
- Ports: These are access holes made on abdominal walls to insert trocars
- Instruments: Basic surgical instruments used in a laparoscopic surgery include forceps, scissors, probes, dissectors, hooks, and retractors
- Veress' needle
- Suction apparatus
- **Energy devices:** Diathermy—monopolar or bipolar, ultrasonic shears.
  Or advanced bipolar devices, (vessel sealing).

Sterilization

- Ideally—gamma irradiated disposable set of instruments.
- Ethylene oxide gas for reusable instruments.

A compromised approach often practiced is use of:

- Formaldehyde gas
- Glutaraldehyde solution.

Patient Selection

Indications: Unlimited.
Laparoscopy is being increasingly used to perform more and more types of surgeries.

Contraindications:

- In a patient, unfit for general anesthesia or carbon dioxide insufflation.

- Hemodynamic instability.
- Coagulopathy—uncorrected.
- Unavailability of a laparoscopic surgeon competent in the particular procedure.

Relative contraindications
- Severe cardiopulmonary disease.
- Loss of tissue planes (domain), e.g., multiple previous surgeries, extensive adhesions
- Severely distended bowel and peritonitis.

Procedure
- Anesthesia: General.
- CO_2 pneumoperitoneum
  - Veress needle or "open"—small stab incisions to insert trocar cannula.
- Trocar insertion and port placement
  - Exploration and procedure
  - More trocars and instruments if need be—hemostasis and end of procedure
- Deflation: Release CO_2
- Removal of ports and closure of wounds.

Triangulation
- Working on principle of triangulation.
- The camera port is placed centrally with working ports on either side to help the long armed instruments converge at the organ or site without collision.

Note: A urinary catheter keeps bladder empty and helps monitor urine output.
- **Positioning of patient.**
- **Supine (American) position**—supine patient. Surgeon stands on the sides (and the team too)
- **French position for upper abdominal surgery**
  - Legs are separated and knees are fixed like in a lithotomy position.
  - The position allows the surgeon to operate from between the legs.
- **Lithotomy position**—for laparoscopic with pelvic procedures perineal approach.
- **Lateral decubitus position**
  - For thoracoscopic or retroperitoneal procedures.
- **Safety straps**—to secure the patient to the table, help tilting the patient.

Surgeon's ergonomics
Position of monitor, table height and port placement should allow the surgeon to operate without stran and fatigue.

A preoperative safety and equipment checklist is essential prior to any laparoscopic operation.

Preoperative Assessment
To assess patient's ability to withstand procedure and anesthesia (open or laparoscopy).

Applications of Minimally Invasive Surgery
Diagnostic Laparoscopy
- Gynecological practice: Infertility/pelvic disease/endometriosis
- Abdominal trauma
- Staging/biopsy of tumors
- Peritoneal disease, ascites
- Omental/lymph node biopsy
- Undescended testis.

Therapeutic Procedures: Endless List
- Most operations for disorders of digestive organs and urogenital system are tackled by laparoscopic or retroperitoneoscopic MIS.
- Extra abdominal surgeries include sub-fascial endoscopic perforator surgery (SEPS) for varicose veins, thoracoscopy; mediastinoscopy, MI CABG.
- MI parathyroid surgery and thyroidectomies.
- Arthroscopy and intra-articular joint surgery.

Postoperative Care
- Analgesia for pain in the wound and shoulder.
- Antiemetics and antibiotics, early feeding and early mobilisation.
- Anticoagulants thromboprophylaxis with low molecular weight heparin (enoxaparin).

Complications

> Q. Enumerate complications of laparoscopic surgery.

Per-operative
- **Entry—injury**
  - **Visceral/vascular**
  - By needle/trocars/instruments
  - Thermal/energy sources.
- **Bleeding**

- **Septic**
  - Peritoneal
  - Trocar wound
  - **Iatrogenic**—atypical mycobacteria
- **Pneumoperitoneum:** High intra-abdominal pressure and low venous return. Ventilatory deficit, sympathetic stimulation.
- **CO_2 (hypercarbia)**—parasympathetic stimulation, cardiac arrhythmias, CO_2 retention, CNS depression.
- **Anesthesia-related**.

Postoperative
- Thromboembolism
- Cardiorespiratory events.

CONVERSION TO OPEN SURGERY

- May be necessary anytime during the surgery due to technical, hemodynamic, anesthetic difficulties or hypercarbia.
- Hence a blanket informed consent must be taken from the patient and relatives before hand for conversion to open laparotomy, in case of necessity.

Innovations and advances
• Single incision laparoscopic surgery (SILS)
• Natural orifice transluminal endoscopic surgery (NOTES)
• 3D laparoscopy
• Robotic laparoscopic surgery

Q. What are the advantages and disadvantages of minimally invasive surgery?

Advantages of Minimally Invasive Surgery

Minimal Incision and Maximal Access

Figures 16.2 and 16.3 depict the advantages of minimal access surgery.

Advantages and Disadvantages of MIS

Refer below to "sumamry—minimally invasive surgery".

Summary—Minimally Invasive Surgery

Definition and principles
- Endoscopic viewing of internal organs and structures to perform surgeries
- Without large incisions of access
- Involves general anesthesia and positioning
- Entry through needle or trocar
- Insufflation with CO_2 to create working space within the cavity
- Placement of ports to insert laparoscopic camera and instruments
- Careful dissection, retraction and procedures with the additional help of energy devices and suture material staples
- Deflation and removal of pots w
- Closure of port wounds.

Surgery follows principle of triangulation with laparoscope at top and instruments at sides.

Indications: Endless and growing to involve all organs and systems.

Contraindications
- Patient unfit for general anesthesia
- Severe cardiopulmonary disease
- Coagulopathies uncorrected
- Loss of tissue domain, severe sepsis (e.g., peritonitis)

Complications
- Related to anesthesia
- Carbon dioxide retention (hypercarbia)—cardiovascular, neurological and respiratory
- Surgery—entry trauma to organs, vessels and bleeding
- Thermal injuries—due to energy devices—diathermy and vessel sealants
- Septic—to peritoneal
- Ports sites—atypical mycobacterial infections of ports.

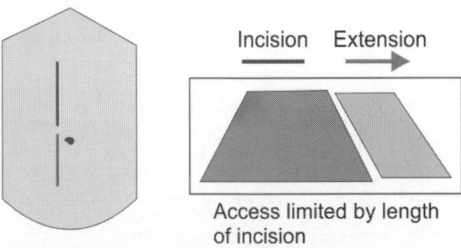

Fig. 16.2: Large incision

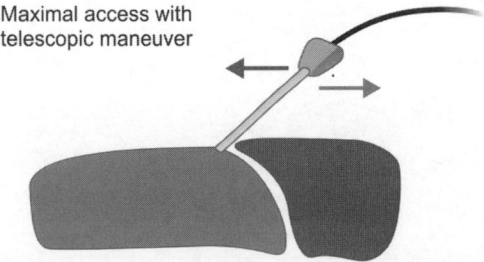

Fig. 16.3: Minimal incision

Advantages
- Better visualization and maximal access to inner tissues at surgery
- Small wound—less pain
- Less infection
- Faster recovery and earlier return to work.

Disadvantages
- 2D viewing to perform surgery in a 3D field
- Limited depth perception
- Dependence on eye hand coordination
- Inability to extract large specimen.

Should always be ready to convert to open operation.

Bariatric Surgery

SURGERY FOR OBESITY AND DIABETES

- Baro—weight; bariatric surgery—surgery for overweight.
- Obesity and overweight are considered as a disease and in epidemic state.
- The socioeconomic impact of obesity is of concern to all.
- Obesity is associated with increased risk of disease and many disorders.
- To name a few- Atherosclerosis, cardiovascular disorders, cerebrovascular events, sleep apnea syndrome, diabetes, digestive disorders including GERD, gallstones and pancreatitis musculoskeletal disorders, osteoarthritis, immunological disorders, dermatological disorders, polycystic ovarian disease. Obesity is also liked to carcinogenesis in many organs including the breast and pancreas.
- It negatively impacts the cosmetic appeal of the individual and also leads to compulsive eating disorders, depression, behavioral problems, social ostracisation, to mention only a few.

Physiology of hunger and satiety
- Ghrelin from gastric fundus stimulates hunger by stimulating the brain
- Leptin from adipose cells (and also from gastric mucosa) inhibits hunger by a feedback.
- Insulin regulates leptin secretion. Also high glucose levels suppress appetite.
- Circulating ghrelin concentration rises before meal and falls after meal.
- Plasma leptin levels decrease during fasting or energy restriction and increase during refeeding, overfeeding, and surgical stress. Leptin secretion is stimulated by—insulin, glucocorticoids, serotonin, and estrogen. Plasma leptin levels are significantly correlated with body mass index (BMI). Leptin has a crucial role in regulating food intake and energy expenditure.

In obesity, individuals have leptin resistance and the inhibitory signals against appetite fail.

Incretin hormones - GIP and GLP-1
- They are gut peptides, causing the incretin effect
- Secreted after nutrient intake
- Stimulate secretion of insulin and inhibit release of glucagon.

GIP (glucose-dependent insulinotropic polypeptide) from the upper GI tract (K cells) and GLP-1 (glucagon-like peptide-1) from lower (L cells) gut.

Effects of GLP-1(negligible in healthy normal individuals).
- Incretin effect
- Reduction in appetite and food intake—leading to weight loss.

Insulin secretory response to oral glucose is three-fold higher than to intravenous glucose.

Q. Explain the rationale of surgery for diabetes and obesity.

Basis of Surgery for Diabetes and Obesity

In type 2 diabetes: The incretin effect is diminished or no longer present.
- Due to reduced effectiveness of GIP on the beta cells.
- But the incretin effects of GLP-1 are preserved in subjects with type 2 diabetes and the same can be stimulated by certain drugs or delivery of food directly to the distal ileum (rich in L cells) to stimulate secretion of GLP-1.
- This is the basis of surgery for diabetes and obesity to stimulate GLP-1 receptors. It causes hypoglycemia and improves glycemic control and leading to weight loss.
- GLP-1 secretion from the gut seems to be impaired in obese subjects, this may even indicate a role in the pathophysiology of obesity.

Q. Define and classify obesity.

This is given in **Table 16.1**.

Treatment of Obesity

Principle: It involves dietary discipline, lifestyle modification, exercise, medications and counseling. Surgery is the last resort.

Surgical contouring is not obesity surgery and is only a cosmetic correction of shape.

For example, liposuction—to suck out fat cells to reduce subcutaneous adipose tissue.

Abdominoplasty—resection of abdominal wall fat and reshaping.

OBESITY SURGERY

Aim: To achieve sustained weight reduction and improved quality of life.

Indications
- BMI—over 40 kg/m²
- BMI—over 35 with comorbidities, e.g., diabetes, cardiovascular disease.
- When all non-surgical options have failed.
- Type 2 diabetes with BMI above 35 kg/m² (some even accept BMI 30).

Goals
- Sustained weight loss of over 50% over 5 years.
- Improved glycemic control.
- Minimal metabolic and nutritional side effects.

Table 16.1: Classification of obesity.

Obesity	BMI kg/m²	Obesity class	Disease risk
Underweight	<18.5		
Normal	18.5–24.9		
Overweight	25.0–29.9		Increased
Obesity	30.0–34.9	I	High
	35.0–39.9	II	Very high
Extreme obesity	≥ 40	III	Extremely high

Q. Enumerate main types of bariatric surgery.

TYPES OF BARIATRIC SURGERY

- *Restrictive procedures*—restrict the person's ability to eat.
- *Malabsorptive procedures*
  - Induce malabsorption of calories and effect hypoglycemia and weight loss.
  - Also affect increased response to leptin to reduce appetite.
  - Stimulate incretin (proinsulin and antiglucagon) response to cause hypoglycemia.

Restrictive Procedures (Depicted in Figure 16.4)

- **Laparoscopic adjustable gastric band (LAGB):** An adjustable band is applied across the stomach just below the fundus and tightened to make a pouch of proximal stomach and restrict patient's intake.
- **Laparoscopic sleeve gastrectomy**
  - The greater curvature and body are resected vertically and stomach is converted into a tube along the lesser curvature. This will also reduce the capacity to eat and in addition take away the Ghrelin effect by resection of fundus and greater curvature which have K cells.
  - Also glycemic control will be better.

Disadvantage: Stomach dilates over a period and patient eats his "normal" diet.

Malabsorptive Procedures: Includes Restrictive Steps Too

Restrictive steps cut the capacity to consume. Malabsorptive measures cause metabolic effect.

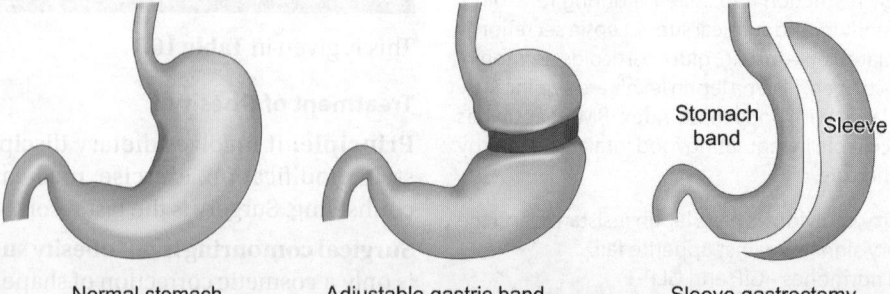

Normal stomach   Adjustable gastric band   Sleeve gastrectomy

Fig. 16.4: Restrictive procedures in bariatric surgery.

Note: Only the most commonly done procedures are mentioned.
- **Roux-en-Y gastric bypass (RGB)** (Refer **Table 16.2** and **Figure 16.5**)

Biliopancreatic Diversion with Duodenal Switch Gastric Bypass (BPD/DS)

This is given in detail in **Table 16.3** and **Figure 16.5**.

Table 16.2: Roux-en-Y gastric bypass (RGB).

Proximal stomach is stapled and divided just below the GE junction to make a small pouch of 40 mL	Restricts capacity Reduces eating capacity	Early fullness No ghrelin effect—appetite lowered
Divide jejunum 120 cm from D-J flexure Anastomose distal end to gastric pouch	Food bypasses duodenum and jejunum to reach ileum	Minimizes calorie absorption from proximal bowel. Avoids mixing of food with bile and pancreatic juice again reducing absorption.
Anastomose proximal cut end to the distal ileum about 100 cm proximal to ileocecal junction	Provides food to mix with juice in distal ileum	Stimulates release of GLP—causes incretin effect—hypoglycemia. Allows mixing of food with bile and allows enterohepatic absorption through ileum of bile salts, minerals and nutrients.

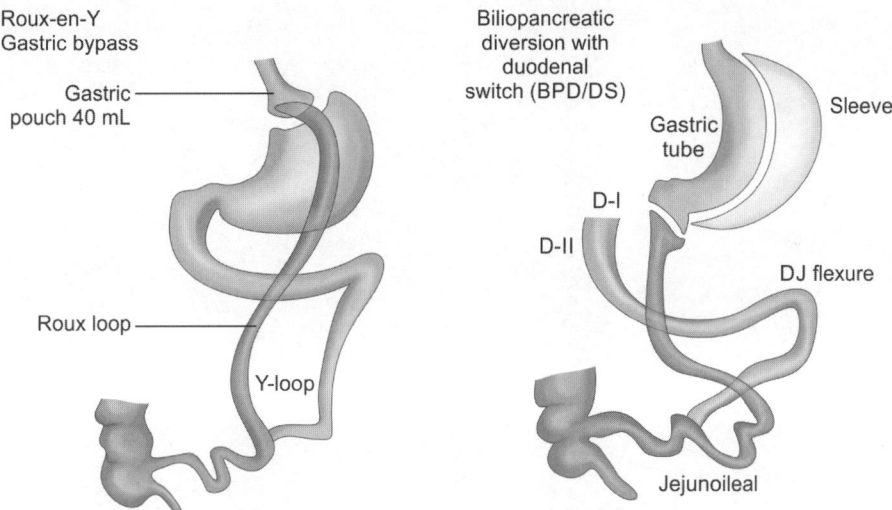

Fig.16.5: Malabsorptive procedures in bariatric surgery.

Complications of Obesity Surgery

Complications

- ***Immediate complications***
  - High risk surgery in obese patients: Including cardiac and thromboembolic accidents. Complications of laparoscopy and anesthesia
  - Electrolyte disturbances
  - Anastomotic leaks and fistulae
  - Sepsis

- ***Long-term complications***
  - Diarrhea
  - Nutritional deficiency: Vitamin B12, iron, minerals, protein calorie, cirrhosis, osteoporosis

- ***Long-term management includes***
  - Preoperative counseling and advice
  - Regular follow up
  - Nutrition, hemopoietic parameters, liver function and electrolyte.

Table 16.3: Biliopancreatic diversion with duodenal switch gastric bypass (BPD/DS).

Sleeve gastrectomy to create tubular stomach (A)	To restrict intake Removes ghrelin secretion	Restricts calories, and digestion anorexia
First part of duodenum divided (B)	Stomach contents don't go through duodenum and jejunum	No digestion with bile and pancreatic juice. No absorption of calories and nutrients from proximal gut
Ileum is divided—proximal (C) and distal end (D)		
Distal end (D) is anastomosed to stomach (A)	Gastric contents enter distal ileum bypassing biliary and pancreatic juice. Instead stimulate leptin and GLP secretion	No digestion and less calorie absorption decrease in the absorption of calories and nutrients (particularly protein and fat, fat soluble vitamins)
Proximal ileal end (C) is anastomosed to distal ileum	Biliopancreatic secretions enter distal ileum	Facilitates enterohepatic absorption of bile salts and nutrients, vitamin e.g., B12. Also stimulates L cells to secrete GLP-1

Chapter 17: Trauma

SU17.1	Describe the principles of first aid.
SU17.2	Demonstrate the steps in basic life support (BLS). Transport of injured patient in a simulated environment.
SU17.3	Describe the principles in management of mass casualties.
SU17.4	Describe pathophysiology, mechanism of head injuries.
SU17.5	Describe clinical features for neurological assessment and GCS in head injuries.
SU17.6	Chose appropriate investigations and discuss the principles of management of head injuries.
SU17.7	Describe the clinical features of soft tissue injuries. Choose appropriate investigations and discuss the principles of management.
SU17.8	Describe the pathophysiology of chest injuries.
SU17.9	Describe the clinical features and principles of management of chest injuries.
SU17.10	Demonstrate airway maintenance. Recognize and manage tension pneumothorax, hemothorax and flail chest in simulated environment.

SU17.1: Trauma and principles of first aid.

SU17.2: Demonstrate the steps in basic life support. Practical class.

Questions:
1. What are the basic principles of first aid?
2. What is "time line" concept in trauma care?
3. What are the steps of first aid. Describe "primary survey".

- **Trauma**—injury—major cause of death and main among younger population.
- **External force causing injury to the body**
  - Accidental
  - Intentional—violence or war
- **Mode of Injury:**
  - Mechanical/thermal/electrical/sonic/light/electromagnetic
  - Chemical/radiation.
- **Impact (Table 17.1):** Depends on intensity and mechanism of trauma and patient factors like age, general health and comorbidities.

Q. What are the basic principles of first aid?

Principles of first aid
It is essentially providing basic trauma life support (BTLS)
- Preserve life—save life resuscitate
- Prevent suffering—pain relief, control bleeds if possible

Table 17.1: Implications of trauma and importance in treatment.

Implications	Importance to the trauma team	Action to save life
Immediate death	–	If possible
Possible early death	Immediate care and prevent death, primary survey	Resuscitate and immediate action
Late death due to secondary complications	Sustain resuscitation and secondary survey	Continue above and plan treatment

- Prevent further Injury—resuscitate and evaluate—shift to trauma care center
- Promote recovery—prevent secondary complications.

Remember

- Life can be saved with timely life support in a majority of cases.
- Most limbs can be saved.
- Outcome is directly related to the speed of providing support and type of injury (e.g., the interval between trauma and death is shortest in airway blockage followed by intra-abdominal bleed, intra-thoracic bleed, intracranial hematoma, and ischemic limbs respectively.
- Initial asessment of injury and associated non-traumatic comorbidities (elderly or diseased) are also deciding factors.

Q. What is "time line" concept in trauma care?

Timeline: The concept of timeline is decisive in trauma management in outcome. Assessment and response should be over within the timeline of a specified trauma for best outcomes—to save life and to prevent irreversible damage or permanent disability.

The first aid providers are generally not doctors or nurses (barring exceptions) and they cannot prescribe medicine nor can declare a death.

Their job is to:
- Assess the situation and act quickly.
- Ask for help—call for an ambulance/hospital.
- Safety for the trauma victim and self
- Shift the injured to a safe place—hospital or a care faciltiy
- Record events and report to authority.

Q. What are the steps of first aid? Describe "primary survey".

Steps

Emergency Medical Services (EMS)

History—from the victim or from an eye witness
- Assessment—examination—all injuries and victim's condition
- Stabilization and monitoring
- Treatment—until medical team arrives
- Transportation (shift) to hospital, call the doctor—under monitoring.

Primary Survey

To **find and act** on immediate threats to life "ABCDE"
- Airway and cervical spine
- Breathing and ventilation
- Circulation and bleeding control
- Disability—mainly neurological
- Exposure to environment.

Airway

Ensuring a patent airway saves many a life. This could be:
- Tongue falling—pulling it off the throat.
- Clearing the throat of secretions.
- Positioning of the patient (head down, lateral or prone) may help.
- Endotracheal intubation (if trained).
- Tube cricothyrotomy.
- Needle tracheotomy.

Breathing

- Pneumothorax—identify breathlessness and immobility of a hemithorax.
- Needle decompression—2nd space mid clavicuar or 4th space—mid axillary line
- Tube thoracostomy (intercostal drainage) in the hospital.

Chapter 17: Trauma

Hemorrhage
- Control with pressure, tamponade, elevation, tourniquets to limbs
- Maintain circulation with an intravenous line and saline drip on the way to hospital.

CPR – Cardiopulmonry Resuscitation
- External cardiac massage 60 to 65 per minute
- Synchronised with mouth to mouth breathing—4:1 ratio.

Immobilizing the Patient
Avoid further damage while transporting the patient:
- Avoid flexing the neck and stabilize it with a splint in head and neck injuries;
- Splinting of limbs, chest and back.

The first aid team provides the record of its account to the trauma team for further management (on site or in trauma centre).

Advanced trauma life support (ATLS) protocol follows—once the patient reaches the trauma center.

> **SU17.3:** Describe the principles in management of mass casualties.

MASS CASUALTIES

Causes
- Natural disasters (flood, cyclones or tsunami or earthquake)
- Accidents—train or road accidents, air crash.
- Man made disasters like, terror acts.
- Wars (separately dealt with)

Need coordinated efforts of medical team, civil administration, police, fire and disaster management force.

Problems
- Large number of casualties—requiring care and help—medical and basic humanitarian needs like food, water and shelter.
- Accessibility of the site of disaster
- Infrastructure—loss of road, communication, power, and more.
- Action—the availability and readiness of the team, ability to reach and provide care, limitation of the peripheral centres and financial constraints.

Standard Principles of Action
Establish chain of command and communication. Assess the gravity of damage. Act fast to minimize loss of life. Triage of the victims and start emergency treatment (see below) concurrently with evacuation of victims from the site.

Mobilize resources and coordinate with relief agencies.

How to Manage?
Casualties are Generally in Four Groups
1. Dead
2. Immediate threat to life
3. Major injuries
4. Minor injuries

Coordination is important to achieve the best within the *time line of injuries*.
- Priority—the primary purpose of triaging.
- Respective specialities are involved as per the triage recommendations.
- Evacuation of the victims to safety—by air or road ambulances.

Coordination with security and transport along with good communication between the leader and respective team heads is crucial.

> **Q. What are the triage categories in situations of mass casualties?**

Triage categories—four

Red-I: Immediate treatment can save life
Yellow-II: Urgent treatment—within hours can save life
Green-III: No urgency—can wait for hours before treatment (lower priority)
Black-IV: Moribund—unlikely to benefit from treatment–death imminent.

Record and report the triage categories—for legal and management purpose.

Evacuation of victims to peripheral hospitals.

Treatment
- **First aid**—wound dressing, splinting or minor suturing.
Tetanus prophylaxis—toxoid and anti-tetanus globulin—500 mg intramuscular.

- **Life saving interventions:** To prevent further deterioration before shifting to centers with definitive care.
  - For example, endotracheal intubation, tracheostomy
  - Intercostal tube to drain hemothorax, or to release air from pneumothorax release of compartment pressure
  - Pericardiocentesis—for cardiac tamponade
  - Fasciotomy in limb or drain in abdomen, controlling the bleeding points.
- **Surgery for non-life-threatening injuries:** Wound toilet, debridement and suturing; reduction and splinting of fractures.
- **Definitive treatment:** With respect to the specific injuries of respective organs and systems under respective specialities.

WAR SURGERY: MASS INJURIES DUE TO WAR (CONFLICTS)

- Small group or mass casualties – may include supporting medical teams too.
- Injuries due to transmission of high energy from weapons cause severe degree of tissue destruction and vary in pattern.
- Triage is most important to minimize loss of life with principles of trauma life support and disaster management.

> **Q. Describe the "staged approach in surgery" for war injuries.**

Surgery involves a **staged approach from basic field unit to the speciality center. Medical Team is engaged in multiple role units:**
- **Role I**: Unit for—primary health care, specialised first aid, triage, resuscitation and stabilisation.
- **Role II**: Unit for holding—intermediate level care—mostly inpatient. After casualties are evacuated from primary units.
  - From here, casualties go back to (1) field or (2) are shifted to 3rd level centers (Role III)
  - The unit performs—triage of casualties, resuscitation and treatment of shock.
  - Damage control surgery (DCS) and a limited period admission. Holding when required.
- **Role III**: General speciality level diagnosis and surgery.
- **Role IV**: Definitive care and speciality level surgical facilities away from field.

> **Q. Damage control surgery (DCS). (Short Question)**

DAMAGE CONTROL SURGERY (DCS)

Concept: Staged approach to minimize continued threat to life, thus aiming at restoration of physiology and ensure safe and effective restoration of anatomy.

War trauma is complex (e.g., abdomino-thoracic and vascular trauma) and the facilities in the battle field are inadequate for effective application of treatment including the definitive surgery. The poor condition of casualties due to the hemorrhagic shock, looming sepsis and secondary organ damage, makes victim unfit for the definitive surgery.

A staged approach (proposed by Rotondo et al) has better and improved results than the one stage definitive surgery.

Damage control resuscitation (DCR) runs along with DCS.

The principles of DCR:
- Secure hemostasis
- Transfusions, avoid crystalloids
- controlled (permissive) hypotension
- Management of acute traumatic coagulopathy (ATC)—recognition and correction.

Steps of DCS

- Assessment of severity of injuries
  - Planning DCS and DCR
  - Rapid sequence anesthesia early rewarming
  - Early shifting to the operating room.
- Immediate surgery—limited to save life (laparotomy/thoracotomy): To control bleeding, packing and temporary closure of wounds.
- Continued resuscitation and restoration if physiological and biochemical state.
  - This is done in the ICU.
- Definitive surgery for injuries (re-exploration in theater): This may be done in stages if needed, depending on patient's condition.

The Benefits v/s Harmful Effects of DCS

Selection of cases is important—to avoid under or over application of DCS.

Chapter 17: Trauma 137

Advantages
- Saves life by restoring physiology and limiting damage done by injuries.
- Unsafe surgery is made safer and more effective in an unstable patient.
- Stabilized patent can be shifted to higher level care after initial damage control and stabilization.

Disadvantages
- Requires more time for treatment
- Staged approach requires more resources and staff.

Students are advised to refer to forensic medicine book for blast injuries and bullet injuries.

Neurotrauma

SU17.4: Describe pathophysiology, mechanism of head injuries.

The timely attention and care play a vital role in minimizing the damage from head injuries which are among the most common cause of death and disability.

PATHOPHYSIOLOGY OF HEAD INJURY

- Brain cannot sustain hypoxia for long periods; continuous supply of oxygenated blood is vital.
- Raised intracranial pressure compromises cerebral perfusion and leads to cerebral ischemia, brain swelling and further increase in pressure with brain damage.
- Mean arterial pressure (**MAP**)—90-110 mm Hg
- Intracranial pressure (**ICP**)—5-15 mm Hg
- Cerebral perfusion pressure (**CPP**)—75-105 mm Hg - (**MAP – ICP = CPP**)
- CBF is about 55 mL per minute/100 grams of brain—ischemia results if CBF falls below 20 mL/min.
- CPP is autoregulated by baroreceptors to ensure continuous cerebral blood flow (CBF).

Q. Discuss the compensatory mechanisms to neutralize the raised intracranial pressure. What is the Monro-Kellie doctrine?

Compensatory mechanisms to neutralize the raised pressure lead to further damage.
- **The Monro-Kellie doctrine:** Brain is nearly incompressible and skull is a rigid box.
- Increase in the pressure(ICP) is compensated for by draining out of CSF and venous blood.
- Further increase in ICP will also compromise CBF leading to ischemia and edema of brain.
- Ischemia can lead to cell infarction of part of brain and permanent damage.

Continued increase in ICP leads to herniation of:
- Uncus of temporal lobe through tentorium cerebelli (compressing 3rd cranial nerve) and
- Cerebellar tonsils through foramen magnum—compressing brain stem and respiratory and vasomotor centers of the medulla, causing coning and death.

Coning signs: Cushing's Triad—hypertension, bradycardia and irregular respiration.

Q. Mechanism of increased intracranial pressure following head injuries.

- Primary trauma—causing intracranial bleeding/hematoma.
- Reactionary brain edema following injury and bleed.
- Ischemia of brain due to compensatory decrease in cerebral perfusion pressure and oxygenation.
- Secondary changes—that follow trauma
  - Increase in size intracranial hematoma, brain, sepsis.

Q. Classify head injuries based on mechanism of injury.

Mechanism and classification of Head injuries
- **Mechanism of the occurrence of trauma:**
  - **Accelerating**—hit to the static head by a moving object; a moving object hits a person at rest.
  - **Decelerating**—hit against a static object, e.g., hit against a wall or tree in a road traffic accident or hit the floor in a fall.
- **Nature of wound:**
  - **Closed**—injury without an open wound
  - **Open**—injury with an open wound over the head.

Open Head Injuries

- Penetrating injuries (rod/projectile/or a tree branch)
- A blunt injury (fall/hit) - acceleration or deceleration injuries.

These may be with an external wound **with or without a fracture** of skull bone.

Q. What is a contrecoup injury?

Nature of Internal Damage

- **Coupe:** Damage occurs on the side of impact of injury, (e.g. A hit on Rt temporal causes a hematoma on the same side).

- **Contre-coupe:** The damage is sustained by the part of brain on the side opposite to the side of trauma, (e.g. a hit on occiput causes a hematoma in anterior cranial fossa contrary to the expected bleed under the occiput).

TYPES OF HEMATOMAS IN HEAD TRAUMA

Extracranial
- Subcutaneous, subaponeurotic, subgaleal
- Sub-pericranial—usually with a fracture of skull bone.

Intracranial
- Acute extradural (epidural)—rupture of vein or artery
- Acute subdural hematoma—venous bleed or an underlying brain hematoma.

Intraparenchymal Hemorrhage
- **Intracerebral/cerebellar/brainstem hematoma**—associated with severe brain injury.
- **Intraventricular hemorrhage:** Lateral ventricles/third or fourth ventricle. Always associated with brain injury.

An open wound provides access to the external physical and microbial contaminants and it has an increased risk of intracranial infection.

Q. Black Eye. (Short note question)

Collection of blood around the orbit in subcutaneous plane in the periorbital loose areolar tissue.

Causes
- Unilateral black eye—orbital fractures
- Bilateral black eye—subgaleal hemorrhage, fracture of base of skull—ethmoidal and sphenoidal fractures.

Differential diagnosis: Sub conjunctival hemorrhage.

Pathology of Intracranial Hemorrhage

Acute Extradural Hematoma (EDH)
Between skull and dura. Due to rupture of an artery, vein or venous sinus—commonly they have a skull fracture.

There is an initial hemorrhage—contained, followed by:
- Compensatory mechanism to control ICP (Monro-Kellie doctrine)
- A delayed decompensation and rapid deterioration.

Q. The lucid interval. (Short note question)

Lucid interval: The period between the initial impact and decompensatory state is the compensated state, which is called the lucid interval. Initial loss of consciousness followed an apparent normal state erroneously thought to be post-concessional state but followed by rapid deterioration due to enlarging extradural hematoma.

Acute Subdural Hematoma (A-SDH)

Caused by ruptured vessels of cortical surface of brain, following an accelerating or decelerating injury. Significant associated brain injury is always present.

The loose subdural space allows the hematoma to expand of over the brain surface leading to raised ICP and rapid deterioration similar to extradural hematoma. But, there is no lucid interval.

Acute subarachnoid hemorrhage: They bleed into CSF or may form a localized hematoma these are mistaken for a spontaneous (aneurysmal) subarachnoid hemorrhage and collapse.

Q. Chronic subdural hematoma. (Short Question)

CHRONIC SUBDURAL HEMATOMA (C-SDH)

Usually seen in elderly with a trivial injury which is often forgotten. The atrophic brain causes stretching of veins between cortex and dura, which rupture easily in trauma. Also anticoagulant therapy, if any makes them more vulnerable.

There is a contained small hematoma in subdural space which liquefies over next two weeks and fails to undergo resolution.

This is followed by:
- Osmotic absorption of fluid into the collection over the weeks or months into an expanding

intracranial collection causing neurological deterioration.
- Chronic subdural hematomas actually a misnomer as contains fluid more than blood.

Cerebral Contusion
- Parts of brain in contact with the skull are vulnerable to contusions;
- For example, inferior temporal or frontal lobes—abutting the anterior or middle fossae.
- May be coup or contrecoup
- The contusion resolves over 7 o 10 days; but may cause brain edema and raised ICP.
- Cerebral dysfunction, varying from confusion to coma—seen during this period.

Diffuse Axonal Injury

It is a primary brain injury—without obviously visible changes.

Clinical states following head injuries (described in the next section).

> SU17.5: Describe clinical features for neurological assessment and GCS in head injuries.
> SU17.6: Choose appropriate investigations and discuss the principles of management of head injuries.

Other Questions
1. Describe Glasgow Coma Score (GCS).
2. Discuss pathogenesis of head injury
3. Describe the principles of treatment of head injury.

CLINICAL ASSESSMENT OF HEAD INJURY

History

From a conscious patient (not always possible) or eyewitness to the injury.
- Mechanism of injury, time and place.
- Loss of consciousness, vomiting, seizures, headache.
- Previous episodes and illness.

Primary Survey

ABC—airway, breathing and circulation—must be ensured.

- Record vital signs—pulse rate, respiration and blood pressure
- Look for general condition and
- Blood sugar levels checked for hypoglycemia
- Check pupil size and response
- Glasgow Coma Scale score
- Check for focal neurological deficits—as soon as possible.

Secondary survey—after initial stabilization of patient (refer below).

Intubation is done if necessary.

Suture the external wounds and control bleeding.

> **Q. Describe Glasgow Coma Score.**

Described in **Table 17.2**.

Glasgow Coma Scale—Total score: E-1-4, V-1-5, M-1-6 = 15 (Table 17.2)

Remember: In Head Injuries
- **Tachycardia and/or hypotension**—indicate bleeding in abdomen, chest or a major fracture.
- **Bradycardia and hypertension** - warns of intracranial bleed.

Further Management: Investigation and Specific Management

After primary survey and basic management, head injury is classified as per GCS and injuries evaluate blood parameters for —coagulopathies, hemodynamics, and system functions.

CT head—plain study:
- For GCS below 13 at presentation and below 15 after 2 hours
- Repeated vomiting, seizures, loss of balance
- Fractures—skull and spine
- Focal neurological deficit
- Retrograde amnesia of over 30 minutes
- CSF rhinorrhea, nasal bleed blood in ear, bilateral black eye
- Senior citizens
- High velocity injuries or fall from high levels
- Suspected lucid interval.

Hospitalization indicated—for all moderate and severe injuries

Table 17.2: Glasgow Coma Scale scoring.

Eyes		Verbal response		Motor response	
Open spontaneously	4	Normally oriented and converses	5	Obeys commands	6
To verbal command	3	Confused	4	Localizes to pain	5
To painful stimulus	2	Inappropriate/words only	3	Withdrawal/flexion	4
Do not open	1	Sounds only	2	Abnormal flexion	3
		No sounds	1	Extension	2
				No motor response	1
		Intubated patient	T		

Classification of head injuries – after Glasgow Coma Scale (GCS) Score	
Minor	GCS 15 with no loss of consciousness (LOC)
Mild	GCS 14 or 15 with LOC
Moderate	GCS 9–13
Severe	GCS 3–8

- Mild injuries—with vomiting, seizures, loss of balance, continues drowsiness.

Secondary Survey

A thorough search made for injuries missed before resuscitation.
- Depressed fractures, skull base fractures, bleed from nose, ear.
- Bruise over mastoid area Battle's sign, eye and periorbital areas.

Assess for other associated injuries
- Particularly cervical spine and entire spine
- Abdomen and thorax
- Major limb fractures.

Late CT scans—after 8 hours/2 days/3 weeks to watch for and identify secondary changes and resolving or expanding subdural hematomas.

MRI—helps in picking a SDH better than CT, which may not pick a hematoma small and close to inflamed dura.

Q. Describe the principles of treatment of head injury.

PRINCIPLES OF TREATMENT OF HEAD INJURY

- Assess and classify initial damage—evaluate, history, GCS score and CT
- Prevent secondary brain damage—and facilitate recovery

    Primarily by preventing rise in intracranial pressure (ICP) that leads to ischemia by reducing cerebral perfusion pressure (CPP).

Medical Management

- Under active monitoring with GCS scores and scans as needed.
- It is instituted in concussions, contusions and most small subarachnoid bleeds
- Also in CSF rhinorrhea or otorrhea for 1–2 weeks.
- Control of intracranial pressure
  - Diuresis—mannitol.
  - Steroids—dexamethasone.
  - Avoid hypotonic solutions (against brain swelling)

Surgery

- Surgical intervention
  - To reduce ICP—decompressive drainage of collections and ventricles.
  - To evacuate hematomas—EDH, SDH, intraparenchymal clots
  - To control hemorrhage
  - Depressed fractures—to elevate or remove part of depressed skull fracture.
  - Continued CSF rhinorrhea or otorrhea to prevent meningitis.

  Urgent intervention
  - If patient develops signs of raised ICP—continuing or worsening of headache, vomiting, seizures, focal neurological deficits, falling consciousness levels, worsening of GCS score.
  - CT or MRI evidence of expanding intracranial clots.

- Control of seizures:
  - Phenytoin and/or levatiracetam.
- Watch for pituitary dysfunction—and sodium and water imbalance.
  - Syndrome of inappropriate antidiuretic hormone (SIADH)—common after head injuries—leads to hyponatremia due to water retention.
  - Watch for hypernatremia due to deficiency of antidiuretic hormone (ADH)
- Analgesia—acetaminophen or a NSAID. Opioids are generally avoided.
- Nutrition
- **Antibiotics:** For open head injuries, CSF rhinorrhea/otorrhea.

Definitive treatment is instituted as per the clinical state and specific injuries:

Clinical States after Head Injuries

Concussion
- No demonstrable brain damage. Cerebral function suspended for a short period.
- Clinical features
- Loss of consciousness—a few seconds to minutes.
- Vomiting, vertigo, headache, seizures.

Amnesia—memory loss.
Post traumatic amnesia—variable duration after initial loss of consciousness.
Retrograde amnesia—loss of memory for the period preceding trauma.
- Longer the retrograde amnesia worse is the long-term recovery.

Brain Contusions
Pathology discussed in the previous section.
- Expectant management with monitoring.
- Surgical decompression to reduce ICP.
- To evacuate a resolving intraparenchymal bleed to reduce brain edema.

> **Q. Acute extradural hematoma (pathology discussed in previous section). (Long answer question)**

Lucid interval
- Pathology discussed in previous section under extradural hematoma
- Typically seen in about 30 to 40% of acute extradural hematomas

Clinical features
- Initial loss of consciousness., seizures, vomiting.
- **Lucid Interval:** Recovery to near normal state—there may be headache mistaken as post concussion effect; there is no clinical neurological deficit.
  - This is due to compensation of ICP by Monro-Kellie doctrine.
- This is followed by rapid deterioration (Decompensation and raised ICP)
  - Falling level of consciousness
  - Contralateral hemiparesis due to expanding hematoma shifting the brain to opposite side
  - Ipsilateral papillary constriction followed by dilatation (3rd nerve at tentorial herniation)
  - Coning (Cushing's triad) of hypertension, bradycardia and irregular respiration.
  - Comatose state.

Lucid interval is also seen in psychiatric patients, who are normal between episodes of exaggeration of mental deterioration.

Treatment—1. Immediate evacuation by burr hole or craniectomy; 2. Sealing the bleeding vessel.
Prognosis—very good with timely intervention.

Acute Subdural Hematoma
- Generally *severe underlying brain injury*
- Profound loss of consciousness and rapid deterioration of clinical state
- No lucid interval seen
- Localizing signs—may or may not be present
- *CT-* shows crescentic hyperdense shadow (hypodense in chronic SDH)
- *Small SDHs* are managed by expectant treatment for spontaneous resolution.

Emergency Evacuation
- In case of neurological deterioration and in large hematomas.
- Craniotomy or craniectomy needed to control bleeding and secondary brain damage.
- Prognosis related to primary brain injury.

> **Q. Chronic subdural hematoma. (Short notes)**

- Generally seen in elderly persons, often taking anticoagulants or antiplatelet drigs and who have a shrunken brain. A minor head injury causes a small hematoma which enlarges slowly by osmosis of fluid from vessels.
- After weeks or months, (uncommonly even after years) of the trauma, they deteriorate
- Variable fluctuating levels of consciousness

- Behavioral changes mistaken for depression or mental illness
- Phase of decompensation—with deterioration of consciousness
  - Focal deficits followed by coma.
- CT—a crescentic hypodense shadow (hyperdense in acute subdural hematoma)

Treatment
- Needs urgent evacuation.
- Burr hole or craniectomy.

Prognosis is excellent.

Interdisciplinary Procedures

- CSF rhinorrhea/otorrhea—may need ENT surgeon's for microscopic procedures.
- Hemotympanum—to be evacuated in petrous bone fractures.

Sequelae of Head Injuries

- Postconcussive syndrome
- Headache, memory and cognitive impairments
- **Rehabilitation**—multi-disciplinary approach.

SU17.7: SOFT TISSUE TRAUMA.

Short question
1. What are the severity grades of soft tissue injury?
2. What is "PRICE" protocol in soft tissue injuries?
3. What is "no HARM" protocol?

Q. What are the severity grades of soft tissue injury.

Soft Tissue Injury: Types, Causes and Treatment

Soft tissue trauma refers to injuries to the muscles, nerves, ligaments and tendons (soft tissues of the limbs and pelvis).

Short Question

Types based on severity: Grade 1, Grade 2 or Grade 3
- Grade 1:
  - Tissue fibres get overstretched
  - Pain and swelling. Heal over a period of time with rest and symptomatic treatment
- Grade 2: Partial tear of fibers
  - Pain, swelling and partial disability
  - Healing time is 6 weeks to 12 weeks
  - Treatment: Rest and symptomatic treatment
- Grade 3: Total rupture of the soft tissue.

The injuries may be:
- Penetrating,
- Blunt impact
- Crushing

The injuries may cause:
- A contusion, and hematoma
- Profuse hemorrhage and shock
- Vascular injuries
- Nerve injuries
- Secondary complications
  - Compartment syndromes
  - Vascular occlusion and gangrene
    - Arterial thrombosis
    - Venous thrombosis.
  - Myoglobinemia and acute kidney injury.
  - Infections—gas gangrene and tetanus
- Long-term
  - Lymphedema venous insufficiency
  - Secondary arterial insufficiency.
- Loss of limb function (muscle/joint).

Approach to Soft Tissue Trauma

Primary Survey

- Emergency first aid and assessment
- Resuscitation along ATLS guidelines—ABCDE: Airway with cervical spine precautions; Breathing, Circulation, Disability, Exposure.

Secondary Survey

- The secondary survey is the identification of all injuries via a head-to-toe examination.
- The history mnemonic—AMPLE - T:
  - Allergies, Medication, Prior medical history, Last meal, Events leading to the injury, T-tetanus immunization.
- This is followed by a regional examination starting from the head and face including all parts of body extremities.
- Evaluation and treatment of associated injuries.

Tertiary Survey—Done 24 hours after Admission

This is to detect the injuries that may have been missed earlier. It requires a repetition of the primary and secondary surveys and of all laboratory and imaging studies.

SOFT TISSUE INJURIES

- Subcutaneous
- Subfascial
- Ligament injuries—with or without instability of joint
- Vascular injuries
- Nerve injuries.

Muscle Injuries

- Gr I—strains—a stretch or a tear at junction with tendon—tenderness present
- Gr II—direct injury to muscle against a bone—damaging fascia, muscle and blood vessel. Contusion of muscle with an intra or intermuscular hematoma or hemorrhage
- Gr III—complete disruption of muscle. The muscle avulsion may be with arterial or venous tear or an expanding hematoma leading to distal ischemia and gangrene of limb.

Nerve Injuries

The reader is referred to orthopedics textbook for details.

> **Q. What is PRICE protocol in soft tissue injuries? What is no HARM protocol?**

Management of Soft Tissue Injuries

PRICE Protocol

- **P**rotection
- **R**est
- **I**ce—for cooling and hemostasis
- **C**ompression and containing hematoma
- **E**levation

No HARM protocol:
NOT DONE in first 72 hours of injury:

- **H**eat—increases bleeding and worsens hematoma
- **A**lcohol—affects pain perceptions and patient worsens, unawares.
- **R**e-injury—any activity aggravating the injury.
- **M**assage—adds more damage.

Severe pain after 24 hours needs evaluation.

- Nerve conduction studies help to differentiate myopathy from neuropathy; localize nerve dysfunction, e.g., carpal tunnel syndrome and to assess severity/prognosis.
- Magnetic resonance imaging (MRI), for imaging soft tissue is useful but has high false positive rate.
- Ultrasonography for muscle hematoma
- Doppler study for detecting to assess venous thrombosis or arterial occlusion.

Specific Treatment for Soft Tissue Injuries

Contusion of muscle: Rest and compression with elevation of extremity under.

- Active observation for worsening.
- Antibiotic if there is any open wound.
- Tetanus prophylaxis.

Surgery: To let out the hematoma in case of:

- Nerve or vessel injury or compression.
- Expanding hematoma and signs of compartment syndrome.
- Significant distal neurological or vascular deficit, and loss of function.
- Signs of infection.

Muscle lacerations

- Immediate exploration, evacuation of hematoma and suturing.
- Associated vascular injury and nerve injuries are managed as needed.

Compartment syndrome

Immediate exploration to evacuate hematoma and adequate multiple fasciotomies.

Nerve injuries

- Primary repair for neurotmesis after evacuation of hematoma.
- Evacuation of hematoma only for injuries with intact nerve sheath.

Arterial injuries: Refer chapter on vascular injuries.

- Angiography is performed to check for any arterial disruption.
- Periarterial hematomas evacuated and artery repaired.

Venous injuries are difficult to manage as they are prone for thrombosis—of deep veins.

- Heparinization is required to prevent any deep venous thrombosis.

Chest Trauma

> 17.8 and 17.9 are discussed together in continuity.
> 17.10 is DOAP session to be learnt in wards.
> Principles of management of pneumothorax, hemothorax and flail chest are briefly discussed.

PATHOPHYSIOLOGY OF CHEST INJURIES

Chest injuries may be isolated or more often with injuries to other organs—spine, abdomen, head, neck and extremities.

Junctional Zones

- Thorax and root of neck
- Thorax, diaphragm and abdomen.

All chest injuries are managed along ATLS guidelines first aid, BTLS, triage and ATLS.

Mechanism

Penetrating
- Trauma—criminal acts like—stabs. Accidental fall or penetration of sharp objects.
- War injuries—bullet and bionet injuries.

Blunt
- Road accidents—steering wheel injures, entrapment between the vehicles
- Fall from height
- Crush injuries as in disasters—earthquakes, entrapment under a collapsed building
- Mob violence—with blunt weapons.

Types of Injuries

- **Contusions** of lung, pericardium. Myocardium—due to compressive force from broken rib cage or sternum).
- **Lacerations**.

Classification of Injuries (Anatomy Based)

Chest wall—contusions or laceration
- Rib cage—rib fractures—single/multiple
  - Flail chest

Thoracic contents
- Lung—contusion or laceration.
- Bronchus—avulsion or tear

- Mediastinum
- Pericardial hematoma and tamponade
- Heart—penetrating wounds and contusions to myocardium
- Aortic arch and thoracic aorta
- Superior vena cava and innominate veins.
- Inferior vena cava and azygos vein—tear
- Thoracic duct—disruption
- Esophagus—tear, laceration, rupture or disruption.

Diaphragm
- Rupture or tear along with herniation of abdominal organs.
- Common to see associated injuries to liver or spleen and abdominal viscera.

Classification of Chest Injuries

American College of Surgeons Committee on Trauma based on the impact of chest injuries linked to their clinical morbidities:
- Immediately life threatening
- Potentially life threatening

> **Q.** The deadly dozen of chest injuries (ACS–committee on trauma).

Refer **Table 17.3** for the "deadly dozen" of chest injuries.

Morbid physiology of chest injuries—depends on type of injury and organ involved.

Table 17.3: The deadly dozen of chest injuries (ACS committee on trauma).

Immediately life threatening	Potentially life threatening
Airway obstruction Pericardial tamponade Tension pneumothorax Massive hemothorax Open pneumothorax Flail chest	Aortic injuries Myocardial contusion Tracheo-bronchial injuries Rupture of diaphragm Esophageal injuries Pulmonary contusion
Detected during primary survey and managed as emergency	**Detected during secondary survey and managed accordingly**

Immediate Dangers and Complications

- **Acute cardiac arrest**—vasovagal impact of injury to chest.
- **Hypoxia** and CO_2 retention (hypercarbia)
  - Caused by respiratory distress due to airway obstruction
  - Compressive force of a fractured rib cage
  - Hemothorax, pneumothorax
  - Tension pneumothorax with or without an open sucking wound
  - Flail chest
  - A traumatic diaphragmatic hernia.
- **Hypovolemic/hemorrhagic shock**—due to blood loss—great vessels or pulmonary.
- **Acidosis:** Respiratory acidosis followed by metabolic acidosis.

Intermediate and Secondary and Late Complications

- Cardiac arrhythmias
- Septic complications
  - Infection of blood by bronchial or esophageal contents or external matter
  - Empyema, lung abscess, bronchopleural fistula
- Mediastinitis
- Esophageal fistula.

Clinical Features of an Internal Bleeding

Source of bleeding: External injury, thoracic, abdominal, pelvic and extremities.

History

- Penetrating injury—stab or missile/bullet
- Overt and continuous bleeding
- Injury site close to major vessel.

Signs of Bleeding

- Rising pulse rate, low pulse volume
- Falling systolic blood pressure, later diastolic too
- Rising respiratory rate
- Low urine output
- Lactic acidosis (serum lactate levels).

Management

First aid, basic life support, assessment, stabilisation, investigation, specific treatment.

Initial Treatment

- ATLS principles of ABCDE
- Airway, breathing, circulation, disability (neurology), environment and exposure of patient.

Investigations: In Emergency Room

- Blood—hemoglobin, hematocrit, blood group.
  Blood gas analysis—for arterial gas levels PaO_2 and $PaCO_2$ and acidosis.
  Tests for vital organ functions—heart, liver, kidney
- Ultrasound—e-FAST
  Extended focused assessment with sonography for trauma (eFAST)
  For quick and accurate detection of:
  - **Hemopericardium**
  - Hemothorax (blood in pleura), hemopericardium and hemomediastinum. Abdomen—subdiaphragmatic, paracolic and pelvis
  - Diaphragmatic tears and hernia
  - Liver and splenic tears/contusions
  - Free air.
- **Chest X-ray**—can help diagnose pneumothorax, hemothorax and rib fractures. But can be confusing too, as it is taken in supine position.

> **Q. Intercostal drain under water (tube thoracostomy). (Short note)**
>
> - Through the 4th intercostal space mid axillary space
> - Indication—an unstable patient—when in doubt
> - Diagnostic to find and measure bleeding
> - Therapeutic and life saving
> - In massive hemothorax
> - Tension pneumothorax
> - X-ray or e-FAST shows free gas or fluid in pleural cavity

CT scan of chest and abdomen—at the earliest. Most useful, to detect tears of major structures, fractures and collections as well as air.

CT angiography—for detecting (and controlling) focal bleeding in a stabilized patient in preparation for thoracotomy.

Conservative Management of Chest Injuries

- 80% managed with a tube thoracostomy and resuscitative support to tackle bleeding, collections and free air.
- Sucking open chest wound: These are not closed until a tube thoracostomy is performed to prevent converting a pneumothorax into a tension pneumothorax.
- Monitor—hemodynamics, blood gases, output.
- Analgesia—NSAID. Opiates avoided unless neurotrauma is excluded.
- Antibiotics—usually cloxacillin + penicillin or broad spectrum.
- Tetanus prophylaxis—ATG 500 mg intramuscular and tetanus toxoid subcutaneously.
- Oxygen—nasally or endotracheal.

Thoracotomy (or Sternotomy)

- Emergency room surgery—thoracotomy/sternotomy (for mediastinal structures)
- Planned (semi-elective) thoracotomy or sternotomy—refer below.

Q. Emergency department thoracotomy (EDT). (Short note)

Emergency department thoracotomy (EDT)
- Also called resuscitative thoracotomy.
- Required in about 20% of cases.

Goals
- Internal cardiac massage—for cardiac arrest during resuscitation or
  - Before entry to emergency room.
- Relieve cardiac tamponade
- Control of intrathoracic hemorrhage—heart, lung, vessels or abdominal bleed in chest.
- Control of air leaks
- Restoration of cardiac output—by cross-clamping the thoracic aorta
  - To sustain blood supply to heart and brain and to control bleed from distal source

Indications for EDT: Emergency department thoracotomy
- Over 1500 cc blood drained at first insertion of intercostal drainage (ICD) tube. Subsequent bleeding in excess of 200 mL/hour for three hours.
- Penetrating trauma with unstable hemodynamics—systolic pressure 60 mm Hg or less.
- Hemopericardium and pericardial (cardiac) tamponade.
- Major vessel injuries if patient is unstable.
- To cross clamp thoracic aorta—to sustain blood to heart and brain and to control distal bleed—abdominal or lower limbs.

Any stabilized patient is shifted to a major operation theatre for a more planned (semi) emergency thoracotomy (sternotomy and laparotomy if need be).

Indications
Potentially life threatening conditions
- Open pneumothorax (with bleed)
- Tracheobronchial trauma
- Diaphragmatic hernia
- Esophageal perforation
- Thoracic duct tear
- Associated liver and splenic trauma.

Planned Thoracotomy

Goals
- Definitive correction of specific injuries—depends on the organ injured.
- Treatment of complications.

Indications
- Bronchopleural fistula, esophageal fistula, persistent chylothorax, empyema thoracis
- Collapse of lung, stove in chest.

Q. Short notes on VATS (video assisted thoracoscopic surgery) in chest trauma.

Indications
- Retained hemothorax or pneumothorax
- Persistent air leak
- Post-traumatic emphysema, after a properly placed intercostal drainage tube
- Drainage of lung abscess, and early empyema
- Removal of foreign body
- Diagnostic uncertainty.

Not indicated in life threatening emergency situations.

Treatment for specific conditions—discussed next section.

Rehabilitation

Physiotherapy
Follow up for late complication.

Specific Problems after Chest Trauma
- Rib fracture
- Flail chest
- Pneumothorax and hemothorax
- Tension pneumothorax
- Post-traumatic empyema
- Post-traumatic lung abscess.

Medical complications (excluded from this discussion)
- Pneumonitis, acute respiratory distress syndrome (ARDS), air embolism
- Coagulopathies—disseminated intravascular coagulation (DIC).

Q. Rib fractures. (Short answer question)

Common after blunt trauma.

Sites
- At the point of traumatic impact,
- Angles of ribs, costochondral junction and costovertebral articulation.

Unilateral or bilateral or with sternum and or thoracic spine
- Single rib or multiple ribs
- Single site or multiple sites

Impact—local—hematoma
- Underlying lung contusion or tear with air leak.
- Damage to intercostal vessels causing hemothorax.

Complications
- Atelectasis and pneumonia, late abscess
- Pneumothorax, hemothorax or hemopneumothorax
- Tension pneumothorax
- Empyema thoracis
- Upper ribs—1 and 2—injury to subclavian vessels and brachial plexus
- Lower ribs—injury to diaphragm, liver, spleen
- Multiple fractures—flail chest (see next section).

Clinical Features
- Pain, swelling and tenderness. Subcutaneous emphysema—crunchy feel of subcutaneous air (crepitus) if there is a lung tear with air leak
- Breathlessness and absence of breath sounds case of pneumothorax
- Chest X-ray and CT are diagnostic.

Treatment
- Single or two ribs—analgesia, oral or thoracic epidural analgesia—infusion and chest physiotherapy.
- The intercostals muscles act as splints and no further treatment is necessary.
- Tube thoracostomy intercostal drainage tube (ICD)—for a large hemo or pneumothorax.
- Surgery—to control of bleeding intercostal vessel or suturing of an open wound.

Q. Flail chest. (Short Answer question)

Flail chest a life threatening emergency condition.

Definition: A condition with an unstable segment of chest wall due to fracture of three or more ribs at at least two sites in each of them. Commonly associated with a pneumothorax too.

Types
- **Lateral** - over shafts of ribs—most common—lateral impact of any blunt trauma—accidents, falls, violence. May be from 2nd to 10th ribs (11 and 12 are floating ribs).
- **Central (Anterior) flail**-bilateral rib fractures with sternum making the flail segment—fractures are generally the costochondral junction. Common in steering wheel injuries.
- **Posterior**—underlying the scapula—generally missed
- **Unilateral**—most common
- **Bilateral**—not uncommon in severe trauma.

Pathophysiology and Morbid Respiratory Physics of Flail Chest

Normally each rib is held together by intercostal muscles—above and below the rib making it move synchronously with respiratory excursions as a cohesive unit of ribs.

Rib cage moves out with inspiration and inwards with expiration.

Flail chest: When more than two ribs break at more than one site each, the intervening segment becomes unstable, separated from the rest of the rib cage. *This is the flail segment.*

Complications

Central flail poses the greatest threat to life due to cardiac arrest or later arrhythmias, injury to heart, great vessels, trachea and bronchi.

Lateral flail: *Paradoxical respiration*—the unstable flail segment moves in passively at inspiration and outward at expiration.

Pendulum movement (of air) lung shrinks with inspiration and the deoxygenated air enters the opposite normal lung (instead of the oxygenated inspiratory air) causing further deoxygenation. The lung expands with expiration, drawing the expiratory air of normal lung adding to further deoxygenation. This back and forth movement of air between the two lungs is called the pendulum movement (like that of a wall clock).

This causes hypoxia and hypercarbia—**cyanosis respiratory failure**.

Mediastinal Flutter

- Compensatory hyperinflation of normal lung and collapse of the damaged side lead to sideward movement of mediastinal contents with often kinking of vena cava and drop in cardiac input.
- This causes sudden cardiac arrest.
- An associated tension pneumothorax often worsens displacement of mediastinal veins.

Clinical Features

Diagnosis is clinical and easy with a high degree of suspicion.
- Paradoxical respiration
- Hypoxic patient with underventilation

Confirmation: Contrast enhanced CT scan, a 3-D reconstruction of the chest wall.

Treatment

Principle: Urgent stabilization of the chest wall to prevent abnormal motion and hypoxia.
- *ICD tube insertion* to drain pleural cavity and *analgesia plus respiratory physiotherapy.* For small flails—3 to 4 ribs and stable patient
- *Positive pressure ventilation*—through endotracheal intubation for hypoxic patients despite analgesia and oxygen support.
   - For large lateral flails and bilateral flails
   - Central flails
- Early stabilization of flail (fixing of rib fracture with wiring at two points)—one at the upper most rib and one at the lower most rib. This brings the whole segment in alignment with the rib cage.
- Supportive measures—antibiotic, ICD drainage of hemo and pneumothorax.
- Active monitoring with oxygen supplementation and correction of hypercarbia and cardiac arrhythmias.

Stove in Chest

- A localized segment of rib cage caves into thoracic cavity due to a severe blunt blow (similar to a depressed skull fracture)
- Underlying lung contusion or lacerations.
- Features mimic those of a small flail chest.

Treatment

- To deal with intrathoracic bleeding or pneumothorax
- Fixing of rib fractures
- Physiotherapy to achieve expansion of the lungs and atelectasis/infection.

Post-traumatic: Pneumothorax and Hemothorax

- Often associated with rib fractures
- Uncommon causes include rupture of intra thoracic structures
- Diaphragmatic rupture along with perforation of hollow abdominal viscus.

Diagnosis: Clinical and Imaging

- e-FAST—asses abdomen and chest
- CT–emergency CT–plain or later with contrast case of internal bleeding.

Treatment

General
- ATLS guidelines to support
- Monitor with oxygen.

Specific
- Intercostal drainage through 4th intercostal space midaxillary line to drain a hemopneumothorax.
- A second tube inserted through 2nd space in the mid-clavicular line for pneumothorax.
- Lung physiotherapy.

Interventional radiology in massive hemothorax
- CT Angiographic control of focal bleeding angio-embolization or coils
- Useful as a preoperative step to an otherwise a hemodynamically unstable patient, before a thoracotomy.

Emergency thoracotomy evacuation of hemothorax and control of bleeder.

Antibiotics.

> **Q. Short notes on tension pneumothorax.**

Caused by rent in chest wall or lung due to:
- Chest wound wider than 60% of trachea
- A lung tear in a penetrating or blunt injury.

Other Causes
- Ruptured bulla, cavity (tuberculosis)
- Lung injuries during placement of CVP catheters for monitoring
- Positive pressure ventilation.

Pathophysiology
- Each inspiratory movement causes air to get sucked into the thoracic cavity.
- *The rent is a 'one-way valve' leading to progressive entrapment of air with no exit.*
- The lung collapses completely due to compression by air.
- The mediastinum is pushed to opposite side.
- Results in compression of the opposite lung and kinking of great veins with decrease in cardiac input causing sudden cardiac arrest.

Clinical Features
- Sudden and increasing dyspnea, tachypnea and restlessness.
- Distended neck veins.
- Hyper-resonant hemithorax with absence of breath sounds.
- Tracheal deviation to opposite side.

Diagnosis: X-ray is confirmatory but should not be waited for.

Treatment
Urgent clinical diagnosis and action saves life: Rapid decompression of the hemithorax on affected side by inserting a needle into 2nd intercostal space in the mid-clavicular line. An intercostal drainage tube (tube thoracostomy) is then inserted into the 4th intercostal space in anterior axillary line.

Surgery for Chronic and Recurrent Pneumothorax

Pleurectomy and Pleurodesis

Usually done by video-assisted thoracoscopic surgery (VATS) or an open thoracotomy.

Principles
- To seal any air leaks from the lung
- Obliterate blebs and bullae
- Ensure the adherence of visceral pleura to the parietal pleura
- Prevent the lung from completely collapsing.

Pleural adhesion (pleurodesis)—can be done by any of the following:
- **Pleurectomy:** Stripping the parietal pleura from the chest wall.
- **Pleural abrasion:** To scrape off the surface of the parietal pleura and induce inflammation.
- **Chemical pleurodesis:** Usually talc is used and is insufflated into the chest cavity.

Potentially Life-threatening Injuries

Disruption of Thoracic Aorta
- Common after fall or motor accidents—causes sudden death
- Usually distal to origin of left subclavian artery
- Survivors have an intact adventitial layer and early intervention can save them.

Chest X-ray
- Wide mediastinum
- 3D CT–confirmation.

Treatment
- Endovascular stenting under angiographic control in selected cases or
- Thoracotomy and definitive repair.

Tracheobronchial Injuries
- Severe subcutaneous emphysema, respiratory distress and failure of lung to expand after a chest tube insertion are suspicious.
- Bronchial intubation (normal side) under vision and urgent sternotomy to repair the lacerations is needed.

Diaphragmatic Injury
- Causes herniation of abdominal organs through the diaphragm.
- Dyspnea, empty abdomen. Dyspnea, bowel sound in chest are often seen
- X-ray and CT are diagnostic.

Treatment

Immediate thoracotomy and repair of diaphragm with repair of thoracic injuries.

Thoracoscopic Repair of Diaphragm

Laparoscopic reduction of contents and repair of diaphragm in hemodynamically stable patients.

Esophageal Injury

Cause: Penetrating (common) or blunt trauma.

Clinical Features and X-ray

Subcutaneous emphysema, pleural effusion, pneumothorax, pneumomediastinum.

Complications

Mediastinitis and empyema, fistula.

Treatment
- Operative repair of the tear and drainage of pleural cavity and mediastinum antibiotic coverage.
- A temporary gastrostomy for feeding.

Post-traumatic Empyema

Management
- Antibiotics
- Early decortication—thoracotomy or minimally invasive thoracoscopic route.

Post-traumatic Lung Abscess

CT-guided aspiration, thoracoscopic drainage, rarely lobectomy.

> **Q. Short note on pericardial tamponade in thoracic trauma—a life threatening condition.**
>
> - Due to steering wheel injuries to sternum causing a tear of pericardial venous tear and a hematoma
> - Or a fracture causing a tear of internal mammary vessel
> - Diagnosis is clinically suspected—by a low blood pressure, pulsus paradoxus, high pulse rate, low pulse volume, raised jugular venous pressure (JVP) and tachycardia with muffled heart sounds and breathlessness
> - Immediate sonography—e-FAST may help diagnosis
> - Chest X-ray shows a widened cardiac shadow
> - Treatment is urgent—early pericardiocentesis (PCC)
> - A wide bore needle is passed through xiphisternal notch upwards and backwards to relieve the tamponade even as preparations are made for an emergency room thoracotomy. Any associated cardiac injury adds to high morbidity and mortality.

Myocardial contusions—*notorious for cardiac arrhythmias.*

Managed under intense monitoring.
- ECG abnormalities.
- Two-dimensional echocardiography—shows motion abnormalities.
- Transesophageal echocardiogram is useful in diagnosis and monitoring.

Section 3

Skin, Face, Mouth, Oropharynx, Salivary Glands, and Jaws

18. Infections and Tumors of Skin
19. Developmental Anomalies of Face, Tumors and Swellings of Gums and Jaws
20. Oropharyngeal Cancer
21. Salivary Glands

Infections and Tumors of Skin

Chapter 18

SU18.1	Describe the pathogenesis, clinical features and management of various cutaneous and subcutaneous infections.
SU18.2	Classify skin tumors. Differentiate different skin tumors and discuss their management.
SU18.3	Describe and demonstrate the clinical examination of surgical patient including swelling and order relevant investigation for diagnosis. Describe and discuss appropriate treatment plan.

SU18.1: Describe the pathogenesis, clinical features and management of various cutaneous and subcutaneous infections.

ANATOMY AND FUNCTION OF SKIN AND ADNEXA

Skin has two layers:
1. Superficial—epidermis (5% of skin)
2. Deep—dermis (95% of skin)

Subcutaneous fat and fibrous tissue are deep to dermis.

Epidermis

Made of keratinized, stratified squamous epithelium by the keratinocytes (epidermal cells), arranged in 5 strata (layers):
1. Basale, 2. Spinosum, 3. Granulosum, 4. Lucidum and 5. Corneum (from deep to superficial)

The **stratum basale** contains keratinocytes and melanocytes (dendritic cells from neural crest).

The **basal keratinocytes** undergo mitosis in statum granulosum; they move superficially to reach stratum corneum losing their nuclei and organelles.

Melanocytes synthesize melanin, brown black pigment, which is transferred into keratinocytes, conferring protection against UV radiation.

Dermis (95% of skin): Has two layers:
1. A superficial papillary dermis—made of delicate collagen and elastin fibers with a network of capillaries and lymphatics.
2. A deeper reticular layer; composed of course collagen, parallel to the skin surface.

Dermo-epidermal junction—wavy arrangement with epidermal rete "pegs" project deep into dermis interdigitating with dermal papillae, which project into epidermis.

Other cells in the skin: Pacinian corpuscles, Langerhans cells (which engulf antigens and expose them to T-lymphocytes), Merkel cells and Meissner's corpuscles.

Skin Adnexa

- Hair follicles, sebaceous and sweat glands—run through dermis and epidermis.
- Keratinocytes are present in the ducts.

Functions of Skin

- Physical barrier against trauma, radiation and pathogens
- Sensory receptors for pain, pressure and movement
- Regulation of temperature and water homeostasis, excretion of water, sodium chloride, urea, potassium, metabolites of

food like garlic, fenugreek and cumin and drugs.
- Endocrine and metabolic functions
- Skin cells contain receptors for, thyroid hormones and neurotransmitters, sex hormones and respond to: Peptides, exposure to sunlight produces cholecalciferol.

INFECTIONS OF SKIN

Q. Short note on hidradenitis suppurativa, erysipelas and cellulitis.

Please refer Page 51 in Chapter 6. for the above.

Q. Short note on impetigo.

- It is a superficial infection of skin with staphylococci, streptococci or both.
- It is highly infectious, and characterised by blisters that rupture and coalesce to form a honey-colored crust and usually affects children.

Treatment
- Washing of the affected part
- Apply antistaphylococcal ointment—mupirocin or fusidic acid.
- Oral antibiotics—amoxicillin clavulanic acid.

Q. Write a short notes on necrotising fasciitis.

An Acute Surgical Emergency

A severe synergistic, polymicrobial infection—streptococci, *Staphylococcus, Escherichia coli, Bacteroides* or Clostridia. *Pseudomonas* and *Proteus* are less commonly seen.

Usually preceded by trauma or septic focus, e.g., abrasions, bites, boils, like perianal abscess or Bartholin's abscess.

Predisposing conditions: Diabetes mellitus; smoking; penetrating trauma; pressure sores; immunosuppression.

Sites affected:
- Lower limb is affected in over 50%.
- Other sites: Upper limbs, chest and abdominal wall (variant - Meleney's gangrene) and perineum (variant: Fournier's gangrene).

Rapid progression to septicemia with very high mortality (30–50%).

Clinical Signs
- Edema extending beyond erythema of skin
- Hardness of subcutaneous tissue and blurring of plane of muscle, on palpation
- Pain—very severe and disproportionate to area of visible affected area.
- Skin vesicles and soft tissue crepitus (gas forming organism)
- *Lymphangitis is generally absent* (contrast for superficial cellulitis.
- *Crepitus* indicates gas forming organisms in the pathogenesis.

Treatment

It is a surgical emergency:
- Intravenous antimicrobials—administration of combination of piperacillin, clindamycin and metronidazole to ensure antimicrobial coverage against both aerobic and anaerobic bacteria).
- Fluid resuscitation
- Active monitoring of hemodynamics
- Blood—cell counts and renal function
- Sonographic evaluation.

Surgical intervention at the earliest—to incise and debride the necrotic tissues
- Local dressing of the affected part.
- Supportive treatment.

LIPOMA

A benign tumor from mature adipose tissue cells.

Sites: Called the ubiquitous tumor—can arise in any part of the body except the brain.

Planes: Subcutaneous, subfascial, intramuscular, submuscular, subperiosteal, submucous, subserous, extradural, subsynovial (intra-articular).
- May run in families as multiple lipomatosis.
- It is a well encapsulated tumor with multiple lobules separated by septa.
- May be mixed with nerve fibers and cause painful lipoma (adiposis dolorosa).

Complications
- Tumor—enlargement and saponification leading to calcification

- Cosmetic disfigurement
- Interference with function—such as joint or in limb
- Pressure effect on neighbouring organs/tissues—nerve, vein, ureter, trachea, viscera.
- Intussusception due to submucous lipoma in the intestines
- Malignant transformation—liposarcoma.
- Clinical features of a subcutaneous lipoma (typical)
- Soft tumor, slips under the palpating finger and is mobile fixity indicates saponification rarely a malignant change.
- Differential diagnosis—a sebaceous cyst (punctum with skin fixed; sign of indentation)
- Neurofibroma—skin is not free, tingling along the course of nerve while palpating.

Treatment

Excision.

NEUROFIBROMA

Benign tumor from the nerve sheath of a peripheral nerve
Neurilemmoma—arises from sheath of Schwann.

Types of Neurofibroma

- Single, multiple neurofibromatosis (von Recklinghausen's disease)
- Plexiform neurofibroma
- Elephantiasis neuromatosa.

Neurofibromatosis

- These Schwann cell tumors due to genetic mitations occur with associated abnormalities (70% autosomal dominant -30%, sporadic).
- Three types—NF-1, NF-2 and schwannomatosis.
- NF-1 (Von Recklinghausen's disease) mutation on chromosome 17. Neurofibromata, café-au-lait spots (flat light brown skin spots) and freckles in axilla and groin often with bone deformities, poor cerebration and hypertension.
- Type 2 with hearing loss, vision loss and difficulty with balance.
- Type 3 causes chronic diffuse pain in body.

Complication

- Pressure effect in large tumors in cranial cavity, spinal column or body cavities or nerve deficit in the nerve of origin.
- Sarcomatous transformation.

Treatment

- Generally observation for complications
- Excision may cause deficit
- Peripheral tumors need excision at the risk of sensory or motor deficit.

Q. Write a short note on hemangioma.

HEMANGIOMA

Plural: Hemangiomata.
- Benign tumor—from endothelium.
- Usually have a birth mark like a patch.
- Sex ratio—3 females: 1 male.

Types

Capillary hemangioma (strawberry nevus)
- Generally grow fast during the first year and then slow down.
- May undergo spontaneous resolution in about 60 to 70% (10% per year upto 7th year).
- Raised over the skin.
- **Sign of blanching:** On finger pressure.

Cavernous hemangioma
- May be seen in extremities, abdomen and viscera, chest, intracranial.
- Sign of compressibility is diagnostic.
- Hemangioma may be associated with neurofibroma, cafe au lait spots.
- Rarely a sarcomatous change may occur.

Vascular malformations
- Generally they are associated with various syndromes.
- Present at birth
- Affect both sexes equally.
- They grow during growing years of the child.
- May also cause corresponding skeletal changes like a local gigantism due to hypertrophy or a small limb due to hypoplasia of bone.
- Stasis of blood may occur, trapping platelets.

Salmon patch
- Large reddish purple birth marks—over neck, face and other areas.
- Usually they resolve by 2 years; others need cosmetic therapy.

Port-wine stain (PWS)
- Capillary malformations due to localized intradermal capillary vasodilatation
- Flat, smooth, purple-stained areas
- Raised over the skin surface (common site) head and neck.

Acquired vascular lesions

Campbell de Morgan spots
- These are arteriovenous fistulae at the dermal capillary level
- In sun-exposed skin of older population.

Spider nevi
- These are angiomata that appear (and may disappear) spontaneously at puberty or in two-thirds of pregnant women, usually disappearing in the puerperium
- The are also seen in patients with chronic liver disease.
- They can be treated with intense pulsed light or pulse dye laser.

Q. Write a short note on pyogenic granuloma.

- Infective lesion but shares histology of hemangioma.
- Usually small—less than 1.5 cm
- Red and soft nodules—pedunculated with superficial ulceration and bleed on touch.
- Diff diagnosis
  - Hemangioma
  - Infected papilloma
  - Skin adnexal tumors
  - Hemangioendothelioma.

Treatment

Excision with a margin of 2 mm surgical excision or removal by laser.

Q. Write a short note on glomus tumor (glomangioma).

- This is a tumor, arising from a subcutaneous arteriovenous shunt
- Commonly seen in the nail bed, many may be invisible
- It is a small purple nodule (less than a centimeter), very painful on minor

Q. Write a short notes on aneurysm.

An aneurysm is a dilatation of a part of artery (Fig. 18.1).

Types
- **True aneurysm:** Dilated part consists of all three layers of artery (*Tunica adventitia, T. media* and *T. intima*).
- **False aneurysm:** Periarterial hematoma with a wall made of a fibrous wall communicating with the arterial lumen.

True Aneurysm
- **Fusiform:** Diffuse dilatation—most common in atherosclerosis.
- **Saccular:** A part of the artery alone makes the wall of the aneurysm.
- **Dissecting:** The blood rips (dissects) through a slit in the arterial intima into the arterial

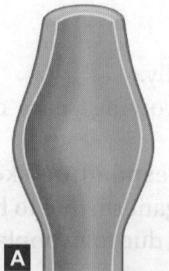 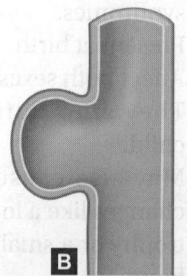 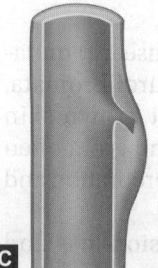 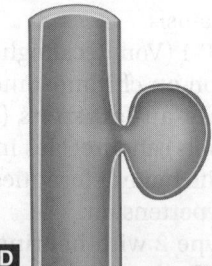

Figs. 18.1A to D: Types of aneurysm: A. Fusiform; B. Saccular; C. Dissecting; D. Pseudoaneurysm.

wall leading to longitudinal split between the layers of the artery.

Mycotic Aneurysm

An infective focus lodges and leads to weakening of arterial wall due to necrosis.

Etiology of Aneurysm
- Atherosclerosis
- **Connective tissue disorder:** Marfan syndrome, Ehler-Danlos syndrome.
- **Chronic frictional trauma:** Scalene syndrome causing a poststenotic dilatation of the artery
- **Pseudoaneurysm:** Caused by arterial trauma.
- **Mycotic aneurysm:** *Aspergillus*, Staphylococci—septic emboli from infective endocarditis, *Streptococci, Salmonella, Proteus* and *Candida*.

Complications
- Thrombosis
- Thromboembolism
- Rupture.

Diagnosis
- Depends on the site and type of aneurysm.
- MRI, Duplex sonography, CT angiography are the investigations
- Angiography (aortography or selective arteriography for specific sites).

Treatment
- Endovascular stenting of fusiform part.
- **Surgical repair:** Resection and graft or endarterial graft.
- Proximal ligation of artery and bypass grafting.

Saccular Aneurysm
- Angiographic—transcatheter placing of wire coils to cause obliteration of aneurysms
- Resection of aneurysm and arterial repair with patch graft
- Endoaneurysmorrhaphy
- **Pseudoaneurysm:** Exploration, evacuation of hematoma and repair of the artery (patch graft).

SHORT NOTES

ARTERIOVENOUS FISTULA (AV FISTULA)

Abnormal communication between artery **and a vein**.

Etiology
- **Congenital:** Arteriovenous malformations, e.g., brain, limbs.
- **Acquired:** Trauma—penetrating or blunt injury—limbs, abdomen.
- **Surgical:** Cimino shunt for long-term hemodialysis (wrist, brachial or femoral).

Pathophysiology
- It is a shunt between a high pressure arterial tree into a low pressure venous system.
- **Arterialisation of veins:** Adaptive dilatation, thickening and tortuosity of veins with pulsation.
- **Thrill and bruit:** Due to abnormal turbulent arterial flow into vein.
- **Local gigantism:** Overgrowth of the part due to excess oxygenated blood—especially congenital.
- **Cardiovascular system.**
  - A-V shunt causes heart to compensate by increasing output and leads to a high output failure.
  - Distal ischemia and gangrene of the limb may happen due to shunting.

Clinical Signs
- Tachycardia
- High systolic pressure
- Late stages: Heart failure
- Local signs
- Local gigantism—large limb due ot the hypertrophy of muscles.
- Pulsatile swelling, local warmth
- Bluish discoloration and arterialized veins over the swelling/thrill and bruit.

BRANHAM'S BRADYCARDIAC SIGN

Compression of the artery proximal to the fistula causes bradycardia and rise of blood pressure due to blocking of the shunting of arterial blood.

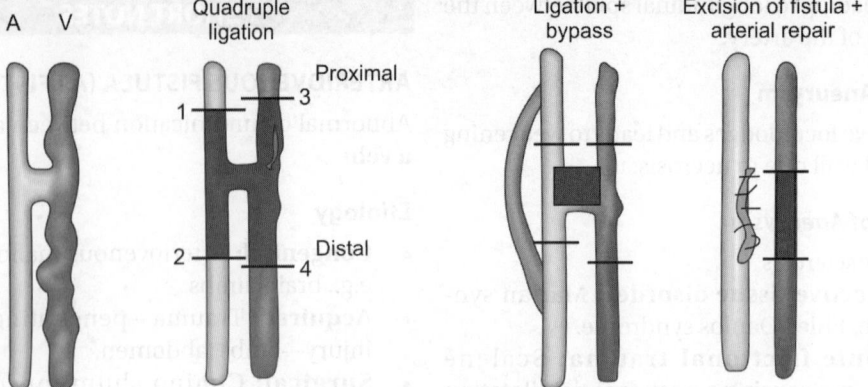

Fig. 18.2: Treatment of arteriovenous fistula

Investigation

- Duplex scanning with Doppler
- MR angiography
- Angiography.

Treatment (Refer Figure 18.2)

Radiological intervention: Angiographic coiling may work in small fistulae.

Surgery

1. Excision (division) of fistula and repair of the artery with synthetic patch (Dacron)
2. Quadruple ligation: In emergency
3. Quadruple ligation with arterial bypass grafting to correct distal limb ischemia.

BENIGN LESIONS OF SKIN AND SUBCUTANEOUS TISSUE

> Q. Write a short notes on Cock's peculiar tumor sebaceous horn.

Epidermal Cysts

Arise from hair follicle (sebaceous or epidermoid cysts) or as inclusion dermoids (inclusion of cutaneous epithelium after trauma).

Sebaceous Cysts (Epidermoid Cysts)

The cysts arise from infundibulum of hair follicle are lined by stratified squamous epithelium,

Sebaceous cysts can occur anywhere except palm and sole, common over back and scalp and scrotal skin. They contain inspissated sebum which is like putty.

Clinical Features

- Spherical swelling fixed to the skin, having a punctum
- Indentable (sign of moulding).

Differential Diagnosis

- A dermoid cyst—no punctum and skin is free.
- Lipoma—skin free, not indentable, slip sign.
- Rarely a sebaceous carcinoma may present as an infected cyst.

Complications

- **Acute:** Infection, suppuration and ulceration or abscess.
- **Koch's peculiar tumor:** Ulceration of infected sebaceous cyst over scalp has appearance of an ulcerated tumor.
- **Sebaceous horn:** Caused by slow accumulation of sebum over the punctum.

Treatment

- Uncomplicated cyst is excised with an elliptical incision to include the punctum.
- Infected cyst—incision and drainage followed by elective excision of cyst after the inflammation has subsided.

Seborrhoeic Keratosis

Syn: Senile keratosis, basal cell papilloma.
- It is a warty lesion may be pigmented and hyperkeratosis
- These vary from muscular to soft, excrescent, warty lesions

- Arising from the basal layer of epidermal cells and contain melanocytes.

Viral Warts
- Due to human papilloma virus (HPV)
- Verruca vulgaris (papillary projections)—warty surface
- Plantar warts
- Condylomata acuminata.

> **Q. Enumerate the tumors of hair follicle. Write a short note on pilomatrixoma.**

Tumors from Hair Follicle

Pilomatrixoma (Calcifying Epithelioma of Malherbe)
Benign tumor from skin hair matrix—undergoes calcification—presents as a hard swelling, sometimes undergoes ulceration—common in children and young individuals.

Tuberous Sclerosis (Adenoma Sebaceum)
Red, popular swellings in face (angiofibromas), common in children.

Trichoepithelioma
Small nodular swellings—near nasolabial fold similar to a basal cell carcinoma.

Trichilemmoma (Nevus Sebaceous)
It is a hamartoma with the appearance of a long vertical wart.

Benign Sweat Glands Tumors

Giant hairy naevus [Syn: Giant congenital pigmented nevus (GCPN)]—premalignant.
- It is a hamartoma of melanocytes which is distributed among the dermatomal limits.
- **Histology:** Similar to a compound nevus but melanocytes are seen in all layers.
- It is premalignant (turning into a melanoma).

Hidradenoma (Cystadenoma)
- It is seen as translucent cystic nodular swelling.
- Syringoma—small soft lesions commonly near naso labial folds.

Benign Vascular Lesions of Skin

Congenital: Malformations and hemangioma.
The endothelial characteristics distinguish a vascular tumor from a malformation.

> **Q. Name the pigmented lesions of the skin. What is a junctional nevus.**

Pigmented Lesions: Melanocytic Lesions

Moles/nevi (naevi)
Aggregation of melanocytes, in the dermis or at the dermo-epidermal junction forming nevus.

Freckle (ephelis)
An area of skin containing a normal number of melanocytes, which produce excessive melanin granules.

Lentigo
- Small and circumscribed pigmented macules
- Excessive exposure to sun increases risk of these lesions.

Compound nevus
- It is a maculopapular, pigmented lesion due to proliferation of melanocytes at junctional area with cell nests in the dermis.
- Mostly seen during growing age.

Intradermal nevus
- It has no malignant potential.
- This is a lesion with dermal clusters of melanocytes.
- Usually seen in adults as a pigmented lesion, fainter in pigmentation than a junctional nevus.

Junctional nevus
- It is more prone to turn into a melanoma.
- Shows proliferation of nevus cells at dermo-epidermal junction, presenting as darkly pigmented macules or papules over the skin or in mucosa.
- The start in childhood or adolescence.
- Progress with ageing to form compound or intradermal nevi.

Atypical nevus (Syn: dysplastic nevus)
It is a premalignant lesion
- Due to irregular proliferation of melanocytes at the stratum basale of epidermis.
- Sporadic or familial.
- Can be multiple (more than 5 increases risk of melanoma).
- Can lead to Familial atypical multiple mole-melanoma (FAMMM) syndrome.
- Usually over 5 mm in size

Three characteristic features of "atypical" nevus:
1. Ill-defined borders
2. "Wavy" or undulating irregular surface
3. Non-uniform pigmentation (variegated).

> **Q. Discuss pathology, clinical types staging and management of malignant melanoma of skin.**

MALIGNANT MELANOMA (MM) OF SKIN

- **Cell of origin:** From melanocytes.
- **Sites:** Skin, mucosa, retina and the leptomeninges.

Etiopathogenesis

- **Genetic syndromes:** MM in first generation relatives seen.
- **Genetic mutations:** BRAF proto oncogene mutation in over 40%.
- **Acquired causes:**
  - Exposure to UVR.
  - White race and overexposure to sun light
  - Immunosuppression increases risk
  - Multiple nevi (predispose)—junctional lentiginous nevi, atypical nevi, giant pigmented congenital naevi.

Pathology

- De novo—80%
- From pre existing nevus—20%.

Phases of Spread

- In situ—atypical melanocytes in dermoepidermal junction with dermis intact.
- Horizontal phase along dermoepidermal junctional plane and dermis may be involved.
- Vertical phase (deeper)—into dermis and subcutaneous fat; lymphatic and blood spread is faster from here.

Macroscopic Types

- Lentigo meligna maligna (LMM) (5–10%)
- Superficial spreading melanoma (SSM) (70%)
- Nodular melanoma (NM) (About 15–20%)
- Acral lentiginous melanoma (ALM)

Special types: Amelanotic melanoma, desmoplastic melanoma.

Special sites: Subungual melanoma, anal melanoma, ocular (choroid plexus) and in meninges.

Clinical Types

Summarized in **Table 18.1**.

Signs of Malignant Change in a Mole

- Change in color, size and shape—irregular edges, elevation, nodularity or ulceration
- Rapid growth, itching, or discharge.
- Satellite lesions.

Subungual Melanoma

Progressive nail fold pigmentation with nail dystrophy. They behave as SSM and not ALM.

Amelanotic Melanoma

- Anaplasia leads to failure of melanin production.

Table 18.1: Summary of pathology and clinical features of melanomas.

	LMM	SSM	NM	ALM
Age Sex Race	Elderly and female White race	Middle age Both sexes Whites more	Middle age Men	No age/sex preference Asian/African
Site	Face neck hand Sun exposed areas	Pre-existing nevus	De novo Trunk, head and neck	Palm sole
Growth and spread	Slow, horizontal Vertical late	Mostly horizontal Late vertical phase	Vertical phase	Vertical phase
Metastatic potential	Less and late	Slow and late	Early and rapid	Variable
Lesion	Pigmented macule	Flat lesion after years in a nevus Nodular later	Short duration and rapid	Mimics pyogenic or fungal granuloma

Chapter 18: Infections and Tumors of Skin

- They are most aggressive and have a poor prognosis.
- Lesions are without pigmentation
- Fleshy lesions, look vascular, without induration.

Summary of Pathology and Clinical Features of Melanomas

Described in **Table 18.1**.

Differential Diagnosis of a Melanoma

- Other pigmented lesions (read previous section)
- Ulcerative lesions
- Squamous cell carcinoma—indurated edges
- Fungal granuloma
- Hematoma.

Prognostic Factors in Melanoma (Given Below in Table 18.2)

B-RAF V600 mutations–locks B-RAF protein signaling, initiation, malignant transformation, progression and metastasis of Melanoma, via the mitogen-activated protein kinase (MAPK) cellular pathway.

TNM staging of Melanoma (based on AJCC Classification) simplified table. This is given in Table 18.3.

Q. Short note on staging of melanoma; what are in transit nodules and satellite nodules.

T – Tumor

- Tis in basal layer of intact epidermis
- T1–T4—based on depth (thickness) of invasion (not size of lesion), viz., T1— < 1 mm, T2—1-2 mm, T3—2-4 mm and T4— > 4 mm.
- Each of these stages—T1-T4 may be subclassified as "a" when ulceration is absent and "b" when ulceration is present.

N – Regional Nodes

- (1) number N0—no nodes, N1—1 node, N2—2-3 nodes and N3, more than 3 nodes. Microscopic or macroscopic (a or b).
- (2) MSI make it Nc (microsatellite, satellite, in-transit).
- Satellite lesions—(Nc) deposits with in 2 cm of lesion—microsatellite or macroscopic satellite nodule—due to dermal lymphatics.
- In-transit metastases—(Nc), skin nodule beyond regional node is Stage M1. Regional spread of tumor via lymphatic vessels in the dermis or subcutaneous tissue, to regional node area.

M

- Extraregional nodes, or skin or other system M1a or b
- Serum LDH level – raised –in M1c.

Table 18.2: Prognostic factors in melanoma.

• Ulceration	• Serum LDH
• Mitoses at microscopy	• Stage— TNM stage
• Breslow's depth	

Table 18.3: TNM-staging of cutaneous melanoma.

	Tis	T1	T2	T3	T4	N0	N1	N2	N3	M
Breslow thickness	In situ	<1 mm	1–2 mm	2–4 mm	>4 mm	0	1 nodes	2–3	>3 nodes	M0–NIL
Ulceration absent	-	T1a	T2a	T3a	T4a					M1a—skin subcutaneous tissue, distant node
Present		T1b	T2b	T3b	T4b					M1b—lungs
MSI • Microsatellite lesions • Satellite nodules • In transit lesions				Absent			"a" if clinically occult "b" clinically detected			LDH normal in M1 a and b
				Present			"c"			M1c LDH high

Staging of Melanoma as per TNM staging (Given in Table 18.4)

Diagnosis and Staging

- Excision biopsy with 2-3 mm clearance (wide and deep) wherever feasible
  Incision biopsy from the large primary lesions. or facial lesion near eye or nose etc
- FNAC from clinically enlarged. regional lymph node field
- **Sentinel node biopsy:** Best predictor of prognosis on nodal disease. Lymph nodes are clinically negative and tumors – T1 > 0.8 mm – T2 low thickness tumors.
  Sonography to study lymph nodes—regional (groin or neck) and extraregional (e.g. abdomen)

Table 18.4: Melanoma stages.

Stage		T	N	M
Stage 0		Tis	N0	M0
Stage I	a	T1a	N0	M0
	b	T1b/T2a		
Stage II	a	T2b		M0
	b	T3b/T4a	N0	
	c	T4b		
Stage III	a-d	Any T	N1–3	M0
Stage IV		Any T	Any N	M1

Table 18.5: Prognosis related to thickness and nodal status.

Breslow thickness	
< 1 mm – 5 year 90%	N + - 30–65%
• 1-2 mm- 60%	• M + <10%
• > 2 mm - 40%	

Q. What is lymphoscintigraphy?

Lymphoscintigraphy—radioisotope injected into space and recorded with gamma camera. For evaluation of in transit nodules and for evaluation of lymph nodes upstream, e.g., retroperitoneal and mediastinal nodes in a case of melanoma of foot.

CT scan—chest and head for metastases.
Bio markers—to study the (B-RAF) and plan treatment.

Prognosis related to thickness (depth of invasion), nodal status and metastases (summarized in Table 18.5).

Treatment of Cutaneous Melanoma

Principles: Early diagnosis and treatment gives best results.
- Surgery is the main modality
- Adjuvant therapy—chemotherapy
- Biological targeted therapy—for mutant.

Surgical Treatment

Surgery for primary lesion:
Wide local excision of the primary lesion with margin of normal skin margin depending upon thickness of lesion.

Primary

Less than 1 mm thick: 1 cm margin
1 mm to 2 mm thick: 1-2 cm margin
More than 2 mm thick: 2 cm margin

Amputation of the limb—for large T4 lesions or N3 lesions with ulceration.

Management of Lymph Nodes

Sentinel Lymph Node Biopsy (SLNB)
- Done with lymphoscintigraphic or blue dye injected guidance
- SNLB is not therapy but a surgical procedure to decide on node clearance
- Indication—T1 and T2 with N0 clinical status.

Lymph Node Dissection (LND) - clearance of the regional lymph node group/s.
- Completion (CLND)—if SLNB is positive.
- Therapeutic (TLND)—for node positive (clinical or FNAC/biopsy proven), e.g., ilioinguinal node dissection (superficial inguinal and deep iliac nodes)
  Indications:
  – Stage II
  – Stage III or IV, after neoadjuvant therapy, for BRAF V600K mutated melanoma.
- Elective (prophylactic)—not preferred for N0 although opinions differ.
- **Metastases**—resection of oligo metastases after neoadjuvant therapy.

Non-surgical Treatment

Nonresectable disease—advanced primary, recurrent disease and presence of satellite or in transit deposits in limbs.

Regional therapy
High dose regional chemotherapy—hyperthermic chamber.
- Methods
  - Isolated limb perfusion (ILP)
  - Isolated limb infusion (ILI) of chemotherapy.

SYSTEMIC THERAPY

- **Immunotherapy**—improved survival by enhancing T-cell–mediated anti tumor immunity.
  Through blockade of inhibitory receptors, CTLA-4 and PD-1
  Monoclonal antibody: Ipilimumab
- **Molecular therapy (targeted therapy)**
  - Over 40% of melanomas show activation of BRAF, a proto-oncogene.
  - Vemurafenib and dabrafenib are small molecule inhibitors of BRAF
  - "BRAF mutation plus" patients respond to these agents.

Local Therapy

- For palliation of in-transit metastases
- Laser ablation
- Electrodessication
- Intralesional therapy
- BCG injection or herpes simplex virus derived vaccine
- Interferon, Interleukin -2 (IL-2).

Malignant Tumors of Skin

- **Epithelial**
  - Basal cell carcinoma—most common skin tumor.
  - Squamous cell carcinoma, 2nd most common, incidence is high in India.
- **Adnexa**
  - Sweat glands—sebaceous carcinoma
  - Eccrine carcinoma spiradenocarcinoma
  - Cylindroma
- **Melanocytes**—malignant melanoma
- **Vascular**—hemangioendothelioma
- **Lymphoma**—NHL mycosis fungoides, sezary syndrome.
- **Metastatic**—from adenocarcinoma, pancreas, stomach, colon.

> **Q. Describe pathology, clinical features and management of basal cell carcinoma. Short note on rodent ulcer.**

BASAL CELL CARCINOMA (BCC)

Most common skin cancer.

Etiology

- Age: 45–80, Sex: More in men
- UV radiation and previous irradiation
- Familial/genetic syndromes.
- Race—whites far more affected than rest
- Site—of preference—face— above along a line joining tragus to angle of mouth.
  Also arise in unexposed parts like trunk (30%).

Pathology

- Slow growing, invade local parts including bones.
- Metastasis rare: Both—lymphatic and hematogenous.
- Basi squamous variety behaves like SCC.

Morphological Types

Localised

- Nodular and nodulocystic (make 90%)
- Rare types; cystic, pigmented, nevoid.

Generalized

- Superficial: Multifocal and superficial spreading
- Infiltrative: Morphoeic, and cicatrizing.

Microscopy reveals—over 25 varieties
- **BCC:** Two types—high risk and low risk.
- **High-risk signs:** Size >2 cm, site –face –near ear, nose (mask area), infiltrative signs, recurrent lesions, h/o previous radiotherapy.

Clinical Features

- Nodular type—elevated, irregular nodule with induration and umbilication.
- Nodulo ulcerative—most common
- "Rodent ulcer" indurated base, and telangiectatic edges.
- "Field fire type"—mostly superficial spread with crusting at original site and active lesion at peripheral edge.

Differential diagnosis: SCC, nodular melanoma seborrheic keratosis.

Management

- A skin biopsy is done to diagnose and stratify the risk—high or low.
- The recurrence risk, high versus low, will determine the treatment plan.

Surgical excision

- For low risk lesions—with a margin of 4 mm
- For high risk lesions—and margin—wider (1.5-2 cm).
- Moh's micrographic surgery is done for high-risk lesions under microscopic control, performed by dermatologists. for cosmetically sensitive areas.

Repeated frozen section and complete margin clearance is the alternative to Moh's method.

Radiotherapy: Good curative results but another cancer is very common after 15 to 20 years. Hence reserved for—old, infirm patients.

> Q. Describe management of squamous cell carcinoma of skin.

SQUAMOUS CELL CARCINOMA

- Second most common skin cancer.
- Arises from stratum basale of the epidermis—or from skin appendage like hair follicle.

Etiology

- U-V radiation—more common in sun exposed skin
- Ionizing radiation.
- Chronic irritation.
- HPV (human papillomavirus)
- Chemicals—arsenicals. Tar (Chimney Sweeper's Cancer).

Premalignant Lesions

- Actinic keratosis
- kerato acanthoma
- Bowen's disease—SCC in situ, scaly lesion at mucocutaneous junction
- SCC may arise - de novo or from chronic wounds, sinus (osteomyelitis), ulcers (venous or traumatic), or from scars—burns or snake bites (**Marjolin ulcer**).

Pathology

Macroscopic types:
- Papilliferous, (proliferative)
- Nodular and ulcerative types
- Verrucous type—is special—locally invasive and rarely spreads by lymphatics.

Spread: Local infiltration and lymphatic. Blood spread is uncommon.

MICROSCOPY

- Epithelial pearls, keratin plugs, dyskeratosis and mitoses with atypical nuclei in epithelium
- Invasive carcinoma—basal layer invaded.
- The tumor expresses cytokeratins.

Broder's grading—on dedifferentiation of cells—low grade, intermediate and high grade

High risk factors: (Poorer prognosis) if:
- Size: Morphology > 2 cm size
- Grade: Broder's grade 2 or higher
- Depth (microscopic) of invasion, > 2 mm
- Perineural and lymphovascular invasion, microscopic tumor invasion in deep and lateral margins of excision specimen.
- Lesion near ear and lip.
- SCC in immunosuppressed individuals
- SCC in scar, sinus, previous lesions has higher metastatic potential.

Pathology of Verucous Carcinoma

- Warty growth dry, exophytic, slow local infiltration
- Lymphatic and blood spread are rare
- Microscopy—well differentiated SCC. Epithelial pearls are not seen.
- Site—oral, sole of foot and penile glans.

Treatment

- Wide local excision of the primary and lymphadenectomy if regional nodes are invaded.
- Radiotherapy—generally not preferred.

> **Short note: Marjolin's ulcer—SCC in a scar (as described by Marjolin)**
> - Commonly seen in scars following burns, healed venous ulcers, scars of snake bite.
> - Scar is avascular and devoid of lymphatics

- Hence it is slow growing, cant spread to lymphatic or neural plane
- Non-metastatic until it reaches margins of the scar.
- After that, it is aggressive and has high metastatic potential.
- Therefore treatment is early diagnosis (Wedge biopsy) and wide excision.

Note: Recent books include SCCs arising in chronic ulcers (e.g., venous ulcers) also in the definition of Marjolin ulcer.

TNM Staging of Squamous Cell Carcinoma (Refer Table 18.6)

SCC- TNM Staging (summarized with WHO classification 2018 – pTNM – pathological).

Clinical Features

- Males more affected than females
- Usually 40 plus
- Types—ulcerative or proliferative.
- Induration is typical.
- **Classical signs:** Irregular shape, everted edges and overhanging margin, **bleeding** touch due to **friability**, **indurated** edges and base.
- **Lymph nodes:** When palpable are hard, nodular and may be fixed.

Differential Diagnosis

- **Malignancies:** Basal cell carcinoma. Amelanotic melanoma.
- **Benign:** Pyoderma gangrenosum; warts, actinic keratosis.

Treatment

These are general principles. The site and region decide specific treatment as applicable.

Surgery

Wide excision of lesion is done.
- T1 – 0.5 cm clear margin
- T2 – 1 cm clear margin
- T3 – lesions need adjuvant radiotherapy.

Radiotherapy

Primary (curative) radiotherapy or adjuvant therapy after surgery for T3 lesions, and when HPE shows perineural invasion/inadequate clearance.

Table 18.6: TNM staging of squamous cell carcinoma.

TX	Primary tumor cannot be assessed
T0	No tumor, Tis - basement membrane intact
T1	Primary <2 cm
T2	> 2 cm upto 4 cm
T3	More than 4 cm wide or deeper than 6 mm
T4	Invades subdermal cartilage, muscle, bone
N0	No lymphatic spread
N1	3 cm single node
N2	3–6 cm: a-1; b- >1 ipsilateral, c-bilateral
N3	> 6 cm, any regional node
M0	Metastases absent
M1	Metastases present
Stage I	T1, N0, M0
Stage II	T2 N0 M0 or T1 N1
Stage III	T1–3, N1 M0
Stage IV	T1–T3, N2c, M0 or
	T4–
	Any T, N3 or M1

Other Therapies

- Cryoablation, photodynamic and laser therapy.
- Topical 5-FU, topical imiquimod

Metastatic SCC

Systemic treatment: Cisplatin 5-FU and bleomycin with EGFR inhibitors (**cetuximab**).

MALIGNANT SOFT TISSUE TUMORS

Q. Short note on dermatofibrosarcoma protuberans (DFSP).

- A cutaneous sarcoma
- Cell of origin—fibroblast in skin.
- Locally invasive and tendency to recur.
- Metastases less common.

Treatment

- **Surgery:** Wide local excision with 2 cm margin
- **Radiotherapy:** Postoperative RT if margins are positive and resurgery is not considered.

- Moh's microsurgery—controversial.
- Tyrosine Kinase Inhibitors
  - Imatinib mesylate
  - Unresectable and recurrent tumor
  - Metastatic disease

Q. Short notes on desmoid tumors.

Desmoid tumors
- Arise from connective tissue
- May be associated with FAP (familial adenomatous polyposis) syndrome in some patients.
- Locally aggressive tumors are non-metastasizing
- Asymptomatic tumors starting as small and growing slowly.

Treatment
- Wide excision large tumors should be excised with margin of 2 cm.
- Radiotherapy—they are radiosensitive, indicated in multimodality treatment.
- Antiestrogen—tamoxifen chemotherapy
- Tyrosine kinase inhibitors (TKI) (e.g., **imatinib, sunitinib**) for unresectable, progressive, or recurrent disease.

Soft Tissue Sarcomas (STSs)

Arise from mesodermal tissues.
Heterogeneous group of malignant tumors—account for about 1% of adult malignancies.
- De novo
- Arising from pre-existing benign tumors—e.g., in neurofibromatosis.

Spread
- Local invasion
- Lymphatic (nodal)—rare
- Hematogenous—common.

Classification of sarcomas—based on cell type of origin and grade.

Most common
- Pleomorphic undifferentiated sarcoma (malignant fibrous histiocytoma)—(40%)
- Liposarcoma (25%).

Others
- Spindle cell sarcoma
- Fibrosarcoma
- Myxosarcoma
- Fibromyxosarcoma
- Rhabdomyosarcoma
- Neurofibrosarcoma
- Malignant schwannoma
- Leiomyosarcoma
- Angio sarcoma—Kaposi's sarcoma, glomangiosarcoma.

Clinical Features

Sites: Commonly intra-abdominal and retroperitoneal. Other sites may include limbs or back.

Presentation
- As an asymptomatic mass
- Due to compressive symptoms (venous, bowel, ureter depending on site)
- Those due to invasion of nerve and muscles
- Due to metastases.

Diagnosis
- Core biopsy—is obtained for histopathology, grading and immunohistochemistry (IHC)
- MRI and CT of the part assess the tumor and its spread
- CT—Chest—for lung metastases (most common).

Staging: The AJCC staging system, is based on tumor size and depth, nodal status, histologic grade, and metastasis.

Prognosis is variable as per the histological grade of tumor.

Treatment

Surgery
- Wide local resection without spillage of tumor cells, if tumor is resectable.
- Re-excision—if HPE shows tumor positive surgical margins, when possible.
- **Limb sparing resection** combined with radiation therapy—for limb lesions.
- **Amputation** is when locally advanced.

Retroperitoneal sarcomas
- Most are liposarcomas
- Vital structures are also involved and this makes treatment difficult
- Organs associated with the tumor should be resected en bloc.

Surgery for small (<5 cm, superficial and low grade tumors).

Radiotherapy and/or chemotherapy.

Neoadjuvant—for large tumors to facilitate an R0 resection.

Radiotherapy
- Concurrent RT—and surgery—for high grade tumors
- Preoperative (neo adjuvant)—large non-resectable tumors
- Postoperative RT—(adjuvant)—residual and recurrent tumors after surgery
- Brachytherapy—for large deep tumors implantation of radio active beads (iridium).

Chemotherapy—variable benefit

Neoadjuvant or postoperative chemotherapy are given—usually with RT

Indication: Advanced, unresectable or metastatic and high risk tumors for recurrence or metastasis.

Chemotherapy: Doxorubicin, epirubicin, and ifosfamide.

Targeted therapy and immunotherapy:
MAbs: Tyrosine kinase inhibitors—pazopanib, olaratumab, anlotinib.

Isolated limb perfusion (ILP) or infusion (ILI) with melphalan to treat un resectable or recurrent STS in limbs.

Prognosis: Overall 3 years survival—30–60% depending upon stage, grade, histo type and treatment efficacy.

Kaposi's sarcoma
- Arises from vascular endothelium
- Proliferation of endothelial cells
- Associated with immunosuppression
- Post-transplant patients, HIV infection
- Clinically—a red indurated plaque is seen. Ulceration is seen later
- Treatment—radiotherapy.

Developmental Anomalies of Face, Tumors and Swellings of Gums and Jaws

Chapter 19

SU19.1	Describe the etiology and classification of cleft lip and palate.
SU19.2	Describe the principles of reconstruction of cleft lip and palate. Define and describe epulis. Describe briefly the swellings of jaw.

SU19.1: Describe the etiology and classification of cleft lip and palate.

CRANIOFACIAL ANOMALIES: THE "OMENS"

- O Orbital alteration
- M Mandibular deformity
- E Ear deformity
- N Nerve involvement
- S Soft tissue alterations.

Van der Meulen et al. classification of hemifacial (craniofacial) microsomia:
This is useful in planning the treatment. Refer **Table 19.1**.

> **Q. Classify the types of developmental abnormalities of the face, mouth and jaws.**

Refer **Figure 19.1** for development of face.

CLEFT LIP AND PALATE

A common anomaly—about 1 in 600 to 700; more in male children.

Etiology

- Genetic factors and environmental factors.
- Isolated or with various other anomalies (150 to 300 identified) in newborn.
- Maternal illness, drugs (phenytoin, steroid, diazepam) and radiation.
- All defects except isolated cleft palate are detected during gestation by 18 weeks by prenatal sonography.

Classification

> **Q. Classify cleft lip and cleft palate.**

Given in **Table 19.2**.

Table 19.1: Classification of hemifacial (craniofacial) microsomia.

Type of anomaly (dysplasia)	Examples
Cerebro-cranial dysplasias	Microcephaly, anencephaly
Cerebro-facial dysplasias	Oculo-orbital and rhinencephalic dysplasias
Craniofacial dysplasias	

- **With clefting:** Mandibulo-maxillary cleft, medial and lateral naso-maxillary cleft.
- **With synostosis:** Craniosynostosis—sutures fused with facial bones.
- **With dysostosis:** Defective development of bones of skull and face.
- **With dysostosis and synostosis:** Syndromic anomalies.
- **With dyschondrosis:** Achondroplasia.

Chapter 19: Developmental Anomalies of Face, Tumors and Swellings of Gums and Jaws

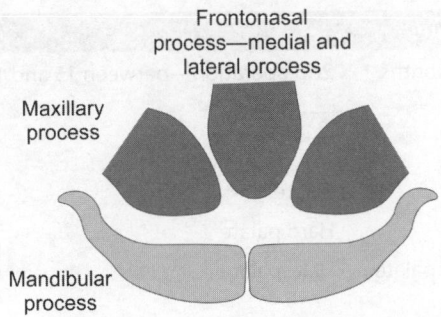

- Frontonasal process—medial and lateral process
- Maxillary process
- Mandibular process
- Median nasal process—from frontal arch→nose tip and bridge
- Lateral nasal process→alae nasi, sides
- Maxillary process—cheeks and upper lips palate—hard and soft
- Mandibular processes—from mandibular arch→lower jaw and lips
- Maxillary arch—jaw, palate and nasal cartilages

Cleft lip and palate of various types are due to defective fusion among the above processes during development of face.

Fig. 19.1: Development of face

Table 19.2: Classification of cleft lip and palate.

1.	Cleft lip (CL)—unilateral or bilateral	15%	Males more	Unilateral cleft lip and palate more on left side
2.	Cleft lip with cleft palate (CLP)	40%	Males more	
3.	Cleft palate (CP) alone • Hard palate only • Both hard and soft palate Separated palatine process from nasal septum and vomer		Females more	Most have associated anomalies
4.	Submucous cleft palate (SMCP)			

Q. What are the problems with cleft lip and palate?

Problems with cleft lip and palate:
- Function of sucking, feeding, nasal regurgitation and swallowing.
- Airway obstruction or aspiration.
- **Speech:** Nasal twang, defective articulation with consonants.
- Cosmesis.
- Growth of facial muscles and skeleton.
- Psychological impact.

Evaluation and principles of repair:
- Identify the defect and associated anomalies.
- Assess muscles of face and mouth.
- Assess the bony anomalies and defects, (e.g. a protrusive premaxilla).

Q. What are the objectives and goals of surgery for cleft lip and palate?

- Proper closure of mouth and swallowing without regurgitation.
- Speech with proper articulation and voice.
- Cosmetic correction to ensure a normal appearance of lip, nose and face.
- Restoration of dentition and facial growth closest to normal range of development.

Principles of Surgery for Cleft Lip and Palate

Surgery involves the reconstruction of the muscles of lip, nose, face and soft palate, which are distorted, displaced, deformed and underdeveloped, to restore normal anatomy, normal function and development of lip, nose, palate and facial skeleton.

Cleft palate repair (palatoplasty): Single or two stage repair, usually done between 6 and 18 months. The two stage approach minimizes dissection and scarring of muscles and mucosa which are brought together.

The surgical principle is—mobilization and reconstruction of functional muscles. There are many different surgical techniques.

Cleft lip repair: Primary repair is performed between 3 and 6 months. It aims at a functional

Table 19.3: Timing of operations for cleft lip and palate.

Anomaly	1st operation— 6 months	2nd operation—between 15 and 18 months
Cleft lip alone—uni/bilateral	Yes	—
Cleft soft palate—alone	Yes	—
Cleft lip with palate	Lip	Palate
Cleft hard and soft palate	Lip and soft palate	Hard palate
Bilateral lip and palate	Bilateral lip and soft palate	Hard palate

oral sphincter and a cosmetic restoration. It may need revision during palate surgery at 18 months.

Secondary (corrective) surgery for cleft lip and palate (first surgery is the best), when required, is done with alveolar bone graft if needed—after 2 years of primary surgery.

Timing of operations for cleft lip and palate are given below in **Table 19.3**.

Secondary Palate Procedures
- Correction of palatal fistula
- Rhinoplasty
- Pharyngoplasty
- Correction of prognathism or micrognathia.

Management of Associated Problems
- Facial growth
- Hearing loss—both sensorineural and conductive defect done in first year
- Speech—nasal twang or articulation problems
- Dental development—orthodontic care.

EPULIS ("EPULIDES" PLEURAL)

Q. Define and describe epulis (short notes).

Epulis is a word from Greek "epi" and "ulon" meaning on the gingival.

An epulis is a swelling of the gingiva having an intimate relation with periodontal membrane or with the periosteum of the jaw. The term is applied to mucosal hyperplasias of the edentulous alveolus. Generally a localized measuring 0.5–2.5 cm, broad based or with a stalk, soft to firm, with a normal to reddish color, depending on the histopathology of the lesion.

- **Incidence:** Not uncommon.
- **Age:** Epulis appears in any age but mostly affects people between 30 and 50 years. Newborns may have epulis like swelling (congenital epulis). Sex: Female predilection.
- **Site:** The gingiva and alveolar mucosa are the most prevalent sites.

Types of Epulis
Described in **Table 19.4** given in next page.

SWELLINGS OF JAW

Q. Enumerate the primary jaw tumors (short notes).

Tumors of Jaw
They may be primary and metastatic.

Odontogenic Tumors
- Benign—epithelial/mesenchymal or mixed (includes benign ameloblastoma).
- Malignant—carcinoma, sarcoma (includes malignant ameloblastoma).

Maxillofacial
- Tumors from bone and cartilage
- **Benign:** Osteoma/chondroma/osteochondroma
- **Malignant:** Sarcomas—osteosarcoma/chondrosarcoma.

Hemato-lymphoid
- Solitary myeloma (plasmacytoma)
- **Non-neoplastic:** Cysts and cyst like lesions
- Developmental—dentigerous cyst
- Giant cell lesions
- Fibro-osseous, osteochondromatous
- Bone cysts.

Chapter 19: Developmental Anomalies of Face, Tumors and Swellings of Gums and Jaws

Table 19.4: Types of epulis, details of pathology and treatment.

Type of epulis	Age /sex	Site of origin	Clinical appearance and treatment	
Congenital	Newborn female	Gum pad—upper gum	Swelling upper jaw over premolar area. Bleeding on touch	Excision
Fibrous	Any age/ sex 30–50	Periodontal membrane	Painless, non-tender, hard, pale pinkish grey swelling, on gum bleeds on touch	Excision (rule out carcinoma)
Type of epulis	**Age /sex**	**Site of origin**	**Clinical appearance and treatment**	
Epulis fissuratum	Elderly edentulous	Vestibular mucosa	Chronic low-grade irritation from an ill-fitting denture	Correction of denture, local hygiene
Granulomatous	Any age	Gum tissue	Made of granulation tissue around a caries tooth. As a fleshy mass in the gum which bleeds on touch	Extraction of the carious tooth and curettage of granulation tissue
Epulis gravidarum	During pregnancy	Gingival mucosa	Bleeding swelling/s	Oral hygiene and symptomatic treatment. It resolves after delivery
Giant cell epulis	30–50	Mandible or maxilla less often	Ulceration of osteoclastoma through mucosa of gum	
Differential diagnosis and variants				
Carcinomatous epulis		Carcinoma of oral cavity		
Fibrosarcomatous		Fibrosarcoma of jaw bone		
Myelomatous		Leukemia		
Metastatic "epulis like"		Carcinoma—lungs, breast, kidney		

Q. Write short notes on dental cyst and dentigerous cysts.

DENTIGEROUS CYST (FOLLICULAR ODONTOME)

Origin and Pathology

- Arises from dental epithelium of an unerupted tooth (premolar or molar), affecting the lower jaws more commonly.
- It is a unilocular cyst with an unerupted tooth within, expanding the outer table of mandible (or maxilla).

Clinical Feature

- A smooth and hard painless swelling in the jaw along with a missing tooth.
- A dental X-ray or orthopantomogram confirms the diagnosis, showing a tooth within a radiolucent lesion in the expanded bone.

Differential Diagnosis

Dental cyst, adamantinoma (ameloblastoma), giant cell tumor (osteoclastoma).

Treatment

- Small lesions—excision of cyst with extraction of the tooth involved.
- Large—marsupialization—opening of cyst, removal of the unerupted tooth and curettage of the contents. The cavity is left to granulate (excision, if the cavity fails to fill).

DENTAL CYST

Syn: Periapical cyst, radicular cyst.

- This lesion occurs due to chronic root abscess of an erupted and dead tooth.
- **Pathology:** The cyst lined by squamous cells and epithelial debris.
- **Clinical feature:** A painful and smooth swelling in the jaw bone in relation to caries.

Differential Diagnosis
Dentigerous cyst.

Complication
- Osteomyelitis of mandible or maxilla.
- Intraoral sinus due to rupture of cyst.

Investigation
Dental X-ray or orthopantomogram.

Treatment
- **Antibiotics:** Amoxyclav 625 mg Q8H for 7 days.
- **Surgery:** Drainage of cyst (or curettage of cavity) and extraction of tooth or root canal treatment.

> Q. Write short notes on adamantinoma.

ADAMANTINOMA
Syn: Ameloblastoma (Note: Important)
- An odontogenic tumor—arising from dental epithelium or dental lamina.
- Age group—mostly 4th and 5th decade with a male preponderance.
- **Sites:** The jaws—mandible five times more often affected than the maxilla.
- **Rare sites:** Base of skull or tibia.
- The ramus of the mandible is involved more frequently than body.
- It is mostly benign, less often malignant; but acts like a locally invasive tumor, usually with multilocular cystic spaces (occasionally unilocular). It does not spread to lymph nodes. However recurrent and malignant adamantinomas spread by blood to lungs.
- **Histopathology:** Shows cords of odontogenic epithelium, ameloblasts, fibrous tissue and reticulum cells as in a basal cell carcinoma.

Clinical Features
- Jaw swelling commonly affecting the mandible involving the angle and ramus.
- It expands the outer table of bone gradually causing a smooth, hard and painless swelling. The inner table is intact and normal. It grows and expands the bone causing crackling of the bony cortex ("egg shell crackling").

Differential Diagnosis
- Giant cell tumor (osteoclastoma) of the mandible—more in the ramus than at angle of mandible; inner table also is affected.
- Dentigerous cyst—contains a dental abscess.
- Giant cell reparative granuloma (Jaffe's tumor)—fibrovascular hyperplasia following of hemorrhage into the marrow.

Investigations
- X-ray of mandible or orthopantomogram (OPG)—show a multiloculated lesion with "honeycomb" appearance and an intact inner table. In case of osteoclastoma—uniformly lytic lesion of bone with multiple large lucent areas are seen.
- CT scan or MRI of the lesion and cervicofacial region is preferred.
- Biopsy from the swelling.

Treatment
Surgery
- If the tumor is small—segmental resection of the mandible.
- If the tumor is large—hemimandibulectomy with reconstruction of the mandible using a fibular free graft is preferred.
- Curettage and bone grafting is not recommended (risk of recurrence).

Oropharyngeal Cancer

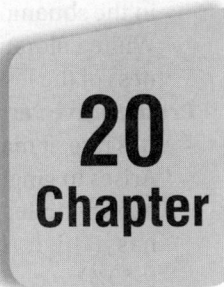

Chapter 20

SU20.1	Describe etiopathogenesis of oral cancer symptoms and signs of oropharyngeal cancer.
SU20.2	Enumerate the appropriate investigations and discuss the principles of treatment.

Q. Short notes on Waldeyer's ring.

Refer **Figure 20.1**.

Waldeyer's Rings

The oropharyngeal lymphatics drain through the Waldeyer's rings to the cervical lymph nodes.

Inner Ring

Anteriorly the adenoids, lymphoid tissue around the eustachian tube and faucial tonsils laterally and lingual tonsil (lymphoid tissue at posterior tongue).

Outer Ring

From anterior to posterior—submental nodes, submandibular nodes, upper jugular nodes, tonsillar nodes and retropharyngeal nodes.

PREMALIGNANT LESIONS OF ORAL CAVITY

Q. Describe pathology and treatment of leukoplakia. (Short note)

Leukoplakia (Leucoplakia)

- A white plaque which cannot be rubbed off.
- It is a clinical term—cannot be correlated with histological changes.
- It may be a single patch or multiple patches.
- Small lesion or large area/s of the mucosa.
- Smooth or wrinkled, cracked (fissures).

Variants of Leukoplakia

- **Speckled leukoplakia**
  - Is a variant with an erythematous base and has the maximum potential for malignant transformation.

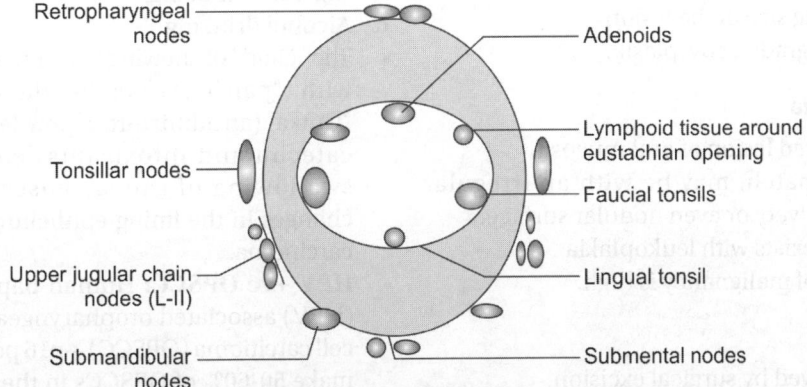

Fig. 20.1: Waldeyer's rings.

- Microscopy—variable dysplastic changes in the squamous epithelium.
- White coloration depends on the thickness of the lesion.
- **Proliferative verrucous leukoplakia**
  - It is rare; it may affect non smokers too.
  - Arises in gingival margins, as multifocal exophytic lesions with leukoplakia. It has a high risk for cancerous change (>50%).
- **Chronic hyperplastic candidiasis**
  - Caused by invasion of the leukoplakia lesion by *Candida albicans*. Has a high risk of malignant transformation.
  - *Clinical features:* Dense plaques of leukoplakia, particularly around the commissures of the mouth.

Treatment

Follow up Regularly

Management:
- Antifungal treatment against candidiasis—2 weeks of systemic or 6 weeks of topical.
- Folic acid and vit B12 supplementation.
- **Biopsy:** Multiple edge biopsies to exclude cancerous change.
- Surgery indicated if lesions persist after 6 weeks
- **Excision:** For single and small lesions—excised.
- **LASER ablation:** For large lesions and multiple lesions.

Factors for Malignant Transformation
- Age of the patient
- Increasing size of the lesion
- Severity/grade of dysplasia.

Erythroplakia
- A bright red lesion of oral mucosa.
- Velvety patch, may be with an irregular shape, velvety or even nodular surface.
- Often coexists with leukoplakia.
- The risk of malignancy is high.

Treatment

Biopsy followed by surgical excision.

> **Q. Short notes on: Oral submucous fibrosis.**

Oral Submucous Fibrosis
- This is characterized by progressive fibrous scarring, formation of fibrous bands beneath the oral mucosa and contractures.
- Microscopy reveals dysplasia.
- It has a high risk of malignancy.

Etiology
- Mainly chewing of tobacco and pan masala and gutka.
- Results in restriction in movement of tongue and mouth opening.

Treatment
- Limit the progression by stopping pan masala or gutka.
- Surgery—to help release the fibrous bands.
- Improves mouth opening but recurrence is common.

ORAL AND OROPHARYNGEAL CANCERS

Incidence of oral cancer in India is very high (about 28-30 per 100,000 population). Oral and oropharyngeal cancers are among the commonest cancers in India and Asian countries making nearly half of world cases. They share a lot of common in etiology and pathogenesis.

> **Q. Write a short note on etiology of oro pharyngeal cancers.**

Etiology

"S—smoking, sepsis, speckled leukoplakia, spirits, syphilis, sharp tooth"
- Cigarette smoking,
- Alcohol drinking.
- The "Quid" of chewing betel nut plus tobacco with ("pan"leaves or "tendu leaves") and "Gutka" (an admixture of powdered tobacco, catechu and intoxicants) chewing and swallowing of saliva causes dysplastic changes in the lining epithelium leading to carcinoma.
- **HPV +ve OPSCC:** Human papillomavirus (HPV) associated oropharyngeal squamous cell carcinoma (OPSCC)—p16 positive; They make 50-60% of OPSCCs in the west. Affect

younger aged and non smoking patients and have a better prognosis than the HPV-ve and p16 -ve cancers.
- Plummer-Vinson syndrome (sideropenic dysphagia) dietary deficiency—vit A, B, iron and chronic glossitis.
- Dental ulcers and poorly designed dentures
- Oral lichen planus (OLP)
- Family history of cancers.

> **Q. Write a short note on enumerate the pre malignant lesions of oral cancers.**

Premalignant Conditions
- Leukoplakia—particularly speckled type.
- Erythroplakia.
- Chronic hyperplastic candidiasis.
- Oral submucosal fibrosis.
- Syphilitic glossitis.

> **Q. Describe pathology and staging of oropharyngeal cancer.**

Pathology
- Pathological microscopic changes in transformation of normal mucosa to carcinoma
- Hyperkeratosis, dyskeratosis and then carcinoma in situ.

Distribution of Oral Cancer
- **India:** Buccal mucosa (65–70% in India, but 20–25% in western world)
- **Tongue:** Most common site (western world)
- Floor of mouth—15%
- Lips, gums and palate are other sites.

Multiplicity
Multiple primary tumors are common—exposure to carcinogens induce diffuse mucosal changes, **"field change"**, a phenomenon causing a migration of clone of mutant cells to other areas of mucosa.

Multiple tumors may be:
- Synchronous (20%)—within 6 months of each other.
- Metachronous (80%)—half of them within 2 years and rest later than 2 years.

Spread
- Local infiltration to adjoining structures—muscles, bones vessels and nerves
- Lymphatic spread and to cervical lymph nodes—usually to levels I, II and III, but skip metastases may be seen in level IV.
- Hematogenous—less commonly (nasopharyngeal carcinoma).

Morphology
- Proliferative type
- Ulcerative type
- Fissure
- Diffuse infiltrative (tongue).

Microscopy: Squamous cell carcinoma in most (low, intermediate, high grade or anaplastic).

Other malignancies in oral cavity
- Adenocarcinoma
- Minor salivary gland tumors
- Melanoma.

Behavior of tumor: Generally—most aggressive in tongue, least in lip, moderately aggressive, in floor of mouth, cheek, gums, and palate.

TNM Staging of Oral and Oropharyngeal Carcinoma – (AJCC Staging)
Refer **Table 20.1**.

Histological Grading
Broder's Grades: I–IV

I—Well differentiated, II—Moderately differentiated, III—Poorly differentiated, IV—Anaplastic.

The Alternate Grading System: Gx, G1–3

Indeterminate—Gx, Low grade—G1, Intermediate—G2, High grade—G3.

Clinical Features and Treatment of Oropharyngeal Carcinoma
Symptoms: Mainly dysphagia or odynophagia, halitosis, aspiration.

Signs: Neck nodes may be present. Signs of pneumonitis may be present.

Table 20.1: TNM staging for oral/oropharyngeal sq cell carcinoma (AJCC 8th edition).

TNM staging is different for HPV +ve and **HPV -ve** cancers (they vary in prognosis)

Tumor "T"

T0: Only for HPV +ve cancer- undetected primary with node metastases - p16 +ve.
TIS: Only applicable for HPV negative
T1: Tumor, 2 cm and thin
T2: Tumor 2–4 cm
T3: Tumor > 4 cm or involves dorsal tongue
T4: Spread to adjacent bone - mandible or maxilla
  – Extra oral -to skin, pterygoids, masticator space or carotid sheath
Note: Depth of invasion (DOI) is a prognostic factor for HPV -ve oral cancers
T1 < 5 mm—thin, T2 5-10 mm (intermediate) T3-DOI > 10 mm

Nodes "N"

HPV +ve (p16+ve)	HPV -ve (p16-ve)
N0	ENE (extra nodal extension -prognostic factor)
N1 ipsilateral node/s < 6 cm	N1- ipsilateral < 3 cm
N2 contra or bilateral nodes < 6 cm	N2a single Ipsilateral < 6 cm
N3 - node/s > 6 cm	N2b - ipsilateral multiple < 6 cm
	N2c - contra or bilateral nodes < 6 cm
	N3 - node/s - >6 cm (N3a/b - ENE negative)
	N3c - extra nodal spread (ENE positive)

Pathological stage: pN0, pN1 < 4 nodes pN2 > 4 nodes (irrespective of side-bilateral or unilateral)

Metastases (M)

M0 – no distant spread
M1 – distant spread – lungs or bones

Stages

HPV positive (p16+VE)	HPV negative- (p16 -ve)
I-T0, T1, T2; N0 N1	I-T1-N0
II-T0, T1, T2, N1-N2; T3, T4, N0, N1	II-T2 N0
III-T3 T4 N2	III-IIIa T3 N0; IIIb T1-3 Ni
IV-Any T, Any N, M1	IVa-T1-4a, N1-2
	IVb-T4b, any N; AnyT, N3
	IVc-Any T, any N, M1

Investigations

- Pan endoscopy of oro-digestive tract with biopsy is done for diagnosis. Includes nasopharyngoscopy.
- CT evaluation of neck nodes and chest.
- Evaluate for HPV virus IHC marker P16.

Treatment

Early Stage

Radiotherapy or LASER ablation of primary lesion - T1- T2 - As curative therapy.

Surgery

- For large lesions and recurrent lesions
- Following neoadjuvant RT CT
- Radio/chemo resistant lesions

Wide resection with reconstructive flaps—myocutaneous or free flaps.

Advanced Stage

- T3 and T4
- Neoadjuvant chemoradiation and surgery—resection with and reconstruction (myocutaneous pedicles or free flaps).

Neck nodes
- Modified radical neck dissection (MRND) ipsilateral or bilateral node dissection for bilateral spread (N2-c)
- Inoperable cases—palliative radiotherapy.

ORAL CANCERS

All oral cancers have common etiological factors, biological behavior and the staging. Therefore the principles of management are essentially the same with modifications in depending on site, stage, grade and functional considerations.

Carcinoma tongue is described in detail as an index; the same principles are applicable to carcinoma of—cheek, gum, lip, floor of mouth and palate.

> Q. Pathology, clinical features and management of carcinoma tongue. (Major question)

Carcinoma Tongue
- Most common oral cancer in west, second commonest in India.
- Males out number females.

Pre Disposing Factors
- Papilloma, HPV, oral syphilis, oral candidiasis, hypovitaminosis B12.
- Premalignant lesions—leukoplakia, erythroplakia, submucous fibrosis.

Pathology
Sites: The distribution of carcinoma tongue is given in **Figure 20.2**.
- Anterior two thirds: 80%
- Posterior: 20-25%.

Lateral side of tongue—most common 45-50%
Tip of tongue   : 10-15%
Dorsum of tongue   : 10-15%%
Ventral side   : 5-6%

Morphology
- Proliferative
- Ulcerative
- Fissure
- Diffuse infiltrative.

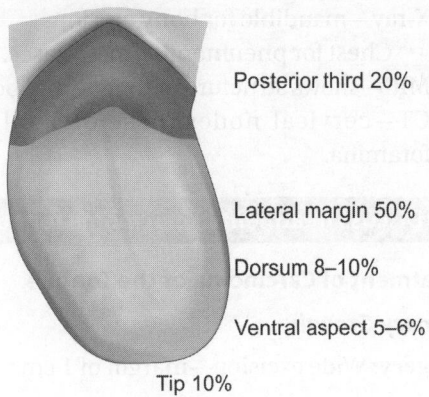

Fig. 20.2: Carcinoma tongue distribution.

Microscopy
- Squamous cell carcinoma—the most common.
- Adenocarcinoma, may arise from minor salivary glands or mucous glands.
- Melanomas.
- Lymphoepithelioma rarely.

Local Spread
- To floor of mouth, mandible
- Palatoglossal fold and oropharynx
- Retromolar trigone.

Lymphatic Spread
- Submental nodes—both sides
- Lateral side—to submandibular nodes and deep cervical
- Dorsum—both sides—deep cervical nodes (level III)
- Posterior two thirds—deep cervical level III and IV.

Clinical Features
- Growth over the tongue, difficulty in eating, swallowing, speech, ear pain.
    - Trismus, ankyloglossia, halitosis.
    - Aspiration pneumonitis.
- **Neck nodes:** Level I,/II, III and IV, depending on the site and stage.
    - Fixed nodes in submandibular triangle with hypoglossal nerve palsy.

Investigation
- Biopsy—from edge of growth.
- FNAC—neck nodes

- X-ray—mandible for bony erosions
  - Chest for pneumonitis/metastases.
- MRI—shows structure of tongue and bone.
- CT—cervical nodes, base of skull and foramina.

Q. Discuss treatment of carcinoma tongue.

Treatment of Carcinoma of the Tongue

Primary Growth

Surgery: Wide excision—margin of 1 cm.

Indications

- Early growth, for T1, T2 tumors
- T3 lesions – lateral side of tongue
- Radioresistant and radio-recurrent lesions, syphilitic seropositive.
- T4—after neoadjuvant—tumor invading bone and floor of mouth and fauces.

Anatomically surgical procedures are as per site of lesions

- Tip of tongue—wide excision
- Lateral side of tongue—wide excision for T1 and T2
- Hemiglossectomy on respective side for T3
- Total glossectomy—for dorsal growth. But the same is generally avoided in view of very high morbidity.
- Wide excision with reconstructive flaps—for posterior third of tongue (reconstruction done to correct defective swallowing function and aspiration).

Radiotherapy (RT)

- **Primary radiotherapy (curative)**—external beam RT—for well differentiated tumors

  Indications:
  - T1, T2 well differentiated (G1/2)
  - In cases where surgery causes—severe morbidity defective swallowing, speech, severe mutilation or disfigurement, e.g., dorsum, posterior third of tongue.
- **Neo-adjuvant** RT—for downstaging of T4 or T3 tumors before surgery.
- **Adjuvant RT** after surgery for T3 tumors.

- **Palliative RT:**
  - External beam RT or brachytherapy.
  - Brachytherapy (iridium-192 or caesium -137 needle implantation)
  - For T4 tumors or tumors of posterior third and dorsum.

Lymph Node Metastases

- **N0:** FNAC and scan negative
  - Elective (prophylactic) node dissection levels I–III
- **N1-N2:** Modified radical neck node dissection-MRND (level I–V)
- **N2C:** MRND on side of growth and selective node dissection (I–III) on opposite side.
- **N3:** Palliative RT + CT.

Q. What is commando operation? (Short question)

Commando Operation

En bloc wide resection of growth and lymph node field on the respective side along with resection of part of mandible in continuity.

Hemiglossectomy, hemimandibulectomy and radical neck node dissection—en bloc

Problems: Mutilation, disfiguring, dysfunction of speech, mastication, swallowing and neck.

This was the standard of care before the current advances modified the approach.

Chemotherapy: Intravenous or intra-arterial.
- No curative role
- Used with RT as neoadjuvant or adjuvant.
- Combination of 3 or 4 drugs
- Cisplatin, bleomycin, cyclophosphamide, adriamycin and 5-fluorouracil.

Targeted therapy with monoclonal antibodies—not proven yet.

Prognosis

Worse than in carcinoma of the lip and the cheek.
5 year survival—St I, II – 70–80%, III – 50%.

Cause of Death

- Aspiration pneumonitis
- Carotid blow out due to nodal infiltration.
- Cachexia.

Carcinoma of Cheek and Buccal Sulcus

- Most common oral cancer in Indian subcontinent (40% of all oral carcinomas)
- **Cause:** Pan masala (betel nut with slakes lime and tobacco) and gutka.
- Males dominate but females also make a big section.

Pathology and epidemiology: Similar to that of tongue cancer, but less aggressive.

- Mandible, masseter and buccinators retromolar trigone are invaded.
- Cervical nodes are affected level I-V.
- Synchronous lesions may often be seen.
- Staging (refer previous section).

Clinical Features

- Trismus, loosening of tooth, halitosis and odynophagia.
- Pain referred to ear (auriculotemporal nerve) due to infiltration of inferior alveolar nerve.
- Oral mucosa always has stains of pan or tobacco, leukoplakia, erythroplakia.
- Irregular thickening of mandible.
- Enlarged cervical nodes.

Staging

Refer Previous Section.

Investigations

- Edge biopsy from lesion and FNAC of node.
- X-ray of mandible or ortho pantomogram to assess bony erosion.
- MRI—is more informative with reference to invasion of bone, nerve and muscles of cheek and also retromolar trigone.
- CT—is useful to evaluate
  - Invasion of skull base area—if tumor extends to in retromolar trigone.
  - Cervical nodes.

Treatment

- **Curative RT**—for T1 lesions, grade I, isolated and without leukoplakia or erythroplakia.
- **Generally surgery is preferred to radiotherapy** as a curative modality.
  Neoadjuvant RT – T4 and T3 lesions near retromolar trigone.
- **T1-2 N0:** Wide excision of primary lesion with margin of 1 cm with
  - **Elective** (prophylactic) node dissection level I, II, III (supraomohyoid)
  - Follow up with serial CT and FNAC for 5 years.
- **T1-2 N1:** Wide excision with **selective** node dissection level I, II, III (supraomohyoid)
- **T3 N0 –or high grade:** Wide excision with modified radical node dissection (level I-V)
- T3 or T4 lesions—require resection of part of mandible or half of mandible too (segmental or hemimandibulectomy).

Wide excision may involve reconstruction of cheek defects with pedicled (deltopectoral) flaps or myocutaneous flaps (e.g., pectoralis major or) and/or bony defects with osteocutaneous free flaps (fibular graft with peroneal artery pedicle).

Palliative Treatment

Neo adjuvant RT + chemotherapy—followed by surgical resection with reconstruction and radical neck dissection.

Carcinoma Lip

- Lower lip (90%) more often involved than upper lip. UV radiation is considered as a cause.
- Visible early and early presentation, easily accessible.
- Least aggressive among oral carcinomas.
- But in upper lip and commissures of mouth
  - These cancers are aggressive and spread to pre parotids nodes, worsening the prognosis.

Treatment

Primary Lesion

- **T1:** Wide excision and primary closure or primary RT (curative radiotherapy)
- **T2:** Wide excision with reconstruction of lip with local flap (to avoid microstomia) or primary RT
- **T3:** Neoadjuvant RT CT and wide excision with reconstruction
- **T4:** Neoadjuvant RT CT and Surgery to remove growth, part of bone and nodal field

Nodes

- **N0:** Observe and follow up for T1 and T2
- **N1:** Selective node dissection level I-III
- **N2:** MRND
- **N3:** Palliative RT CT.

Q. What is retromolar trigone and its importance?

Retromolar Trigone (Retromolar Pad)
- A triangular area of mucosa covering ramus of mandible behind the third molar crowns
- Base – mucosa behind the lower (mandibular) molar
- Apex – maxillary tuberosity
- Lymphatic drainage to Node Level II

Importance—spread to this area marks advance stage and poor prognosis.
- Tumor infiltrates the mandibular ramus, mandibular nerve, palatine branch, and buccinator and superior pharyngeal constrictor, both attached to pterygopalatine raphe.
- Tumor also spreads from here to tonsil and palate glossal folds.
- Early tumors are treated by RT.
- Advanced lesions need neoadjuvant RT/CT and palliative surgery.

MANAGEMENT OF SECONDARIES IN NECK NODES

About 80–85% are from cancers of head and neck of which about 80% are squamous cell carcinomas, while others include salivary tumors, rarer malignancies like sebaceous cancers and sarcomas. About 15% of metastatic neck nodes are due to primary from lungs, breast or abdomen.

Q. Describe the neck lymph node levels in the diagnosis and planning of treatment.

Anatomy of Neck Nodes (Refer Table 20.2)

150 to 200 nodes on each side of neck totalling 300–400.

Conventionally described as: Pre-auricular, post-auricular, occipital nodes; submental and submandibular nodes; jugulodigastric, nodes, upper deep cervical nodes; Jugulo-omohyoid node and supraclavicular nodes.

The level II nodes, (jugulodigastric node, included) drain the following **FIVE "silent"** areas:
- The oral cavity (posterolateral part); oropharynx including the tonsils
- Nasopharynx (including fossa of Rosenmuller)
- Pyriform fossae and supraglottic larynx.

Table 20.2: Neck lymph node groups and levels.
- Level I: Submental nodes - Ia and submandibular nodes - Ib
- Level II: Upper jugular (jugulodigastric) nodes
- level III: Middle jugular group
- level IV: Lower jugular group
- level V: Posterior triangle group
  – Va: Those above course of spinal accessory nerve
  – Vb: Those below the nerve
- Level VI: Anterior compartment group from thyroid cartilage to suprasternal notch.
- Level VII: Is superior mediastinal nodes (not neck)—significance in thyroid cancers.

SCC (squamous cell carcinoma) from the above five primary sites account for nearly 80% of metastatic nodes in cancers of head and neck.

Clinical Examination

History
- History of oral and pharyngeal lesions—odynophagia, dysphagia, halitosis, aspiration, cough.
- Habitual smoking and drinking, chewing of tobacco or products.
- Examination of oral cavity is the first step.

Oropharynx, larynx and the neck should be examined methodically.
- A focus light, a tongue depressor and a laryngoscope preferably a flexible laryngoscope.
- **The neck** is examined for laryngeal movement on deglutition, laryngeal crepitus, lymph nodes with the patient in sitting position.

A methodical examination of oral cavity, oropharynx and neck is performed.
- Other sites are also examined—thyroid, scalp and ear
- About 15–20% of metastatic neck nodes are due to primary from lungs, breast, GI tract and uro-genital tract, which should be examined.

Staging of Nodal Metastases in Neck

Generally applicable to cancers of head and neck **(Refer Table 20.3).**

Chapter 20: Oropharyngeal Cancer

Table 20.3: Staging of neck node metastases.

N-0	No nodes		No nodes
N-1	Single node <3 cm		No nodes
N-2	a	Single node 3–6 cm	No nodes
	b	Multiple discrete nodes 3–6 cm	No nodes
	c	Bilateral nodes, but largest node <6 cm	
N-3		Lymph node larger than 6 cm	

Clinical Presentation of Neck Nodes

Hard, irregular nodes and in late stages, fixed to jugular vein or skin, finally ulceration.

Nodes may be detected as with

- Overt primary—lesion presents with symptoms and signs.
- Silent primary—no symptoms, but detected by examination (silent areas).
- Occult primary—silent primary not detected even by all methods.

Investigations
Search and find the primary:

- Panendoscopy of upper aerodigestive tract to look for primary lesion and biopsy.
- Multiple blind biopsies are taken from "silent" sites if no primary lesion is found.
- X-ray neck and chest—foreign bodies, pneumonitis.
- CT scan of neck and chest—for nodes and lesion in chest. PET CT is useful.
- MRI may be of limited use.
- FNAC (under ultrasonographic guidance, if need be)—from the node is a must to check for metastatic node.

Treatment of Metastatic Neck Nodes

- **Primary lesion**—treated when detected as per stage – curative RT or surgery or palliative RT + chemotherapy.
- **Nodes**—are treated concurrently with primary surgery or following RT (neo-adjuvant).

- **Occult primary with nodes:** If no primary is found, treat the secondaries and observe for the primary to show up—after 6 to 12 months.
- The overall better prognosis of SCC is better than that of other types and that is the rationale of surgical resection of the metastatic nodes with the curative intent (radical) called **radical neck dissection (RND)**.

The extent of lymph node dissection is modified by the site of lesion, grade of tumor and the stage – both T and N, where the morbidity and postoperative functional loss associated with RND are minimized without compromising long-term oncological outcome (radicality and long-term prognosis) of the neck dissection called **modified radical neck dissection**.

> Q. Define radical neck dissection.

> Q. What are the modifications of radical neck dissections?

Types of Radical Neck Dissections (RND)

Radical neck dissection (RND) on each side (right and left) involves:
- Removal of all lymphatic tissue, vessels (except carotids), nerves (except vagus nerve), fat, muscle and fibro-fatty tissues of neck on one side, in an area between trapezius posteriorly, strap muscles anteriorly, mandible superiorly and clavicle inferiorly, in a plane superficial to the prevertebral fascia behind upto and including investing layer of cervical fascia (with sternomastoid belly with spinal accessory nerve).

Note:
- This procedure removes lymph nodes in levels I to V.
- Level VI is not a part of standard RND.
- Here the **carotid artery and vagus nerve are the only major structure preserved.**

Modified Radical Neck Dissection (MRND)

The following **three structures—one, two or all three** are preserved and the modified procedures

are classified as MRND—type I, II or III, by careful dissection to avoid morbidity.
1. Spinal accessory nerve (N)—paralysis and wasting of trapezius.
2. Internal jugular vein (V)—especially bilateral- intracranial venous drainage MRND type II)
3. Sternomastoid muscle (M)—loss of shape of neck and weakness on the side.

Type I: N preserved.
Type II: N and V preserved
Type III: N, V and M are preserved

> Q. Write note on selective neck dissection.

Selective Neck Dissections

One or more group of nodes are selectively removed to clear the expected field of the spread of respective cancer depending upon the site and extent of primary.

Indications
- Early N stage (N1-2b) nodes
- Not indicated for N2c and N3, high grade SCC, aggressive salivary carcinoma, or medullary thyroid cancer.

Types of Selective Neck Dissections
- Antero-lateral neck dissection (supraomohyoid dissection) removal of levels I, II and III.
- Lateral neck dissection—levels II–V
- Posterolateral neck dissection—level V a and V b along with levels III and IV.
- Central dissection—levels VI and VII.

Extended neck dissection: When dissection goes beyond the standard boundaries, e.g., central dissection (level VI, VII with selective lateral dissection II–V.

Commando operation: En bloc resection of primary tumor with surrounding tissues and nodal field in neck in continuity.

Elective neck dissection: A selective node dissection or MRND is done for N0 disease (when clinical and imaging reports fail to detect significantly enlarges nodes).

Indication: Aggressive tumors –high grade SCC of tongue, palate or any T3/T4 SCC, melanoma, adenocarcinomas.

Palliative debulking has no role.

External carotid ligation is done for bleeding lesions of oropharynx or oral cavity.

Radiotherapy
For Primary
- External beam irradiation
- Curative for primaries of oral and oropharyngeal growths in early stage
- Neoadjuvant RT is given with concurrent chemotherapy for downstaging the tumor before surgery.

For Neck Nodes
- Radiotherapy
- Adjuvant therapy after neck dissection in N2c or N3 lesions.
- Palliative radiotherapy with chemotherapy for fixed nodes.
- Brachytherapy (implantation of iridium needles)—for palliative therapy in N3 disease.

Chemotherapy
- Neoadjuvant—with radiotherapy.
- Adjuvant or palliative along with radiotherapy.
- Drugs used—combination of 2 or 3 among – cisplatin, bleomycin, cyclophosphamide, 5-fluorouracil, doxorubicin, vincristine.

End stage neck nodes
Cause of death:
- Aspiration pneumonia.
- Bleeding due to erosion of nodal disease into carotid or one of the branches.
- Respiratory obstruction due to pressure on trachea.

> Q. Short note topics of oral cavity.

- **Sublingual dermoid**
- **Ranula**
- **Cancrum oris**
- **Epulis**

Oral Ulcers

Painful Ulcers

Vincent's Angina (Stomatitis) – "Trench Mouth". Acute necrotizing ulcerative gingivitis (ANUG).

Etiology

Vincent's (twin) organisms: *Spirochaeta vincenti* and *Bacillus fusiformis* and anaerobes may be associated with stress or immunocompromised states) HIV/steroids.

Starts from gingival ulceration progressing to painful ulcers of oral cavity upto oropharynx including tonsils. Necrosis of mucosa and sloughing may happen.

Clinical Features

- Pain, foul smell, fever
- Ulceration and necrosis of mucosa.

Treatment

- Penicillin, preferably intravenous crystalline penicillin 20 lakh units Q6H
- Warm gargles, nutritional support.

Herpetic Ulcers

Multiple painful, shallow.

Dental Ulcers

Painful and against an ill fitting dentures.

Tuberculous Ulcers

Painful ulcers, more near tip of tongue, bluish overhanging margins.

Secondary Syphilis

Snail track ulcers of secondary syphilis. Mucous patches often seen.

Painless Ulcers

- **Syphilis (rare now):** Primary – chancre – indurated single ulcer – tip or sides Tertiary – gumma – punched out margin – dorsum.
- **Carcinoma:** Ulcerative type – indurated ulcers – anywhere
- Sarcoma with ulceration.

Q. Short notes on cancrum oris.

Cancrum Oris

Syn: Noma—greek word meaning greedy eating.
- An infective condition of oral mucosa, which spreads rapidly to cause progressive necrosis and gangrene of full thickness of muscles and skin of cheek and lip.
- Often it leads to an oro cutaneous fistula through cheek.
- It is due to synergistic infection (anaerobic and aerobic organisms of oral flora) usually seen in ill nourished children and
- Adults with severe debilitation or immunosuppression (HIV or following acute infections like enteric fever and viral exanthemata).

Clinically: It presents with severe toxemia.

Treatment

- Antibiotics—penicillin or piperacillin aminoglycosides anti-anaerobic medicines (metronidazole)
- Blood transfusion and fluid resuscitation
- Extensive necrosectomy to remove infected tissue
- Supportive parenteral nutrition
- Elective reconstructive surgery after recovery.

Prognosis—high mortality.

Similar condition is also reported pudendal areas.

Q. Short note on macroglossia.

Macroglossia (large tongue)
Causes: Given below in **Table 20.4**.
Problems—speech and swallowing drooling, aspiration.

Table 20.4: Causes of macroglossia.	
• Hypothyroidism—cretinism	• Plexiform neurofibroma
• Hemangioma	• Unusually, congenital a-v malformation
• Lymphangioma	• Primary amyloidosis

Salivary Glands

Chapter 21

SU21.1	Describe surgical anatomy of the salivary glands, pathology, and clinical presentation of disorders of salivary glands.
SU21.2	Enumerate the appropriate investigations and describe the principles of treatment of disorders of salivary glands.

SU21.1: Describe surgical anatomy of the salivary glands, pathology, and clinical presentation of disorders of salivary glands.

SU21.2: Enumerate the appropriate investigations and describe the principles of treatment of disorders of salivary glands.

SURGICAL ANATOMY OF SALIVARY GLANDS

- Major salivary glands—2 parotids, 2 submandibular and 2 sublingual gland on each side
- Minor salivary glands—about 800-1000 in aerodigestive tract.
- Ectopic/aberrant salivary gland tissue—commonly in submandibular space.

Function: Secretion of saliva—1000-1500 mL per day. Approx 65-70% is from the submandibular gland in unstimulated state and 25% from parotids; at least 50% is from parotid in stimulated state (e.g. chewing/eating).

Saliva is alkaline, contains calcium, salivary amylase an lipase.

Parotid secretion is more serous—approx. 20% = 300 mL to 750 cc when stimulated.

Submandibular glands secrete viscid saliva approx. 65% (>700-800 mL).

Sublinguals also secrete 10% (75 mL) - viscid saliva minor glands account for 10% (60-70 mL).

Parotid Salivary Glands

Two glands—a right and a left.

The parotid is situated in the wedge between the mandible and the mastoid, enclosed by the cervical fascia which splits into a superficial layer, thick and tough, the parotid fascia, attached to the zygomatic arch, and a deep, thin and ill defined layer, separating the gland from the submandibular space. Part of the gland extends (tail) into the upper neck.

Q. Faciovenous plane of Patey.

The gland is divided into a superficial lobe (about 80% of gland) and a deep lobe (20% of the gland) by the faciovenous plane of Patey—made of the facial nerve and its branches along with the retromandibular vein.

The nerve runs superficial to the posterior facial vein. The external carotid branches into the superficial temporal artery and maxillary artery deep to the vein. This plane is crucial in surgical dissection of the gland.

The superficial lobe lies on the masseter, angle of mandible, below ear lobule and in front of mastoid. The tail is in upper neck over sternomastoid belly.

The deep lobe is wedged in a space:
- Posteriorly—with mastoid (covered by sternomastoid and stylohyoid muscles)

- Anteriorly—mandible with masseter and pterygoid
- Medially—the pharyngeal wall (lateral to tonsillar fossa) and internal carotid artery.

Parotid duct, about 5 cm, runs through the gland forwards to pierce the buccinator muscle to open into the mouth opposite the upper second molar tooth.

The facial nerve, from stylomastoid foramen enters the gland and divides as below:
- **Temporofacial:** Branches are—temporal, zygomatic and buccal
- **Cervicofacial:** Branches—marginal mandibular and cervical.

Nerve supply: Secretomotor fibers - run through auriculotemporal nerve, which carry the parasympathetic fibers from otic ganglion.

Sympathetic is from plexus around external carotid.

Lymphatic drainage: The parotid drains into intraparotid nodes and into preauricular nodes. Further drainage is into deep cervical nodes—Level II and III.

The surface anatomy of the gland is important in clinical diagnosis of parotid diseases.
The gland is like a pyramid with the base superficial and tip in deep in the groove.
- The pyramid base is made by joining four points
- A point anterior to tragus—superiorly
- Mastoid process—posteriorly.
- A point 2 cm below and behind the angle of mandible inferiorly.
- A point at the junction of anterior two thirds and posterior third of a line between angle of mouth and ear lobule. And the parotid duct marked on the surface by the line making the middle third of the line above.

Submandibular Salivary Glands

The gland is in submandibular triangle bound by mandible and digastric bellies.

This gland is hugs on to the free border **of mylohyoid muscle, which divides the gland into again two parts—superficial and deep,** the deep part being palpable with a finger (index) on the floor of the mouth and the other index over the skin over the submandibular gland.

Wharton's Duct

Each gland has a submandibular duct (5 cm), running from deep lobe forwards to open into floor of mouth through the papilla on either side of frenulum linguae.

Facial artery—runs in a groove on posterior aspect of gland before it crosses mandible.

Nerves

Lingual nerve, and the submandibular ganglion, run close to superior aspect of deep lobe gland

Hypoglossal nerve runs on floor of triangle, deep to gland.

Lymphatic drainage: Level I B and II, the lymph nodes are close to gland in the space. In disease, they are inseparable from the gland.

Nerve supply: Secretary fibers are from submandibular ganglion through lingual nerve.

Sublingual Glands

One gland on each side is in sublingual space deep to mandible, sharing the space with deep part of submandibular gland, lymph nodes and about 10–20 minor salivary glands.

The duct of sublingual (Bartholin duct) drains into Wharton's duct.

Minor Salivary Glands

About 800–1000 small salivary glands are dispersed throughout the submucosa of aerodigestive tract (oral cavity, pharynx, larynx, trachea, lungs, and middle ear cavity), mostly concentrated along the mucosa of buccal cavity, lips, tongue, palate—soft and hard, and floor of mouth.

Minor salivary gland tissue is not seen on conventional imaging, but is seen only when replaced by tumor or benign processes, most commonly mucus retention cyst.

DISORDERS OF SALIVARY GLANDS

Sialorrhoea (sialorrhea): Excess salivation (**Note: Drooling** is due to abnormal closure of mouth and inability to swallow).

Causes of Sialorrhea

- Diseases—neurological (e.g., cerebral palsy, mental retards)
- Drugs—sialogogues.

Treatment—anticholinergics—atropine derivatives like propantheline.
- Rarely sialoadenectomy.

> Q. Write a short notes on xerostomia.

XEROSTOMIA

Dry mouth—decreased salivation.

Causes of Dry Mouth
- Dehydration
- Anxiety and depression
- Drugs—antidepressants, anticholinergics
- Disease—autoimmune disorder like Sjogren's
- Post-radiation (for head and neck).

> Q. Write a short notes on ranula.

CYSTS: RANULA

An extravasation cyst arising from the sublingual gland with the mucous contents causing a transparent swelling on floor of mouth, looking like "frog belly".

Types
- **Simple ranula:** In the floor of mouth—deep to mylohyoid
- **Plunging ranula:** Mucous contents extravasate and pierce through the the mylohyoid edge to superficial plane into the neck—it is not a true cyst (no epithelial lining).

Clinical Course of a Ranula
- Spontaneous resolution
- Enlargement—causing difficulty in speech and eating.
- Bleeding due to rupture and erosion into lingual artery.

Differential Diagnosis
- Sublingual dermoid cyst and a lipoma.
- Plunging ranula—resembles a lymphangioma or lymph cyst with clear fluid.

Ultrasonography and MRI are useful in diagnosis.

Diagnostic aspiration of yellowish content is done orally to exclude a lymph cyst.

Treatment
- Surgery—intraoral approach
- Marsupialization (deroofing and opening the cyst wall into oral mucosa)
- Resection of sublingual gland with the ranula—complex surgery.
- Incision and drainage – also done but it has risk of recurrence.

Plunging ranula is aspirated and drained intraorally as there is no epithelium in its wall.

Disorders of Minor Salivary Glands
- Cysts—they are "extravasation " type cysts due to secretion against pressure on the duct.
  Sites: Commonly—in lips, gums or palate.
- Treatment - excision.

Tumors: Benign and malignant.

Sites: Upper aerodigestive tract but commonly in lips, and palate.

Size varies. Bluish and opaque.

Rubbery consistency or hard and ulcerated in malignancy.

Treatment
- **Small:** Benign tumor—excision biopsy.
- **Larger than 1 cm:** A punch biopsy done to confirm benign or malignant
- Wide excision with mucosal flap reconstruction.

SUBMANDIBULAR SALIVARY GLAND AND PAROTID DISORDERS

> Q. Write a short note on sialectasis.

- State of dilatation of the ductal system commonly affects parotid.
- Generally bilateral and generalized. But it may be rarely focal.
- The ducts are dilated with formation of pouches resulting in stasis of saliva and concretion of calcium salts in the ducts leads to inflammation, fibrosis and strictures.
- The gland develops recurrent infection, worsening the changes—fibrosis
- Calculi may be seen in the ducts.

Clinical Features

- Episodes of pain and swelling of gland often with fever.
- Worsening of the pain during eating, due to stimulation of salivation.
- Tenderness over the area of gland.

X-ray and ultrasonography help detect calcification.

MRI scan—shows ducts and parenchyma.

Sialography: It helps in depicting the ductal system with obstruction and calculi or strictures, But it may lead to flaring of inflammation and should hence done after acute inflammation has subsided.

Principles of treatment

It is difficult to cure—due to the nature of pathology.

- Treat the acute episodes
- Anti-inflammatory drugs
- Promote salivary flow by message over the cheeks.
- Oral hygiene.

After the acute episode – treat any correctable pathology like a strictureplasty of the parotid duct.

Q. Write a short note on sialography.

A diagnostic contrast dye study to depict the ductal system and to evaluate the obstructive lesions in the ducts of salivary glands and also salivary fistulae.

MRI is used for diagnostic work while sialography helps documentation of strictures and stones.

Contraindications

- Acute infection in the gland.
- Hypersensitivity to the dye.

Steps

- Identify and cannulate the opening of the respective salivary duct opening in the mouth.
- Inject 2 to 5 cc of water soluble dye (not oil soluble) into the duct.
- Shoot X-ray pictures.

Complications

- Wrong cannulation.
- Acute parotitis or submandibular sialadenitis and secondary sepsis.

SALIVARY CALCULI

Q. Write short note on salivary calculi.

- More than 85% are in submandibular salivary duct due to: 1. Viscid saliva, 2. Stasis
- Uncommonly seen in parotid duct.
- There may be more than one calculi.
- Calcium salts form the calculi, obstructing salivary flow and induce inflammation in the parenchyma (sialadenitis).

Clinical Features

- The patient presents with pain and swelling over the gland, which is worse on mastication.
- Often the pain is colicky ("salivary colic")
- The calculus may be palpable on floor of mouth and distinguished from a lymph node by bidigital palpation.

X-ray—large calculi are radiopaque.

MRI—shows calculus and ductal picture.

Treatment

Submandibular Salivary Calculi

Acute inflammation is treated by antibiotic and local warmth.

Removal of Calculus

- Non-surgical interventions are not indicated when a stricture is present, e.g., endoscopic lithotripsy to fragment and retrieve of stone fragments.
- Surgery:
  - Intraoral route—opening the duct close to gland and laying it open into the oral cavity with care to avoid damage to lingual nerve.
  - Resection of the submandibular gland (sialadenectomy) is done for a calculus in main gland or for a diseased gland.

Calculi in parotid duct: Usually associated with a stricture of Stensen's duct.

- **Surgery:** To remove calculus along with excision of stricture of the duct or to open the strictured segment.

Salivary Fistula

It is parotid fistula most of the times.

Etiology
- Following surgical incisions or trauma or rupture or draining of parotid abscess.
- Major fistula arises from Stenson's duct and minor fistula from parenchymal ductules.

Clinical Presentation
- Opening internally—salivary leak into mouth
- External—over the facial skin—leaking saliva.

Treatment
- Sialography depicts the duct and fistula tract
- Antibiotics to treat infection
- Anticholinergics to reduce salivary secretion.
- Radiation is not a preferred modality.
- Usually parenchymal fistulae heal. Ductal fistulae may heal if there is no stricture.

Surgery
- The conservative measures fail.
- There is a clear tract and fistula with major leaks.

Principles
Lay open the tract, excise the stricture and resuture the open end of the duct to the mucosa of the cheek to create a new parotid papilla into mouth.

ACUTE SIALADENITIS AND PAROTID ABSCESS

Acute Sialadenitis

Etiology
- Viral—mumps—hematogenous infection
- Bacterial – retrograde infection
- Organisms get access to duct—facilitated by poor oral hygiene, immunocompromised states,
- Viral exanthemata, postoperative state, generalized debility, diabetes, radiotherapy, HIV, suppuration and abscess formation are common.

> Q. Write a short note on clinical features of acute sialadenitis.

Acute Submandibular Sialadenitis

Clinical Features
- Painful submandibular swelling and swelling in floor of mouth.
- Fever, dysphagia and dysarthria.

Signs—high temperature, tenderness, redness over the region.
- Inflamed opening of Wharton's duct.
- Edematous chin.
- Double chin appearance due to spreading of edema downwards.
- Duct is inflamed and swollen.

Complications
- Ludwig's angina.
- Abscess of submandibular area.

Treatment
- Antibiotics—cloxacillin and metronidazole.
- Anti-inflammatory drugs—ibuprofen or diclofenac.
- Associated systemic disorders like diabetes are treated.
- Oral hygiene.

Calculus removed after acute condition subsides.

Chronic submandibular sialadenitis—typically pain increases after food intake and swelling enlarges.
- Diff. diagnosis—neoplasm, lymphadenopathy—tuberculosis, lymphoma
- Investigation—ultrasonography, FNAC to rule out tumor or specific pathology.
- Treatment—excision of the submandibular salivary gland.

ACUTE BACTERIAL (SUPPURATIVE) PAROTITIS AND PAROTID ABSCESS

> Q. Diagnosis and management of parotid abscess.

Acute infection due to infection along the duct from oral cavity.

Pathology—refer above.
- The swollen parotid is within the tough parotid fascia and hence under increased pressure.
- Commonly leads to abscess formation and it may rupture.

Clinical Features
- Very severe pain over parotid.
- Fever, trismus and difficulty to swallow.
- The patient is febrile.
- Locally the parotid area is swollen—a diffuse and ill-defined swelling over the surface area of parotid (entire gland affected). Severe tenderness is seen.
- But no fluctuation is demonstrable.
- The parotid papilla is edematous and red, may extrude a bead of pus.

Complications
Rupture, fistula, septicemia.

Investigations
- Blood—WBC counts, sugar
- Ultrasonography
- MRI

Treatment
- Oral hygiene, hydration, analgesics
- Antibiotics: Antistaphylococcal (cloxacillin or piperacillin) and against oral organisms (metronidazole).

Surgical drainage—for abscess—incision and drainage under general anesthesia.

Should not wait for fluctuation.

Follow imaging guidance
- Surgical incision is in front of tragus through skin and then the sinus forceps are thrust into open transversely (never vertically) to avoid damage to facial nerve.

Complications
- Parotid fistula formation.
- Facial nerve damage.
- Frey's syndrome may develop as a late complication.

Chronic parotitis: Usually due to stricture of Stensen's duct.

Clinical features—pain during mastication, swallowing—hard and fixed.

Diff diagnosis: Tumor of parotid.
- Surface anatomy shows the way:
  - Due to diffuse nature, parotitis corresponds to the shape of parotid gland.
  - A tumor is focal and hence distorts the shape of the gland on the surface.

Treatment
- Sialogogues and maintain oral hygiene.
- Analgesics and steroid in extreme situations.

> **Q. Write a short note on Frey's syndrome.**

FREY'S SYNDROME (AURICULOTEMPORAL SYNDROME)

This condition follows injury to twigs of auriculotemporal nerve in facial trauma or surgery (e.g., on parotid).

The patient gets "gustatory sweating"— sweating, erythema, and flushing over cheek and forehead during chewing.

It is due to stimulation of sweat glands, abnormally innervated by regenerating auriculotemporal branches (post-trauma), when stimulated by food. The parasympathetic fibers regenerate and connect with sympathetic fibers for sweating.

Starch iodine test—paint the symptomatic area with iodine, apply dry starch over the area after iodine dries, watch for appearance of blue color due to sweating, stimulated by salivary stimulation.

Treatment
Many settle with reassurance and conservative measures.
- Anticholinergics.
- Antiperspirants, usually containing aluminium chloride
- Botulinum toxin injection into the affected skin is the most effective.

Interventions and Surgery
- Denervation by tympanic neurectomy.
- Auriculotemporal nerve avulsion.
- Interposition of temporal fascia, fascia lata, or sternomastoid muscle flap as a barrier to prevent abnormal innervation of skin by parasympathetic fibers.

Granulomatous sialadenitis
Tuberculous, non **tuberculous** mycobacterial, sarcoidosis, mycotic granuloma, collagen disease like Wegener's granulomatosis.

> Q. Write a short notes on sialosis.

SIALADENOSIS (SIALOSIS)
- Bilateral symmetrical, non-inflammatory salivary gland swelling—particularly parotid gland, association with - alcoholism, diabetes mellitus, endocrine diseases, pregnancy, drugs.
- Age 40-65 Years
- Treatment is to correct associated condition like alcoholism and diabetes.

Sjögren's Syndrome (Short Notes)
An autoimmune disorder—due to progressive destruction of salivary and lacrimal glands.
- Primary Sjogren's—without associated autoimmune or connective disorder. **More severe**.
- Secondary Sjogren's—associated with SLE, polymyositis or thyroiditis, rheumatoid arthritis.

More females than males affected (ratio 10:1). Microscopy of salivary and lacrimal glands: Progressive lymphocytic infiltration and destruction of acinar cells with proliferation of duct epithelium.

Complications
- May develop lymphoma (more in primary). Non-Hodgkin's B-cell lymphoma.
- Oral candidiasis.
- Secondary bacterial sialadenitis.

Clinical Features
- Keratoconjunctivitis sicca (dry eyes)
- Xerostomia (dry mouth)
- Diffuse enlargement of parotids, submandibular glands and lacrimal gland.
- It is more severe and progressive and in primary type while it is associated with thyroiditis and arthritis in secondary type.

Treatment
Mainly symptomatic and supportive. No known treatment to check progress.
- Eye care—artificial tears.
- Salivary substitutes.
- High water intake.

Watch for complications and treat them accordingly.
- Eye
- Lymphoma.

> Q. Describe pathology of tumors of salivary glands. (Long Answer)

> Q. How do you evaluate malignant tumors of parotid? (Long Answer)

CLASSIFICATION OF SALIVARY GLAND TUMORS (REFER TABLE 21.1)
Salivary Gland Tumors
Distribution: 70-80 % in parotid, 15-20% in submandibular and vary uncommon (<2 %) rare in sublingual and minor glands.

Incidence of malignancy 10-20% on parotid, 50-60% in submandibular, 80-85% in sublingual glands and over 90% in minor salivary glands.

Parotid tumors: The parotid gland is the most common site for salivary tumors.

Clinical Features of Salivary Tumors
Parotid Tumors
- About 80% of tumors arise in the superficial lobe, present as slow-growing, painless swellings below and in front of the ear, raising the lobule of ear, In the upper neck (tail of gland) and 10% arise in deep lobe as para pharyngeal mass.
- Oral examination—reveals a swelling of soft palate—pushing the tonsil medially.

Remember: 80-90% for parotid.
- 80-90% of tumors are benign.
- 80-90%—they arise from superficial lobe.
- 80-90%—pleomorphic adenoma.

Features of Malignancy
- Rapid growth and pain referred to ear.
- **Hard** tumor, fixity to muscle or skin, **facial nerve weakness**, lymph nodes

Table 21.1: Tumors of salivary glands.

Benign

Epithelial (90%): Adenomas.	Nonepithelial (stromal tumors)
Monomorphic adenomas • Adenolymphoma (Warthin's tumor). • Oncocytoma (oxyphil adenoma) • Basal cell adenoma	Hemangioma, lymphangioma Neurofibromas and neurilemmoma
Pleomorphic adenoma—most common tumor	

Malignant tumors

Epithelial—carcinomas	Lymphomas: Non-Hodgkin lymphoma (NHL)

• Mucoepidermoid carcinoma
  – Most common malignancy
• Adenoid cystic carcinoma-
  – Very aggressive 10%
  – Common in minor salivary glands
• Acinic cell carcinoma: 1–2%
• Adenocarcinoma
• Squamous cell carcinoma 2%
• Carcinoma in a pleomorphic adenoma
• Undifferentiated carcinoma
	• More common in parotid than submandibular gland.
	• Sjogren's syndrome and HIV have a high association.
	Metastatic (secondary) tumors
	• Tumors of head and neck region; and bronchus
	• Skin, melanoma

- Low grade tumors may not show these signs in early stage.

Submandibular Salivary Tumors

50–60% are malignant.

Benign—usually pleomorphic adenomas.
- Present as mass in submandibular gland
- Bidigitally palpable in floor of mouth when deep lobe is affected.

Diff diagnosis—lymph node swellings.

Malignancy—suspected in cases with
- Fixity to mandible or skin, lymph nodes palpable
- Nerve palsy—hypoglossal or in marginal mandibular nerve distribution.

Sublingual Salivary Tumors

- 80–90% are malignant
- Rubbery mass, purple or pale
- Hard, large and ulcerated mass is always malignant.

Benign Salivary Tumors

> Q. Write a short notes on Warthin's tumor (adenolymphoma).

Warthin's Tumor (Adenolymphoma)

Syn: Papillary Cystadenoma Lymphomatosum

- Exclusively a parotid tumor.
- Monomorphic benign adenoma.
- Postulated to be due to entrapment of jugular lymph sacs in the developing parotid gland.
- Arises from lower part or tail.
- Single or multiple.
- Bilateral tumors are common.
- High association with smoking and those with exposure to radiation.
- May be associated with malignant tumors.

Histology

"Adenolymphoma " denotes:
- Encapsulated lymphoid tissue in stroma
- A double layer of columnar epithelium projecting as papillae into the cystic spaces.

Clinical features

- Age: 45–60 years.
- Sex: Male 4 times more than females.
- Soft tumor in lower part of gland.

Diff. diagnosis

Cystic tumors—mucoepidermoid or adenoid cystic carcinoma.

Investigations

- Ultrasonography **and FNAC.**
- Technetium-99 pertechnetate scintiscan—it shows as a "hot spot".

Treatment

- Partial (superficial) parotidectomy.
- Enucleation of the tumor (only if FNAC proven).

Q. Write a short note on mixed tumor (pleomorphic adenoma)

Pleomorphic adenomas make:
- 80% of all parotid tumors
- 80% arise in from parotid
- 80% arise from superficial lobe
- 80% in lower part of superficial lobe, 10% in deep lobe and 10% in tail and accessory lobe.

Pathology
- Origin—myoepithelial cells and ductal cell.
- Tumor encapsulated with finger extensions into neighboring gland.
- Often seen in deep lobe also.
- Histology—pseudo-amyloid stroma combined with glandular pattern.
- Variable firm to hard mass from parotid lower part as described under clinical features.
- Slow growth over years into very large size.
- May turn malignant—invading the facial nerve, skin and masseter.

Clinical features:
- A swelling in parotid area—small to large—smooth or lobulated.
- Retromandibular groove is full, ear lobule is raised.
- Swelling cannot be pushed above zygomatic arch (curtain sign).
- Deep lobe tumors—tonsil pushed medially and uvula displaced.
- Malignancy suspected if the there is fixity to skin, masseter or facial nerve weakness.

Diagnosis: Clinical history and examination.
- FNAC—helps, trucut biopsy—proves type of malignancy in case of suspicion.
- MRI—to study the extensions of tumor into other parts of gland and ensure complete removal.
- Open biopsy—never done—spillage of cells causes recurrences.

Treatment
- **Superficial lobe tumors:** Conservative superficial parotidectomy (also called conservative partial parotidectomy when a part of superficial lobe is removed, e.g., warthin's tumor limited to lower part).
- Extracapsular partial parotidectomy—tumor with margin of normal parotid tissue excised without dissecting facial nerve.
- **For deep lobe tumors:** Conservative total parotidectomy.

Types of Parotidectomy

Conservative Parotidectomy

Refers to conservation of **facial nerve**.
- **Superficial:** Removal of **superficial** lobe—for benign tumors in superficial lobe.
- **Total:** Removal of **entire gland** without sacrificing the nerve.

Radical Parotidectomy

Refers to sacrificing the facial nerve for tumor clearance involves resection of the entire gland with adjoining structures like muscle, part of bone and lymph nodes.
- **"Enucleation"** only for proven benign monomorphic tumors like Warthin tumor or lipomas. Partial parotidectomy—part of the gland (superficial) for proven localized tumor.

Extracapsular Partial Parotidectomy

Facial nerve not dissected.
- Focus is on boundaries of tumor and dissection is performed outside the tumor margin along with a margin of healthy tissue without spillage of tumor cells.
- Suitable for benign tumors of lower part of gland or tail and low grade malignancies.

Advantages: Low risk of facial nerve injury. Over dissection avoided.

Disadvantage: Not suitable for high grade malignancies—as it fails oncological clearance.

Complications of Parotidectomy

- Facial nerve damage
- Frey's syndrome
- Scarring
- Sialocele and salivary fistula
- Facial numbness
- Anesthesia over the ear lobe due to transaction of great auricular nerve
- Recurrence of tumor – more due to missed extensions of the pleomorphic adenomas

Mixed tumors of submandibular glands are less common.

The need to be treated with a submandibular salivary gland excision (sialadenectomy).

PRIMARY MALIGNANCIES OF SALIVARY GLANDS

Generally Less Aggressive

- Mucoepidermoid carcinoma—low grade
- Acinic cell carcinoma
- Adenoid cystic carcinoma.

Generally Aggressive

- Mucoepidermoid carcinoma—high grade
- Carcinoma in a pleomorphic adenoma
- Adenocarcinoma
- Squamous cell carcinoma
- Undifferentiated (anaplastic) carcinoma
- Lymphoma.

General Features: Salivary Carcinomas

Pathology: All tumors spread locally to neighbouring structures and through lymphatics to the regional nodes.

- Carcinomas of submandibular gland are more aggressive than those of parotid.
- Sublingual and minor gland cancers are highly aggressive.
- Invasion of nerve, skin and muscle and bone—depends on pathology.

Clinical features include features of tumor: Hardness, fixity and spread.

- Nodes—regional
- Nerve weakness or palsy—facial nerve—trunk or branches in parotid, hypoglossal in submandibular and sublingual gland tumors.

Staging: TNM Staging of Carcinomas of Salivary Glands (Refer Table 21. 2)

Investigations

- FNAC—to evaluate pathology
- Trucut biopsy may be needed in confirming types
- CT—helps in evaluation of deep lobe of parotid and submandibular glands and neck nodes and also bone erosion, skull foramina.
- MRI—helps in evaluation of nerves—facial in parotid tumors, hypoglossal, lingual and marginal mandibular nerves. Also it helps in looking for involvement of masseter, bone and infratemporal fossa.

Table 21.2: TNM staging of carcinoma of salivary glands.

• T1 <2 cm • T2–2-4 cm • T3 > 4 cm or minimal extraglandular spread • T4 > T4a - 4 cm—spread to nerve, muscle or bone • T4b—fixity to carotid sheath, base of skull, pterygoid plate	**N–N0** • N1 <3 cm • N2—node with extranodal extension or multiple nodes < 3 cm • N3—6 cm one or more
M0–M1—metastases	
Stage: Stage 0 - Tis N0 M0 Stage I - T1 N0 M0 Stage II - T2 N0 M0 Stage III - T3 N0 M0; T1–3. M0 I Stage IV - IVa - c, T4a, or T4b/N3 and M1	

TREATMENT OF SALIVARY MALIGNANCIES (GENERAL)

Surgery is the Sheet Anchor – is Curative

Conservative total parotidectomy

T1, T2, T3: Low grade tumors.

Extracapsular wide excision of salivary tumors—gaining popularity.

This is suitable for small, early stage and low grade tumors.

Radical total parotidectomy is indicated in all tumors—T1-3 with high grade; all T4a tumors; squamous cell carcinoma.

Tumors with propensity for neural spread like adenoid cystic carcinoma or adenocarcinoma.

Postoperative irradiation

- T3, T4 tumors, squamous cell carcinoma.
- All high grade tumors—after radical parotidectomy.
- High grade mucoepidermoid tumor.
- Residual tumor and inadequate resection margins.

Radical neck dissection—usually done when there is spread to neck nodes.

Q. Short notes on muco-epidermoid carcinoma.

Muco-epidermoid carcinoma
- Most common of the carcinomas. (10 % of all tumors and 20 % of carcinomas)
- Most common—parotid. Next is submandibular.

Pathology—soft tumor with solid and cystic spaces. Microscopically
- Low grade—mucin secreting with good prognosis
- High grade—epidermoid cells—with poor prognosis. More often submandibular gland.
- Intermediate grade—also described.

Low grade—slow local, lymphatic spread
- Also hematogenous spread (in high grade)
- Nerve involvement generally late.

Clinical presentation
- Common in children and younger age groups. Elderly are also affected.
- Presents like a soft or cystic swelling mimicking a Warthin's or a pleomorphic adenoma.
- Lymph nodes may be enlarged but facial nerve weakness is late.

Diagnosis
- Ultrasonography to study structure of the tumor and gland
- FNAC—for diagnosis
- Trucut biopsy—for histological diagnosis and grading
- CT neck—evaluate the nodes and deep lobe of the gland for tumor

Treatment

Mucoepidermoid of parotid: Low grade tumors:
- Conservative total parotidectomy- And postoperative irradiation of the field of tumor.
- Radical parotidectomy: High grade tumor (trucut biopsy): With selective neck dissection level I-II, III and IV for high grade.

ADENOID CYSTIC CARCINOMA (CYLIDROMATOUS CARCINOMA)

- Second most common salivary cancer after mucoepidermoid
- But it is the commonest among salivary cancers in submandibular, sublingual and minor salivary glands.
- More common in females, age 40-60 years.
- It is slow growing and hence considered as a low grade tumor.

Early perineural spread—facial nerve and mandibular nerve branches
- Very high incidence of spread through periosteum and medullary plane of bone
- It has a high propensity for recurrence.

Hematogenous spread: To lungs, bones and liver. These are slow to grow.

Treatment
- Wide or radical excision of submandibular or/and sublingual glands.
- Radical parotidectomy—for parotid tumors.
- Modified radical or selective neck dissection
- Postoperative radiotherapy.

Local recurrence is common.

Prognosis:
Relatively good survival—about 65-70% survive 5 years after treatment.

ACINIC CELL TUMOR
- Uncommon tumor (about 2%)
- Mostly in parotid gland (90%)
- Sex: Females more often affected
- Age: Elderly 50 to 70 years.

A slowly growing tumor, and is placed under a low grade malignancy.

Variable consistency with cystic areas, microscopically made of spaces with acinar appearance.

Treatment
- Conservative total parotidectomy
- Postoperative radiotherapy.

MALIGNANCY IN A MIXED TUMOR (MMT)
- Third most common (8-10%), about 2-3% turn malignant
- Has a very poor prognosis
- It is among the most aggressive parotid cancers
- Histologically it may show epithelial and mesenchymal appearance (carcinosarcoma).

Clinical Features

A longstanding parotid tumor changes its course and develops rapid growth, fixity, pain, facial nerve weakness, spread to lymph nodes, and often hematogenous spread.

Treatment
- Radical parotidectomy is only option.
- Palliative radiotherapy may be given, with poor results.

Squamous Cell Carcinoma, Anaplastic Carcinoma and Adenocarcinoma
- Uncommon but highly aggressive malignancies of salivary usually submandibular glands.
- Radical excision of gland with surrounding structures is performed if feasible.
- Palliative radiotherapy followed by surgery is performed for inoperable tumors.
- Prognosis is poor.

MINOR SALIVARY GLAND TUMORS
- These tumors make 10% of salivary tumors—commonly seen in palate and lip/cheek
- 90% are malignant (only 10% are benign pleomorphic adenomas)
- Mostly adenoid cystic carcinomas.

Clinical Features
- A submucous swelling, rubbery and ulcerated.
- Spread to hard palpate, maxilla and infratemporal fossa occurs early.
- Lymph nodes may be enlarged.

Differential Diagnosis
Oral squamous cell carcinoma.

Diagnosis
- A punch biopsy or excision biopsy in small tumors less than 1 cm.
- FNAC of the lymph node
- CT scan head and neck

Treatment
Benign tumors—excision.

Malignant tumors
- Tumors less than 1 cm in size
- Wide excision with 1 cm margin.

For larger tumors and deep fixed tumors
- Radical excision may include maxillectomy or palatal excision with reconstruction or dental implants for maxillary and palatal defects.
- Lymph node block dissection of the neck is done if involved.

Section 4

Endocrines and the Breast

22. Thyroid and Parathyroid
23. The Adrenals Glands
24. The Pancreas - Exocrine and Endocrine
25. The Breast

Chapter 22
Thyroid and Parathyroid

SU22.1	Describe the applied anatomy and physiology of thyroid.
SU22.2	Describe the etiopathogenesis of thyroidal swellings.
SU22.3	Demonstrate and document the correct clinical examination of thyroid swellings and discus the differential diagnosis and their management.
SU22.4	Describe the clinical features, classification and principles of management of thyroid cancer.
SU22.5	Describe the applied anatomy of parathyroid.
SU22.6	Describe and discuss the clinical features of hypo - and hyperparathyroidism and the principles of their management.

SU22.1: Describe the applied anatomy and physiology of thyroid.

Q. Describe development of thyroid

Embryology of thyroid is depicted in **Figure 22.1**.

EMBRYOLOGY

Thyroid gland develops from the thyroid diverticulum arising from the foramen cecum, between first and second pharyngeal arches. The diverticulum, continues as thyroglossal tract, descending behind and through the hyoid bone (see above) upto the thyroid cartilage level, just to the left of midline to give rise to the isthmus and two lateral lobes. The pyramidal lobe connects the isthmus with tract.

Congenital Anomalies

Agenesis of thyroid—absence of thyroid tissue—causes failure of development—physical and mental—cretinism.

ECTOPIC THYROID AND THYROGLOSSAL CYST (REFER COMPETENCY SU22.2)

Thyroid gland (thyreos—means a shield) is butterfly shaped, having two lateral lobes, an isthmus covering the cricoids and upper 4-5 tracheal rings. It weighs about 20 to 30 g. The gland has a true capsule and a false capsule made of pretracheal fascia from cervical fascia. Posteriorly the ill defined loose pretracheal fascia has condensation on each side to fix the gland to the trachea (Berry's ligaments) and cricoid. The gland is has 20-40 follicles in each lobe in a fibrous

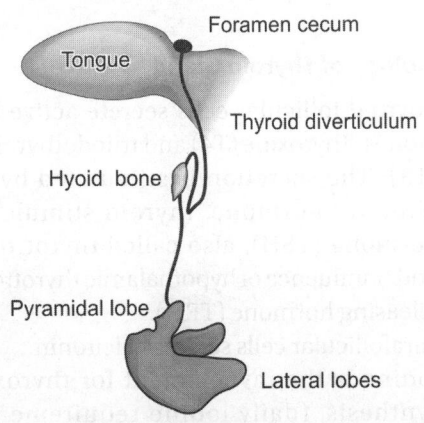

Fig. 22.1: Embryology of thyroid.

stroma and also the parafollicular cells (calcitonin producing-C cells). The follicles have glands with a secreting epithelium, filled with colloid and thyroglobulin, which binds to the hormones.

Parathyroid glands—(refer section on parathyroid).

Arterial Supply

- Superior thyroid artery from external carotid artery.
- Inferior thyroid artery is a branch of thyrocervical trunk of subclavian artery, and
- Thyroidea ima—a branch directly from thoracic aortic arch is seen in some. Both superior and inferior arteries have extensive branching within the glandular capsule keeping the gland highly vascularized.

Venous Drainage

Superior thyroid veins accompany the artery to drain into internal jugular veins on respective side, while the middle thyroid vein joins the IJV directly. Inferior thyroid veins, right and left, drain into respective brachiocephalic vein.

Lymphatic Drainage

Intrathyroid and subcapsular network of lymphatic vessels drain into pretracheal and para tracheal nodes and nodes along the veins (central compartment – level VI). These drain into substernal part of mediastinum (level VII). Lateral drainage is to the deep cervical nodes along the internal jugular vein (levels 2, 3 and 4 and thence to posterior triangle (level 5).

Nerves Related to Thyroid

External laryngeal nerve, supplying the adductors of vocal cords, is close to the superior pole on sides of thyroid cartilage. Recurrent laryngeal nerve supplies the abductors of cord. The left nerve loops around the aortic arch in mediastinum and right nerve, around the right subclavian artery before running into the neck.

Applied Anatomy

- Lateral lobes vary in size and disease and my enter retrosternal or intrathoracic space.
- Pyramidal lobe may be missed during thyroidectomy leaving residual gland or disease.

Arteries

- Superior thyroid artery is ligated close the upper pole of gland to avoid damage to external laryngeal nerve?
- **Inferior thyroid arteries:** Recurrent laryngeal nerves are safeguarded by ligating the arteries away from gland in a subtotal thyroidectomy. But devascularization of parathyroid can be avoided by ligating the artery on the gland, distal to the parathyroid branches.
- The nerve dissected carefully along its course near or through the ligament of Berry in total thyroidectomy.
- A non-recurrent laryngeal nerve is often mistaken for a horizontally running vessel and easily damaged during surgery.

Veins

- Short middle thyroid vein—may tear and leave a direct rent on internal jugular vein, causing serious hemorrhage.
- Slipped inferior thyroid vein stump retracts into superior mediastinum and causes hemorrhage from brachiocephalic vein.

Lymphatic

Lymphatic network in the gland causes spread of papillary carcinoma within gland to contralateral lobe.

Physiology of Thyroid Gland

- Thyroid follicular cells secrete active hormones. Thyroxine (T4) and triiodothyronine (T3). The secretion is stimulated by the pituitary hormone, thyroid stimulating hormone (TSH), also called thyrotropin, under influence of hypothalamic thyrotropin releasing hormone (TRH).
- Parafollicular cells secrete calcitonin.
- Iodine is the raw element for thyroxine synthesis, (daily iodine requirement is 0.1 mg.)

Steps

- Iodide trapping (inorganic iodide) from the blood into follicle.
- Oxidation of iodide to iodine—in follicle—by thyroid peroxidase enzyme.
- Binding of iodine with tyrosine to form mono and diiodotyrosine (MIT and DIT).
- Coupling of monoiodotyrosines and di-iodotyrosines to form T4 and T3.
- Binding of hormones to thyroglobulin in the follicle.
- T4 and T3 are released into the circulation and are bound to albumin, thyroxine binding prealbumin (TBPA) and thyroxine binding globulin (TBG).

T4—1% free and 99% is protein bound.

- After release, T4 is converted to T3 by deiodination, for facilitating quick onset of action of T3 in hours(4 hrs) unlike slow acting T4 (4 days).
- Thyroid hormones are metabolized in liver.
- Iodine is retrieved from circulating iodinated tyrosines (e.g., T1, T2) by deiodination (by the enzyme iodotyrosine dehalogenase in the kidney) and sent back to the iodine pool of the thyroid for synthesis of thyroxine.

The normal levels of thyroid hormones are given in **Table 22.1**.

Functions of Thyroid

- Sustains basal metabolic rate.
- Helps growth—physical and mental.
- Sensitizes peripheral adrenergic receptors to catecholamines
- Has chronotropic and inotropic effect on heart
- Helps respiratory drive of medullary centre.
- Glycogenolysis to increase blood sugar levels
- Stimulates turn over of bony calcium.

Table 22.1: Plasma levels and half life of thyroid hormones.

	Plasma half life (approx.)	Normal blood levels
T4	1 week (5–7days)	5.4–11.5 mcg/dL
T3	1 day	80–220 ng/dL
TSH	1 hour	0.4–4.0 mIU/L (1.8–3 optimum)

> SU22.2: Describe the etiopathogenesis of thyroidal swellings.
>
> SU22.3: Demonstrate and document the correct clinical examination of thyroid swellings and discuss the differential diagnosis and their management (considered together—SU 22.3 is essentially for bedside demonstration; the principles and rationale are described)

CONGENITAL THYROID DISORDERS

Ectopic Thyroid

- Seen in infancy, childhood and adolescence
- Along the course of the thyroglossal tract
- Or away from the tract
- Due to partial or total failure of descent of thyroid diverticulum.

> Q. Short notes on lingual thyroid.

- Mass of thyroid tissue at base of tongue foramen.
- It may be the only existing thyroid tissue or a residual thyroid tissue with normal thyroid being present.

Complications

- Respiratory obstruction, hindrance to swallowing, speech
- Hypothyroidism
- Ulceration and bleeding
- Papillary carcinoma.

Differential diagnosis: Tumors and cysts of tongue.

Principles of Management

- Look for normal thyroid tissue in neck in addition to lingual thyroid. Ultrasonography—of neck and Tc labeled Iodine scintiscan.
- Exclude malignancy—FNAC from lingual thyroid, high serum thyroglobulin levels.
- Look for hypothyroidism thyroid hormone profile—low T4/T3 and High TSH.

Treatment

- **L-thyroxine:** If malignancy is ruled out and TSH levels are elevated.

- 50–100 mcg/day orally with monitoring of TSH levels can cause regression.

Surgery: Resection of lingual thyroid—indicated in:
- Respiratory obstruction,
- Repeated episodes of bleeding
- Interferes with speech and swallowing
- carcinoma suspected or proved.

Median ectopic thyroid—rests along line of thyroglossal tract. Normal thyroid may be absent at times.

Lateral aberrant thyroid—thyroid rests in posterior triangle of neck. These are usually metastases from microscopic undetected papillary carcinoma of thyroid gland.

Q. Write note on thyroglossal cyst.

THYROGLOSSAL CYST (REFER FIGURE 22.2)

Cystic swelling—due to remnants of thyroid follicular epithelium along thyroglossal tract forming into cyst (tubuloembryonic cyst).

Pathology
- Contains epithelial cells and colloid, lined by thyroid epithelium.
- Normal thyroid may be absent due to arrest of descent in a small section of patients.

Complications
- Infection, hemorrhage into cyst
- Rupture and formation of thyroglossal fistula
- Papillary carcinoma thyroid in a thyroglossal cyst.

Clinical Features
- Presents in childhood or early adult life (teenage and 20s)—females more often affected
- Forms a midline cystic swelling.
- Moves upwards on deglutition and also on protrusion of tongue.

A fistula presents as a sinus in the midline with the track running up the thyroglossal tract including hyoid bone through the mylohyoid muscle, opening into mouth at foramen cecum.

Diff. Diagnosis
- Subhyoid bursa (more a horizontal swelling)
- Lymph nodes in submental triangle

Investigations
- Thyroid hormone levels in serum—to look for hypothyroidism
- Ultrasonography and guided FNAC—to exclude carcinoma.
- Iodine-123 or Technetium-99 scintiscan—detects functioning thyroid in the neck.

Treatment of Thyroglossal Cyst

Sistrunk's Operation
Surgical excision of cyst along with the entire thyroglossal tract from neck upto floor of mouth *including the body of the hyoid bone* in which

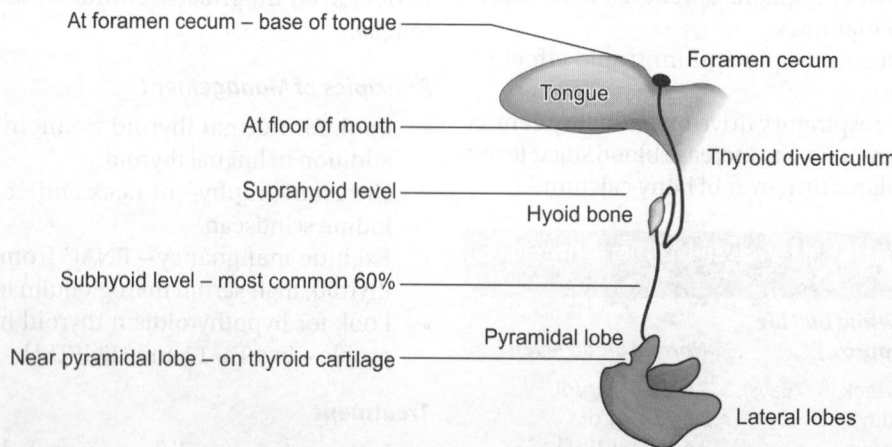

Fig. 22.2: Positions of thyroglossal cysts

the developing thyoglossal tract gets entrapped during the descent of tract.

Any part of the tract left behind can lead to a fistula.

> Q. Classify goiter, discuss goitrogenesis, complications and management of nodular goiter

GOITER (GOITRE) ANY ENLARGEMENT OF THYROID GLAND

Classification of Goiters

- Simple goiter (normal thyroid function—euthyroid)
- Toxic goiter
- Neoplastic goiter
- Thyroiditis
- Others

Simple goiter: Diffuse (euthyroid) or nodular
- **Diffuse:** Hyperplastic (pregnancy/physiological/puberty), colloid goiter
- **Nodular:** Solitary/multinodular goiter.

Toxic goiter

- Diffuse toxic goiter (Graves' disease)
- Multinodular
- Toxic adenoma (autonomous toxic nodule)

Neoplastic

- **Benign:** Adenomas—follicular adenoma, Hurthle cell adenoma.
- **Malignant:**
  - Differentiated—papillary/follicular carcinoma
  - Undifferentiated—anaplastic carcinoma
    * Medullary carcinoma (C-cells)
    * Metastatic
    * Melanoma and sarcoma (rare).

Thyroiditis (inflammatory goiter)

- Subacute granulomatous thyroiditis (de Quervain's thyroiditis)
- Autoimmune chronic lymphocytic thyroiditis (Hashimoto's disease)
- Fibrosing—Riedel's thyroiditis
- Infective—Acute bacterial thyroiditis, viral thyroiditis and chronic tuberculous.

Others

- Familial goiter—peroxidase deficiency
- Drug induced goiter
- Amyloid goiter.

Clinical Terminology: Clinical Palpation Plus Ultrasound Imaging

- Diffuse goiter
- Discrete nodule—single nodule/swelling
- Dominant nodule—a single palpable nodule; but multiple impalpable nodules detected by imaging
- Multinodular goiter—clinically detectable nodules.

Etiopathogenesis of Thyroid Swellings

Neoplastic goiter—please refer Competency SU22.4—Thyroid cancers.

Simple and Nodular Goiter

Goitrogenesis: (Simple and toxic goiter)
Basically low levels of active circulating thyroid hormone causes elevated TSH, which stimulates the gland causing compensatory hyperplasia and enlargement of the gland.

- Congenital and inherited causes—deficiency of thyroid peroxidase causes failure of conversion iodide to iodine and defective hormonogenesis.
- Endemic goiter—caused by:
  - Iodine deficiency—in water in hilly areas. (Western ghats of India).
  - Iodine excess also causes goiter (e.g. Hokkaido Goiter of Japan) due to **Wolf-Chaikoff effect—blocking** the oxidation of iodide to iodine and also release of thyroid hormone from follicles into circulation.
- Drug Induced goiters, e.g., anti TB drugs like PAS, antithyroid drugs, lithium
  - Perchlorate and thiocyanate inhibit iodide trapping;
  - Thiouracil and carbimazole interfere with oxidation of iodide to iodine as well as forming iodotyrosines (MIT, DIT).
- Pregnancy and adolescence—due to increased physiological need of thyroid hormone.

Pathogenesis of Goiter

- High levels of TSH stimulates the gland parenchyma causing hyperplasia.
  This leads to diffuse enlargement with uniformly active follicles (diffuse hyperplastic goiter).
  Thyroid cell membrane has estrogen receptors and females get goiters more often than men.
- When TSH levels fluctuate according to demand, irregular stimulation of gland leads to asymmetrical hyperplasia. Some areas have active follicles and a few inactive. The active areas develop hemorrhage and necrosis of cells amidst the surrounding active follicles forming the early nodule.
  Many such necrotic areas with inactive follicles coalesce to form the nodule.
- Nodules may be cystic—inactive with colloid or active and solid nodule; the internodular tissue remains with active follicles.
- The process gets replicated leading to multiple nodule formation.

Toxic Goiter

- Generally, stimulation by thyroid stimulating antibodies, excess of Iodine intake or high level TSH causes excess of thyroid hormone, causing hyperthyroidism and toxicity.
- In the nodule the hyperplastic internodular thyroid follicles are active and nodules inactive.

Immunological Stimulants (Thyroid-stimulating Antibodies)

- A group of IgG immunoglobulins (thyroid stimulating immunoglobulins - TSI)
- They bind to the TSH receptors on the follicular cell membrane.
- They have action of 16–24 hours and hence called long acting thyroid stimulating (LATS) antibodies, responsible for thyrotoxicosis.

Autonomous toxic nodule (toxic adenoma)—is a distinct entity not due to TSI. The thyroid tissue in the nodule assumes autonomous function, independent of TSH regulation.

Other specific pathologies causing goiters—thyroiditis and neoplasia

DIFFUSE HYPERPLASTIC GOITER AND NODULAR GOITER

Complications

Mechanical Effects on Trachea and Esophagus

Respiratory obstruction (most common): Dyspnea and dysphagia (less often) due to displacement and compression of trachea and esophagus.

Extension into retrosternal space and thorax causes respiratory distress, compression of great veins (visible while raising arms to touch the ears—Pemberton's Test).

There may be deviation of carotid artery.
Hemorrhage into a nodule is common—causing painful sudden enlargement of nodule often with pressure effect on trachea.
Cystic degeneration and calcification.

Effects on function: Hyperthyroidism and secondary thyrotoxicosis in about 30%.

Carcinoma: It is a less frequent complication of nodular goiter, (generally follicular but papillary carcinoma too).

INVESTIGATIONS FOR THYROID DISORDERS

1. Assess Thyroid Function (Refer Table 22.2)

Serum TSH: Level indicates state of thyroid function (if pituitary is normal)
Serum – T-4 and T3 total and free.
In hypoproteinemia, total T4 may be low but free T4 will be indicative of thyroid status.

> Q. Sonographic diagnosis of thyroid swellings, what is TIRADS?

2. Ultrasonography: Most Important Investigation

Done with high frequency probe of 7 to 8 M Hertz: To study structure of gland and nodules,

Table 22.2: Thyroid function states.

Serum levels	TSH	T4 total	T3
Euthyroid	Normal	Normal	Normal
Hyperthyroidism	Low	High	High
Hypothyroidism	High	Low	Low

Table 22.3: TIRADS.		
TIRADS (Thyroid Imaging Recording and Data System)—sonographic stratification of thyroid swellings—for risk of malignancy.		
TIRADS		
1.	Normal thyroid imaging	Reassure
2.	Benign swelling aspects	Observe
3.	Probably benign aspects	Re image or FNAC if >2.5 cm
4.	Low suspicious aspects	FNAC for >1.5 cm
5.	High suspicious aspects	FNAC

papillary tumors show microcalcification and increased vascularity and macroscopic capsular breach, enlarged nodes are diagnostic of malignancy. Sonographic findings suspicious of malignancy include -micro calcification, hypoechoic nodules, irregular margins of nodule, oval –taller than wide lesion.

TIRADS (Thyroid Imaging Recording and Data system)—(**refer Table 22.3**) Sonographic stratification of thyroid swellings—for risk of malignancy.

Q. Write a short note on fine needle aspiration cytology in thyroid disorders.

3. Fine Needle Aspiration Cytology
- FNAC should be used, ideally under ultrasound guidance on all nodules that look suspicious of a malignancy at ultrasonography
- FNAC is accurate in finding a papillary carcinoma but not follicular cancers, which are diagnosed by histological criteria, like capsular and vascular invasion by tumor.

Q. Write a short note on thyroid scintiscan.

4. Thyroid Scintiscan
Radioactive isotope scans—isotope take up is assesses by the gamma radiation it emits. Take up - increased in "hot nodules" with no take up in surrounding parenchyma, nil in cold nodules and normal or low in "warm nodules".

Iodine isotopes—I-123 (short half life in hours) for diagnosis, I- 127 used less often.

I-131 (long half life 7 to 10 days)—generally for therapeutic ablation and not for diagnosis.

Technetium 99—has affinity for thyroid and is often used.

5. CT scan—to assess retrosternal and intrathoracic goiter and lymph nodes.

6. Thyroid antibodies in serum—anti-thyroid peroxidase antibodies (TPO Ab) and anti-thyroglobulin antibody to differentiate from autoimmune thyroiditis.

Treatment
Hyperplastic goiter: TSH suppression by L-thyroxine 50–75 mcg/day causes regression of goiter in many cases.

Surgery
Indications: Respiratory obstruction, toxicity and cosmetic disfigurement.

Total thyroidectomy and thyroxine replacement 100 to 150 mcg/day for life (with TSH monitoring).

Subtotal thyroidectomy: If thyroid tissue is in tracheoesophageal groove is normal.

Multinodular goiter: Needs thyroidectomy.

Total thyroidectomy
It is the standard of care with lifelong thyroxine replacement. It avoids recurrence, but has higher risk of hypoparathyroidism and damage to recurrent nerve.

Subtotal thyroidectomy
Removal of all portions of gland having nodules, leaving behind enough tissue in tracheo esophageal groove (approx 8 g of tissue) for meeting normal thyroxine needs.

Advantages: Avoids life long thyroxine replacement, low risk of of damage to parathyroid and recurrent nerve damage.

Disadvantages: Risk of recurrence of nodules. Re-thyroidectomy has a higher risk of injury to recurrent nerve and the parathyroids.

TOXIC GOITRE (TOXIC GOITER)
Causes of Toxic Goiter
- Diffuse toxic goiter – Grave's disease (exophthalmic toxic goiter)

- **Toxic multinodular goiter: Plummer's disease**
- **Autonomic toxic nodule (toxic adenoma).**
- **Hyperthyroidism due to other causes**
  - Iodine given for endemic goiter (Jod Basedow thyrotoxicosis)
  - Thyroxine given to suppress TSH in a goiter (thyrotoxicosis factitia)
  - Ectopic thyroxine production- ovarian teratoma—secreting beta HCG that stimulates receptors in thyroid follicles.
  - Early phase of thyroiditis due to cell damage and release of hormone.

Drugs, e.g., amiodarone.

> Q. Etiopathogenesis of toxic goiter, management of Grave's disease.

Grave's disease: Three features—
1. Thyrotoxicosis, 2. Goiter, 3. Exophthalmos.

Etiopathogenesis: 50% are familial.
Autoimmune immunity—through thyroid stimulating immunoglobulins (TSIs) including long acting thyroid stimulator (LATS).
- Act on the TSH receptor on the thyrocyte of the follicle as TSH receptor antibody/(TSH R – Ab), stimulate the follicular cells causing hyperplasia and hypertrophy leading to diffuse goiter and hypersecretion.

Other substances like exophthalmos producing factor (EPS)—cause.
- Exophthalmos due to retrobulbar deposition of myxomatous tissue and displacement of eyeball. Dermopathy—due to pretibial myxomatous tissue.

Pathology and Clinical Features

Thyrotoxicosis is a clinical entity: It includes features of hyperthyroidism and of causes other than hyperthyroidism.

Primary thyrotoxicosis: Clinical features of thyrotoxicosis appear concurrently with goiter.

Secondary thyrotoxicosis: Thyrotoxicosis develops in a previously euthyroid patient with a long-standing multinodular goiter.

Hyperthyroidism
- Hypermetabolic state—lose of weight with increased appetite, intolerance to warmth
- Catecholamine hypersecretion—anxiety, high systolic blood pressure and tachycardia
  - Tremors and emotional lability
- Cardiopathy—conduction defects tachyarrhythmias leading to cardiac failure
- Myopathy—proximal muscle weakness and wasting
- Osteopathy—osteoporosis
- Enteropathy—diarrhea.

Features not due to hyperthyroidism

Ophthalmopathy (Grave's ophthalmopathy)
- Mild proptosis—staring look.
- Moderate—diplopia and inability to wink- extraocular muscle dysfunction.
- Severe—extraocular ophthalmoplegia, congestive—chemosis exposure keratitis and corneal ulcers papilledema.

Dermopathy - Pretibial myxedema, Dupuytren's contracture.(rare)-TSI levels are high

Acropachy: Clubbing of fingers and toes.

> Q. Diagnosis and management of toxic nodular goiter. (Long question)

TOXIC MULTINODULAR GOITER (PLUMMER'S DISEASE)

Features of hyperthyroidism are due to hyperfunctioning of the internodular hyperplastic tissue. Rarely some nodule may turn autonomous secreting thyroid hormones.
- TSI and EPS have no role here. Hence exophthalmos is rarely seen.
- Cardiopathy, which sets in early and with catecholamines causes cardiovascular complications.

Clinical Features
- Features of hyperthyroidism (refer previous section)
- Features of a multinodular goiter.

Cardiopathy
- Early—tachycardia followed by missed atrial beats
- Paroxysmal atrial tachycardia
- Later atrial fibrillation
- AV conduction block and cardiac failure.

Q. Autonomous toxic nodule (toxic adenoma). (Short notes).

- These are secreting solitary hyperplastic adenomas, independent of TSH regulation leading to severe hyperthyroidism.
- Generally they secrete more of T 3 than T 4. and TSH is almost reduced to nil.
- Genetic mutation of TSH receptors is reported in some.

Clinical feature: Generally—a clinically discrete nodule with hyperthyroidism.

Q. Write a short note on retrosternal goiter.

- Goiter may extend into superior mediastinum from one of the lobes retaining its blood supply from the parent gland.
- Clinical types—plunging and intrathoracic.
- This causes compression of trachea and great veins too.
- Respiratory distress may be postural—mild or severe or at times life threatening, when there is hemorrhage into these nodules in mediastinum.

Clinical Features of Diffuse and Nodular Goiters (Discussed along with Toxic Goiter)

History Taking

- Painless long-standing neck swellings in younger patients (but may present later also).
- Females outnumber males by 3:1.
- History of geographic endemicity and family history of goiters.
- Also history of goitrogenic drug intake and dietary factors may be revealed.

Symptoms of pressure on trachea and esophagus—dyspnea, stridor and dysphagia.

Change of voice or loss of voice indicates malignancy

Symptoms of hyperthyroidism—like loss of weight despite increased appetite, intolerance to heat, excessive sweating, palpitation, insomnia, anxiety.

Symptoms of hypothyroidism—gain in weight despite loss of appetite and intolerance to cold weather, loss of hair.

Menstrual irregularities are common with thyroid dysfunction—scanty flow in thyrotoxicosis and menorrhagia in hypothyroidism.

Clinical Examination

- Swelling in front of neck, moving up on deglutition.
- A retrosternal extension is shown by a goiter obliterating suprasternal notch and
- Pemberton's sign—venous congestion upon raising of both arms to touch ears.
- Palpation: smooth surfaced or nodular goiter—discrete or multinodular. Hard irregular goiter with fixity indicates malignancy. Tenderness is suggestive of acute hemorrhage into a nodule or thyroiditis. Warm and with bruit in toxic goiters.
- Deviation of trachea and carotid pulsation.
- Nodules and impalpability of carotid pulsation indicates infiltration of carotid sheath by cancer.

Signs of Hyperthyroidism and Toxicity

- Pulse rate (sleeping pulse is reliable as patient is at rest): Tachycardia
- Crile's grading—pulse rate 90–00/min in mild, 100–110/min in moderate and above 110/min in severe thyrotoxicosis.
- Blood pressure—higher systolic pressure—wide pulse pressure.
- Cardiovascular—missed beats, atrial fibrillation (pulse deficit) and congestive failure.

Q. Write a short note on eye signs in thyrotoxic ophthalmopathy.

- Naffziger's sign—projection of eyeball beyond orbital margin.
- Stellwag's sign—staring look, absence of blinking.
- Von Graefe's sign, lid lag.
- Moebius' sign inability to converge.
- Joffroy's sign—an absence of wrinkling of forehead.
- Features of muscle wasting, dermopathy (pretibial myxedema) and acropachy.
- Hyperreflexia is seen in hyperthyroidism and hyporeflexia in hypothyroidism.

Q. Differentiating clinical signs between primary and secondary thyrotoxicosis.

This is summarized below in **Table 22.4**.

Signs of retrosternal nodule or intrathoracic goiter—deviation of trachea, Pemberton's test and percussion over manubrium for dullness.

Malignancy is an infrequent complication of multinodular goiter but may be missed for latter.

Tracheal Fixity and Hardness of a Goiter

- Malignancy—solitary nodule in follicular cancer, generalized in anaplastic.
- Thyroiditis—usually de Quervain's goiter is tender, hard and fixed.
- Hashimoto's thyroiditis—may be fixed, with or without nodules with features of hypothyroidism. In early phase—transient thyrotoxicosis may be seen (Hashitoxicosis).
- Riedel's thyroiditis—presents with hard, small thyroid with progressive tracheal obstruction.
- Hemorrhage and calcification in a long standing goiter—fixity is postinflammatory reaction.

Lymph nodes to be examined: Prelaryngeal, pretracheal and paratracheal nodes are not easily palpable (due to the enlarged thyroid covering the nodes). Suprasternal space may have enlarged nodes (L-VI) and jugular nodes are commonly involved and looked for—at levels II, III, IV and V-b.

Abdomen should be palpated for hepatosplenomegaly and ovarian masses.

Investigations

- **Serum thyroid function**—low TSH levels and high levels of T3 and T4.
- **Ultrasonography**
  - Shows nodules with scanty colloid and internodular hyperplasia in toxic nodular goiter.
  - Accurately differentiates a multinodular goiter presenting as a clinically solitary nodule (the "dominant nodule") from a true solitary nodule (discrete nodule).
- **Radioisotope scintigraphy: Iodine I-123** - shows uptake patterns
  - Mainly indicated to differentiate autonomous toxic nodule from toxic nodular goiter.
  - Autonomous toxic nodule—increased take up (hot nodule) with absence of take up in rest of the gland.
  - Toxic nodular goiter—internodular tissue shows take up with no take up in the nodule/s.
  - Diffuse increase in take up in Grave's disease.
- X-ray of neck and chest—anteroposterior and lateral views to check for tracheal deviation/compression and mediastinal shadows (intrathoracic and retrosternal goiters)
- CT—to look for intrathoracic goiter.
- Laryngoscopy—indirect or flexible direct laryngoscope to check vocal cords for pre existing vocal cord palsy due to earlier illness before surgery.

Table 22.4: Primary thyrotoxicosis as compared to secondary thyrotoxicosis.

	Primary thyrotoxicosis	*Secondary thyrotoxicosis*
Toxic symptoms	Precede or appear with a diffuse goiter, involving whole gland	Preceded by a long-standing multi-nodular goiter
Age group	20 to 30	40 plus
Toxicity	More severe at first presentation	Milder or moderate at presentation
Eye signs and exophthalmos	Diagnostic of Graves' disease	Rare
Cardiovascular system	Uncommonly involved	Commonly involved
Pre tibial myxedema	Common	Uncommon

TREATMENT OF THYROTOXICOSIS (VERY IMPORTANT TOPIC)

Primary Thyrotoxicosis: Grave's Disease

Principles of treatment: Control of hyperthyroidism: General symptomatic and supportive treatment and treatment of complications.

Control of Hyperthyroidism

Antithyroid Drugs
- Generally Carbimazole—20 mg to max 80 mg per day in divided doses.
  It blocks formation of iodo-tyrosines and peripheral conversion of T4 to T3. Clinical effects noted only after 3 weeks. Dose increased at monthly intervals until necessary clinical and biochemical control is achieved; continued for at least one year upto a maximum of 2 years.
  Drug discontinued if:
  - It fails to show effect after 3 months.
  - It shows adverse effects—leukopenia.
- Methimazole—5 to 10 mg daily—If carbimazole therapy fails or causes adverse effects. Also it is safer in pregnant patients.
- Propylthiouracil and methylthiouracil—drug of choice in pregnancy.
- Potassium thiocyanate.
- Lithium salts (in resistant severe cases). Sodium iodide infusion is used for rapid control of toxicity in thyroid storm.

Radioactive Iodine Ablation (RIA) with Iodine I131.
- Treatment of choice in all cases where antithyroid drugs fail and cases recurring after antithyroid drugs. Not preferred in pregnant women.
- Also indicated in recurrent thyrotoxicosis after surgery for Grave's disease.
- Treatment of choice in autonomous toxic nodule.

Surgery: Total thyroidectomy with thyroxine replacement performed—after preoperative control of clinical toxicity with antithyroid drugs.

Indications for surgery: Failure of antithyroid drugs or their adverse effects; patient unsuitable or not willing for radioiodine ablation and very large goiter.

Supportive and symptomatic treatment
- Beta blockers—to control symptoms of hyperthyroidism rapidly
- Sedatives and anxiolytics—nitrazepam.
- Hydration.

Treatment of complications
For example, exophthalmos: Orbital decompression-lateral or superolateral (Rowbotham).

TREATMENT OF TOXIC (MULTI) NODULAR GOITER

- Treatment of toxic nodular goiter is surgery viz., total thyroidectomy.
- Medical therapy is for controlling thyrotoxicosis preoperatively and making the patient fit for a safe anesthesia and surgery.

Preoperative Treatment

Control of hyperthyroidism—antithyroid drugs as described for primary thyrotoxicosis
- Carbimazole, methimazole or thiouracil.
- Usually this takes about 2 to 3 months.
- Symptomatic control of hyperthyroidism—beta blockers—propranolol or metoprolol.

Surgery
- Total or subtotal thyroidectomy.
- Total thyroidectomy is preferred to subtotal thyroidectomy currently to avoid recurrent goiter and thyrotoxicosis.
- Postoperative thyroxine replacement after 2 weeks, for life (about 100 to 150 mcg/day).

Treatment of Autonomous Toxic Nodule

Treatment of choice is radioactive iodine ablation with Iodine – I-131.

Surgery: Thyroid lobectomy

Surgery is indicated for large goiters and in the pregnant. It is performed after preoperative control of hyperthyroidism with antithyroid drugs.

> **Q. Write a short note on thyroid storm (thyrotoxic crisis).**

- A life threatening clinical emergency—during the course of Thyrotoxicosis or

- During and after thyroidectomy due to very high levels of active thyroid hormones in the circulation.

Pathology

Hypermetabolic state, high levels of circulating catecholamines and thyroid hormones.

Precipitated by

- Anesthesia and surgical trauma—any surgery in a patient with uncontrolled thyrotoxicosis during after thyroidectomy.
- Any infection, trauma or certain drugs like diuretics.

Clinical Features

- Hyperpyrexia (over 105-106 °F/40°C), dehydration
- Anxious state, cardiac arrhythmia.

Treatment: Emergent and Active

- Rapid correction of dehydration and hyperpyrexia.
- Intravenous fluids with glucose and saline tepid sponging with ice packs
- Hydrocortisone—intravenous—100-200 mgs Q 8 H.
- Rapid reduction of circulating thyroid hormones—by blocking release of hormones and also blocking their production.
  Plasma exchange therapy is also practiced for rapid reduction of thyroid hormones, as a bridge to surgical treatment.
  Intravenous sodium Iodide (1 to 2 g) infusion.
- Reversal of effects of catecholamines—infusion of beta-blockers propranolol or metoprolol with active monitoring.
- Cardiac failure and atrial fibrillation: Diuretics, digoxin
- Sedation and supportive oxygen
- **Antithyroid drugs:** Carbimazole 60 mg daily (for long-term control)

This is followed by elective thyroidectomy in cases other than the post thyroidectomy storm.

> Q. Write a notes on (1) De Quervain's thyroiditis, (2) Hashimoto's thyroiditis and (3) Riedel's thyroiditis.

THYROIDITIS

de Quervain's Thyroiditis (Acute Granulomatous Thyroiditis)

- Considered as of viral etiology.
- Common among age group of 20 to 40 with female preponderance.
- May follow a common cold or respiratory infection.

Phases

- **Hyperthyroid phase:** Lasts for 4 to 6 weeks. It is due to release of thyroid hormones from the damaged follicular cells (not a true hypersecretion).
- This is followed by a phase of euthyroid state—lasting for about 4 weeks
- Later a hypothyroid state follows. A full recovery is rule after 3 months but mild hypothyroidism may persist in some patients.

Treatment: Symptomatic

- **Antithyroid drugs:** Carbimazole prevents peripheral conversion of T4 to T3.
- Beta blockers.
- NSAIDs—like diclofenac and naproxen.
- Prednisolone 10 mg twice daily for 2 weeks and tapered over next 2 weeks.
- Thyroxine supplementation in hypothyroid state with monitoring of TSH.

No role for surgery.

Riedel's Thyroiditis—uncommon condition. Progressive fibrosis of gland, capsule and surrounding fascia resulting in fixity of thyroid gland to trachea and respiratory distress and also entrapment of carotid sheath and recurrent laryngeal nerve.

Exact etiology is unknown.

Association seen with mediastinal and retroperitoneal fibrosis and primary sclerosing cholangitis.

Differential diagnosis

Anaplastic carcinoma.

Treatment—For Release of Tracheal Obstruction

- Thyroid isthmusectomy (Lahey's operation)
- Empirical steroids, and thyroxine supplementation.

HASHIMOTO'S THYROIDITIS

Syn: Chronic lymphocytic thyroiditis

- A condition due to autoimmune antibodies against thyroid peroxidase and thyroglobulin.
- Resulting follicular cell destruction causes initial release of hormones and transient and generally mild hyperthyroidism (Hashitoxicosis).
- Late hypothyroidism sets in later due to cell destruction.

Complications: Hypothyroidism

- Association (or predisposing to) with papillary carcinoma and malignant lymphoma.
- Microscopy—focal destruction of follicles and infiltration with lymphocytes.
- Askanazy cell (a type of giant cell) is diagnostic of Hashimoto's thyroiditis.

Clinical Features

- Age group commonly 20-40 years, more common in females.
- Thyromegaly—a lobular or nodular enlargement of thyroid and rarely with fixity.
- Clinical features of hypothyroidism—commonly subclinical but often frank.

Diagnosis

- **Blood levels:** Raised TSH, decreased thyroid hormones.
- **Raised serum levels of Anti TPO (thyroid peroxidase) syn:** Antimicrosomal antibodies (AMA) And also antithyroglobulin antibodies—in active phase of thyroid cell lysis.
- FNAC—Askanazy cells and lymphocytic density.

Treatment

- Thyroxine supplementation with TSH monitoring.
- Follow up—clinical and biochemical—TPO antibodies

- Serum thyroglobulin levels—to check for papillary cancer.

Surgery—infrequently indicated in:

- Rapid enlargement of goiter with respiratory obstruction
- Suspicion of malignancy—rapid growth—high thyroglobulin levels, FNAC.
- Generally a subtotal thyroidectomy is preferred to avoid severe hypothyroidism.

THYROIDECTOMY: DEFINITIONS

Thyroid lobectomy—one lateral lobe and isthmus with pyramidal lobe. Indicated in proven solitary nodule, cysts, benign adenoma, autonomous toxic nodule. Currently the term is used synonymously with hemithyroidectomy.

Done in—benign adenoma, multinodular goiter confined to one lobe and isthmus.

Isthmusectomy: For tracheal decompression in Riedel's thyroiditis.

Subtotal thyroidectomy:

- Most of thyroid removed leaving behind just about 8 g of postero inferior part of gland (for producing normal thyroid hormones) with intact parathyroids and recurrent nerve.
- Indicated in benign thyroid conditions like diffuse goiters, multinodular goiters (nontoxic).

Total thyroidectomy: Figure 22.3 shows operative specimen of total thyroidectomy for a multinodular goiter. All thyroid tissue removed taking care to preserve nerve and parathyroids.

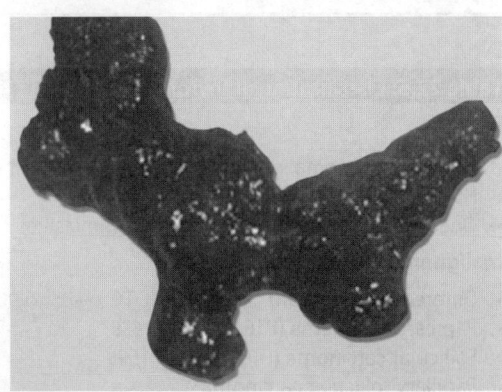

Fig. 22.3: Multinodular goiter with retrosternal nodule.
(For color version see Plate 1)

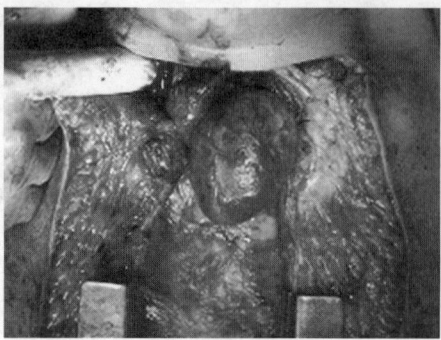

Fig. 22.4: Intrathoracic goiter.
(For color version see Plate 1)

Indications: All malignancies. Generally Graves' disease and toxic multinodular goiter. Near total thyroidectomy—very little tissue in trachea esophageal groove left behind—to protect recurrent nerve and parathyroids.

Completion thyroidectomy

- A resection of remaining part of thyroid after a previous thyroidectomy.
- It is done in cases where a preoperative diagnosis is a benign disease and microscopic examination shows carcinoma.
- Also in recurrent toxic nodular goiters or goiters in the residual thyroid gland compressing the trachea—a rethyroidectomy is done.

Median sternotomy for retrosternal and intrathoracic goiters, as shown in **Figure 22.4**.

> **SU22.4:** Describe the clinical features, classification and principles of management of thyroid cancer.

THYROID MALIGNANCIES

Incidence of thyroid cancers approx 30–35 per million population per year.
Sex incidence—three times more in female.

Pathogenesis

- Genetic factors: Dysregulation of mitogen activated protein kinase (MAPK) and phosphatidyl inositol-3 kinase (PI3K)/AKT pathways.
- *NRAS* mutation activates PI3K-AKT pathway; and deletion of pTEN gene lead to follicular cancer.
- BRAF mutations are linked to papillary cancer. RET/PTC3 mutations seen in aggressive cancers.
- **Familial syndromes:** Cowden Syndrome—carcinoma thyroid breast and hamartomas.
- Medullary carcinoma thyroid is often familial.
- Exposure to radiation in papillary cancer.
- **TSH stimulation:** Association of endemic goiter with follicular cancers
- Autoimmune thyroiditis has high risk of developing lymphoma.

Classification of Thyroid Neoplasms

Refer **Table 22.5**.

DIFFERENTIATED THYROID CARCINOMA

Papillary Thyroid Carcinoma (PTC)

- Most common, 90% have a slow course and good prognosis.
- Seen more in younger age, 20–40, (males at an older age).

Table 22.5: Classification of thyroid neoplasms.

Benign	
• Follicular adenoma, colloid adenoma is the most common • Hurthle cell adenomas • Oncocytic and embryonal (potentially invasive)	
Malignant	
• Differentiated thyroid carcinoma (DTC)—85 to 90% • Papillary carcinoma (PTC)—65 to 75% • Follicular carcinoma (FTC)—10 to 15% • Papillary follicular carcinoma • Hurthle cell carcinoma (variant of follicular) • Undifferentiated (anaplastic) carcinoma—5 to 10%	Medullary thyroid carcinoma (MTC)—arise from C-cells—2.5 to 3% Others: • Lymphoma (2 to 3%), sarcoma • Metastatic—(rare) from melanoma, kidney, breast

- It is often of multicentric origin. It Is TSH dependent tumor.

Spread
- **Local:** Intrathyroidal and extrathyroidal infiltration (into trachea, carotid sheath and recurrent nerve).
- Lymphatic spread to pre-tracheal, para-tracheal and mediastinal (central compartment of neck) and thence to deep cervical nodes along jugular vein Levels II, III and IV (and V-b).
- About 35% of patients have micro metastases before imaging can detect them (N – 0 stage).
- **Blood spread:** Distant metastases are rare except in aggressive variety (tall cell type).

Papillary microcarcinoma (PTC)—tumor size less than 10 mm, detected at imaging or in resected specimen of thyroid for benign disease.
- Two thirds of them do not progress. Long term survival is good.
- Micrometastases may be there, but rarely progress.

Treatment
- Thyroidectomy and thyroxine to suppress TSH and observation for progression.
- Some prefer to advise surgery only if the disease progresses on follow up.

Histological grade: Low grade and high grade.

Microscopy:
- Cells show with intranuclear cytoplasmic inclusions, called 'Orphan Annie eye' nuclei;
- Psammoma bodies and cystic spaces with papillary projections are characteristic of PTC.

Papillary Anaplastic Carcinoma

PTC can turn anaplastic with bad prognosis (due to blood spread).

> **Q. Write a short note on follicular carcinoma (FTC).**

- More aggressive than a PTC. Seen in slightly older patients with more males.
- Multifocal tumors are rare.
- Lymphatic spread is rare.
- Blood spread is **early and frequently** to bones causing vascular "pulsatile" metastases in skull and long bones.
- Clinically, it presents as a solitary (discrete) nodule, hard and fixed in some.
- It may also arise in a multinodular goiter.

Histology
- Capsular invasion and vascular invasion (absent in follicular adenoma)
- Tumor may be high grade and low grade.
- FNAC (cytology) **can** only detect follicular neoplasm **and cannot** differentiate follicular carcinoma from follicular adenoma. Trucut biopsy can detect a carcinoma by histology.
- Papillary follicular carcinoma is a variant which is behaviorally like a papillary cancer.
- Hurthle cell carcinoma (oxyphil cell)—is rare variant of follicular carcinoma and has a worse prognosis due to its high incidence of multifocality and early blood spread.

Anaplastic Carcinoma
- Arising—de novo or in previous papillary carcinoma
- It grows rapidly and infiltrates into trachea, nerve and carotid sheath. It also has a high propensity for hematogenous metastases.
- Poor prognosis (less than 10 percent survive 3 years).

> **Q. Write a short note on medullary thyroid carcinoma (MTC) (treatment discussed after DTC).**

MEDULLARY THYROID CARCINOMA (MTC)
- Arises from parafollicular (C cells) accounts for 3–5% of thyroid cancers.
- These involve germline mutation of RET proto-oncogene in familial MTC and somatic mutations in KRAS and HRAS in case of sporadic MTC. 80% are sporadic and 20% are familial.
- May be associated with multiple endocrine neoplasia syndromes
- MEN-IIA (MTC, parathyroid adenoma and pheochromocytoma)
- MEN-IIB—with mucosal neuromas and marfanoid features.

- The tumor may also be multicentric.
- It shows early spread to lymph nodes and also through blood stream.

Histology
- Shows "amyloid stroma" with malignant cells.
- It tests positive for calcitonin at immunohistochemistry.

The tumor secretes calcitonin and also 5-HT (serotonin), prostaglandin, ectopic ACTH and vasoactive intestinal polypeptide (VIP).

Tumor markers
Calcitonin and carcino embryonic antigen (CEA).

Clinical Features and Diagnosis
- Age group—mostly 40-50 years but early age in familial cases.
- Tumor presents as a nodular or lobular goiter with lymph nodes.
- Features of metastasis—bone, lungs, and liver
- Diarrhea and flushing (30%) are seen
- When associated with MEN II syndrome, there are features of hyperparathyroidism, hypertension, pheochromocytomas and mucosal neuromas with marfanoid habitus.

Investigations for Diagnosis
- Elevated serum calcitonin levels.
- Detection of mutation in RET proto oncogene in familial MTC and mutation in KRAS/HRAS in sporadic MTC.
- Serum CEA levels.

Treatment of MTC
- Treatment is total thyroidectomy with central compartment dissection and unilateral or bilateral modified radical neck dissection to get the best chances of cure.
- Follow up with serum calcitonin and CEA levels for recurrence of tumor or metastases.

Symptomatic Treatment
- Antiserotonin agents—cyproheptadine and methysergide to control flushing
- Antidiarrheals are necessary—loperamide, ramosetron.
- There is no role for radioiodine therapy and TSH suppression here.

Thyroxine replacement: L-thyroxine 100 to 150 mcg daily done postoperatively for life and calcium supplementation.

Prognostic Factors in Differentiated Carcinoma Thyroid
Age, size, stage and histology are important in stratifying them as high and low risk tumors.

High-risk Factors
- Age above 55 years in females and 45 years in males
- Size above 4 cm and extrathyroidal spread
- High grade histology—like vascular invasion in FTC and nodes in PTC.

Differentiated Thyroid Carcinoma (Papillary and Follicular Carcinoma)
Refer **Table 22.6**.

Table 22.6: Staging of differentiated thyroid carcinomas.

Staging based on AJCC recommendations (simplified for ease of remembering)

Tumor - size number (single or multiple) and local spread.

T1—less than 2 cm (T1a—micropapillary carcinoma size less than 1 cm)

T2—2-4 cm

T3a—larger than 4 cm but intrathyroidal (capsule intact)

T3b—minimal extrathyroidal (extracapsular) spread.

T4a—spread to adjacent structures—trachea, rec. laryngeal nerve, esophagus, skin and intrathyroidal Anaplastic carcinoma.

T4b—mediastinal vessels, carotid sheath, pre vertebral fascia, mediastinal vessel and extrathyroidal anaplastic carcinoma.

N- nodes—levels, VI and (pretracheal and prelaryngeal) and VII (mediastinal) and lateral

N0—node negative, N 1 node positive

M—metastases – M0 and M1

Staging

Differentiated carcinoma low risk—< 55 years female and < 45 years male—2 stages
Stage I—any T any N, M0 and
Stage II—any T- any N, M1
Differentiated thyroid cancer—high risk– > 55 years female, > 45 years male—4 stages
Stage I—T1, N0
Stage II—T2–3, N0
Stage III—T1–3, N1, M0
Stage IVa—T4A, N0–1 with M
Stage IVb- T4b, N0-1, M0
Stage IVc—any T, any N, M1
All anaplastic cancers are—stage IV a, b, c
ST IVa—T4a, any N, M0
ST IVb—T4b, Any N, M0
ST IVc—metastatic

TREATMENT OF THYROID CANCERS

Treatment of medullary thyroid carcinoma is already discussed.

Treatment of Differentiated Carcinoma—Papillary Carcinoma

- Diagnosis: Triple assessment—clinical, sonography and FNAC.
- Staging: CT helps assess the lymph nodes, mediastinum and thorax.
- Laryngoscopy—to assess vocal cords.

Treatment

Surgery

- **PTC with N0:** Total thyroidectomy and elective central compartment dissection to clear the lymph nodes in level VI and VII.
- Node positive (N-1) cases—add selective node dissection central compartment and (levels II, III, IV AND Vb)—unilateral or bilateral as per finding.

Postoperative–Radioiodine Ablation Therapy

- Radioiodine (I-123) scan after 4-6 weeks or TSH levels reach above 20 mIU/L.
- Radioiodine ablation (I-131)—if residual thyroid or nodal metastases—show take up.
- **Thyroxine for life**—TSH suppressive doses of L- thyroxine (generally 200 to 300 microgram daily. (TSH -level should be below 0.1 mIU/L) and thyroxine replacement too.

Follow up: Thyroglobulin levels in serum (below 25 to 30 ng/mL)

Carcinoma detected in histology specimen after hemithyroidectomy for benign disease:

- Re-exploration and completion thyroidectomy should be done with central compartment dissection.

T 4 and N1 with fixed nodes—external irradiation after thyroidectomy.

Follicular Thyroid Carcinoma (FTC)

Total thyroidectomy is the standard treatment.

Histological surprises: If FTC is reported in lobectomy done for a nodule reported as benign – the following are options:

- Low-risk tumor
    - T1–T3a, M0 disease in a young females below 40 years, tumor histology with minimal capsular invasion.
    - Observe with thyroglobulin levels at six monthly intervals.
- High-risk tumor
    - T3b or T4, any sex, tumor histology showing vascular invasion and capsular invasion.
    - Re-exploration and completion. Total thyroidectomy: Because, it has high-risk of hematogenous metastases, which should be ablated by radioiodine I-131.
    - Any residual thyroid will take up the radioiodine and prevent ablation of metastases.
    - Total thyroidectomy removes all thyroid tissue and ensures ablation of metastases.

TSH suppression (postsurgery or radioiodine ablation): FTC is a TSH dependent tumor, responds well to suppressive dose of L-thyroxine along with monitoring of thyroglobulin levels in serum.

Metastases: Radioiodine ablation—metastases in bone are treated with radio iodine.

Recent advances

- Lenvatinib—4 mg daily.
- It is a tyrosine kinase inhibitor drug and is indicated in treatment of all differentiated

thyroid cancers (papillary and follicular carcinoma) that are progressive, recurrent, metastatic and resistant to radio iodine ablation.

Anaplastic Carcinoma
- Generally poor prognosis and rapid progress.
- Palliation too is difficult—includes tracheostomy or bronchostomy with external irradiation.

Treatment of Medullary Thyroid Carcinoma
Refer previous section under pathology.

> **Q. How do you investigate and manage a discrete (clinically solitary) thyroid nodule? Long answer question:**

MANAGEMENT OF DISCRETE (SOLITARY) THYROID NODULES
Diagnosis

Triple assessment (clinical, ultrasound and cytological) helps plan further treatment
- History and clinical examination
  - H/o exposure to radiation, radiation exposure and family history of cancers.
  - History of taking goitrogenic drugs or iodine.
  - Details of neck swelling and its impact on breathing, voice and swallowing.
  - History suggestive of hyperthyroidism and hypothyroidism
- Examination of the goiter and lymphatics field
  - Central neck, mediastinum and lateral and regional lymphatics
  - *Systemic examination:* Cardiovascular, neurological and abdominal.
- Laryngoscopy to assess vocal cords.
- Features of bony metastases are seen in follicular tumors.
- **Blood examination:** Thyroid function—mildly raised TSH may be seen.
- Ultrasonography—most accurate in assessment of nodule/s and tumor features.
- USG based categories—benign, indeterminate and malignant (**Refer Table 22.7**)

Benign lesions—colloid nodule, cyst, adenomas are usually treated for symptoms and potential to turn malignant.
- Observation and thyroxine—for small colloid nodules, and for Hashimoto's goiter with hypothyroidism.
- Surgery is for relief of pressure symptoms of airway or gullet or for cosmesis.

Indeterminate or malignant lesions need specific treatment.

Investigation:
- Ultrasound—differentiates solitary (discrete—isolated, making two thirds) from dominant (visible among multiple nodules, accounting for one third).
- FNAC detects cancers other than follicular carcinoma.
- Thyroid function—to assess for hyperthyroidism.
- Contrast enhanced CT of neck and chest—to evaluate for lymph node spread, airway

Table 22.7: Algorithm for solitary thyroid nodule.

Thyroid nodule → low TSH → Evaluate for hyperthyroid state → hyperthyroidism

	Thyroid scintiscan I 123—normal (warm) or low (cold) uptake			Hot nodule	
Normal or high TSH ↓	Ultrasound evaluation ↓			**Treat hot nodule** **Radioiodine ablation or surgery**	
No Nodule	Nodule				
High TSH **Treat** **hypothyroidism**	TIRADS Gr FNAC	Benign 1 and 2 -No FNA	Indeterminate 3 if >2.5 cm FNAC	Suspicious 4 FNAC	Cancer 5 FNAC

tracheal obstruction in mediastinum and also metastases in thorax—for lymphadenopathy and mediastinal/thoracic shadows.
- Radioiodine uptake scan—done in a case of nodule with a hyperthyroid feature
- A functioning nodule takes up iodine (hot nodule)—is rarely malignant.
- Cold nodule—may be in neoplasm with 30 to 40% risk of cancer.

Features of High-risk of Cancer in a Solitary Nodule

- Solitary nodule, > 4 cm, hard, fixed, male sex.
- Tirads grade 4 and 5 and lymphadenopathy.
- FNAC—follicular neoplasm.

Differential Diagnosis of Solitary Nodule

- Follicular adenoma/carcinoma
- Cyst
- Toxic adenoma

Treatment

Benign: Dominant nodule—subtotal or total thyroidectomy for multinodular goiter.
Solitary nodule (isolated nodule): If benign—thyroid lobectomy.
Nodules suspicious of cancer are subjected to total thyroidectomy.

Cancer—total thyroidectomy with central compartment dissection in papillary cancer
- Total thyroidectomy in follicular cancer
- Total thyroidectomy with elective modified radical neck dissection level 2 to 5 + 6 and 7.

Toxic Adenoma (Autonomous Toxic nodule)

- Radioiodine ablation: Small < 4 cm).
- Thyroid lobectomy after control of hyperthyroidism for those with large adenomas, with compressive symptoms or not willing for radioiodine.

PARATHYROIDS

> **SU22.5: Describe the applied anatomy of parathyroid.**

Four parathyroid glands—two (superior and inferior glands) on each side are situated behind thyroid lobes. They are brownish yellow, each weighing between 30 to 50 mg inferior glands larger than superior.

Embryology: Parathyroids develop between gestational weeks 5 to 12.

Each superior parathyroid arises from dorsal part of fouth pharyngeal pouch
It is more constant in position at the cricothyroid articulation dorsal to recurrent laryngeal nerve.

The inferior gland arises from the third pharyngeal pouch (along with thymus), and descends in the neck resulting in a variable and inconstant position—but ventral to the recurrent nerve.

Each gland lies enclosed in a fatty envelope movable over the thyroid capsule.

Blood supply: Each gland gets a separate branch from inferior thyroid artery and has venous drainage into internal jugular vein independently on each side.

Microscopy

Parathyroids contain chief cells secreting parathormone (PTH) and oxyphil cells (clear cells).

Parathormone (PTH) secretion is stimulated by low calcium levels and high magnesium levels.

Physiology of Parathyroid

Calcium is an essential cation:
- For cardiovascular rhythm, cellular activity (membrane potential), neuromuscular activity, coagulation factor, and bone structure in elemental and dynamic form.
- Dietary calcium, drugs and disease may increase calcium levels.

Parathormone (PTH) is an aminopeptide with a half life of 4-5 minutes—having a biologically.

- Normal serum parathormone (PTH) levels—10-60 pg/mL.

Action of PTH—primarily increases circulating calcium levels.
- Mobilisation of calcium from the bone (resorption) (acts on osteoblasts and osteoclasts) and
- Increases reabsorption of calcium from renal tubules and increases excretion of phosphate.
- Enhances absorption of calcium from the gut.

Normal serum total calcium level 8.5-10.5 mg/dL (2.2-2.5 mmol/L). 45% of calcium is in ionised form and 55 % is bound to serum albumin, (total calcium may be low in persons with low serum albumin (catabolic state, sepsis, liver disease).

PTH is balanced by calcitonin secreted from C-cells of the thyroid glands.

> **SU22.6: Describe and discuss the clinical features of hypo and hyperparathyroidism and the principles of their management.**

HYPOPARATHYROIDISM

Hypoparathyroidism—PTH levels are below 10 pg/mL (normal levels 10-60 pg/mL).

Types

Transient—lasting for less than 6 months, (more common)

Permanent—lasts beyond 6 months. Low Calcium (below 8 mg/dL), high phosphorus levels.

Etiology

- Parathyroidectomy, (includes inadvertent removal in thyroidectomy).
- Devascularization of the glands during surgery like thyroidectomy.

Hungry Bone Syndrome

Here the patient develops profound and immediate hypocalcemia following removal of parathyroids (a drop in immediate postoperative PTH level to below <1.5 pmol/L).

Mechanism

- The bones, starved of calcium due to the disease take up circulating calcium very rapidly leading to severe shortage of circulating calcium (aided by calcitonin reversing PTH action). Also low albumin levels contribute.
- Needs per operative anticipation and emergency calcium infusion with Vit D injection and monitoring.

Q. Write a short note on on tetany.

Clinical Features of Hypoparathyroidism

Typically Tetany in Classical Form

Mild to Moderate

- Carpal and pedal spasm. Tightening a BP cuff causes carpal spasm (Trousseau's sign), laryngeal strider, Chvostek's sign—tapping over side of face (over) facial nerve causes twitching
- Circumoral tingling, numbness, paresthesia.

Severe: Muscle Spasm

- **Respiratory muscle:** Stridor and suffocation. May cause death.
- Convulsions.
- Blurred vision due to intraocular muscle spasm.

Differential Diagnosis of Tetany

- Hypoparathyroidism
- Deficiency of vitamin D
- Respiratory alkalosis—hyperventilation causes a relative fall in ionic calcium
- Metabolic alkalosis (e.g., pyloric stenosis—due to vomiting of gastric acid
- Acute pancreatitis, chronic renal failure
- Massive transfusion (citrate overload).

Treatment

- Severe symptoms—corrected by intravenous calcium gluconate 1 g in 10 mL over 10 minutes followed by a slow infusion of 1 mg/kg body weight/hour.
- Monitor heart and breathing.
- Repeated measurement of serum calcium
- Intravenous magnesium infusion is added

Followed by oral therapy: At the earliest for 2 to 3 months.

- Oral calcium 1-2 g (elemental calcium) and Vitamin D3 are started at the earliest.
- Calcitriol (active form of Vit D3, normally formed in kidney) is preferred.
- Magnesium gluconate tablets 500 mg orally.

Weaning succeeds in temporary hypoparathyroidism but not if permanent.

Q. Write a short notes on pseudohypoparathyroidism.

PSEUDOHYPOPARATHYROIDISM

- Genetic disorder due to—mutation in GNAS 1 gene. Body fails to respond to PTH levels. Low calcium and high phosphorus levels in plasma and high PTH
- Clinical features—all features of hypoparathyroidism, weakness, short stature, short metacarpals, drowsiness. Blurring of vision and even cataract.

Treatment

- Symptomatic and supportive
- Genetic counseling.

Q. Write a note on hyperparathyroidism.

HYPERPARATHYROIDISM (HPT)

Classification: Three Types

1. **Primary HPT: (PHPT):** Primary hypersecretion of PTH and hypercalcemia.
2. **Secondary hyperparathyroidism:** Parathyroids oversecrete to compensate for low calcium secondary to renal loss of calcium and hyperphosphatemia.
3. **Tertiary hyperparathyroidism:** In a case of secondary HPT, parathyroids start hypersecreting autonomously or develop one or more adenomas, causing hypercalcemia.

Generally seen in postrenal transplant patients or in those on long term hemodialysis.

PRIMARY HYPERPARATHYROIDISM (PHPT)

Hypercalcemia with high parathormone levels in blood.

Causes

- Parathyroid adenoma (mostly single(about 70 to 75%)
- Parathyroid hyperplasia (multiple glands)—about 20 to 25%
- Parathyroid carcinoma—less than 1%.

Sporadic cases form the majority.
Familial cases—with MEN Type I ot MEN type II.
Age—5th and 6th decade.
Sex—females far more than males (3:1).

Pathology and clinical features (due to hypercalcemia)

Summary: "Bones, stones, abdominal groans and psychic moans".

Presentation

- Asymptomatic—often detected incidentally at bone densitometry and hypercalcemia.
- Chronic—typical features.
- Acute crisis.

Bones

- Skull bones—"salt and pepper erosions".
- Long bones and carpal bones—subperiostal bone reabsorption
- Osteitis fibrosa cystica (X-ray findng) and
- "Brown tumors" at cut section (due to hemorrhage into lesions

Renal stones: Renal stones, most common among clinical symptoms neuromuscular dysfunction and muscle weakness.

Acute pancreatitis (life threatening and severe) or **chronic calcific pancreatitis**

- Intestinal hypoperistalsis with constipation
- Peptic ulcers.

Psychiatric symptoms and depression.

Band keratopathy—if found, is pathognomonic of PHPT.

Differential Diagnosis of Hypercalcemia

Causes of Hypercalcemia

- Primary hyperparathyroidism
- Secondary and tertiary hyperparathyroidism
- Thyrotoxicosis pheochromocytoma
- Granulomas
- Sarcoidosis, tuberculosis
- Paget's disease of bone

- Dietary—calcium excess, milk-alkali syndrome
- Drugs—hypervitaminosis D and A, lithium
- Aluminium intoxication.

Malignancies

- Skeletal metastases.
- Myeloma, lymphoma, leukemia.
- Breast, lung, kidney, SCC of head and neck, genital tract.
- Ectopic PTH like substance produced by cancers renal failure.

Diagnosis of Primary HPT

Always by biochemical test (and not by imaging) by finding elevated plasma levels of parathormone (PTH). The other tests include:

- Elevated ionized calcium and total calcium
- Low phosphorus—provided serum Vit D and creatinine levels are normal.
- Elevated 24 hour urinary calcium levels.
- Elevated bony alkaline phosphatase level—warns of a hungry bone.

Localisation studies only after biochemical confirmation of diagnosis.

Non-invasive Radiology

- Ultrasonography—largely helpful
- **4D - computed tomography (CT) scanning** very accurate, but high radiation exposure.

Nuclear medicine-based studies (Sestamibi scanning)

Invasive Imaging

- Ultrasound or CT-guided fine-needle aspiration with PTH assay.
- Parathyroid angiography
- Selective jugular venous sampling for the PTH gradient.

Useful in recurrent cases—for locating a missed gland at re-operation.

> Q. Sestamibi scan in parathyroid disorders.

Nuclear Medicine-Based Studies (Sestamibi Scanning)

- Sesta- methoxy -isobutyl isonitrile (MIBI)) for parathyroid localization by accumulating in mitochondria of oxyphil cells of parathyroid.

- False positives–solid thyroid nodules, (Hurthle cell nodules)—with high oxyphilic content.
- 99Tc-pertechnetate is thyroid-specific and helps in subtraction scan.
- Or SPECT (Singe photon emission computed tomography).

Treatment

Surgery (parathyroidectomy - minimally invasive or open method).
- For all symptomatic PHPT
- Asymptomatic PHPT—with calcium levels elevated, younger than 50 years, renal and skeletal findings.

Parathyroidectomy—is done for a solitary adenoma localised preoperatively:
- Bilateral neck exploration and resection of all parathyroids with reimplantation of half of the gland into a sternomastoid belly—indicated in cases of diffuse parathyroid hyperplasia and in cases where preoperative localization of tumor has failed.
- Intraoperative venous sampling to confirm falling PTH level following resection of gland helps confirm resection of gland adenoma.
- Post operative calcium monitoring and possibility of long term calcium supplementation should be kept in mind.

ACUTE HYPERCALCEMIC CRISIS

Potentially lethal emergency.

Etiology
- Primary hyperparathyroidism
- Metastatic carcinomatosis, ectopic PTH secreting tumors—pancreas, breast.

Clinical features
- Sudden outburst of hypercalcemia.
- Serum total calcium of over >3.5 mmol/L (13 mg dL)
- Calcium level above >4.5 mmol/L (17–18 mg/dL) can lead to coma and cardiac arrest.
- ECG shows -Prolonged P–R interval with a shortened Q–T interval prior to cardiac arrhythmias.

Treatment—promoting renal excretion of calcium
- Hydration with normal saline followed by loop diuretic (frusemide)
- Hemodialysis or hemofiltration may help in reducing calcium level quickly
- Calcitonin—to reduce osteoclastic release of calcium from bone and increase renal excretion along with
- Hydrocortisone—to enhance action of calcitonin and reduce intestinal absorption of calcium
- Bisphosphonates—disodium pamidronate 60 mg—intravenous slowly over 2–4 days (max 90 mg)—to block release of bone calcium (slow action and until them calcitonin)
- Mithramycin, intermittent doses

SECONDARY HYPERPARATHYROIDISM

Renal failure causes hyperphosphatemia and reduced absorption of calcium from GIT leading to chronic hypocalcemia which stimulates PTH secretion and parathyroid hyperplasia in all four glands, often nodular. Also seen is metastatic calcification in the skin and muscles or viscera. Bone is osteoporotic.

Refractory to Medical Therapy
- Anemia which is resistant to erythropoietin stimulation.
- Bone, joint, muscle symptoms; progressive ectopic calcification.
- Dilated cardiomyopathy with cardiac failure.

Serum phosphate level is higher (>6.g/dL); with low serum vitamin D.

Serum calcium is normal or low; high intact PTH >500 pg/mL.

Treatment

Medical
- Supplementation of calcium and vitamin D.
- Calcimimetic drug, e.g., cinacalcet, which stops stimulation of parathyroids by high phosphate levels.
- Dialysis and renal transplantation.

Surgery: Total parathyroidectomy with auto-transplantation of half of a gland.

Indications
- Failure of vitamin D therapy to restore PTH levels.
- Failure of calcimimetic drugs or intolerance to these drugs.

- Severe bony changes (fibrosa cystic), incapacitation, cardiomyopathy.
- Calciphylaxis.

Calciphylaxis: A condition with significant mortality in secondary HPT.
- Disseminated vascular and cutaneous calcifications and necrosis seen.
- Low serum levels of a calcification inhibitory protein, α-2-Heremans–Schmid glycoprotein and abnormalities in smooth muscle cell biology in the uremic patients.

Pathology
Calcific uremic arteriolopathy (tunica media) presents with expanding painful cutaneous purpuric lesions, leading to necrosis and gangrene.

Treatment
- Hemodialysis
- **Wound care:** Hyperbaric oxygen, sodium thiosulphate to the necrotic areas.
- Emergency parathyroidectomy.

Parathyroid Carcinoma
Rare Malignancy

HRPT2 mutations causing inactivation of parafibromin contribute to forming of parathyroid carcinoma. Parafibromin—helps in of cellular transcription and histone modification.

Clinical diagnosis
Difficult as it mimics PHPT.
- Patients are younger, neck mass is felt in 50% of cases, and calcium levels are usually very high (above 14 to 16 mg %) and also are PTH levels
- All cases are symptomatic of hypercalcemia, crisis is common.
- Metastases are seen in bone, lungs and liver.

Work up
- Biochemical confirmation—serum calcium and PTH
- Localisation—4D CT
- FNAC
- Markers—parafibromin and protein gene product 9.5 (PGP 9.5).

Treatment
- Surgery—en bloc resection of parathyroid gland without spilling cells (practically—it is thyroid lobectomy on the affected side)
- Resurgery for recurrent or residual disease
- Medical management of hypercalcemia and bone disease as supportive.
- Mithramycin

Prognosis
With early surgery—80% survive for 5 year and 50% for 10 years.

Chapter 23: The Adrenal Glands

SU23.1	Describe the applied anatomy of adrenal glands.
SU23.2	Describe the etiology, clinical features and principles of management of disorders of adrenal gland.
SU23.3	Describe the clinical features, principles of investigation and management of adrenal tumors.

SU 23.1: Describe the applied anatomy of adrenal glands.

APPLIED ANATOMY OF ADRENAL GLANDS

- Two adrenal (suprarenal) glands—right and left.
- Each abutting superior pole of the respective kidneys separated by perinephric fat within Gerota's fascia (capsule) like a cap.
- Right side—behind inferior vena cava and liver, lateral to right crus of diaphragm.
- Left side—lateral to aorta, left crus of diaphragm, close to pancreatic tail.

Arterial Supply on Each Side

Superior, middle and inferior adrenal arteries arising from—inferior phrenic artery, abdominal aorta and renal artery respectively, form a subcapsular network to supply the gland.

Veins

- Right side—a single vein drains into inferior vena cava. (Variation—2–3 veins).
- Left side—drains into renal vein.

Lymphatic Drainage

- Right—para-aortic and paracaval nodes.
- Left—along renal vessel onto para-aortic nodes.

Morphologically

Each gland weighs about 4–5 grams and has a cortex and a medulla.

Embryologically

Cortex develops from mesoderm and medulla from neuroectoderm, following migration of neural crest cells.

Histology and Function

Q. Describe function of adrenal glands.

Cortex has Three Layers

1. Zona glomerulosa—this layer secretes aldosterone, the mineralocorticoid—regulated by renin angiotensin system and potassium levels in blood.
2. Zona fasciculata and
3. Zona reticularis.
   - Secrete glucocorticoids—cortisol. Under ACTH control from pituitary secretes.
   - Ketosteroids—DHEA (dehydroepiandrosterone) and its sulphate DHEAS; (under gonadotropic influence).

Medulla

Histology: Contains fat and yellow chromaffin cells forming part the sympathetic nerve plexuses—secretes catecholamines, adrenaline

(90%) and noradrenaline (10%) and also dopamine.

> **Q. Describe the surgical importance of anatomy of adrenals.**

Applied Anatomy
- Embryologically medulla is from neuroectoderm
  - Hence seat of multiple endocrine neoplasia syndrome II with other sites.
  - Medullary carcinoma thyroid and cutaneous neuromas.
- Cortex is a mesodermal structure accounting for different tumors from cortical layers.
- Lymphatics along renal vessels explain mediastinal secondaries in carcinoma.
- Hematogenous metastases from neuroblastoma of right adrenal medulla is more often to liver and lungs while the same from left is to orbit and skull.
- Difference in venous drainage
  - Short right adrenal vein draining into IVC poses operative challenge in right adrenalectomy.
  - Left vein draining into renal vein is a challenge in left nephrectomy, may require a concurrent adrenalectomy on account of devascularization of adrenals.
- Surgical approach to adrenal—open or laparoscopic—may be transperitoneal or retroperitoneal.

Applied Physiology
Most tumors of adrenal—cortex or medulla are functional due to their secretory properties and have systemic symptoms.

Medullary chromaffin cells secrete catecholamines. There is reversal of adrenalin to: noradrenaline ratio in tumors like pheochromocytoma or neuroblastoma.

> **SU23.2: Describe the etiology, clinical features and principles of management of disorders of adrenal gland.**

Adrenal glands have functional cortex and medulla secreting different hormones.

DISORDERS OF ADRENAL GLANDS (REFER TABLE 23.1)

Clinical Features
These depend on the type of pathology and its functioning or non-functioning status:
- Asymptomatic mass in abdomen
- Features of metastases—in liver, skull, orbit—proptosis
- Disorders due dysfunction.

Principles of Management
- Diagnosis by history taking, and clinical examination along with imaging and biochemical investigations
- Therapeutic approach—surgery or non-surgical.

> **Q. Short note on incidentaloma.**

INCIDENTALOMA
A mass lesion in adrenal, asymptomatic, detected incidentally at abdominal imaging for other reasons than adrenal symptoms.

Table 23.1: Disorders of adrenal glands.

Disorders without adrenal dysfunction	Disorders with adrenal dysfunction

• Non-functioning adenomas
• Non-functioning cortical carcinomas
• Metastases in adrenal cortex or medulla
• Melanoma
• Medulla-ganglioneuromas
	Cortex
	• Adrenal cortical hyperplasia
	• Cortical adenomas—aldosteronoma
	  – Cushing's adenoma
	  – Virilizing tumors
	Medulla
	• Pheochromocytoma
	• Neuroblastoma

- About 70–75% are non-functioning adenomas
- Functioning (Cushing's) adenoma
- Adrenocortical carcinoma
- Pheochromocytoma
- Aldosteronoma (Conn's)
- Metastases
- Benign soft tissue tumors and cysts.

Risk of malignancy in non-functional mass:
- Size over 4 cm has a risk 25%
- If mass grows over next 6 to 12 months

Treatment of an Incidentaloma
- Actively observe non-functioning lesions—smaller than 4 cm
- Through imaging at 6 monthly interval for 2 years if they don't grow.

Surgery (Adrenalectomy) for
- Functioning tumors
- Malignancy
- All tumors over 4 cm size
- Non-functioning lesion smaller than 4 cm and growing over 6 to 24 months on serial imaging.

Q. How do you investigate an adrenal mass?

INVESTIGATIONS IN ANY ADRENAL MASS
- Is it functional?
- Is it a pheochromocytoma? Is it malignant or potentially malignant?
- Generally a pheochromocytoma is excluded before any invasive investigation is undertaken to prevent a hypertensive crisis.

Biochemical
- Serum catecholamine assay
- Serum levels of metanephrines
- 24 hour urinary excretion of metanephrines
- Urinary—vanillylmandelic acid (VMA levels)
- Serum potassium and sodium levels
- Plasma aldosterone
- Plasma renin activity
- Plasma DHEA and DHEAS or
- Plasma levels of estradiol and 17-OH estradiol.

Imaging Studies

Generally a pheochromocytoma is excluded before any intravascular contrast imaging is undertaken to prevent a hypertensive crisis.

Ultrasonography of Abdomen
- MRI: Angiography of abdomen detects tumor emboli in vena cava
- MRI of head: Detects pituitary tumors
- MRI: Angiography of abdomen—detects tumor emboli in vena cava
- MD CT abdomen and chest—detects metastases—in liver and chest.
- **MIBG scan** (Meta-iodobenzylguanidine)—helps in detecting pheochromocytoma or/neuroblastoma
- NP 59 scan—I-131 labeled—6 beta-iodomethyl nor iodocholesterol scintiscan to localize adrenals in hyperaldosteronism
- PET scan **usually with MIBG**

Biopsy of adrenal mass—**never** done except to evaluate for a metastasis from extra adrenal site—only after excluding a pheochromocytoma.

General Principles of Treatment

Incidentaloma—see previous section.

Disorders of Adrenal Dysfunction
- Once diagnosis made and lesion is localized, the symptoms are controlled with medications, e.g., antidiabetic, antihypertensives and supportive treatment.
- Specific lesions are treated accordingly with surgery.

Q. Short notes on primary hyperaldosteronism.

PRIMARY HYPERALDOSTERONISM (PHA)
- Sporadic or have somatic mutations
- A few are autosomal dominant forms.

Cause
- Unilateral adrenocortical adenoma most common (Conn's adenoma)
- Bilateral micronodular hyperplasia
- Adrenocortical carcinoma.

Clinical Features

- Hypertension at young age 30 to 50 years
- Females affected more than males
- Hypokalemia in most (a few normokalemic)
- High or normal sodium
- Headache and weakness are common.

Biochemistry of Hyperaldosteronism

- High plasma aldosterone
- Low plasma renin activity (PRA)
- Serum sodium—normal or/high
- Potassium—low on most (normal in a few)
- Selective adrenal venous sampling for aldosterone levels—to localize.

Localization studies—MRI/CT, selective adrenal venous sampling and NP 59 scan.

Treatment

For aldosterone secreting adenoma
- Adrenalectomy (laparoscopic or open) after correcting hypertension and hypokalemia.

Spironolactone

Non-diuretic antihypertensives. For cases of bilateral hyperplasia.

> Q. Write a short note on Cushing's syndrome.

CUSHING'S SYNDROME

Causes

- Primary adrenal adenoma
- Adrenocortical carcinoma
- Pituitary adenoma causing bilateral adrenal hyperplasia (Cushing's disease)
- Ectopic ACTH causing bilateral adrenal hyperplasia.

Clinical Features

- General—central obesity, weight gain buffalo hump (lemon on a match stick appearance
- Skin—hirsutism, bruise and striae
- Bone—osteoporosis/fractures muscle weakness
- Muscle—muscle weakness
- Metabolic—hyperglycemia, diabetes, hyperlipidemia
- Cardiovascular—hypertension
- Psychiatry—mania or depression
- Menstrual irregularity/impotence
- Hypokalemia.

Biochemical Investigations in Cushing's Syndrome

- Serum cortisol—high levels
- Loss of diurnal rhythm
- 24 hour urinary cortisol—elevated
- Dexamethasone 2 mg—fails to suppress secretion of cortisone
- Serum ACTH levels elevated in pituitary tumor and Ectopic ACTH syndrome
- Serum—testosterone or 17-hydroxyestradiol (virilising or feminising tumor)
- DHEA and DHEAS (dehydroepiandrosterone sulphate) levels for androgenic tumors.

Medical Therapy of Cushing's Syndrome

Metyrapone or ketoconazole—for suppression of cortisol secretion—this is indicated in pre-operative control of hypercortisolism and in patients, who are unfit for surgical adrenalectomy.

Surgery

Adrenalectomy

- For unilateral adenoma
- For cases of bilateral adrenal hyperplasia with normal ACTH-levels.

Hypophysectomy (Resection of Pituitary)

For ACTH-producing pituitary tumors.

Radiotherapy

Adjuvant.

> Q. Write a short note on adrenogenital syndrome.

ADRENOGENITAL SYNDROME

Causes

- Autosomal recessive condition: Congenital bilateral adrenal hyperplasia due to—deficiency of 21 hydroxylase trait—treated medically by long-term steroid supplementation.
- Sex hormone producing tumors—need adrenalectomy.
  - Virilizing syndrome with ambiguous genitalia, clitoral hypertrophy in female
  - Precocious puberty and early fusion

of epiphyses in male. High levels of testosterone and DHEA in serum and 17 ketosteroids in urine help in diagnosis and MRI imaging of adrenals helps localizing and staging.

Adrenocortical Insufficiency (Addison's Disease)

- Primary adrenocortical insufficiency
  - Disease or loss of adrenal—tumor invasion, tuberculosis, amyloidosis, post partum adrenal hemorrhage, autoimmune disease, post-traumatic surgery, drugs—ketoconazole, metyrapone.
- Secondary—pituitary failure to secrete ACTH
- Tertiary—hypothalamic failure.
  - Deficiency of CRH from hypothalamus
  - Brain tumor, irradiation, head injury.

Corticosteroid Therapy

Clinical features—appear late in the disease (after 90 percent of adrenal cortex is destroyed)
- Symptoms include—chronic weight loss, nausea, anorexia, weakness, hyponatremia, hyperkalemia, hypoglycemia diarrhea or abdominal pain
- Hyperpigmentation of skin.

Acute Addisonian Crisis: Often Life-threatening

Presenting as acute abdomen, fever, hypotension and hyponatremia, hyperkalemia and dehydration with profound shock.

Serum

- ACTH—high level
- Cortisol levels low
- High pro-opiomelanocortin (POMC) levels.

ACTH Stimulation Test (Synacthen Test)

No rise in the low cortisol levels following the administration of ACTH.

Treatment

Acute crisis urgent need to start treatment in:
- Hydrocortisone: Intravenousbolus 200 mg and 100 mg every 6 hours.
- Rapid saline infusion—under monitoring
- Glucose infusion
- Antibiotics to treat associated infection.

Chronic Adrenal Insufficiency

Lifelong replacement therapy with glucocorticoid (daily oral hydrocortisone (10 mg/m^2 body surface) and mineralocorticoid (fludrocortisone 0.1 mg) under supervision.

> **SU23.3:** Describe the clinical features, principles of investigation and management of adrenal tumors.

> **Q. Classify adrenal tumors and describe management of adrenocortical carcinoma.** (Long question)

TUMORS OF ADRENAL

Refer **Table 23.2**.

Table 23.2: Tumors of adrenal gland.

Cortex	Medulla
Non-functioning • Benign: Non-functioning – Adenoma—unilateral/bilateral • Malignant—adrenocortical carcinoma	Ganglioneuroma

Functioning
• Benign
  – Adenoma
  – Aldosterone secreting adenoma (Conn's)
  – Cortisol secreting adenoma (Cushing's)
  – Sex hormone adenoma
  – Virilizing or feminizing
	Pheochromocytoma

• Malignant – Adrenocortical carcinoma (mostly cortisol, some also secrete sex hormones)	Pheochromocytoma Neuroblastoma
Secondaries From breast, lungs, kidney, melanoma	
Benign stromal tumors—lipoma	

Adrenocortical Carcinoma (ACC)

Incidence
- A rare malignancy.
- Females: males 3:2.
- Age: Child hood and between 30 and 50 years (bimodal distribution).

Pathology
- A mass—with local invasion and later lymphatic and blood spread spread.
- A minority are non-functioning.
- Majority are secreting cortisol (most), virilizing hormones or aldosterone.

Staging of Adrenal Tumors
Refer **Table 23.3**.

Clinical Features
Hyperfunctioning tumors (hypersecretion of hormones)
- Cushing's syndrome: Majority of patients present with hypercortisolism.
- Virilizing or feminizing features in some.
- Features of hyperaldosteronism rare.

Non-functioning carcinomas—form a minority
- A mass abdomen.
- Pressure effect of the mass—effect on vena cava and the bowel in front.
- To invasion of nerve.

Incidentalomas (refer previous competency 23.2) form about 25% of all adrenal carcinomas.

Diagnosis
- Plasma: Cortisol, DHEAS
  - Catecholamines or metanephrines to exclude pheochromocytoma.
- Dexamethasone suppression test—excludes pituitary tumor induced Cushing.
- Tumor marker—Ti-67 for risk of recurrence.
- MRI—angiography shows tumor thrombus in vena cava.
- CT—to look for metastases in chest.

Treatment
Surgery
- Wide en bloc resection: For T1-2 and T3—adrenalectomy with nephrectomy with Gerota's fascia and nodes (and spleen on left side) and a tumor thrombectomy of vena cava..
- Tumor debulking—for T4 tumors to reduce hormone excess.
- Adjuvant therapy—mitotane (o,p, DDD) monotherapy or - combination with etoposide + doxorubicin + cis platin.
- Palliative radiotherapy—poor response.

Prognosis—Poor Survival
Only 25% of those with Stage I and II survive 5 years and just 5% of Stage III and IV.

> Q. Write short notes on: (1) Ganglioneuroma, (2) Neuroblastoma, and (3) Pheochromocytoma.

TUMORS OF ADRENAL MEDULLA

Benign
- **Ganglioneuroma**—mostly non-functioning, large abdominal mass, pressure effect on ureter, bowel, vena cava.

Table 23.3: Staging of adrenal tumors.	
T Tumor T-1 tumor less than 5 cm localized to adrenal T-2 larger than 5 cm but localized T-3 extra-adrenal spread but not invading the neighboring structures T-4 invading the local structures	N= N0: No lymphatic spread N-1: Spread to nodes M: Metastases—extra-abdominal nodes or other organs like lungs bone, skull
Stage I: T1, N0, M0 Stage II: T2, N0, M0 Stage III: T3, N0, T-1, T2 NI, M0 Stage IV: T3,4, NI, M0; Any T, NI, MI	

- Diagnosis by imaging.
- Resection of affected adrenals is curative.
- Malignant tumors.

NEUROBLASTOMA

Commonly seen in infancy and children below 5 years.

Site of Origin

- Mainly from adrenal medulla (40%), also from sympathetic chain from orbit to pelvis—paravertebral sympathetic chain—abdomen (30%) and chest (20%), neck and pelvis (10%)
- Generally the tumors secrete catecholamines mainly noradrenaline and dopamine
- Rapidly growing to invade kidney, pancreas and intestines
- Early metastases are seen in liver in right sided tumor (pepper type), mainly infants
- Metastases in skull and orbit with left sided tumors (Hutchinson type), mainly older children
- 60 to 70% present first as metastases.

Diff. Diagnosis

Wilms' tumor and pheochromocytoma.

Diagnosis

- Urinary excretion (24 hourly) of dopamine and noradrenaline vanillylmandelic acid (VMA), homovanillic acid (HVA).
- CT scan or MRI of the chest and abdomen, MIBG scan.

International Staging System

Applies to postsurgery report on residual tissue and metastases stratified as low risk, intermediate and high risk based on age and tumor stage.

Treatment

- Low risk—radical resection
- Intermediate risk—surgery plus adjuvant chemotherapy—(carboplatin, etoposide, doxorubicin and cyclophosphamide.)
- High-risk—neoadjuvant, high-dose combination chemotherapy followed by surgery.
- Spontaneous regression of tumor - rare.

PHEOCHROMOCYTOMA

Arising from adrenal medulla or extra-adrenal (10%) organ of Zuckerkandl, paraganglia–neck, chest or abdomen, bladder neck or renal hilum rarely.

- Sporadic or familial (10%)
- Solitary or multiple (10%)
- Unilateral or bilateral (10%)—familial tumors have a higher incidence of bilaterality.
- Associated with multiple endocrine neoplasia type IIA (10%)—parathyroid, medullary thyroid carcinoma (parafollicular cell carcinoma) and or with cutaneous neuromas (Type IIB).
- Malignant (10%)—bilateral tumors are rarely malignant in MEN II.

Hereditary pheochromocytomas in association with many syndromes due to germline genetic mutations in the, SDHB, SDHC, SDHD, NF1 and RET genes.

Familial paraganglioma (PG) syndrome: Glomus tumors of the carotid body and extra-adrenal paraganglioma.

Multiple endocrine neoplasia type 2 (MEN 2): An autosomal dominant inherited disorder due to germline mutations of the RET proto-oncogene.

Neurofibromatosis (NF) type 1: Pheochromocytomas, and café au lait spots on skin and mucosa.

Von Hippel–Lindau (VHL) syndrome: Pheochromocytoma, bilateral kidney tumors, cerebellar and spinal hemangioblastomas.

Pathology

Refer to operative photograph of adrenal pheochromocytoma in **Figure 23.1**.
- Soft tumor with capsule, yellow on cut section
- Most are small (4 cm, rarely large)
- Highly vascular, often with hemorrhage and necrosis
- Malignancy is diagnosed based on pheochromocytoma of the adrenal gland scaled score (PASS) includes the following:
  - Capsular invasion, high count of Ki-67 positive cells, and metastases with chromaffin tissue, commonly to lymph nodes, liver and bone

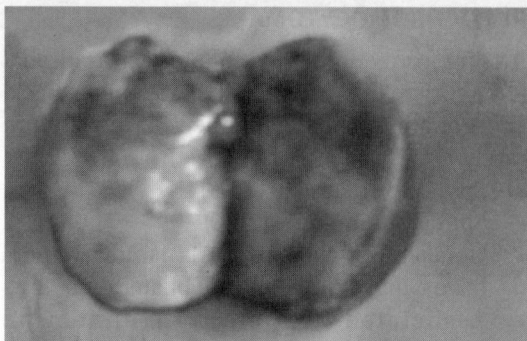

Fig 23.1: Adrenal pheochromocytoma.
(For color version see Plate 1)

- The tumors secrete catecholamines, mainly norepinephrine, (reversal of ratio—epinephrine to norepinephrine from 90:10 to 10:90%), dopamine and sometimes also produce calcitonin, and parathyroid hormone-related protein (PTHrP), ACTH, vasoactive intestinal polypeptide (VIP).

Clinical Features

- **Symptoms and signs:** Initially intermittent—later continuous and severe.
- Age—30 to 50 years.
- Paroxysms of headache, palpitations and sweating, sometimes syncope.
- Others—hyperglycemia, behavioral and emotional upset, weight loss, blurred vision.
- Hypertensive crisis may be life threatening and it may cause sudden death.
- Symptoms are precipitated by exertion, fever, injury; infection, abdominal palpation and surgery, anesthesia and drugs like opiates and antidepressants.

Diagnosis

- Elevated urinary and plasma levels of catecholamine metabolites—metanephrine and normetanephrine, often may need to be repeated twice.
- Localising the tumor—MRI of abdomen (avoid contrast injection to prevent provocation of symptoms).
- 123-I-MIBG (metaiodobenzylguanidine) scan.
- Single-photon emission computed tomography (SPECT).
- Fluorodeoxyglucose (FDG), labeled positron emission tomography (PET), for detection of multiple extra-adrenal tumors and metastases.

Treatment

Diagnosis and localization (as described above).

Optimal control of symptoms with alpha blockers (phenoxybenzamine or metyrapone) and beta blockers (e.g., propranolol). This is followed by:

- Surgery
  - Adrenalectomy—unilateral or bilateral
  - Resection of paraganglioma for extra-adrenal tumors
  - Debulking and metastasectomy for advanced tumors
- Chemotherapy for control of symptoms
  - Mitotane—as adjuvant or palliative.
  - Radiotherapy—131-I-MIBG (or combination)
  - *Targeted therapy:* Tyrosine kinase inhibitors-sunitinib, cabozantinib, axitinib are currently tried.

Post-treatment follow up—biochemical tests and imaging every year for 5 years.

Prognosis

Generally poor in malignant cases—less than 50% survive 5 years in non-metastatic disease.

The Pancreas - Exocrine and Endocrine

Chapter 24

SU24.1	Describe the clinical features, principles of investigation, prognosis and management of pancreatitis.
SU24.2	Describe the clinical features, principles of investigation, prognosis and management of pancreatic endocrine tumors.
SU24.3	Describe the principles of investigation and management of pancreatic disorders including pancreatitis and endocrine tumors.
As there is an overlap of topics in the competencies, a systematic review of pathologies of pancreas are discussed.	

SU24.1: Describe the clinical features, principles of investigation, prognosis and management of pancreatitis.

ANATOMY OF THE PANCREAS

The pancreas is a retort shaped retroperitoneal organ across the 1st lumbar vertebra over to the left. It has a head with uncinate process, a neck, a body and a tail (close to the spleen). It weighs about 80–100 g, measures about 15 cm long, 3 cm wide and 1.5–2 cm thick (can vary).

Arterial Supply

The head and neck are supplied by an arch formed by the superior and inferior pancreaticoduodenal arteries.

Body and tail of the gland are supplied by the splenic artery, which runs along the upper border of the gland.

Venous Drainage

The head region is drained by veins along the pancreaticoduodenal arcade into the superior mesenteric vein and the body and tail of pancreas, by the pancreatic veins into the splenic vein to join the portal vein.

Lymphatic Drainage

The superior and inferior pancreatic nodes around the head, neck, and along the body of the pancreas drain into the celiac above and superior mesenteric and middle colic nodes below and further into the para-aortic nodes.

Embryology of the Pancreas

Figure 24.1 depicts the pancreatic ductal system with embryological basis.

The pancreas develops from the ventral and dorsal pancreatic buds from the caudal end of the foregut in 5th week of gestation. The ventral bud fuses with the dorsal bud due to rotation of the gut in the 6th week. The head and uncinate process with the wide and short ventral duct, develop from the ventral bud. The body and tail with its long duct develop from the dorsal bud. A communication connects the dorsal duct to the ventral duct. The same and the ventral duct form the main duct of Wirsung, which is dilated and joined by the terminal bile duct at the ampulla of

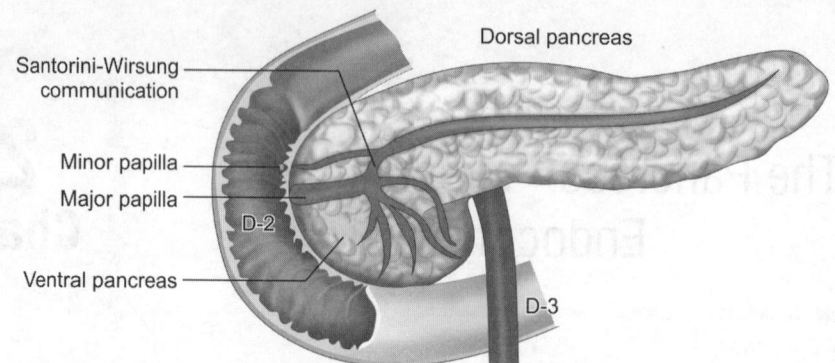

Fig. 24.1: Pancreatic duct system

Vater. The ampulla opens at the duodenal papilla in the second part of duodenum, surrounded by the sphincter of Oddi, that controls the flow of bile and pancreatic juice individually. (Refer pancreas divisum for anomalies).

The acini and the islets of Langerhans develop by the end of third and 4th month respectively.

FUNCTIONS OF THE PANCREAS

Endocrine and exocrine functions.

Exocrine Secretion

Stimuli by vagus → enzyme rich juice (increased volume), pH 8.3, volume: About 1000 to 2000 mL per day.

Control: Secretin and cholecystokinin (pancreozymine) (CCK PZ) from duodenal and jejunal mucosal are released into circulation due to stimulation by acid or food (also gastrin).

Secretin stimulates secretion of bicarbonate rich juice and pancreozymine, of an enzyme rich juice (10–20 g of proteins secreted per day).

Enzymes: Amylase, lipase, trypsinogen, chymotrypsinogen, proelastase, phospholipase, ribonuclease. They get activated in the duodenal lumen.

Endocrine Secretions

A—glucagon, B cell—insulin, G cells—gastrin, D cells—somatostatin, ECL (enterochromaffin-like) cells—histamine, F cells-pancreatic polypeptide.

> **Q. Short note on serum amylase and causes of hyperamylasemia.**

SERUM AMYLASE

- Saccharolytic enzyme from acinar cells (isoenzyme P) with a plasma half life of 2–4 hours and salivary glands (isoenzyme -S). It is excreted in urine.
- **Normal values:** Serum amylase—40–140 IU/L. Urinary amylase—40–400 IU/L.

Elevation of Serum Amylase

Levels over 1000 units is highly suggestive, but not diagnostic of acute pancreatitis. The levels rise within few hours and fall slowly over 4–8 days. Urinary amylase and amylase-creatinine clearance ratio is useful in the diagnosis. But elevated lipase levels are confirmatory.

Other Causes of Hyperamylasemia

- Upper gastrointestinal tract perforation
- Intestinal obstruction
- Mesenteric or visceral ischemia
- Retroperitoneal hematoma
- Ectopic pregnancy
- Renal failure
- Sialadenitis (parotitis)
- Macroamylasemia
- Amylase in secretions: High levels of amylase are found in peritoneal fluid, ascitic fluid in pancreas and also in pseudocyst.

ACR—amylase creatinine clearance ratio > 5% indicative of acute pancreatitis.

Urinary amylase × serum creatinine divided by serum amylase × urinary creatinine × (multiplied by) 100.

Q. Short note on lipase.

LIPASE

- Lipase is secreted by the pancreas, liver and intestines; Normal serum value—0–50 units/L.
- It hydrolyses triglycerides into fatty acids and glycerol.
- Half-life is 10 hours.

Lipase is increased in acute pancreatitis, pseudocyst, chronic pancreatitis, pancreatic cancer, ischemia of bowel, liver diseases, renal failure, liver diseases.

Pancreatic Function Tests

Pancreatic Exocrine Function

- Assessed by stimulating pancreatic secretion and measuring the same.
- Physiological stimulation—by giving a standard meal.
- Pharmacological stimulation—a triple lumen tube is passed to aspirate gastric and duodenal juices before and after stimulation by intravenous injections of secretin and CCK separately. Each time, enzyme and bicarbonate in duodenal juice are measured.

Stool Elastase Content

Low levels of the enzyme elastase indicate chronic pancreatic exocrine insufficiency.

Imaging Investigations

Ultrasonography

Useful in evaluation of obstructive jaundice; to look for dilated bile duct, gallstones, hepatomegaly, or a pancreatic mass and cysts.

Limitation

Gas in front of pancreas and obesity—a poor window for ultrasound.

Q. Short note on role of CT scan in pancreatic disease.

Computed tomography in pancreatic diseases

- Very accurate in assessment of pancreatic pathology.
- Pancreatic protocol—contrast enhanced CT with 3D image reconstruction is performed.
- Plain CT to check for calcified pancreas or gallbladder.
- Rapid injection of intravenous contrast.
- CT scan is done in arterial and venous phase in small slices (2 mm).
- The stomach and duodenum are distended with water to delineate the duodenal loop.
- Diagnostic information available: Pancreatic carcinomas of 1–2 cm in size, endocrine tumors, pancreatitis with necrosis (non-enhancement of contrast), pseudocysts, inflammatory collections.

Therapeutic applications

CT-guided drainage of collections, pseudocyst, true cysts, biopsy (percutaneous Trucut needle).

Q. MRCP (Refer section obstructive jaundice).

Magnetic Resonance Imaging

- Clear delineation of the pancreas, pancreatic duct and bile duct and fluid collections.
- Magnetic resonance cholangiography and pancreatography (MRCP) has almost replaced diagnostic ERCP.
- Non-invasive and less expensive.
- Also ductal obstructions can be evaluated by screening the pancreatic duct after intravenous injection of secretin, which should result in emptying of the duct.

Q. ERCP-also refer under chapter on bile duct.

Endoscopic Retrograde Cholangiopancreatography (ERCP)

- ERCP is performed using a side-viewing fiberoptic duodenoscope.
- The contrast is injected into the biliary and pancreatic ducts after cannulating the ampulla of Vater. The biliary and pancreatic ductal anatomy is displayed on X-ray screening.

- In pancreatic carcinoma, narrowing or obstruction of the main pancreatic duct (MPD) or distal common bile duct (CBD).
- **Narrowing of both ducts:** Double duct sign.

Chronic Pancreatitis: Stricture and dilatation of pancreatic ducts—main and side ducts, ductal calculi and communication with cysts and bile duct strictures.
- Plain X-ray shows calcifications and calculi.
- Sampling of bile or pancreatic fluid for analysis, culture or cytology.
- Brush cytology from strictures.
- Biliary and pancreatic stenting.

Endoscopic Ultrasonography
- Endoscopic ultrasound (EUS) has a high-frequency ultrasonic transducer at the tip of an endoscope.
- The pancreas and its surrounding vasculature and lymph nodes are assessed.
- Useful in identifying small tumors, missed at CT or MRI and in displaying the relationship of the tumor to major vessels and duct (helps in deciding on an enucleation of tumor).

> **Q. Short note on annular pancreas.**

ANNULAR PANCREAS
A congenital anomaly where in the ventral pancreatic component undergoes malrotation during 5th week of intrauterine life and fails to rotate and migrate fully to fuse with the dorsal component of the pancreas. A collar of pancreatic tissue is seen around the second part of the duodenum. It is often associated with congenital duodenal stenosis or atresia and in children with Down syndrome.

Clinical Presentation
- It is asymptomatic in many and in others it may present with duodenal obstruction.
- Adults (make two thirds) present as duodenal obstruction or pancreatitis; infants (one third) present with bilious vomiting.
- X-ray—double bubble appearance (a bubble each in 1st and 2nd part of duodenum).
- CT scan or MRI—will be diagnostic.

Treatment
- Duodenoduodenostomy—(First part of duodenum to third part) or duodenojejunostomy.
- Pancreaticoduodenectomy (Whipple's)—in adults if there is recurrent pancreatitis.

> **Q. Short note on pancreas divisum.**

Pancreas Divisum
A congenital anomaly of the pancreatic ducts. The dorsal duct (Santorini) fails to fuse with main duct (Wirsung) and opens independently as an accessory duct into the duodenum through the minor papilla above the main duodenal papilla. Thus dividing the pancreas into two independent draining units. The relatively larger body and tail region are drained by narrow accessory duct. This causes ductal hypertension leading to recurrent attacks of pancreatitis.

Diagnosis
- MRI/MRCP—depicts the ductal anatomy and state of the papillary obstruction and gland.
- ERCP

Treatment
- Endoscopic—minor papillotomy and stenting of the Santorini's duct.
- **Surgery:** If repeat endoscopic interventions fail to prevent recurrent pancreatitis and pancreatitis has left the pancreas structurally damaged.
- **Surgical options:** Pancreaticojejunostomy (bypass to relieve ductal hypertension).
- Rarely a pancreatic head resection (Whipple or Begar procedure).

MUCOVISCIDOSIS (CYSTIC FIBROSIS—CF)
An autosomal recessive inherited disorder of mucus secreting glands of bronchioles, sweat glands and the pancreas, liver and the intestines due to a mutation on the CFTR (cystic fibrosis transmembrane conductance regulator) gene on chromosome 7. This gene creates a cell membrane protein that helps to control the chloride movement across the cell membrane.
- There is an elevation in the concentration of sodium and chloride in the sweat leading to salt loss and dehydration (often fatal).

- The mucus is extremely viscid causing clogging of the lumina of ducts and bronchioles.
- Pancreatic duct is blocked causing ductal dilatation and fatty infiltration of exocrine acini, leading to chronic pancreatitis and malabsorption.
- The liver—biliary cirrhosis (due to biliary clogging) and portal hypertension.
- Skin—loss of salt through sweat, high sodium in sweat and dehydration (may be fatal).
- Respiratory tract—bronchiectasis, recurrent infections.

Clinical Features

Newborn
- Neonatal intestinal obstruction.
- Meconium peritonitis (Refer under peritoneum).

Infant
- Voracious appetite but marasmic.
- Abdominal distension, and steatorrhea.
- Bronchiectasis.

Older Child
- Stunted growth, poor appetite, greasy foul smelling stools (steatorrhea).
- Recurrent respiratory infections (bronchiectasis).
- Hyponatremia and hypochloremia portal hypertension.

Adult
- Pancreatic exocrine insufficiency—fat malabsorption. Steatorrhoea from birth. Bulky and oily offensive stools. Diabetes mellitus may occur in older patients.
- Chronic respiratory disease (bronchiectasis) and finger clubbing.
- Sialosis (enlarged salivary glands) and recurrent infections.
- Eye—vitreal opacities.

Diagnosis: Elevated sodium content in sweat.

Treatment

Respiratory system:
- Infections—treatment and prevention of recurrent infections.
- Bronchiectasis—medical protocols followed
- Nutrition; Diet—high in protein and sugar content, low on fat.
- Supplementation: Vit D (10000 units daily) and Vit A—20000 units daily.
- Pancreatic enzyme supplementation—preparations with pancreatic lipase 20000 to 30000 units per meal.

Mode of Death
- Respiratory infections, heat exhaustion.
- Electrolyte loss, dehydration and arrhythmias.

PANCREATIC FISTULA

Etiology
- Trauma—penetrating or blunt.
- Surgery—splenectomy, enucleation of tumors, pancreatic anastomosis.
- Post pancreatitis—ductal disruption, after drainage of pseudocysts.

Types
- External—to skin
- Internal—into viscera—colon, duodenum, jejunum and ileum.

Clinical implications: Skin excoriation and digestion. Loss of electrolytes.

Investigations
- Amylase content in the fistula output.
- CT fistulography and ERCP.

Treatment
- Correction of electrolyte loss.
- **Skin care:** Zinc paste. Tube drain to collect secretion.
- **Suppression of pancreatic secretion:** Octreotide—100 mcg subcutaneous—twice a day.
- **Nutrition:** Parenteral nutrition or nasojejunal feeding
- ERCP and pancreatic ductal stenting if there is ductal block.
- **Surgery:** To resect the tail in traumatic necrosis and disruption of distal duct.
- Internal drainage of internal pseudocysts.
- **Internal fistulae:** Laparotomy, resection of the segment of bowel.
- Pancreatic resection in major fistulae.

Q. Etiopathogenesis, pathology and complications of acute pancreatitis.

PANCREATITIS

Note: Acute and chronic—do not refer to duration or chronicity of the condition.

Classification: Marseilles Classification

- **Acute pancreatitis (AP) and relapsing pancreatitis:** Inflammatory state which heals without residual morphological changes to pancreatic structure.
- **Chronic pancreatitis (CP)—with or without relapsing acute exacerbations:** The condition is associated with irreversible morphological changes due to fibrosis of parenchyma and/or ducts—causing loss of function and/or pain.

ACUTE PANCREATITIS (AP)

Acute inflammatory condition of pancreas with parenchymal damage and elevated levels of pancreatic enzymes in blood and urine.

It is postulated that an acute attack, first or relapsing may be an early phase of chronic pancreatitis in some.

Etiology of Pancreatitis (Refer Table 24.1)

Pathophysiology of acute pancreatitis

A complex process—not fully explained.
- Intra ductal hypertension due to obstruction to pancreatic duct (biliary stones, ascaris or tumors) and spasm of sphincter of Oddi by any cause.
- Toxic injury by alcohol or drugs, viral infection causes cell damage in duct and acini to trigger the process. Other mechanisms may be involved in autoimmune diseases or metabolic causes.

The events subsequent to acinar damage

Autodigestion: Damage to the intracellular zymogen granules and duct epithelium.

The tissue necrosis causes exudation of a fluid rich in enzymes, vasoactive amines and myocardial depressant factor into the peritoneal cavity, which is absorbed into circulation. This may lead to hemodynamic instability, bacteremia (translocation of gut flora), acute respiratory distress syndrome, gastrointestinal hemorrhage, renal failure and disseminated intravascular coagulation (DIC).

Table 24.1: Etiology of acute pancreatitis.

Etiology

1.	Biliary tract disease	Biliary stones are the most common cause of acute pancreatitis—approx 40%
2.	Alcoholism	Very common 30% approx
3.	Trauma	Iatrogenic—ERCP Surgery—bile duct exploration, gastrectomy, splenectomy Blunt trauma or penetrating trauma
4.	Metabolic	Hypertriglyceridemia Hyperparathyroidism; hypercalcemic conditions. Diabetes porphyria
5.	Infections	Viral—mumps, coxsackie B, mycoplasma, infectious mononucleosis, mycoplasma.
6.	Parasites	Ascariasis, clonorchiasis ductal obstruction
7.	Toxins	Scorpion bite
8.	Drugs	Steroids, ACTH, thiazides, furosemide, azathioprine, 5-ASA, estrogens, sodium valproate
9.	Autoimmune pancreatitis	
10.	Vascular disorders	Ischemia—vasculitis, shock
11.	Pancreatic divisum	
12.	Hereditary pancreatitis	
13.	Idiopathic	

Phases of Acute Pancreatitis

Early phase—7 days: It lasts for 7 days and accounts for a third of all deaths in pancreatitis. There is a systemic inflammatory response syndrome (SIRS)—mild, moderate or severe (refer under pathology of acute pancreatitis).

Late phase—after 7 days to several weeks: Characterized by systemic signs of inflammation, and/or local complications like fluid collections and peripancreatic sepsis. Deaths during this phase are due to septic complications.

Q. Classify acute pancreatitis.

Q. Describe fluid collections in acute pancreatitis.

Pathology of acute pancreatitis

Pancreas; edematous or hemorrhagic/necrotic with surrounding fluid—blood stained.
Peritoneum: Blood stained exudates, fat necrosis with saponification and calcium deposits in omentum, mesentery and parietes, (pleura and pericardium, sub synovial fat of knee).
Associated pathology:
Gallstone, duodenal diverticula, pancreas divisum or other predisposing conditions.

Classification of acute pancreatitis

Defined by three criteria: The early phase features
1. Pain—characteristic of pancreatitis
2. Enzymes elevation of pancreatic enzymes more than 3 times the normal level.
3. CT scan—characteristic findings

Revised Atlanta Classification (2012)—based on clinical, biochemical and CT scan finding.
- Mild acute pancreatitis—absence of local complications; absence of organ failure
- Moderately severe acute pancreatitis—local complications with or without transient organ failure lasting for less than 48 hours
- Severe acute pancreatitis—persistent organ failure lasting for more than 48 hours

Organ failure—defined as a score of 2 or more of renal, cardiovascular or respiratory systems.
Fluid collections—in acute pancreatitis—2012 Atlanta Classification: (Refer **Table 24.2**)

Table 24.2: Fluid collections in acute pancreatitis.

Fluid collections in acute pancreatitis—2012 Atlanta classification

Early phase—within 4 weeks

APFC	ANC (acute necrotic collections)
• Acute peripancreatic fluid collection • Interstitial edematous pancreatitis • Exudation common • No solid encapsulated collection • Homogenous—fluid density	• Acute necrotic pancreatitis • Fat necrosis—pancreatic and/or peripancreatic • Partially encapsulated • Heterogenous collection (debris)

Late phase—after 4 weeks

Pseudocyst	WON—walled off necrosis
Interstitial edematous pancreatitis Homogenous—fluid density has a well defined wall	Necrotizing pancreatitis Heterogenous collection (debris) Encapsulated—well defined wall Fat necrosis—pancreatic and/or peripancreatic

Abandoned terminologies: Acute pseudocyst and pancreatic abscess

Q. Clinical features and complications of acute pancreatitis.

CLINICAL FEATURES OF ACUTE PANCREATITIS

- Age and sex—all ages and both sexes affected.
- Etiology matters and hence common in the age group at 40-50.
- Early stage—only severe symptoms are seen and signs may be absent.

Symptoms

- Pain—epigastric agonizing severity progressively increasing, may be radiating to back.
- "Crescendo type" pain, no remissions.
- Vomiting with severe retching.

Abdominal Signs

- Rigidity—initially upper abdominal later generalized
- Tenderness over the epigastrium may be present but difficult to elicit.
- Ileus—localised or generalized
- Abdominal fluid (flank dullness)
- **Grey Turner's sign:** Hemorrhagic spots and ecchymoses in the flanks (fat necrosis in retroperitoneum and spread across the intermuscular plane.
- **Cullen's sign:** Discoloration around the umbilicus.
- **Foxes' sign:** Ecchymotic areas below the inguinal ligament.
- Abdominal mass—after 2 weeks.

Systemic Signs

- Jaundice—2nd day (edema of head of pancreas)
- Hyperglycemia
- Renal failure—part of (SIRS)
- Hypovolemia—due to third space loss, myocardial depressant factor and low peripheral resistance
- Hypocalcemia and tetany or hypercalcemic crisis (in HPT)
- Respiratory system—asymptomatic hypoxemia (right to left shunt)
- Later—pulmonary edema, (alveolar capillary leak) and respiratory failure
- Cardiovascular system: Hypotension, tachycardia, low volume pulse and shock
- SIRS: Identified—by finding of two or more of the following criteria: Heart rate >90/min, core temperature <36°C or >38°C, respirations >20/min, or pCO_2 <32 mm Hg, and white blood cell count <4000 or >12000/mm³.

Differential Diagnosis of Acute Pancreatitis (Refer Table 24.3)

COMPLICATIONS OF ACUTE PANCREATITIS (REFER TABLE 24.4)

Investigations: For diagnosis (see above), and to assess severity and plan treatment.
- Blood enzymes—amylase and lipase levels
- Blood (parameters)—hemoglobin, PCV electrolytes, gas analysis (oxygen and carbon dioxide) calcium, LFT, renal function
- X-ray-abdomen—gallstone, calcificaton, perforation
- X-ray chest—effusion, pulmonary shadows
- Ultrasound—fluid, edematous gland, gallbaldder and stone
- CT scan—performed after 72 hours for diagnosis and to assess severity by CT staging (Refer **Table 24.5**). Also it helps to assess patients with signs of progressive clinical deterioration, organ failure, sepsis and for localized complications—fluid collection, pseudocyst or a pseudoaneurysm.

EUS and MRI—at a later stage to assess the late changes.

Table 24.3: Differential diagnosis of acute pancreatitis.

Differential diagnosis	
• Acute coronary syndrome • Perforated peptic ulcer or any hollow viscus • Gallstone colic	• High intestinal obstruction • Diabetic ketoacidosis (diabetic abdomen)

Table 24.4: Complications of acute pancreatitis.

Local	Systemic
• Pancreatic—fluid/necrosis(see next) • Peritonitis • Pseudoaneurysm of splenic artery • Secondary hemorrhage into peritoneal cavity • Thrombosis of splenic and portal veins • Necrosis of transverse colon • Duodenal ileus	• Respiratory failure—acute respiratory distress syndrome (ARDS) • Renal failure • Cardiopathy • Encephalopathy and psychosis • Hypocalcemia and tetany or hypercalcemic crisis (in acute hyperparathyroidism) • Metastatic fat necrosis • Late diabetes mellitus

Table 24.5: CT SI (CT severity index).

CT SI (CT severity index): The Balthazar criteria for severity CT findings:

CT score 0-4 (nil, edema, peripancreatic changes—mild to severe, multiple collections/gas)

Necrosis score 0-4-6 (0-none/<1/3 /<50% />50% of pancreatic necrosis).

Severity index SI = CT score +necrotic score:

0-3 mild. 4-6—moderate and 7-10—severe pancreatitis

ERCP—urgent ERCP acute gallstone pancreatitis—for relief of biliary obstruction to remove a CBD stone and to relieve ascending cholangitis.

Clinical prognostic scores include Ranson criteria, Glasgow prognostic criteria.
APACHE II classification system, and Balthazar CT-enhanced scoring system.

Q. Glasgow prognostic criteria in acute pancreatitis (AP).

Glasgow scoring is simple and reliable to follow and preferred (Refer **Table 24.6**).

Q. Management of acute pancreatitis.

MANAGEMENT OF ACUTE PANCREATITIS

Aim: Assess and act to assist in recovery, anticipate complications—abort or antagonize them
- Analgesia
- Aspiration of gastric contents (to avoid pancreatic stimulation through secretin)
- Adequate fluid and electrolyte
- Anti-secretary measures
  Anticholinergics, e.g., hyoscine bromide or aprotinin
- Against acid—proton pump inhibitors (omeprazole or pantoprazole)
  Octreotide—(somatostatin analogue) infusion or subcutaneous 50 to 100 mcg Q8H.
- Antibiotics—only in sepsis.

Ancillary Aid
- Assisted ventilation and oxygen as needed
- Monitoring of CVP (central venous pressure) and PCWP (pulmonary capillary wedge pressure) by placing a Swan-Ganz catheter)
- Plasma expanders are not of proven value
- Closed peritoneal lavage—to wash away peritoneal fluid
- Dialysis in renal failure and hypercalcemia
- Inotropes and cardiotropic drugs as needed.

Action
- Emergency ERCP and relief of biliary obstruction in gallstone pancreatitis
- Nasojejunal feeding tube insertion for early enteral feeding after 48 hours.
- Diagnostic laparoscopy—for uncertainty in diagnosis.
- Drainage of peritoneal fluid and lavage.

Antagonising Complications
Active measures to treat the complications.

Table 24.6: Glasgow criteria and Ranson's criteria.

Glasgow criteria for prognosis of AP in first 48 hours of admission.

P	PaO_2: Low < 60mm Hg (8.0 kPa)
A	Age: High (>55 years)
N	Neutrophilia: High (>15000/cu mm)
C	Calcium: Low
R	Renal function: Low—urea >44 mg/dL (16 mmol/L)
E	Enzymes: High—LDH >600 IU/L
A	Albumin: Low <3.2 g/dL (32 g/L)
S	Sugar: High—blood glucose >180 mg/dL (>10 mmol/L)

Ranson's criteria—2 assessments required and timing may not be accurate at admission.

Five parameters are assessed on admission, and the other six at 48 hours post-admission. One point is given for each positive parameter for a maximum score of 11. (10 in the modified criteria). Five parameters are assessed on admission and the other 5 at the 48-hour mark.

On admission (5 highs)
- Age: Older than 55 years
- WBC count greater than 16,000 cells/cmm
- Blood glucose greater than 200 mg/dL (11 mmol/L)
- Serum AST greater than 250 IU/L
- Serum LDH greater than 350 IU/L

At 48 hours, (6 lows)
- Serum calcium less than 8.0 mg/dL (less than 2.0 mmol/L)
- Hematocrit fall greater than 10%
- PaO_2 less than 60 mm Hg
- Low renal fuction—BUN increased by 5 mg/dL or more (1.8 mmol/L or more) despite intravenous (IV) fluid hydration
- Base deficit greater than 4 mEq/L
- Sequestration of fluids greater than 6 L

Systemic Complications
- Multidisciplinary management in ICU.
- Intensive care monitoring with life support and organ specific support.
- Treatment of coagulopathies and DIC.
- Inotropes, hemofiltration in renal failure, ventilator support, cardiac arrhythmias.

Indication for surgery: Deterioration due to necrotic pancreatitis; patients with severity index (CTSI) of over 5-6 surgery performed after resuscitation and stabilisation.

Surgery: Emergency pancreatic necrosectomy and peritoneal drainage.

LOCAL COMPLICATIONS AND MANAGEMENT
The local complications carry a significant morbidity and mortality.

Repeat CT scan is done in presence of:
- Persistent or recurrent pain.
- Worsening of Clinical status and organ dysfunction.
- Signs of sepsis.
- Re- elevation of amylase.

ACUTE PERIPANCREATIC FLUID COLLECTION (APFC)
They are sterile and resolve generally and are monitored.

Indication for Intervention
Large collections with pressure effects and pain or signs of sepsis supervene.
Ultrasound guided percutaneous transgastric aspiration and drainage.

STERILE AND INFECTED PANCREATIC NECROSIS
Pancreatic necrosis (a diffuse or focal necrosis)—CT scan shows non-enhancement.

Acute Necrotic Collection (ANC)
This is collection with fluid and necrotic material—inside and outside the pancreas without a definite encapsulation or wall. Sterile to start with, they often get infected due to bacterial translocation.

Walled Off Necrosis (WON)
- Over the next 4 week period the ANCs develop an inflammatory capsule like wall and evolve into a WON (Walled Off Necrosis).

Indications for intervention in ANC and WON: Signs of sepsis in a sterile ANC
- CT (or ultrasound) guided aspiration.
- **Fluid:** Sent for culture and sensitivity, irrigation and drainage of the collection with widest possible pig tail drain and regular saline irrigation through the drain.
- Nutritional support is essential. The parenteral nutrition and nasojejunal feeding are options.

Surgery: Pancreatic necrosectomy and irrigation/drainage
- If the patient deteriorates despite adequate repeat aspiration and drainage.
- Laparoscopic approach or laparotomy
- Debridement of necrotic pancreatic and peripancreatic tissue, cholecystectomy (for gallstones) and a feeding jejunostomy—for early enteral nutrition.

Closure technique: To allow a repeat necrosectomy in the unpredictable course of the condition. The techniques include closed drainage, continuous lavage through a drain in peritoneum, repeated explorations and necrosectomy with lavage (laparostomy).

Zipper laparostomy: Abdominal wall and wound closed and this zipper is opened every 2-3 days for irrigation and necrosectomy as and when needed. Infected necrosis (infected ANC or WON)—formerly called pancreatic abscess.
Pus in relation to pancreas—intra and/or extra-pancreatic.

Treatment
- Guided percutaneous drainage by placing wide drains and antibiotic.
- Open drainage by surgery—for inaccessible collections, worsening after aspiration.

Pancreatic Ascites
Peritoneal collection, rich with pancreatic enzyme. Associated with disruption of pancreatic duct. Aspiration reveals high amylase content.

Treatment

- Suppression of pancreatic secretions—nasojejunal feeding or a feeding jejunostomy.
- Injections of octreotide (somatostatin analogue) to suppress pancreatic secretion.
- ERCP and stenting of pancreatic duct.

> **Q. Describe etiopathology, diagnosis and management of pseudocyst of pancreas.**

PSEUDOCYST OF PANCREAS

A pseudocyst is a collection of amylase-rich fluid enclosed in a well-defined wall of fibrous or granulation tissue.

Etiology

Following an attack of mild acute pancreatitis, or may be seen in recurrent attacks associated with chronic pancreatitis.

Pathology

Pseudocyst lies outside the pancreas (rarely inside) and is considered as a matured state of an unresolved APFC (acute peripancreatic fluid collection). It takes at least 4 weeks from the onset of acute pancreatitis for a pseudocyst to evolve.

Sites of the Pseudocyst

- Lesser sac (in relation to body and project between stomach and liver)—pushing the stomach behind and down
- Between the stomach and colon—pushing the stomach forwards and above (the most common)
- Behind the transverse colon towards infracolic peritoneal cavity
- Near the head—paraduodenal
- Near the tail—as mass far lateral.

Complications

- Infection, peritonitis and systemic sepsis.
- Rupture into the peritoneal cavity.
- Pseudoaneurysm of splenic artery and catastrophic hemorrhage.

Clinical Features (Most Typical Form)

- Epigastric mass—with band of resonance over the mass (stomach) and transmitted. Aortic pulsations felt over the mass.

Differential Diagnosis

1. Liver abscess, 2. Aortic aneurysm, 3. Mesenteric cyst.

Management

Investigation: To differentiate a pseudocyst from an APFC and an IPMN (mucinous neoplasm) and treatment accordingly.

Investigation

- Ultrasound
- CT scan
- MRCP/MRI to identify communication of the cyst with ductal system (chronic pancreatitis)
- EUS and aspiration of fluid for carcinoembryonic antigen (CEA)—to exclude a mucinous neoplasm (IPMN) particularly one near the head (CEA of above 400 ng/mL is suggestive of an IPMN).
- Cytology of aspirated fluid: For malignant cells of a mucinous neoplasm.

Treatment

Pseudocysts generally resolve and some undergo complications.

Intervention is performed for those with high risk of complications.
- Pseudocyst exceeding 6 cm in size.
- Pseudocysts unresolving even after 12 weeks (generally 6 weeks).
- Pseudocysts in association with chronic pancreatitis.

Interventional options: Percutaneous image guided, endoscopic, surgical
- Percutaneous transgastric— drainage under image guidance is done. (A direct aspiration has risks of a pancreatic fistula and high recurrence).
- Endoscopic
  - Endoscopic transgastric cystogastrostomy (tube placed between the cavity and stomach)
  - ERCP stenting of pancreatic duct to drain a chronic communicating pseudocyst.

Surgery: Laparoscopic or open laparotomy approach.

- Internal drainage of pseudocyst: Preferred.
  - Cysto gastrostomy
  - Cystojejunostomy.
- **External drainage of pseudocyst**—but it has high risk of pancreatic fistula.
  - Hence an interno-external drainage is preferred for an infected pseudocyst—wherein a tube drain is placed across the stomach into the cyst cavity and brought out through the abdominal wall and it can be removed after adequate drainage and collapse of the cyst.
- **Pancreatic drainage or resectional (major) surgery:** Indicated in—recurrent pseudocysts and pleural effusions with irreparable ductal disruptions, viz., lateral pancreaticojejunostomy, distal pancreatectomy or pancreaticoduodenectomy.

> **Q. Etiology of chronic pancreatitis.**

CHRONIC PANCREATITIS

Chronic inflammatory pathology with progressive destruction and fibrosis of pancreatic tissue. The condition has a very high association with a carcinoma of pancreas—generally body/tail.

Etiology and Pathogenesis (Refer Table 24.7)

Pathology

- Inflammation and swelling to start with: It progresses to induration and scarring leading to atrophy—first the acinar cells and last the islet cells
- The scarred parenchyma gets calcification and ducts get clogged with calculi
- **Ducts:** Distorted—dilated and interrupted by strictures
- Intraductal calculi.

Histology

Lobules—ductular metaplasia and atrophy of acini, hyperplasia of duct epithelium and interlobular fibrosis.

> **Q. Clinical presentation of chronic pancreatitis.**

- **Pain**—deep epigastric or deep in the back. Episodic initially (mistaken for peptic ulcer) and progressive unrelenting later
- **Vomiting**
- **Exocrine pancreatic deficiency**—steatorrhea. Vitamin D deficiency duodenal ulcer (Bicarbonate deficiency in pancreatic juice)
- **Endocrine** deficiency—diabetes
- **Jaundice**—scarring in head may cause entrapment and obstruction of lower CBD
- **Carcinoma**
- **Complications**—recurrent pancreatitis, recurrent peudocysts, pleural effusions or fistulae.

General Course of the Disease

- **Stage A:** Pain (80–85%)—recurrent/acute/episodic pain/weight loss

Table 24.7: Etiology and pathogenesis of chronic pancreatitis.

TIGAR-O risk factor classification 2001	
T: Toxic	Alcohol/tobacco/dietary toxin/drug
	Metabolic - hypercalcemia, hyper lipidemia/lipoprotein lipase deficiency
	Tropical - ? Tapioca rich food (cassava family)
I: Idiopathic	Idiopathic—early/late onset
G: Genetic	Mutations—cationic trypsinogen gene (PRSS 1)
	Autosomal recessive—cationic SPINK 1
A: Autoimmune	Autoimmune or immunologic—primary AIP/with Sjogren/Crohn's
R: Recurrent	Recurrent and severe acute/ischemic/post-radiotherapy
O: Obstructive	Pancreas divisum/annular pancreas; stenotic papilla/duodenal obstruction—post-trauma/pancreatic ductal stones/choledochocele

- **Stage B:**
  - Progressive pain—more severe/prolonged
  - Impaired pancreatic function
  - Complications—pseudocyst/cholestasis/segmental portal hypertension
- **Stage C:** End stage
  - Pain less severe
  - Severe deficiency—exocrine/diabetes
  - Local complications—pseudocysts/obstructive.

Investigations

- Stool (fat content)—most reliable for exocrine deficiency (3 day stool sample)
- Pancreatic function test—secretin stimulation test or Lundh test (stimulating the pancreas to test for secretory response and aspirating the duodenal juice
- X-ray of the abdomen—shows calcification or calculi along the pancreatic area (30 to 60%)
- Ultrasonography—to detect pseudocysts, dilated ducts and mass in head or body/tail
- Also to evaluate jaundice
- MRI and MRCP—to study the duct and parenchyma
- Endoscopic ultrasound—helps assess ductal pathology and masses in head region
- CT with CT angiogram—to study portal or splenic vein thrombosis
- ERCP- shows ductal morphology—multiple strictures and dilatations—typical "**chain of lakes**"
- EUS-FNAC of head cysts or CT/US guided FNAC for body or tail
- Serum CEA and CA 19-9—for carcinoma pancreas/IPMN.

Differential Diagnosis

- Pain—gallstone disease, peptic ulcer, ischemic bowel
- Steatorrhea—sprue or malabsorption states
- Diabetes—diabetes mellitus.
- Jaundice—pancreatic head cancer or lower CBD disease
- Psychiatric illness—mistaken for mental illness.

Treatment

- **Exocrine deficiency:** Pancreatic enzyme supplementation—preparations with lipase 15000 to 25000 units with each meal.
- **Endocrine:** Treatment of diabetes—insulin required in most.

Treatment of Pain

Medical, endoscopic, nerve blocks and surgery.

Medical

- Analgesia—graded scale
- Starting with non-narcotic—paracetamol and NSAID
- Narcotics—opioid or tramadol, fentanyl patches for severe (prone for narcotic addiction).

Endoscopic Therapy

Endoscopic retrograde cholangiopancreatography (ERCP)—sphincterotomy (Oddi) and further procedure: For ductal obstruction (PD and CBD) and strictures.

- **Pancreatic ductal stenting**
  - For draining a chronic pseudocyst recurrent pseudocysts
  - For short strictures and papillary stenosis
  - For fistula, pancreatic ascites pancreatic pleural effusion due to a disrupted duct
  - Endoscopic pancreatic lithotripsy and stone retrieval.
- **Stenting of CBD to relieve jaundice.**
- ERCP (stenting of minor papilla)—for pancreas divisum.
- EUS (aspiration of a cyst in head region).

Non-surgical Interventions

Neural blocks—CT guided splanchnic nerve block.

SURGERY IN CHRONIC PANCREATITIS (REFER TABLE 24.8)

See **Figure 24.2** showing pancreatic ductal calculi at imaging, and **Figures 24.3** and **24.4** showing operative extraction of pancreatic ductal calculi.

- For pain
- Obstruction—biliary or duodenal
- Ductal rupture—fistula or ascites
- Cancer.

Table 24.8: Surgery for chronic pancreatitis.

Surgery: Indications

Pain: Intractable
- Pancreatic duct—stenosis/multiple stricture
- Head—calcified/calculi
- Pancreas divisum

Lateral pancreatico- jejunostomy and Frey's head coring
- Do -

Obstructive complications—post fibrotic
- Bile duct
- Duodenal
- Segmental portal hypertension—splenic vein

- Choledochojejunal anastomosis
- Duodenojejunal anastomosis
- Splenectomy

Ductal rupture
- Pseudocyst, pancreatic fistula/pancreatic ascites

- Distal pancreatectomy

Cancer

- Radical resection—Whipple/total pancreatectomy or distal pancreatectomy

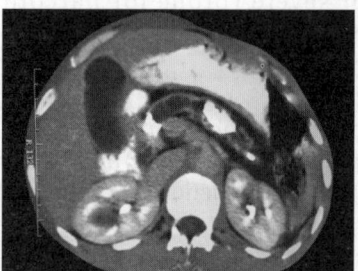

Fig. 24.2: CT-pancreatic calculi—dilated PD

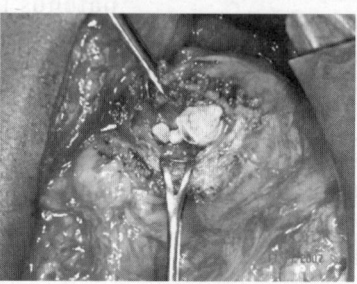

Fig. 24.3: Pancreatic stone retrieval
(For color version see Plate 2)

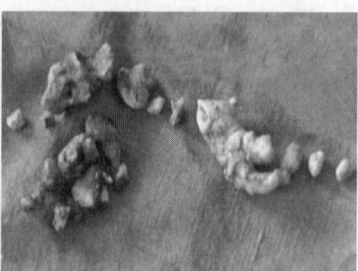

Fig. 24.4: Pancreatic stones removed from head to tail
(For color version see Plate 2)

PANCREATIC TUMORS: EXOCRINE AND ENDOCRINE

SU24.2: Describe the clinical features, principles of investigation, prognosis and management of pancreatic endocrine tumors.

SU24.3: Describe the principles of investigation and management of pancreatic disorders including pancreatitis and endocrine tumors.

TUMORS OF THE PANCREAS

Classification

Exocrine Tumors

Malignant
- Adenocarcinoma (75% of all cancers of pancreas)
  - Ductal carcinoma—adenocarcinoma or mucinous carcinoma
  - Acinar carcinoma—cystadenocarcinoma or solid carcinoma
- Squamous cell carcinoma
- Adenosquamous carcinoma
- Pancreatoblastoma

Benign
- Benign cystadenoma—mucinous (commonest), serous
- Mucinous ductal ectasia of pancreas common in head, can turn into malignancy)
- Papillary cystic tumors—intraductal papillary cystic mucinous neoplasms or serous neoplasms teratomas.

Endocrine Tumors—Pancreatic Neuroendocrine Tumors (PNET)
- Gastrinoma (G-cells)
- Somatostatinoma (D-cells)
- Insulinoma (beta cells)
- Glucagonoma (A-cells)
- Vipoma-pancreatic cholera (Verner-Morrison syndrome)
- Non-functioning neuroendocrine tumor (PNET)

Mesenchymal tumors: Sarcomas
Lymphomas
Secondary tumors (metastatic tumors)

Cystic Neoplasms of the Pancreas

Types
- Cystadenoma—mucinous (commonest) or serous cystadenoma
- Mucinous ductal ectasia of pancreas (common in head, affects elderly males, high-risk of turning malignant)
- Papillary cystic tumors
- Teratomas, etc.

Mucinous Cystic Tumors
More common in females, arising from body or tail, present as large cystic masses with pain, mistaken for a pseudocyst. They may be malignant and show a high CEA levels in serum or aspirate from the cystic mass.

Serous Cystic Tumors
Mostly benign.

> **Q. Intraductal papillary mucinous neoplasms (IPMNs).**

Intraductal Papillary Mucinous Neoplasms (IPMNs)
- It is common in 6th and 7th decade; equal in both sexes.
- A neoplasm with tall, columnar, mucin containing epithelium with or without papillary projections.
- IPMNs may be benign, borderline or malignant—through to an adenoma-carcinoma sequence.

Types
- Main duct (75%)
- Branch duct
- Multifocal in head and body
- Combined main and branch duct.

Details
- Main duct IPMN with dilatation of duct with mucosal bulge through ampulla (70% malignant).
- Branch-duct IPMN—side branches of main duct communicating to main duct.
  - Here the duct is not dilated
  - Seen mainly in uncinate process.
- Multifocal IPMN—in head, neck and body;
- Combined IPMN—from both main duct and branch ducts.

Clinical Presentation
- May be pain or as pancreatitis
- Cystic lesions mainly head or in the body
- EUS- aspiration cytology helps diagnosis
- CEA may be elevated.

Treatment
- Resection: For tumors
  - \> 3 cm—cytology is suspicious of cancer
  - < 3 cm—with benign looking features are followed up for progression.

EXOCRINE PANCREATIC TUMORS

Carcinoma of the Pancreas (Must Know)
Risk factors for the development of pancreatic cancer (Refer **Table 24.9**).

> **Q. Describe pathology and clinical features of carcinoma of pancreas.**

Pathology of Adenocarcinoma of Pancreas

Distribution of Carcinoma Pancreas
- **Head:**
  - 2/3s (70%) of all tumors arise from 1/3 of the gland
  - 2/3—head proper
  - 1/3—periampullaryv (23%)
- **Body and tail:**
  - 1/3 (30%) of tumors arise from 2/3s of gland.
  - 2/3—body proper 15%
  - 1/3—tail 7-10%
- **Diffuse gland involvement:** 8-10%

Genetic Mutations in Pancreatic Carcinoma
Multiple mutations are noticed—inherited and acquired throughout aging.
- K-ras oncogene: 90% of tumors show a mutation in this.
- The HER2/neu oncogene, homologous to the epidermal growth factor receptor (EGFr), is overexpressed.
- Multiple tumor-suppressor genes are deleted and/or mutated in pancreatic cancer (e.g., p53, p16) and BRCA2 in some cases.

Table 24.9: Risk factors for the development of pancreatic cancer.

Epidemiological factors	Genetic factors and family history
• Age (peak incidence 65–75 years) • Male gender • African race: Environment/lifestyle • Cigarette smoking • Diabetes mellitus • Chronic pancreatitis (5- to 15-fold increased risk)	• Familial adenomatous polyposis—risk of ampullary/duodenal carcinoma • Lynch syndrome (HNPCC) hereditary non-polyposis colorectal cancer • H/O pancreatic cancer in family—risk higher by 15–50 times more. • Germline BRCA2 mutations seen in some cases • Hereditary pancreatitis (50- to 70-fold increased risk) • Peutz–Jeghers syndrome • Familial breast–ovarian cancer syndrome • Familial melanoma

Q. Pancreatic Intraepithelial Neoplasia (PanIN)

Pancreatic Intraepithelial Neoplasia (PanIN)—precursor lesions of pancreatic carcinoma

Three stages of pancreatic intraepithelial neoplasia:
1. PanIN 1: No dysplasia
2. PanIN 2: Moderate dysplasia;
3. PanIN 3: Carcinoma in situ

Importance of PanIN
- These lesions show the same oncogene mutations and loss of tumor-suppressor genes (like the finding in invasive cancers). These are considered as precancerous and at this stage a cancer can still be prevented or cured and hence studied.

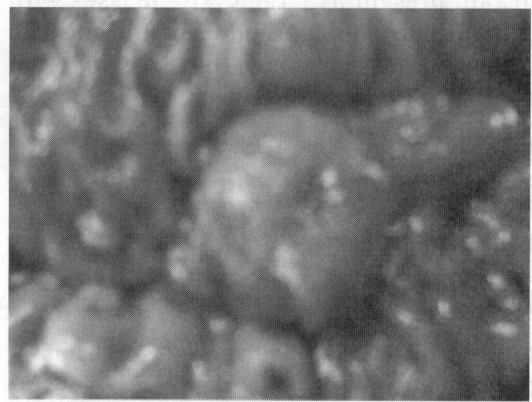

Fig. 24.5: Ampullary tumor.
(For color version see Plate 2)

Q. What is a periampullary carcinoma? Describe the pathology, clinical diagnosis of pancreatic carcinoma.

PATHOLOGY

Figure 24.5 shows an ampullary carcinoma in an operative specimen.
- **Adenocarcinoma:** In head of pancreas or ampulla or periampullary region
  - Most arise from the duct epithelium (85%)
  - Yellowish white mass—in head, neck and ampulla. Ductal/glandular differentiation with desmoplastic stromal reaction
  - Infiltration of nerves and lymphovascular invasion
- **Periampullary carcinoma**—arises from tissue within 2 cm of the ampulla of Vater
  - Includes ampulla of Vater
  - Duodenal mucosa around the papilla
  - Lower CBD and pancreatic tissue—duct
  - Parenchyma of pancreas surrounding the ampulla of Vater.

They cause obstruction of bile duct and early jaundice and hence detected early. The cancers from the lower CBD and duodenal mucosa have a better prognosis than those from the ampulla of Vater or the head tissue.

Spread of the Tumor

Local Invasion
- Head—duodenum, CBD, pylorus, transverse mesocolon at middle colic vessels retroperitoneal structures and splenic vessels.
- Transperitoneal implantation—ascites and pelvic deposits.

Vessels

- Superior mesenteric vein and artery; Portal vein.
- Middle colic vessels; Gastroduodenal vessels and hepatoduodenal ligament.

Lymphatic Spread

- Head subpyloric and suprapyloric nodes—pancreaticoduodenal nodes, nodes along hepatic artery and nodes along splenic artery form body and tail
- Celiac, para-aortic are the next level nodes
- Blood spread—liver, lungs, bone skin.

STAGING OF PANCREATIC CANCER
Refer **Table 24.10**.

TUMOR NODE METASTASIS STAGE (REFER TABLE 24.11)

- Pancreatic carcinomas have a poor prognosis due to late diagnosis (10% are detected in stage I and II and 30% in stage III).

Table 24.11: Stages of carcinoma pancreas.

I.	T1	N0	M0
II.	T2	N0	M0
III.	T3	N0	M0
	T4	N0	M0
	Any T	N1	M0
IV.	Any T	Any N	M1

Clinical Features

- 50–70 years age group is the commonest, sex.
- Jaundice, pain, abdominal mass, weight loss. Diabetes may be the features.

Jaundice

- Head lesions present with jaundice early.
- Painless, progressive and obstructive type.
- **Intermittent:** Some patients with periampullary carcinoma may have intermittent jaundice, due to sloughing of the growth with temporary relief of jaundice.
- Pruritus, dark urine.

Table 24.10: Summary of TNM staging of pancreatic carcinoma.

Summary of TNM staging (ACS - AJCC)

Tumor (T)

TX		Tumor cannot be assessed
T1	Intrapancreatic	Tumor- 2 cm - limited to the pancreas
T2	-Do-	Tumor- 2–4 cm - --- do ----
T3	Large/CBD/DUO	Tumor ->4 cm; or invading the duodenum or common bile duct
T4		Tumor invading adjacent organs (stomach, spleen, colon, adrenal or large vessels (celiac axis or the superior mesenteric artery)

Regional Lymph Node (N)	Nodes involved
NX	Cannot be assessed
N0	Nil
N1	1–3
N2	4 or more nodes

Distant Metastasis (M)	
M0	No distant metastasis
M1	Distant metastasis
M1a	Hepatic only
M1b	Extrahepatic—lung, ovary, peritoneum, bone, extra-regional lymph node.
M1c	M1a + b

- Pale stools—due to obstructive jaundice.
- Body and tail—lesions present with pain and mass.

Pain
- Dull ache—radiating to the back—or at times colicky
- Weight loss—seen in 90%. It may be the sole presenting feature in some
- Anorexia
- **Obstruction:** Duodenal or pyloric—causes vomiting.

Presentation as Pain without Jaundice
- Intractable pain in a middle aged person, felt in L1–L2 vertebral level.
- Partly relieved by bending forwards
- **Weight loss**
- Jaundice—due to liver metastases—in portal fissures or parenchyma—in body and tail growths.

Abdominal mass—large mass in epigastrium—hard, nodular and deep—retroperitoneal.
Ascites—due to peritoneal metastases.

Hepatomegaly
- Smooth—uniform, painless hepatomegaly—due to biliary obstruction—in head lesion—90%
- Nodular irregular hard enlargement due ot multiple metastases—seen in 60% of lesions in the body and tail of pancreas.

Gallbladder
- Enlarged gallbladder (in 80% of head carcinoma).
- With a smooth enlarged liver and jaundice is typical of carcinoma of head of pancreas.
- **Courvoisier's law** defines—it is not due to stone in CBD.

Others
- **Trousseau' sign:** Migratory superficial thrombophlebitis (recurrent attacks in different veins of the body)
- Recently diagnosed diabetes mellitus in a middle aged person.
- Unexplained attack of pancreatitis.
- Supraclavicular node.

Differential Diagnosis
Jaundice
- Hepatocellular jaundice
- Pancreatitis
- Stone in common bile duct (CBD)
- Tumors or strictures of CBD
- Mirizzi syndrome
- Stricture/stenosis of sphincter of Oddi.

Pain and Weight Loss
- Carcinoma stomach
- Pancreatitis
- Ischemic bowel.

> **Q. Management of carcinoma of pancreas.**

Investigations
- Blood tests—to confirm obstructive jaundice—LFT
  Tumor markers: CA 19-9, CEA and alpha-fetoprotein (AFP)
- **Ultrasonography**
  Dilated duct, head mass or a body lesion, nodes,
  liver—texture and intrahepatic bile ducts, metastatic deposits
- **CECT**—contrast enhanced CT scan—pancreatic protocol.
  - Plain CT
  - Post injection of dye—arterial phase CT
  - Venous phase CT
  - Distension of stomach and duodenum with air.
- **MRCP**—to study ductal status—pancreatic and biliary—obstruction
- **MRI/MR angiography** to identify vascular encasement (SMV/SMA).
  Also to delineate the peripancreatic nodes and liver deposits
- **Endoscopic ultrasound (EUS)** and FNAC or Trucut biopsy of solid lesions
  - Aspiration of cystic tumors—in head and lower CBD.
- **ERCP**—to identify small ampullary lesions
  - Biliary stenting—to relieve post obstructive cholangitis.
  - Elevated level of bilirubin over 15 mg

- **Diagnostic laparoscopy**—prior to a planned major surgical resection to identify small peritoneal or omental metastases often missed by scanning modalities and avoid a major operation.

TREATMENT OF CARCINOMA OF PANCREAS

Surgical resection is the only hope of cure in pancreatic cancers of all types.

Curative resections are indicated for:
- Stage I and II carcinomas/imaging shows resectable tumor
- All periampullary cancers
- Cystic neoplasms (even very large)—as they have a better prognosis after surgery
- Neuroendocrine tumors
- Rare tumors of pancreas.

Palliative surgery for inoperable lesions—relief of jaundice and gastroduodenal obstruction.

Surgery

Carcinoma Head and/Periampullary Carcinoma

Q. Short note on Whipple's operation.

Whipple's operation: Radical pancreaticoduodenectomy (PD)

Parts removed:
- Head and uncinate process (divided at the neck) along with the entire duodenum
- Gastric antrum
- The CBD and gallbladder
- Peripancreatic, pericholedochal, paraduodenal and periportal nodes.

Reconstruction to restore gastrointestinal continuity:
- Pancreatic neck anastomosed to jejunum (or gastric stump)
- Common hepatic duct end to jejunal loop
- Gastric stump—to jejunal loop.

Modification
- Pylorus preserving pancreatoduodenectomy (PPPD) (Traverso-Longmire operation)
- Similar to Whipple's; but the pylorus is preserved by dividing the first part of the duodenum and anastomosing the duodenal cuff (instead of the gastric stump) to the jejunal loop.

- This is said to preserve pyloric sphincteric function for better gastric function.

Carcinoma of Body of the Pancreas
Total pancreatectomy.

Carcinoma of Tail
Distal pancreatectomy (pancreas to the left of the superior mesenteric vein is resected).

PALLIATIVE SURGERY

Triple Anastomosis
- To relieve jaundice—choledochojejunostomy (or cholecysto jejunostomy)
- To relieve gastric outlet obstruction—gastro jejunostomy
- To prevent cholangitis after the anastomosis—jejunojejunostomy (diverts food off bile): 6 months of adjuvant chemotherapy with—gemcitabine and/or 5-FU.

Chemoradiotherapy combination of chemo with radiation to the tumor bed particularly in patients with involved (R1) resection margins. Folfirinox—a combination of three 5-FU/leucovorin, irinotecan, and oxaliplatin—is now commonly used as first-line treatment for metastatic pancreatic adenocarcinoma.

Targeted Therapy
- **Monoclonal antibody:** Erlotinib in combination with gemcitabine—poor results.
- **PARP Inhibitor:** Olaparib is used for pancreatic cancers associated with germline (hereditary) BRCA mutation.

PALLIATION IN PANCREATIC CANCER

Surgery (See Above)
Surgical bypass or ERCP stenting for relief of jaundice or or gastrojejunostomy for duodenal obstruction.

Pain Relief
- Graded stepwise analgesia—non-opioid to opioid
- Coeliac plexus block—CT guided
- Splanchnicectomy—thoracoscopic
- Enzyme replacement for steatorrhoea
- Diabetes—management and control
- Counseling and morale boost.

ENDOCRINE TUMORS OR PANCREAS NEUROECTODERMAL TUMORS (PNET)

- The islet cells, making the endocrine pancreas, are from from neural crest cells and are referred to as **amine precursor uptake and decarboxylation cells (APUD)**.
- Tumors can arise in multiple sites from these cells causing the multiple endocrine neoplasia (MEN) syndromes, classified as MEN-I and MEN-II.
- The MEN-I syndrome: Association of pituitary tumors, parathyroid hyperplasia (or adenoma) and pancreatic neoplasms.

> **Q. Classification of pancreatic neuro endocrine tumors (pNETs).**

Pancreatic neuroendocrine tumors (pNETs) (Refer **Table 24.12**)
- Functional if they are associated with a clinical syndrome
- Nonfunctioning if not associated with clinical symptoms.

The majority of pancreatic neuroendocrine tumors pNET (PET) are non-functional and malignant.

Diagnostic Imaging for Pancreatic Endocrine Tumors

Multidetector CT scan with four phases of contrast is **test of choice**.
- Fine cuts through the pancreas and liver.
- pNETs are generally seen enhancing with contrast.

EUS: Helps identify tumors smaller than 1 cm (CT may miss)

Radiolabeled octreotide scan: Intravenous radionuclide is selectively taken up by somatostatin.
- Receptors(SSTR), detected by whole-body radionuclide scanning.

Other tests for localizing primaries and detecting metastases (not done usually):
- Angiography
- Selective venous sampling.

General Management of pNETs
- **Diagnosis:** The key is identifying the specific clinical syndrome.
- **Confirmation:** By measuring serum levels of the elevated hormone.
- **Localization:** By imaging.
- **Surgical remedy:** Complete resection for cure or debulking for controlling symptoms for nonresectable tumor. Curative complete resection for cure or palliative debulking for controlling symptoms for nonresectable tumor.
- Chemoembolization of liver metastases.

Principles of Surgery for pNET

Radical surgery with curative intent is done for resectable tumors including those with spread to nodes and oligometastases (less than three).

Debulking of tumors (cytoreduction)—also helps as these tumors are slow in progressing.

Local ablative therapies include:
- Radiofrequency ablation (RFA)—most popular
- Cryotherapy

Table 24.12: pNETs.		
Type of cell	*Secretion*	*Tumor - pNET*
Alpha cell (A cell) 25%	Glucagon	Glucagonoma
Beta cell (B cell) 50%	Insulin	Insulinoma
Delta cell (D cell) 10%	Somatostatin	Somatostatinoma
F-cells (secrete) 5 HT	Pancreatic polypeptide (PP)	PPoma
Cells not present normally		
D1 cells	Vasoactive intestinal polypeptide (VIP)	VIPoma
G- cell	Gastrin	Gastrinoma

Transarterial chemoembolization (TACE)—palliation in patients with liver metastases.

Platinum-based chemotherapy—for high-grade (poorly differentiated) pNET capecitabine and temozolomide—for well-differentiated pNET.

Treatment of of Specific PNETs

All general principles described are applicable (additional reading "Good to know").

DIAGNOSIS AND TREATMENT OF PNETs

Q. Short note on insulinoma.

- **Insulinoma:** The commonest among pNETs.
- **90% of insulinomas are benign:** Solitary and sporadic.
- 10% are malignant, or multiple or associated with MEN-I.

Whipple's Triad

The triad consists of:
- Symptomatic fasting hypoglycemia.
- Blood glucose level <50 mg/dL.
- Relief of symptoms with the administration of glucose.

Palpitations, trembling, diaphoresis, confusion seizure, and "behavioral change".

Serum insulin levels are elevated which causes elevation of serum C-peptide levels.

Localisation: CECT, EUS and biopsy.

Treatment: Surgery
- **Enucleation:** Done for most insulinomas.
- **Resection:** A distal pancreatectomy or pancreaticoduodenectomy
  - For tumors located close to the main pancreatic duct
  - Tumors larger than 2 cm in size.

GLUCAGONOMA

Triad
- Peptic ulcer
- Diabetes
- Necrolytic migratory erythema.

Present as large tumors in the body and tail of the pancreas and metastases.

Mild diabetes in association with dermatitis—the lower abdomen, perineum, perioral area, and feet, enlarged tongue. The rash in glucagonoma is due to catabolic effect of glucagon causing low levels of amino acid and malnutrition.

Glucagon levels >500 pg/mL

Treatment

Surgical resection after control of the diabetes and parenteral nutrition, octreotide—for palliative suppression of glucagon.

SOMATOSTATINOMA

Most arise in the pancreaticoduodenal groove—in the ampulla and periampullary area (60%).

Clinical features include:
- Abdominal pain (25%)
- Jaundice (25%) due to bile stasis
- **Somatostatinoma triad** - viz., cholelithiasis (gallstone), steatorrhea and diabetes mellitus.

Elevated serum somatostatin levels, are seen (usually >10 ng/mL).

Treatment

Most present with metastatic disease for palliative approach.

But complete excision of the tumor and cholecystectomy is done wherever possible.

VIPoma (WDHA Syndrome—Werner-Morrison Syndrome)

- Watery diarrhea
- Hypokalemia
- Achlorhydria.

Commonly seen in body and tail, often with spread outside.

Diagnosis
- Serum VIP levels, measured on multiple occasions
- CT scan—to localize most VIPomas
- EUS is the most sensitive modality

Treatment

Most are advanced at diagnosis and hence palliative debulking operations help in controlling symptoms. Hepatic artery embolization is tried for metastases.

Gastrinoma—Refer Chapter on Stomach

Non-functioning pNETS
- 30% are malignant
- Others can turn malignant and metastasize.
- The management is same as for the functioning tumors.

- Immunohistochemical markers for diagnosis:
  - Synaptophysin, chromogranin A (CgA)
  - Neuron-specific enolase.

Clinical features include weight loss and vague pain and exocrine pancreatic insufficiency.

Prognosis
The 15-year survival rate for patients with tumors without liver metastases is about 80%, patients with liver metastases 20–50% survive 5 years.

Chapter 25

The Breast

SU25.1	Describe applied anatomy and appropriate investigations for breast disease.
SU25.2	Describe the etiopathogenesis, clinical features and principles of management of benign breast disease including infections of the breast.
SU25.3	Describe the etiopathogenesis, clinical features, investigations and principles of treatment of benign and malignant tumors of breast.
Skill Assessment	
DOAP sessions on radiodiagnosis, SU 25.4 and SU25.5 clinical training	
SU25.4	Counsel the patient and obtain informed consent for treatment of malignant conditions of the breast.
SU25.5	Demonstrate the correct technique to palpate the breast for breast swelling in a mannequin or equivalent.

SU25.1: Describe applied anatomy and appropriate investigations for breast disease.

DISEASES OF BREAST

Anatomy of Breast

Breast is a modified sweat gland.

Embryology of Breast (Refer Figure 25.1)

Ectoderm—ductal and acinar epithelium.
Mesoderm—supporting tissue—fibrous stroma.
- Breast develops along mammary ridge (the **milk line) running from**—axilla to groin.
- The ridge remains only in pectoral region in human (unlike animals).
- Ridge projects slightly on skin and deeper in gland—into ducts and acini.

Congenital Anomalies of Breast

- Amazia (amastia) absence of breast/s.
- Polymazia (polymastia)—multiple breast/s —accessory breast tissue along milk ridge

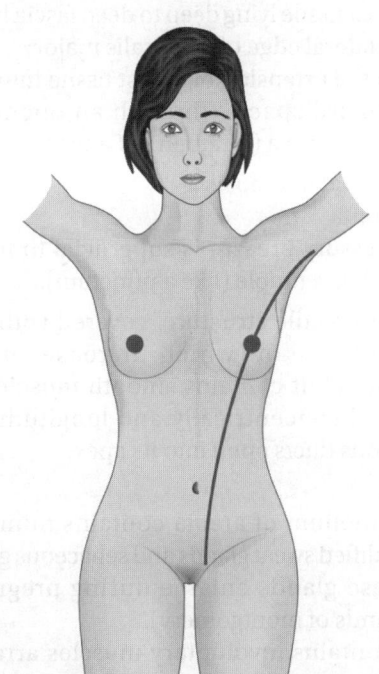

Fig. 25.1: Mammary ridge.

- Accessory nipple
- Polythelia—only rudimentary breasts with multiple nipples—over breast
- **Athelia:** Absence of nipple.

Anatomy

Breast is a subcutaneous gland between skin and pectoral fascia, extending from 2nd to 6th rib vertically and from side of sternum to mid axillary line. It lies over the pectoralis major medially and serratus anterior laterally. The nipple and areola are in the 4th intercostal space.

The breast is made of parenchyma containing 10 to 100 lobules, supported by fibrous stroma. Each lobule is cluster of alveoli, drained by a lactiferous duct.

Acini: An acinar lobule is drained by a terminal duct, making a terminal duct lobular unit (TDLU). These ducts join to form a lobar duct (small ducts). The lobar ducts join to form 15 to 20 major ducts, which come together and drain individually through the nipple.

Fibrous stroma and fat—fills gaps between parenchyma.

Axillary tail of spence

- Breast tissue lying deep to deep fascia behind the lateral edge of pectoralis major
- It is the extension of breast tissue into axilla upto 3rd space—through an opening in axillary fascia (foramen of Langer).

Differential diagnosis

- Lipoma
- Accessory breast—is superficial to muscle and has a nipple (like a punctum).

Nipple: Erectile structure, covered with thick pigmented skin (which increases during pregnancy). It contains smooth muscle fiber arranged concentrically and longitudinally, lactiferous ducts open into its apex.

Areola

- Epithelium of areola contains numerous modified sweat glands and sebaceous glands.
- These glands enlarge during pregnancy (glands of montgomery).
- It contains involuntary muscles arranged in concentric rings as well as radially in subcutaneous tissue.

Q. Retraction of breast surface in carcinoma.

- **Retraction of skin** (dimpling in cancer)—due to involvement of ligaments of cooper (skin to pectoral fascia)
- **Retraction of nipple**—infiltration along milk ducts
- **Retraction of pits of hair follicles**—due to blockage of lymphatics draining the dermis causing edema of the intervening skin—gives "orange peel" appearance **(peau d'orange).**

Q. Write a short note on retracted nipple.

- Congenital retraction of nipple—usually bilateral, may be unilateral too.
- Inflammatory retraction of nipple duct ectasia and chronic periductal mastitis
- Tuberculosis or post-treatment—TB, breast abscess.
- Carcinoma (see above)—infiltration along lactiferous duct
  A history of recent retraction and of circumferential retraction or with a lump.

Blood Supply of Breast

Arteries

- Lateral thoracic artery (from 2nd part axillary)
- Perforating cutaneous branches from internal mammary artery to spaces 2, 3, 4.
- Lateral branches of intercostal arteries 2, 3, 4.

Venous Drainage of Breast

Superficial veins radiate from breast accompany lymphatics to axillary, into mammary and intercostal vessels.

Q. Short note on Mondor's disease.

- Superficial thrombophlebitis of breast veins
- Superior epigastric vein, thoracoepigastric vein and lateral thoracic vein are affected
- It is a self limiting condition—with pain and tenderness over the discolored, thrombosed chord like veins seen as palpable over the breast
- Differential diagnosis: Carcinoma

Q. Short note on lymphatic drainage of breast.

- Lymphatics from the skin and the **subareolar plexus of Sappey drain**—radially to axillary

and supraclavicular nodes and to opposite side through 1st interspace.
- Parenchymal lymphatics drain directly outwards >75% to axillary nodes.
- Internal mammary lymphatics—deeper, medial and lateral parts of breast drain along perforating branches of internal mammary artery. The posterior intercostal lymphatics follow branches of intercostal arteries.
- **Deeper breast lymphatics:** Perforate the pectoral fascia—to interpectoral nodes.
- To opposite side.
- To rectus sheath and subdiaphragmatic lymphatic plexus.

Lymph Nodes

Axillary Nodes – 5 Sets (Mainly)
- Anterior—along lateral thoracic vein over the 3rd rib - (syn: Pectoral.nodes).
- Posterior—posterior fold along subscapular vessels
- Lateral—along axillary vein
- Central—in fat of upper axilla—intercostobrachial nerve may pass through it.
- Apical—"infraclavicular" in the clavipectoral groove along axillary vein.

Other Nodes
- Supra clavicular nodes
- Internal mammary nodes
- Interpectoral nodes (Rotter's)
- Posterior intercostal nodes (rarely).

The Axillary Fascial 'Tent'
- Axillary lymph nodes are enclosed by layers of fascia, resembling a tent
- **Anterior:** Pectoralis minor muscle and clavipectoral fascia fusing with axillary vessels.
- Posterior—subscapularis
- Medial—chest wall, ribs, intercostals and serratus anterior muscles
- Apex—upwards and medially—all layers of fascia fuse.

Surgical Importance
Entire tent along with should be removed in block dissection.

Surgical Classification of Axillary Nodes (Refer Figure 25.2)
Three levels in relation to pectoralis minor:
1. **Level I:** Below P. minor—lateral, central and subscapular nodes.
2. **Level II:** Behind P. minor—anterior and lower apical nodes.
3. **Level III:** Above border of muscle—apical nodes.

EVALUATION OF BREAST DISEASES
Refer **Table 25.1**.

> **Q. What is triple assessment for breast diseases.**

Triple Assessment
- Clinical examination
- **Imaging:** Mammography/USG/MRI/CT
- **Pathology:** FNAC/biopsy—needle/wedge/excision.

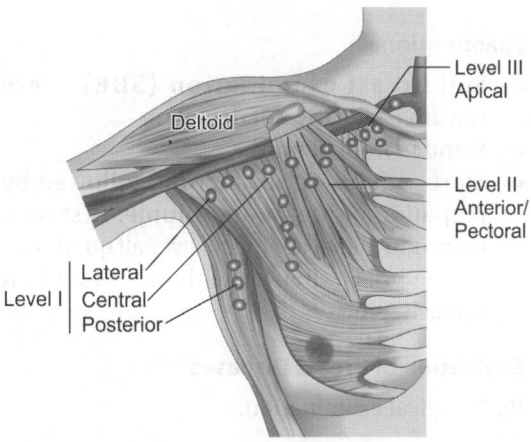

Fig. 25.2: Axillary lymph nodes.

Table 25.1: Ductal system related to breast disorders.

Larger duct Smaller ducts • During development • During involution	Duct papilloma, duct ectasia Fibroadenoma Cyst and sclerosis plus adenosis
From intralobular tissue Terminal duct lobular unit (TDLU)	Majority of carcinomas arise from these

Clinical Examination

Age

History (discussed under respective pathologies)
- Breast lump or mass
- Breast pain or discomfort
- Nipple discharge.

Q. Enlist breast cancer risk factors.

The risk factors for breast cancer are:
- Female 40 plus, h/o estrogen pills.
- Genes expressed: BRCA1 or BRCA2
- Two or more first degree relatives with breast cancer
- Personal history of breast cancer
- High breast tissue density
- Biopsy confirmed atypical hyperplasia
- High dose radiation to chest
- High levels of estrogens

Nipple Discharge

Serous, blood stained or serosanguineous.

Examination

- **Self breast examination (SBE)**—very sensitive for early self detection
- Stand in front of mirror
- Start with breast inspection, followed by palpation of breast and nipple, first with palm and then with fingers over all quadrants of one breast. Repeat with other hand on opposite side.

Evaluation of Breast Diseases

Radiological examination.

Q. Write a short note on mammography.

MAMMOGRAPHY

- Low dose X-ray of soft tissue
- Cranio caudal and mediolateral views
  Uses low dose of radiation (0.1 rad) and it is not proven to escalate breast cancer risk.
- A positive result is only suggestive of carcinoma.
  It is complimentary to other investigations like a biopsy and not confirmative of any disease.

Finding in cancers: (+) fine stippling of calcium –suggestive of carcinoma.

Indications

- Mammographic screening for individuals under category of "high-risk" carcinoma.
- Early detection of an occult carcinoma before reaching 5 mm.
- Indeterminate mass—a solitary lesion suspicious of a neoplasm.
- Large breast with impalpable nodules and for multifocal lesions in planning BCS and in Lobular carcinoma.
- Evaluation of contralateral breast (before and after ipsilateral treatment).
- Follow up—post mastectomy and irradiation.

Recommended Program of Using Mammography

- Daily self breast examination after 20 years.
- Baseline mammography 35–40 year on.
- Annual mammography > 40 years of age.

Q. What is BIRADS?

BIRADS is detailed in **Table 25.2**.

USG: Sonomammography

Useful in young women with dense breasts below 30–35 years of age (mammograms are difficult to interpret). Combined mammography and sonomammography complement each other in BIRADS.

Table 25.2: Breast imaging report and data system (BIRADS).

Assessment	Category	Recommendation
0	Needs additional imaging	Ultrasound or additional views
1	Negative mammography	Annual
2	Benign finding	- Do -
3	Probably benign	Follow up
4	Suspicious abnormality	Consider biopsy
5	Highly s/o malignancy	Biopsy
6	Known carcinoma	

- Differential diagnosis to evaluate a cystic v/s solid component of a lump
- Detects duct papillomas
- Diagnosis, treatment and follow up of abscess
- Guidance for FNAC and core biopsy.
- Localizes impalpable lumps.
- Ultrasound of the axilla—for guided biopsy of needle in diagnosed cases of carcinoma breast.

Limitation
- Not useful as a screening tool.
- It is operator dependent.

MRI Breast
- To detect a tumor and to assess the extent of disease.
- To detect multicentric disease.
- To assess the contralateral breast.
- When a mammogram, sonogram and clinical findings are inconclusive.
- To assess chest wall involvement.
- To differentiate scar from tumor recurrence.
- Evaluation of breast with implants.
- To evaluate axillary nodes—in patients with axillary metastases, occult primary or recurrent disease after treatment.

CT Scan
- To detect metastases—skeletal and visceral—chest and abdomen (liver, pelvis).
- Pathological fractures.

Ductography
- Inject radio-opaque contrast media into the mammary duct
- To evaluate discharge from nipple
- Detection of ductal tumors.

PET scan: FDG—labelled positron emission tomography—for detecting and localizing metastasis, monitoring the response to treatment and early detection of recurrrence/metastasis.

Limitation of PET/CT for breast imaging—poor detection rate for small breast carcinomas., False positives in healing wounds.

Biopsy: Positive Result is Diagnostic
- **Fine needle aspiration cytology:** High sensitivity to diagnose; but cannot differentiate invasion of vessels and lymphatics (needs histology)
- **True-cut or core biopsy:** Considered the standard of care—accurate diagnosis, histo types and grade, histochemistry for hormone and growth receptors.
- **Incision biopsy:** Only in ulcerated lesions or in paget's disease.
- **Punch biopsy:** Also taken from center.
- **Excision biopsy:** Simple excision biopsy usually done for benign lumps and avoided where malignancy is suspected.

Wide lump excision: For lumps suspicious of malignancy, with inconclusive report of biopsy. Incision should be placed over the lump in such way that, it can be included in an ellipse of skin over a subsequent mastectomy specimen (if the biopsy report shows malignancy).

The lump is resected with a margin of at least 2 mm of healthy breast tissue around the lump. This can be curative in a breast conservative surgery.

Sentinel lymph node biopsy (SLNB): Refer section under treatment of non invasive breast cancer.

> **SU25.2:** Describe the etiopathogenesis, clinical features and principles of management of benign breast disease including infections of the breast.
>
> **SU25.3:** Describe the etiopathogenesis, clinical features, investigations and principles of treatment of benign and malignant tumors of breast.

BENIGN BREAST DISEASES

> **Q. Short note on classification of benign breast disorders.**

Classification of Benign Breast Diseases

> **Non-breast disorders** (costochondritis—any cause e.g., Tietze's disease)
> - Injury
> - Inflammation/infection
> - Tumors and cysts of skin over breast

Congenital breast conditions:
- Inverted nipple
- Supernumerary breasts/nipples

ANDI (aberrations of normal development and involution): Currently this term is being given up
Lactation-associated: Galactocele lactational abscess

Q. Describe management of discharge from nipple.

Etiology of nipple discharge: Refer Table 25.3 given below.

Management of Nipple Discharge

Evaluation
- Triple assessment
    - History and physical examination
    - Sonomammogram (below 30 years of age).
    - Mammogram (above 30 years of age)
- MRI to evaluate duct dilation, duct papilloma or parenchymal lesions
- Ductography
- Cytology of discharge.

Treatment for Nipple Discharge
- Benign lesions of duct:
    - Microdochectomy excision of the unit of lactiferous duct and lobar unit
    - Cone excision of the major ducts Syn: Hadfield's operation, Subareolar resection
      Indication: Multiple ductal discharge or uncertainty or inability to localize the discharging duct.
    - Lumpectomy when a lump associate with discharge is identified.

- Carcinoma (ductal) with discharge—treated as per breast cancer protocol (discussed under breast carcinoma).

Galactorrhea
It is milky discharge not related to breastfeeding.
- **Physiologic galactorrhea**—milk produced by continued mechanical stimulation of nipples after cessation of lactation and resumption of menstruation.
- **Drug induced galactorrhea**—caused by depletion of dopamine by drugs:
    - Tricyclic antidepressants, diazepam, methyldopa, domperidone, levosulpiride, metoclopramide, pro-estrogenic drugs like—digitalis, frusemide.
    - Discharge is generally bilateral and not blood mixed or stained.
- **Spontaneous galactorrhea**
    - Due to pituitary prolactinoma—in a nonlactating patient
    - May be associated with amenorrhea
    - **Diagnosis:** High serum prolactin level, CT scan or MRI scan of the pituitary gland
    - **Treatment:** Tablet bromocriptine
      Surgery: To resect the prolactinoma or hypophysectomy.

Q. Describe the etiology, pathology, clinical diagnosis and management of acute mastitis and breast abscess.

ACUTE MASTITIS AND BREAST ABSCESS

Acute Diffuse Mastitis
Acute Breast Abscess
- Lactating
- Non-lactating.

Table 25.3: Causes of discharge from nipple.

Discharge from surface	Discharge from multiple ducts
• Paget's disease • Eczema	• **Blood:** Carcinoma, fibrocystic disease, duct ectasia • **Purulent:** Infection—acute, chronic • **Brownish/greenish**—duct ectasia
Discharge from single duct	• **Serous:** Fibrocystic disease; duct ectasia, carcinoma
• **Blood stained:** Duct carcinoma, duct papilloma, duct ectasia • **Serous- or greenish:** Fibrocystic disease; duct ectasia, carcinoma	• **Milk:** Lactation, pituitary tumor (prolactinoma) hypothyroidism

Chronic Abscess

- Antibioma
- Tuberculous, actinomycotic.

Acute Bacterial Mastitis

- Over 70% are associated with lactation
- Often associated with retraction of nipple and cracked nipple
- Others—with trauma—infected hematoma
- Spontaneous, periductal mastitis.

Acute Lactational Mastitis

- Commonly hospital acquired
- *Staphylococcus aureus* is the usual organism
- Milk plays a rich bacterial culture medium.

Pathogenesis

Source of infection: The infant's mouth colonized by bacteria. Frequently by hospital strains.
- During breastfeeding, the bacteria from the infant's mouth enter the lactiferous apparatus
- This leads to ascending infection and blocking of lactiferous duct, causing stasis and suppuration.
- Multiple micro abscesses form and coalesce to form a large abscess, often with multiple septae. or abscesses.

Pathology - Breast Abscess (Refer Fig. 25.3)

- Subareolar
- Intra mammary (parenchymal)
  - Acute suppurative
  - Chronic—tuberculosis (rare), actinomycosis
- Retromammary - pus in the space between breast and pectoralis major or deep to the muscle. It is mostly due to tuberculous pus from caseation in intercostal or internal mammary nodes, osteomyelitis of rib or a vertebra.

Clinical Features

- Stage of mastitis
- Stage of abscess formation.

Stage of Mastitis

- Acute fever and pain in breast, redness, mostly in a lactating women.
- The nipple may be cracked or retracted.
- Warmth, severe tenderness and induration over the involved part of breast.
- Nipple may be enlarged, red and edematous.

Differential Diagnosis: Inflammatory Carcinoma Breast

Stage of Abscess Formation

- Profound induration is the key sign, not fluctuation.
- All signs of mastitis, given above and profound induration indicate formation of an abscess.
- One should not wait for sign of fluctuation which is a sign of parenchymal destruction, entirely preventable. It is important to save and preserve breast tissue (ultrasound is useful).

Investigations

- **Blood test:** High leukocyte count and ESR, blood sugar to exclude diabetes.
- **Ultrasonography:** To evaluate for abscess.

Complications of Acute Breast Abscess

- Rupture leading to mammillary fistula
- Superficial skin necrosis—necrosis of nipple areolar complex
- Chronic abscess
- Antibioma.

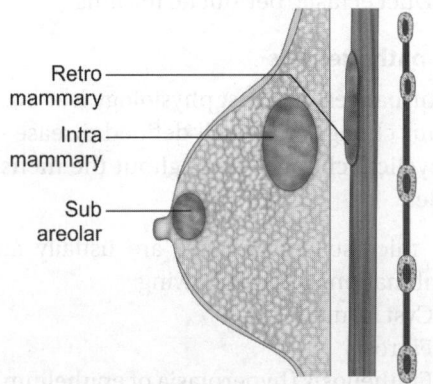

Fig. 25.3: Types breast abscesses.

Treatment

Stage of Mastitis

- Cloxacillin—oral or intravenous 500 mg every 6 hours.
- Symptomatic—paracetamol.
- Manual expression of milk on affected side.
- Follow up for progression to abscess—clinical and sonographic.

Treatment of Acute Abscess

- Ultrasound to detect and localize pus.
- Aspiration and early drainage under general anesthesia.
- Incision over point of maximal tenderness.
- Breaking of all septae to drain the loculi of pus, counter incision at dependent site and insertion of drain to facilitate free drainage.
- Suppression of lactation—with bromocriptine tablet.
  - *Pros and cons:* Helps early healing of abscess; but lactation rarely resumes following suppression and the infant needs milk supplements.

Treatment of Complications of Acute Breast Abscess

Chronic abscess—forms due to inadequate drainage and improper antibiotics.
Treated by drainage and curettage.

Antibioma

- Organisation of an abscess undrained and treated with antibiotics forms thickened walls—to form **a painless and hard lump**.

Differentiate from carcinoma—FNAC/MRI.

Treatment: Excision of lump.

Mammillary Fistula

- Usually follows rupture of a lactiferous duct in a subareolar abscess.
- MRI and ductogram helps delineation of the affected ductal unit.
- **Treatment:** Resection of the affected ductal unit.

Excision of lactiferous duct complex (Hadfield's operation): Excision of all the subareolar ductal complex when multiple ducts are affected or the diseased duct is not identified.

Granulomatous mastitis

- The cause may be immunological or tuberculosis and sarcoidosis.
- Sudden onset of a painful breast mass.
- May ulcerate through skin with redness.
- Partial resolution and recurrence with antibiotics.

Differential diagnosis

- Abscess
- Carcinoma

Diagnosis—core needle biopsy.

Management

- Antibiotics and drainage of abscess.
- Supportive; NSAID.
- Immunosuppression steroids or azathioprine are used. Methotrexate is also used.
- Surgery is only for residual lesions.
- Anti tuberculous treatment—when proved.

> **Q.** Write a short note on aberrations of normal development and involution (ANDI).

ABERRATIONS OF NORMAL DIFFERENTIATION AND INVOLUTION (ANDI)

The term ANDI is being given up currently. It includes the following:

- Cyclical nodularity and mastalgia
- Cysts
- Fibroadenoma
- Duct ectasia/periductal mastitis.

Etiopathogenesis

Disturbances in breast physiology leading from minor changes to a well defined disease—due to cyclical changes throughout the menstrual cycles.

The microscopic changes are usually any or combinations of the following:

- Cyst formation
- Fibrosis
- Epitheliosis (hyperplasia of epithelium)
- Papillomatosis.

Classification (Based on Pathology)

- Non-proliferative lesions—no high risk of carcinoma
  - Cysts/apocrine metaplasia—duct ectasia
  - Mild duct hyperplasia; calcifications; fibroadenoma
- Proliferative breast disease—mildly increased risk
  - Sclerosing adenoma
  - Radial and complex sclerosing lesions
  - Florid duct hyperplasia
  - Intraductal papilloma
- Proliferative disease with atypia—moderately increased risk
  - Atypical ductal hyperplasia
  - Atypical lobular hyperplasia

Non-proliferative Lesions

Q. Write a short note on fibroadenosis.

Syn: Chronic cystic mastitis

Fibrocystic disease, fibroadenosis, Schimmelbusch's disease.

Most common breast lesion in age group of 30-40 years.

Etiology (exact etiology unclear): Increased levels of estrogen and hyperresponse from some parts of the breast.

Histologically—epithelial and fibrous elements cyst formation, fibrosis, epitheliosis and papillomatosis.

Clinical Features

- **Complaints:** Lump, lumpiness, mastalgia and nipple discharge (each, alone or combined)
- **Pain**
- **Generally cyclical (non-cyclical in some).**
- **Lump** or lumpy feeling usually with bilateral pain in breasts.
- Unilateral or bilateral-rubbery in consistency, not encapsulated.
- **Nipple discharge**—greenish or serosanguinous seen in 15 percent of patients.
- **Examination** reveals bilateral tenderness on palpation and diffuse and ill defined lumps. Size changes may be observed; can be tender → related to menstrual cycle.

- **Note:** Schimmelbusch disease: classic diffuse cystic disease.

  Bloodgood cyst: (Short notes)—single, tense, large blue domed cyst.

MASTALGIA

- Cyclical—younger and premenopausal women—as in fibrocystic disease.
- Non-cyclical mastalgia—common in perimenopausal (occasionally in post menopausal women)
- Association is seen with ANDI and periductal mastitis.

Differential Diagnosis of Mastalgia

- Referred pain—from chest wall, back or neck—a musculoskeletal.
- Uncommonly in carcinoma.

Differential Diagnosis of Fibroadenosis

- Carcinoma
- Fibroadenoma—well localized and encapsulated
- Duct ectasia
- There is a risk of carcinoma or some coexist with carcinoma.

Investigation

- Sonomammography and mammography
- Image guided FNAC from areas with less stroma.

Treatment of Cystic Mastitis (Fibroadenosis) and Mastalgia

- Conservative for small and not very painful and tender lesions -
- Reassurance against fear of cancer
- Oral analgesics, oil of primrose, Vitamin E
- Danazol—alleviates moderate to severe painful and tender lesions.
- Synthetic FSH and LH analogue—suppresses FSH and LH
- Tamoxifen (less commonly used).

Mastalgia: Treatment Tips

- Reassurance against fear of cancer
- Advise supportive breast wear during daytime

Cyclical mastalgia is treated by adjustment and symptomatic treatment according to period of mastalgia.

Surgery
- Excision for bloodgood cyst.
- Excision of lumps and nodules with mammographic changes suspicious of malignancy.

BENIGN TUMORS OF THE BREAST

Q. Write a short note on fibroadenoma.

Well circumscribed lesion, movable, smooth, lobulated, encapsulated, painless, not associated with nipple discharge.

Etiology
Hormonal imbalance often blamed. Affects the female in the age group of 16 to 35.

Pathology
- Well circumscribed lump or multiple lumps frequently bilateral.
- Consists of an encapsulated tumor—microscopy shows epithelial and fibrotic elements of varying proportions.

Types of Fibroadenoma

Intracanalicular (Soft) Fibroadenoma
- Epithelial hyperplasia in the ductal lumen less fibrous elements
- Hence called soft fibroadenoma inswert seen in usually those above age of 30 to 35 year
- Risk of carcinoma—low but real.

Pericanalicular (Hard) Fibroadenoma
- Fibrosis around the ducts dominates the picture with less or little epitheliosis
- Seen in teen age and twenties
- More often bilateral and multiple
- Least risk of carcinoma.

Clinical Features
- Painless, lump or lumps in breasts, frequently bilateral.
- Hard or firm lumps, freely mobile within breast parenchyma (breast mouse).
- Size does not regress after menstruation.
- **Investigation:** Sonomammography, FNAC.
- Excision biopsy (rule out malignancy).

Diff. diagnosis: 1. Fibroadenosis, 2. Phyllodes tumor, which mimics a large soft fibroadenoma.

Treatment
Excision of lump or lumps (fibroadenomata)
- A circum areolar incision—for small and subareolar lumps.
- A submammary crease incision (Gaillard Thomas incision).

Q. Write a short note on intra-ductal papilloma of breast.

Proliferation of the ductal epithelium; 75% occurs beneath the epithelium.

Clinical Feature
Bloody nipple discharge—commonly bright red
- With palpable mass—indicates an intra-ductal papilloma (95% chances)
- Without a palpable mass—possibility of malignancy is increased.

Diff. Diagnosis
- Fibroadenosis
- Carcinoma.

Investigations
- Ductography
- MRI.

Treatment
- **Palpable mass:** Excision biopsy
- **Non-palpable mass:** Wedge resection of the nipple/areola based on ductographic result or positive bloody discharge
- Microdochectomy—resection of the unit of duct (containing the tumor) with the lobule.

Paget disease of the nipple: Refer carcinoma breast (next section).

TREATMENT ALGORITHM FOR BREAST LUMPS

After Triple Assessment
- **Triple assessment:** Clinical examination, imaging—sonomammography
- Needle or core biopsy.

Cystic Lump

Disappears after Aspiration

- Clear fluid aspirate—patient is sent away.
- fluid aspirate with multiple colors—the patient is advised review for reappearance of lump or nipple discharge.
- If bloodstained fluid is aspirated—a core biopsy is done
- There is a Residual after aspiration—a core biopsy is done.

Solid Lump

- Benign—excision.
- Atypical—core biopsy to exclude or classify the malignancy.
- Malignant—treat for cancer as per protocol.

Q. Write a short note on phyllodes tumor.

Syn: Serocystic disease of Brodie or cystosarcoma phyllodes.

These are locally invasive tumors. Age—mostly between 30 and 40 years of age.

Pathology

- Large knobby surfaced tumors with no true capsule.
- Mainly fibrous tissue.

Histology

- Fibrous tissue, pseudo gelatinous and edematous areas.
- Cystic areas are due to necrosis and infarct degenerations
- Greater mitotic activity than in fibroadenoma (more than 3 mitoses per HPF).

Grading: Based on mitotic figures (denotes faster growth).

Low grade (benign) - 80%—generally large bulky lesions **(tear drop appearance)**

High grade (make 20% have high potential for malignant sarcoma)—high mitotic figures.

Sarcoma criteria: Malignant component is dependent on:
- Number of mitotic figures/hpf
- Vascular invasion
- Lymphatic invasions
- Metastases (lung—hematogenous).

Differential diagnosis

Giant fibroadenoma—hard and smoother, encapsulation, low mitotic activity.

Clinical features

- They present as a rapidly growing large tumor with an uneven and bosselated surface.
- As the tumor grows, it casues pressure necrosis of overlying skin causing ulceration with the skin edges being free from tumor. The are mobile tumors.

Diff. diagnosis: Carcinoma—hard and fixed tumor, skin fixed to any ulcerated part.

Treatment: Surgery is the mainstay:

Benign phyllodes: Excision biopsy:
- Benign - no further treatment, observe
- **Wide local excision preferred** to excision, enucleation avoided.

Total Mastectomy or Modified Radical Mastectomy (MRM)
- For high grade (malignant type), massive tumors
- Recurrent tumors

Postoperative radiation is also carried out.

Q. Write a short note on mammary duct ectasia.

Syn: Plasma cell mastitis, comedo mastitis and chronic mastitis.

Sub-acute inflammation of the ductal system usually beginning in the subareolar area wth ductal obstruction.

Clinical Features

- Usually present as a hard mass beneath or near areola often with either nipple or skin retraction due to increase fibrosis
- Nipple discharge—may be present—serous or greenish or brownish
- Appears during or after menopausal period—history of difficulty of nursing
- **Histology:** The ducts are dilated and filled with debris and fatty material with atrophic epithelium. Sheets of plasma cells in the periductal area.

Differential Diagnosis
- Carcinoma breast
- ANDI—fibroadenosis/cystic mastitis.

Investigation
- Sonography
- FNAC.

Treatment
Excision biopsy of the lump.

GALACTOCELE
- Cystic or solid mass with or without tenderness
- Occurs during or after lactation
- Due to obstruction of a duct distended with milk.

Treatment
- With abscess → incision and drain
- Solid mass → excision biopsy.

Fat Necrosis
Traumatic Fat Necrosis
- With or without history of trauma
- Uncommonly—metastatic fat necrosis—in acute pancreatitis.

Clinical Presentation
- As a solid mass, hard and sometimes irregular (due to organized necrosis and hemoatoma) usually asymptomatic or with pain
- If may calcify later.

Differential Diagnosis
- Carcinoma breast
- Investigation: Sonography and FNAC.

Treatment
Excision biopsy.

Q. Write a short note on gynecomastia.

Unilateral or bilateral hypertrophy of the **male breast**, with characteristics of female breasts.

Etiology
- Idiopathic—most common
- Age—usually the breasts enlarge at puberty.

Deficiency of testosterone: Causing estrogen dominance.
- Anorchism
- Leprosy; bilateral testicular atrophy.
- Bilateral orchiectomy
- Treatment of carcinoma of prostate with hormone ablation (stilbestrol therapy)
- Feminising tumors (teratoma) of testis, Ectopic hormone producing bronchial tumors, adrenal estrogenic tumors and gonadotrophic tumors of pituitary.

Associated with chronic liver disease
- Cirrhosis—failure of the liver to metabolise estrogens.
- **Drug induced:** Spironolactone, digitalis and cimetidine.

Chromosomal syndromes
- Klinefelter syndrome—47XXY trisomy
- Gynaecomastia may occur in patients with Klinefelter's syndrome.

Symptoms
- Mainly low esteem and shy boys.
- Bilateral breast enlargement with lumps.
- Pain—is a common symptom.

Evaluation
- Serum levels of testosterone, FSH, LH, estradiol.
- Liver function
- Evaluation with sonography of liver, adrenals and testicles.
- Rare cases of Klinefelter syndrome may require chromosomal study.

Treatment
Idiopathic Cases in Adolescence
- In the absence of any abnormality, patients are best reassured and advised proper clothing.
- Pain may be treated by simple paracetamol or a NSAID.

Surgery: Indications
- Unbearable pain
- Psychological impact
- Cosmetic consideration.

Procedures
- Bilateral excision of the breast tissue.
- Subcutaneous mastectomy with preservation of nipple and areola.
Incision: Bilateral submammary incisions.

For Secondary Gynecomastia
Treatment of any tumors or known treatable causes, e.g., testicular tumors or adrenal tumors. Change of therapy for drug induced gynecomastia.

CARCINOMA BREAST

> Q. Write a short note on etiological factors in breast carcinoma.

Etiological Factors
- **Geographical:** Breast cancer affects all populations accounting for 2-5% of all deaths in women (higher incidence in affluent countries).
- **Age:** Most cases present at 45 to 50 years
  - Any age above 20 years can be affected and the incidence increases with age—as high as about 1 in 5 at the age of 90.
- **Gender:** 99% occur in females.
- **Genetic:** Specific genetic-mutations—account for 5% of all cancers. Family history breast cancer increases the risk of cancer by 3 to 5 times.
  - BRCA1 (very high incidence)—chromosome 17q (30% of all breast carcinoma) and about 40-50% life time risk of ovarian cancer.
  - BRCA 2—chromosome 13 q (about 3-5% of cancers) more among male.
  - Abnormal PALP-2 (partner and localizer of BRCA-2) gene—increases breast cancer risk by 5-10 times the average.
  - PALP-2 is a gene that helps producing a protein that works with BRCA-2 protein to repair the damaged DNA and stop tumor growth. Also, TP53 gene mutation and loss of protein pRb1 are seen in aggressive tumors.

Association with other cancer syndromes
- *For example:* Cowden's syndrome - an autosomal dominant syndrome (bilateral breast lesion, cutaneous facial lesion, GI polyps, brain, thyroid tumors.
  - Hereditary nonpolyposis colorectal cancer (HNPCC)—lynch syndrome (cancers in colon, pancreas, uterus, ovary, kidney or breast in families.
- **Endocrine:** Higher incidence of breast cancer in the following situations:
  - *Estrogens:* Estrogen pills or endogenous
  - *Nulliparous women:* More common and late pregnancy after 35 yeas.
  - Early menarche and late menopause
  - HRT (hormone replacement therapy)—given in the post menopausal on a long-term—is associated with a higher incidence of breast cancer.
- **Protective effect** breast feeding.
  - Early pregnancy and child birth.
- **Diet and life style**
  - Obesity is considered a risk factor.
  - Smoking is a risk factor.
- **Ionizing radiation:** Exposure to ionizing radiation—increases the risk of breast cancer.

> Q. Write a short note on pathology of carcinoma breast.

Cell of Origin
Duct carcinoma (DC) and lobular carcinoma. Combined ductal and lobular carcinoma (e-cadherin antibody positive).
- **Ductal carcinoma—85%** DC—arises from duct epithelium—from major lactiferous ducts to terminal duct lobule unit (TDLU)
- **Lobular carcinoma—15%** LC—lobular acinar epithelium—often multifocal (multiple in same quadrant) or multicentric (different quadrants) and bilateral.

Sub-types
Classical—better prognosis.
Pleomorphic type—worse prognosis.

Noninvasive (in situ): Basement membrane intact. They make about 15-20% of all cancers.

Invasive cancer: Basement membrane is breached by tumor cells.

The Spread of Breast Cancer

Local Spread
Invasion of other portions of the parenchyma, skin, pectoral muscle and chest wall.

Lymphatic Metastasis
Lymphatic spread: Through subareolar plexus and intra mammary lymphatic network.
- Primarily to the axillary nodes (75 to 80%) and the internal mammary lymph nodes—especially tumors in the posterior one-third.
- Lymph node metastases represent both the chronological and the biological behavior of the tumor and a predictor of metastatic potential of tumor.
Hence their prognostic significance.

Pleural Effusion
- Through internal mammary lymphatics
- Most common metastatic presentation in chest.

Hematogenous metastasis
Sites:
- Bone—lumbar vertebrae, femur, thoracic vertebrae, rib and skull.
- Skeletal metastases are osteolytic.
- Liver, lungs and brain
- And less commonly the ovaries and the adrenal glands.

Histological grading: Also predicts approximate clinical behavior.

Well differentiated, intermediate and poorly differentiated.

Numerical grading system: Grade I, II, III based on the scoring of three individual factors—Nuclear pleomorphism, tubule formation and mitotic rate.

Grades
I—Well differentiated group
II—Intermediate differentiation
III—Poorly differentiated group.

Histological Classification
General adenocarcinoma (non-special type)—(80%) poor prognosis.

Special types: Better prognosis (20%)
- Mucinous (colloid)
- Medullary
- Tubular
- Cribriform
- Papillary.

Molecular and Hormone Receptors
Estrogen receptors and progesterone receptors (ER and PR): These are hormone responsive tumors and this factor is made use of to plan treatment. Generally better prognosis with hormone responsive tumors.

> Q. Write a short note on Her-2/Neu receptor.

Human epidermal growth factor receptor-2 Neu oncogene (Neuropilin 21)

Syn: c-ErbB-2 (cell surface **erythroblastic** oncogene B2).
- A member of the epidermal growth factor receptor (EGFR) family—a tyrosine kinase receptor—involved in cell growth regulation.
- Associated with ER negative, high grade tumors.
- It is measured by immunohistochemistry.
- Overexpression of HER2/neu is seen in about approximately 30% of patients with breast cancer.
- The same is a poor prognostic factor, indicates high risk of metastasis, early recurrence and decreased overall survival.
- Patients with HER2/neu-amplified (HER2+) tumors are treated with targeted monoclonal antibody therapies, such as **trastuzumab** (**herceptin**) or **pertuzumab**. Pertuzumab, in combination with trastuzumab and docetaxel is effective in prolonging progression-free survival in metastatic HER2+ breast cancer.

Ki-67—indicates the pace of tumor growth, representing the **fraction of actively dividing cells in the growth phase.** When it exceeds 20% it indicates an aggressive tumor calling for an aggressive chemotherapy, particularly the HER2 negative cases.

High proliferation index >5% cell in S-phase of growth cycle.

Classification/stratification based on molecular markers: Prognostication and planning the treatment are done by Immunohistochemistry to check hormonal receptor status, HER2-Neu and Ki 67 index.

Gene array based classification of breast cancer—five major subtypes (Refer **Table 25.4**)
- Involves analysis of 21 genes
- Helps in predicting recurrence, metastatic potential
- Planning and choosing the therapeutic regime.

> **Q. Non invasive breast cancer (in situ carcinoma).**

In situ carcinoma is pre invasive cancer (the epithelial basement membrane not breached).
- Ductal carcinoma in situ (DCIS) or lobular carcinoma in situ (LCIS)—high chance of multifocal and bilateral.
  Predictors for an invasive carcinoma (about a fourth of them turn malignant).

Lobular Carcinoma: LCIS
- Noninvasive (in situ): Considered more as a premalignant than a true carcinoma
- But pleomorphic type is aggressive and classical type is less aggressive.
- Multifocal and bilateral tumors are common.
- Invasive type is more aggressive, more often bilateral or multi focal.
  MRI breast helps in evaluation for multiple tumors.

Duct Carcinoma in Situ (DCIS)

DCIS is treated as a malignancy because it has the potential to develop into an invasive breast cancer.

Physical examination is usually unrewarding, it is mostly detected at mammography as clusters of micro calcifications.

Pathology
- **Multifocal** two or more lesions > 5 mm apart within the same quadrant
- **Multicentric**—in different quadrants.

Histology
- **Five subtypes:** 1-4: Non-comedo types: Papillary, micropapillary, solid, cribriform, and 5: comedo (necrosis).
- The high-grade subtype is often associated with microinvasion, a higher proliferation rate, aneuploidy, gene amplification, and a higher local recurrence rate.

Classification of DCIS—Van Nuys system.

Treatment of Noninvasive Carcinoma
- Complete excision of tumor and observation.
- Tamoxifen or aromatase inhibitors for ER and PR positive tumors.
- Trastuzumab as adjuvant or for recurrence in HER -2 Neu or c-erbB-2 positive tumors.

Table 25.4: Gene array based classification of carcinoma breast.

Gene array based types	ER	PR	HER2 Neu	Prognosis	Response to treatment
Luminal A approximately 50%	Positive	Positive	Negative	Better	Hormone
Luminal B approximately 15% and luminal B-like (more aggressive)	Positive	Positive	Negative "B" Positive "B-like"	High grade	Chemo
Triple negative breast cancer (TNBC) basal like—15–20% BRCA 1	Negative	Negative	Negative	Poor	Chemo plus PARP inhibitors
HER-2 receptor positive (HER2 rich)— brain metastases risk—10%	Negative	Negative	Positive	Poor	Chemo + M Ab
Miscellaneous (many subtypes)	Positive		Negative or positive		

TNM Classification of Breast Carcinoma

Refer **Table 25.5**.

T– Primary tumor
- **Tx**: Primary tumor cannot be assessed
- **T0**: No evidence of primary tumor
- **Tis**: Carcinoma in situ—intraductal carcinoma (DCIS), lobular carcinoma in situ (LCIS)
- **Tis Paget**—Paget's disease of the nipple with no tumor.

T1 Tumor of **2 cm or less**; skin not involved:
T1 mi - <0.1 mm, T1a <0.5 cm, T1b 0.5–1, T1c 1–2 cm

T2 Tumor **2 to 5 cm** in size

T3 Tumor greater than **5 cm** in size.

T4 Tumor of any size with any of the following—skin infiltration dermis, nodules, ulceration, Peau d'orange, skin edema, invasion of pectoral muscle or chest wall.
- **T4a**: Chest wall—beyond muscle invasion
- **T4b**: Skin - fixity, nodules, peau d' orange
- **T4c**: T4a + b
- **T4d**: Inflammatory carcinoma

N: Lymph node metastases
Nx: Regional lymph node cannot be assessed
N0: No regional lymph node metastasis
N_1 Clinically palpable: Mobile axillary node(s) level I, II.
- N1 mi: micro mets in nodes; size 2 mm or less.

N_2: Clinically palpable Fixed axillary nodes level I, II
- **N_2a**: Palpably, fixed, axillary nodes level I, II
- Or internal mammary nodes but not both
- **N_2b**: internal mammary nodes without clinical axillary node involvement.

N_3 Nodal metastases—advanced state. Or with arm edema.
- **N3a**: Metastasis in ipsilateral infraclavicular lymph node(s)—level III.
- **N3b**: Ipsilateral internal mammary lymph node(s) and axillary lymph node(s)—level I and II
- **N3c**: Spread to in ipsilateral Supraclavicular nodes.

M: Metastases
Mx: Presence of distant metastasis not known
M_0: No distant metastasis
M_1: Metastases—distant and in contralateral breast/axillary nodes.

Prefix "c": Clinical staging; "p" for pathologist's staging and "y" for staging after neo adjuvant therapy and " r" for recurrent tumor.

Table 25.5: AJCC staging of breast carcinoma (abridged).

Stage		T	N	M
0		Tis	N0	M0
I	IA	T1	N0	M0
	IB	T0-T1	N1mi	
II	IIA	T0-T1	N1	M0
		T2	N0	
	IIB	T2	N1	
		T3	N0	
III		T0-T3	N2	M0
	IIIA	T3	N1	
	IIIB	T4	N0	
		T4	N1-N2	
	IIIC	Any T	N3	M0
IV		Any T	Any N	M1

AJCC/UICC Stage Group (Refer **Table 25.5**) (American Joint Committee on Cancer/Union Internationale Contre le Cancer)

Clinicopathological Types
- Atrophic scirrhous type—elderly ladies, slow growing hard lumps and with slow spread and late metastatic potential.
- Scirrhous type (60–65%)—most common type, age 40–60, hard tumors, cut surface cutting like an unripe pear, more aggressive and tendency for early invasion and metastasis.
- Medullary (about 10%)—rapidly growing soft tumors (encephaloid), propensity for early metastasis; has a poorer prognosis.
- Colloid—soft tumors with rapid spread.
- Inflammatory carcinoma—presents like acute mastitis and has the worst prognosis.

Clinical Features
Lump—painless to start with in over 90%, growing progressively—in accordance with the tumor biology. The incidence of the tumor in relation to the quadrants of the breast is given in **Figure 25.4**.
- **Upper outer:** 60%, upper inner 12%
- **Central:** 12–15%

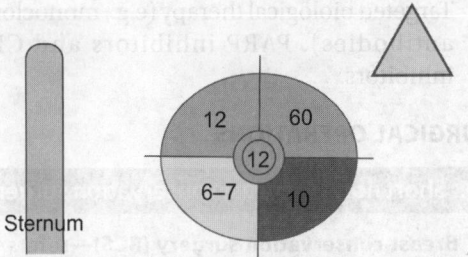

Fig. 25.4: Incidence of carcinoma breast.

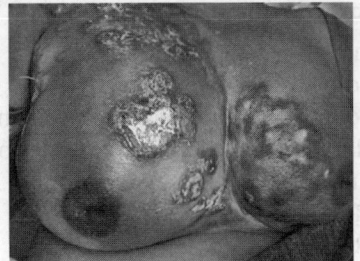

Fig. 25.5: Cancer en cuirasse.
(For color version see Plate 1)

- Inner upper 12%, inner lower—about 5–7%
- Fixity to skin, muscle and chest wall in late stages.
- Nipple discharge—seen in 10–15%, (generally in a duct carcinoma).

Skin Signs

- Tethering (early infiltration)
- Puckered (tumor invasion of Cooper's ligaments)
- Nipple may be retracted (lactiferous duct infiltration)
- Peau d'orange—a sign of dermal lymphatic obstruction previous section
- Ulceration
- **Cancer en cuirasse (Refer Figure 25.5):** Woody hard induration with nodules and ulceration
- Fixity to pectoral muscle and axilla are seen in advanced growths.

Axilla: Nodes enlarge as tumor spreads.

Systemic spread to:
- Pleural cavity and lungs, chest wall, spine and long bones.
- Abdomen (ascites), hepatomegaly and ovarian masses.
- Features of associated cancers.

Q. Paget's disease of the nipple.

- Paget's disease of the nipple—starts from an underlying breast carcinoma and presents as an eczema—like condition of the nipple and areola, not responding to local remedies.
- The nipple gets eroded and destroyed by the progression of the lesion.
- Subsequently, the underlying carcinoma shows itself clinically.

Differential diagnosis: Nipple eczema.

Diagnosis: Biopsies taken front the nipple.

Microscopy: Large, ovoid cells with abundant, clear, pale-staining cytoplasm in the Malpighian layer of the epidermis.

Differential Diagnosis

Lump in the Breast

- Fibrocystic disease
- Periductal mastitis
- Fat necrosis
- Organized hematoma
- Antibioma
- Tuberculosis and granulomatous mastitis.

Nipple Discharge

- Duct papilloma
- Duct ectasia
- Fibroadenosis.

MANAGEMENT OF CARCINOMA BREAST

- **Management includes:** Diagnosis, treatment, follow up, rehabilitation and genetic counseling.
- Diagnosis (refer previous section).
- Triple assessment (refer previous section).
- Clinical examination.
- **Imaging:** Mammography, sonography, CT MRI/PET CT).

Pathology

FNAC/biopsy—needle/wedge/excision.

Markers: ER, PR, HER2/neu, Ki -67, S-phase cell (proliferation index).

Genetic mutation studies—BRCA I and II mutations, PALP-2 abnormalities.

Indicators of Poor Prognosis

- Tumor size 4 cm and more
- Histological—grade III (high)
- Histology—lymphovascular invasion (LVI)
- Axillary nodes—more than 4 nodes positive, (> 8 node positive is still worse)
- ER, PR negative
- HER 2 positive
- Triple negative (ER/PR/HER2-neu—all negative)
- High proliferation ratio (> 5% cells in S-phase, Ki 67 >20%).

TREATMENT OF CARCINOMA BREAST (REFER TABLE 25.6)

Multidisciplinary after diagnosis and staging. Treatment planning involves surgeon, radiologist, pathologist, medical and radiation oncologist.

Carcinoma Breast
See **Table 25.6**.

TREATMENT MODALITIES AND THEIR ROLE

Locoregional Therapy
- Surgery
- Radiotherapy.

Systemic Therapy
- Chemotherapy
- Hormone therapy
- Targeted biological therapy (e.g., monoclonal antibodies). PARP inhibitors and CDK inhibitors.

SURGICAL OPERATIONS

> **Q. Short note on breast conservation surgery.**
>
> **I. Breast conservation surgery (BCS)—refers to conservation of nipple and areola.**
> - Always followed by post operative radiotherapy to the residual breast and chest wall.
>
> **Types**
> - **Wide lump excision (WLE):** Resection of tumor with a margin of at least 2 mm (5 mm generally) of healthy breast tissue—indicated for—noninvasive carcinoma, Tis, T1,T2.
> - **Partial mastectomy or quadrantectomy**—for lumps confined to a quadrant.
> - **Nipple sparing (subcutaneous) mastectomy** (entire breast parenchyma and lactiferous duct system upto the nipple removed preserving the nipple and areolar complex).
>
> **Indications:** LCIS, multifocal, pleomorphic, high grade DCIS, tumor larger than 4 cm.
>
> **Contraindications for BCS**
> - All tumors with poor prognostic indices (see previous page)
> - High tumor to breast ratio
> - Patients who can't receive or those don't agree for, postoperative radiotherapy.

Table 25.6: Broad classification and principles of management.

1. Noninvasive carcinoma	DCIS, LCIS	Local treatment + HT if ER positive
2. Invasive breast carcinoma		
Early breast carcinoma: EBC (confined to origin and can be cured)	T1–2, N0–1,M0; T3, N0, M0	Aggressive locoregional treatment adjuvant systemic therapy
Locally advanced breast carcinoma LABC (has spread beyond origin, risk of systemic spread)	Any T,N2/3 N0, T3 N1 M0, T4 any N M0	Neoadjuvant therapy and local surgical control.
Metastatic breast cancer (gross systemic spread)	Any T, Any N, M-1	Systemic therapy, local salvage
Recurrent breast cancer (systemic cancer recurs locally)		Treatment at par with metastatic ca

II. Total Mastectomy

Resection of entire breast tissue including parenchyma, lactiferous ducts and nipple areolar complex along with skin over and surrounding the area of tumor.

Indication
- Noninvasive carcinoma which is considered unsuitable for BCS (see above).
- Early breast cancer T1 T2 N0 SLNB negative with favorable prognostic indicators.

III. Modified Radical Mastectomy

> Q. Modified radical mastectomy.

Resection of: Entire breast with tumor including nipple and areola along with skin overlying and surrounding area of tumor and pectoral fascia—along with axillary lymphatics—all lymph nodes level I, II (level III when triple assessment shows N2) and fibro-fatty tissue and vessels. Structures preserved: Axillary neuro vascular bundle, nerve to serratus anterior and nerve to latissimus dorsi. (Halsted's classical Radical mastectomy included resection of both pectoral muscles—major and minor and upper digitations of serratus anterior).

Indications
- Early breast cancer EBC - N-1 tumor.
- High grade tumors with LVI or other indicators of poor prognosis.
- Locally advanced breast carcinoma (LABC)—stage II B, III A.
- Post-neoadjuvant therapy—for IIIB, IIIC and for T4 disease for loco regional control.

Complications of a Radical or Modified Radical Mastectomy
- Seroma 50–70%
- Bleeding and hematoma.
- Flap necrosis and wound/infection
- Injury to axillary vein
- Thrombosis of axillary vein
- **Lymphoedema** (common)—upper limb edema, pain, nodules, ulceration and rarely lymphangiosarcoma.
- Neurological:
  - Numbness—medial upper side of arm—to intercostobrachial nerve division.
  - Winged scapula—injury to long thoracic nerve
  - Injury to thoraco dorsal nerve—weakening of latissimus dorsi.
- Stiffness and dysfunction of shoulder.

IV. Skin Sparing Mastectomy

Here all the breast tissue is resected along with nipple and areola, preserving the skin of the breast to the maximum extent.

- Useful for breast reconstruction or implants and also for early post operative radiotherapy.

Indications for Skin Sparing Mastectomy
- T3 tumors
- Centrally situated tumor
- Paget's disease.

Note: Skin sparing mastectomy is not a breast conservative surgery (nipple areola not conserved).

V. Toilet Mastectomy (Salvage Resection)

For palliation—post-neoadjuvant therapy

Here a resection is done after neo adjuvant therapy without clearing the tumor bed—leaving behind residual tumor (micro or macroscopic).

Indication
- For local control of residual tumors T4 stage along with RT and systemic therapy.
- As a palliation against pain, discharge, bleeding, smell of ulceration large T4 tumors after neoadjuvant RT/CT.

SURGERY FOR AXILLARY NODE METASTASES

> Q. Short note on sentinel lymph node biopsy (SLNB).

> Q. What is a sentinel lymph node.

Breast cancers spread by along anatomically specific lymphatic drainage. Most of the lymph (about 80%) drains sequentially into the axillary nodes, and about 20% to internal mammary nodes, irrespective of the site of tumor.

Hence the micrometastases to the axillary node can be predictably traced to the primary draining lymph node among the axillary nodes, draining the breast, which receives metastatic cells from the primary tumor. The same is called the **sentinel node**.

Application of sentinel lymph node biopsy

- In a clinically non invasive tumor, a positive SLNB makes upstages a noninvasive (NO) to invasive carcinoma (N1 mi) and treatment plan changes.
- A negative SLNB helps avoid full axillary dissection for unproven metastases, thereby avoiding the postoperative morbidities including arm edema.
- If it is negative prognosis is better and treatment is as for noninvasive carcinoma.

Indications

DCIS
Invasive carcinoma—N0 node status—in early breast cancer (T1, T2, T3 with clinical N0 stage).

Procedure

- By injecting isosulfan vital blue dye (2.5-7.5 mL) into or near the tumor (peri-tumor area) or into subareolar plane (subdermal plexus).
- The node is mapped and localized by tracing the dye into the axillary fat after 10 to 12 hours at surgery (axillary exploration). The blue discoloration of the lymph node by the dye denotes the sentinel (guard) node and the same.
- **Radioactive tracers:** Alternatively 99m Technitium sulphur colloid dye (6 hours before surgery) or radioisotope labelled albumin (one mCi on previous day)—visualization of sentinel node with a hand held gamma camera.
- The same axillary node, along with the surrounding nodes (3-4) is resected at surgery and subjected to histopathology.

Q. Short answer on axillary lymph node dissection.

Axillary lymph node dissection (ALND)

ALND is an adjunct to a mastectomy or BCS. Lymph node status is the single most important marker for metastatic potential and prognosis.

Aim of axillary surgery: To stage the disease or/and to treat the axillary disease.

Treatment of the axilla—helps control local recurrence but does not affect long-term survival,
- Presence of axillary metastases make an indication for chemotherapy or tamoxifen/aromatase inhibitors in hormone receptor-positive patients.
- Combination of ALND and radiotherapy increases the risk of edema of arm and chest wall and is used only in cases with high-risk of locoregional recurrences.

Procedures for axillary nodes:

- Sentinel node biopsy (see above)
- Axillary node sampling: For impalpable nodes detected by ultrasound or PET.
  - A group of at least 8 nodes are removed at surgery.
- Axillary lymph node dissection (ALND): Node level I and II:
  - Ddone for N 1 disease and in SLNB positive cases as completion ALND
  - A minimum of 14 nodes are removed to help staging —more than 4 nodes positive call for a more aggressive therapeutic approach.
- **Complete axillary clearance ALND—level I, II and III:** Done for N2 disease—local control of disease along with neoadjuvant or adjuvant chemotherapy or targeted therapy as needed.

Q. Radiotherapy in breast carcinoma.

Radiotherapy

Aim: Locoregional control of disease or prevent recurrences.

Indications: (1) to breast, (2) to axilla, (3) to chest wall, (4) to metastases.
- **Irradiation to the breast:** After breast conservation surgery (BCS) to the residual breast.
- **Irradiation to the chest wall:**
  Post-mastectomy RT:
  – For tumors with stage T3 and T4
  – Tumor positive margins after mastectomy at histopathology
  – Large numbers of positive nodes
  – Extensive lympho vascular invasion (LVI)
  – **Tumor stage—T4A, 4C and 4D (inflammatory carcinoma):** Neoadjuvant—RT before salvage surgery. or Palliative RT
  – Local recurrence: To chest wall as a part of multimodal therapy
  Accelerated partial breast irradiation (APBI)
  – In tumors—stage T1 N0 invasive ductal carcinoma in patients aged above 60 years.
  – External beam RT, intracavitary RT or interstitial RT (brachytherapy).
- **Irradiation to the axilla:**
  – RT is given as alternative to axillary node dissection (ALND) if SLNB is positive after a BCS is done for T1, T2.
  – Invasive cancer: After ALND (level I, II)
    • If more than 4 nodes are positive for metastases
    • Primary tumor is report as high grade with LVI
  – Recurrent axillary disease—as a part of multimodality treatment.
- **Irradiation to metastases:** Skeletal metastases, for pathological fractures of long bones and spinal metastases.

HORMONE THERAPY

For hormone responsive tumors testing positive for ER and PR.

Indications

DCIS or LCIS with hormone receptor (ER PR) positive cases—adjuvant to surgery.

Early Breast Cancer
- **Pre menopausal:** Tamoxifen 20 mg daily for 5 years.
- **Postmenopausal women:** Aromatase inhibitors:
  – Letrozole 2.5 mg/day or Anastrozole 1 mg/day for 5 years.

LABC (HR positive): Hormonal therapy given after Neo adjuvant therapy and surgery.

Drugs used are:
Tamoxifen 20 mg/day for 5 years—in pre menopausal women.
Follow up to identify any endometrial cancers in these groups.

Aromatase inhibitors (AI) with Bisphosphonates: In post menaopausal women for 5 years.
- Anastrozole 1 mg/day and
- Letrozole 2.5 mg per day or exemestane 25 mg/day.

Bisphosphonates (e.g., etidronate and nalondronate) are given with an AI to reduce the severity of osteoporosis caused by aromatase inhibitors.

Medical oophorectomy: LHRH analogues.

CHEMOTHERAPY

> **Q. Role of chemotherapy in treatment of breast cancer.**

Role—only in invasive breast carcinoma.

Adjuvant Chemotherapy

Postoperative systemic therapy: To control or prevent systemic disease and prevent loco regional recurrence.
- All high grade tumors and those with LVI
- Tumors with node positivity
- All tumors with indicators of poor prognosis
- Hormone nonresponsive and HER 2 negative tumors.

Neo-adjuvant Chemotherapy (Administered Prior to Surgery)
- To downstage an advanced tumor and make it amenable for a tumor clearance

- For preoperative systemic control of disease
- Downstage selected tumors to get them to qualify for BCS.

Palliative Chemotherapy
- Advanced tumors
- Metastatic tumors
- Recurrent disease.

Combination chemotherapy:
Refer Table 25.7

Rationale: Cells division is subject to phases of cell cycle—S phase, G1, G2 and M phase.
- Combination of cell cycle specific and nonspecific agents act at different phases of cell cycle and a better tumor control than with a single agent.
- The toxicity of a single drug is minimized by optimal smaller doses of multiple drugs.

Current Regimens (Refer Table 25.8)

Anthracycline regimens, non-anthracycline regimes and taxane based.

BIOLOGICAL THERAPY (BT)

Syn: Targeted therapy with antitumor receptor antibodies.

Q. Trastuzumab (Herceptin).
- It is a monoclonal antibody that blocks HER-2/Neu receptors to block growth of cancer cells. Her-2/Neu receptor is tyrosine kinase receptor and Trastuzumab inhibits the c-ErbB2 (growth factor)receptor.

Pertuzumab—similar to trastuzumab.

Margetuximab is the newer lgG monoclonal antibody against HER-2/Neu receptors.
- Dose is 4 mg/kg as loading; 2 mg/kg as maintenance for 1 year. It is cardiotoxic.

Lapatinib ditosylate is a dual tyrosine kinase inhibitor which inhibits HER-2/Neu and EGFR by inhibiting autophosphorylation, it also crosses blood brain barrier.

Oral drug—used in combination with oral capecitabine to treat metastatic breast carcinoma.

Molecular therapy: PARP Inhibitors - to block DNA repair genes and allow cancer cell apoptosis among BRCA mutant cancers.

CDK inhibitors - Palbociclib - in HER 2 negative HR positive tumors.

Table 25.7: Chemotherapeutic agents in treatment of carcinoma of breast.

Nonanthracyclines:	Taxanes:
Cyclophosphamide, methotrexate, 5-Fluorouracil. Gemcitabine, (3rd level), Capecitabine (oral equivalent of 5-FU)	Docetaxel, Paclitaxel Nanoparticle albumin-bound paclitaxel (nab-paclitaxel)
Anthracyclines: Adriamycin (doxorubicin), epirubicin	

Table 25.8: Chemotherapy regimens.

Regimen			
CAF	Cyclophosphamide	Adriamycin (Doxorubicin)	5-Fluorouracil
CEF	Cyclophosphamide	Epirubicin	5-Fluorouracil
TAC/AC	Taxane (Docetaxel/Paclitaxel)	Adriamycin	Cyclophosphamide
CMF	Cyclophosphamide	Methotrexate	5-Fluorouracil
For HER2 +ve tumors	AC followed by paclitaxel + trastuzumab		
	Docetaxel + trastuzumab with CEF		

TREATMENT OF NON INVASIVE BREAST CANCER

Confirmation of diagnosis:
- **Palpable lump**—core biopsy—histology, hormone and molecular markers.
- **Non-palpable lesions**—stereotactic needle biopsy and marking under image guidance.
- **Blood:** Liver function test, Chest X ray.
- Mammography to study remaining part of breast and contralateral breast.
- **MRI breasts in of LCIS:** To look for multiple foci or bilaterality.

Treatment of Noninvasive Carcinoma is Surgical

Plan 1: Breast Conservative Surgery (BCS) followed by Radiotherapy to chest wall.
- **Single lesion:** Wide lump excision (WLE)—excision of the lesion with a 2 mm margin of healthy tissue.
- **For multifocal lesion:** Nipple sparing mastectomy (all breast tissue with lactiferous apparatus is resected sparing nipple and areola)—more in LCIS.
- **Bilateral suspicious foci:** Bilateral nipple sparing mastectomy—LCIS.

Plan 2: Total Mastectomy

Indications: Aggressive tumors.
- Histological high grade or high growth index (Ki 67 >20%)
- High tumor to breast size ratio
- DCIS—high grade or large tumor size
- LCIS—pleomorphic type. E-cadherin antibodies positive
- Multifocal lesions
- Patient cannot receive post operative radiotherapy to residual breast tissue and chest wall after BCS (by preference or coronary disease or previous irradiation).

Axillary node management:
- Sentinel node biopsy done to exclude micro metastases
- If SLNB positive—upstage to treatment for invasive carcinoma (refer invasive carcinoma)
- SLNB negative—nothing more need be done

Postoperative radiotherapy: To residual breast and chest wall to prevent recurrence.

Systemic therapy:
Chemotherapy—no role for chemotherapy
Hormone responsive (ER positive) tumors
- Tamoxifen 20 mg daily—for premenopausal patients for 5 years.
- Aromatase inhibitors (Letrozole 2.5 mg/day or anastrozole 1 mg/day) for postmenopausal for 5 years.

Targeted therapy—monoclonal antibody (Trastuzumab).
HER +ve tumors (treated as invasive carcinoma) and for recurrences.

TREATMENT OF INVASIVE CARCINOMA OF BREAST

Early Breast Cancer (EBC)—T1, T2 N0–N1, T3 N0, M0.

Aim
- Cure—to ensure a long-term loco regional and systemic disease free state.
- Preserve shoulder function and contour.
- Preserve breast cosmesis and function.

Work up
- Diagnosis of primary—core needle biopsy—histo typing, receptors molecular markers.
- Mammography—remaining breast and opposite breast.
- Ultrasound abdomen, pelvis
- Chest X-ray.
- CT- scan of chest—if liver function tests show any abnormality.
- Axillary nodes N1—FNAC stereotactic biopsy for clinically non-palpable nodes
- N0—SLNB
- Bone scintiscan

If patient had bone pain and elevated levels of calcium and alkaline phosphatase.

Treatment
Surgery mainstay—for local clearance.

Adjuvant therapy
- Radiotherapy.
- **Systemic therapy:** Hormonal, chemotherapy, monoclonal antibody.

Surgery for Early Breast Cancer (EBC)

Low grade tumors without favorable indicators of poor prognosis (refer previous section).
- Breast conservation surgery (BCS) plus SLNB followed by radiotherapy to breast for tumors —T1,2 ,N0.
- ALND done if SLNB turn positive.
- BCS plus axillary lymph node dissection (ALND) and RT to breast—T1, T2, N1.
- If ALND reports over 4 nodes positive for tumor, axillary irradiation is considered.
- Skin sparing mastectomy: For central tumors, low grade plus ALND.
- Total mastectomy with SLNB for N0 stage and ALND for N1 stage in patients with:
  - Multifocal/multicentric, lobular carcinoma
  - Lymphovascular invasion (LVI), high grade tumors
  - High tumor to breast ratio
  - Is nonfeasibility or refusal (patient's choice) of postoperative RT after BCS.
- Modified radical mastectomy:
  - For high grade tumors, LVI, multifocal lobular carcinoma and N1 node.

Adjuvant Therapy

Radiotherapy (external beam):
- To residual breast after BCS
- To chest wall after mastectomy: If specimen has inadequate tumor clearance margins
- To axilla—if over 4 nodes are positive after ALND.

Hormone responsive tumors (ER positive):
- Tamoxifen 20 mg for premenopausal ladies
- Letrozol 2.5 mg/day for postmenopausal ladies for 5 years.

Chemotherapy: Refer table in previous section for details of regimes.
- For all node positive cases
- High grade tumors
- Tumors with LVI.

Chemotherapy Regimens (Given in Table 25.8)

FAC or FEC

CMF: For frail and elderly patients or cardiac cripples.

TAC: Generally for extensive axillary disease.
- High grade tumor with unfavorable prognostic indices (Ki—67 above 20%).
- **HER2 + cases:** Trastuzumab with AC regime.

TREATMENT OF LOCALLY ADVANCED BREAST CANCER (LABC)

Invasive breast cancer
- Infiltrating ductal (about 80%)
- Infiltrating lobular (5% to 10%)
- Medullary (5% to 7%)
- Mucinous (3%)
- Tubular (1% to 2%).

Philosophy of treatment:
- LABC is systemic disease, potentially metastatic or one with undetected metastases.
- Hence it is treated as a systemic disease along with locoregional control of the disease.
- Includes tumors—all T4, T3 N1, any T with N2 or 3.

Aims of treatment:
- Adequate loco regional control to prevent recurrences.
- Prevent occult metastases from growing to overt state.

Work Up
- **Tumor diagnosis:** Core needle biopsy, receptor and molecular markers.
- Chest X-ray
- Ultrasound—abdomen pelvis
- CT scan—chest and abdomen
- Bone scintiscan
- FDG - PET scan—to detect undetected metastases in bone, liver and lungs
  - Debated by fraternity over its false positives.

Treatment: Neo adjuvant therapy and surgery
- Except for T3 N 1 stage, where most centres still prefer surgery and adjuvant therapy.
- **T3 N1:** Modified radical mastectomy followed by adjuvant therapy (CT/RT/BT).

Note: Neoadjuvant therapy:
- Non-surgical therapy to gain control over potential or hidden metastases.

- To down stage loco regional disease and make it amenable for surgical resection for local clearance of the tumor.

T4 with any N, T3 N2, any T with N3 disease
- NACT and MRM/toilet mastectomy followed by RT to chest wall. NACT regimen—AC or FAC.
- HER2 +ve—patients receive trastuzumab for 1-2 years.
- ER +ve—receive-tamoxifen or letrozole as the case may be.

Q. What is mastitis carcinomatosa.

INFLAMMATORY CARCINOMA OF BREAST

Syn: Mastitis carcinomatosa.
Highly aggressive cancer.

Clinical features:
- As a painful, swollen breast with tenderness,
- Warmth, erythema with cutaneous oedema, Peau d'orange (cancer cells block the subdermal
- Lymphatics) underlying mass (in 70%) and axillary lymph nodes (50%)
- Usually a major part of the breast is involved.
- Over a third have metastases at diagnosis at first presentation.

Differential diagnosis: Acute mastitis and abscess.
FNAC or a core biopsy are confirmatory—showing undifferentiated carcinoma.

Diagnosis: Skin punch biopsy

Treatment: Neoadjuvant (aggressive) chemotherapy with radiotherapy.

Surgery: "Toilet mastectomy" for local control debulking of tumor - no clearance.

Prognosis: Overall poor, but marginal improvements seen after neoadjuvant therapy and salvage surgery, median survival is about 2 years; 5 years survival just 5%.

Triple Negative Breast Cancer (TNBC)

Negative for ER, PR and HER Neu receptors. Prognosis is bad. Early metastases. It responds poorly to chemotherapy regimens. Pembrolizumab with paclitaxel is tried for controlling the advanced disease.

TREATMENT OF METASTATIC CARCINOMA BREAST

Rationale
- Systemic therapy to control disease progression
- Palliation of symptoms due to loco regional and metastatic disease
- Efforts to ensure a symptom free survival and progression free disease.

Systemic therapy
Based on tumors biology and histochemistry.

Chemotherapy—usually taxane plus anthracycline regimes (docetaxel plus adriamycin and cyclophosphamide—TAC) or equivalent.

Biological therapy: For patients with HER 2+ ve tumors - Trastuzumab—usually with taxanes.

Hormone responsive—rare at this stage.

PARP inhibitors (e.g., olaparib) used in cases with BRCA 1 mutation positive. It is given as a single drug or in combination with paclitaxel, if anthracycline or taxane based therapy fails to control disease.

CDK inhibitors (e.g., palbociclib) for HR positive HER-2 negative tumors.

Locoregional treatment
- For fungating tumors: Toilet mastectomy plus radiotherapy to chest wall.
- Axillary irradiation—worsens arm edema.

Fractures
- **Long bones:** Fracture fixation and radiotherapy
- **Spine:** Risk of paraplegia—spinal fixation with radiotherapy
- **Brain metastases:** Cranial irradiation
- Pleural effusion; drainage with intercostal drainage and injection of intra pleural cyclophosphamide to achieve pleurodesis.

RECURRENT CARCINOMA OF BREAST

It is considered at par with metastatic disease with a locoregional reappearance and hence treated with systemic therapy along with local measures for disease control.

Locoregional Recurrence

Metastatic workup to exclude visceral or bony disease.

Treatment

Systemic chemotherapy or hormonal therapy or/and biotherapy (targeted therapy) along with locoregional treatment.

Recurrence in the breast after BCT—requires total (simple) mastectomy; survival rates are good.

Recurrence in the axilla—requires surgical resection followed by radiation to the axilla and systemic therapy.

Recurrence in the Chest Wall after Mastectomy

Occurs in 4–5% of patients. A third of these have metastases.

Treatment: Multimodal therapy is essential.

Isolated local recurrence: Excision followed by radiotherapy.

Larger recurrences: Radical chest resection with reconstructive myocutaneous flap closure.

PALLIATION

- Ulcers and discharging growths—local toilet
- Pain—analgesics oral, later patient controlled analgesia
- Nutrition
- Psychotropics if need be
- Fracture fixing
- Pleural effusions—drainage
- Aspiration of ascitic fluid.

REHABILITATION IN BREAST CANCER

Physical rehabilitation - nutrition.

Psychological and Vocational Therapy

Counseling of patient and family members should be a part of management before, during and after treatment.

Section 5

Cardiothoracic and Vascular System

26. Cardiothoracic Surgery
27. Arteries, Veins and Lymphatics

Section

Cardiothoracic Surgery

Chapter 26

SU 26	Topic: Cardiothoracic general surgery: Chest, heart and lungs.
SU26.1	Outline the role of surgery in the management of coronary heart disease, valvular heart diseases and congenital heart diseases.
SU26.2	Diseases of chest wall and the pleura.
SU26.3	Describe the clinical features of mediastinal diseases and the principles of their management.
SU26.4	Describe the etiology, pathogenesis, clinical features of tumors of lung and the principles of management.

SU26.1 Outline the role of surgery in the management of coronary heart disease, valvular heart diseases and congenital heart diseases.

PRINCIPLES OF CARDIOPULMONARY BYPASS

The use of first successful cardiopulmonary bypass (CPB) was done in 1953 by **John Heysham Gibbon**, Philadelphia, USA. It is used for surgical procedure wherever a temporary stopping of heart function is needed without compromising vital organ perfusion.

Uses

- All open heart surgeries
- In cardiopulmonary trauma
- In lung transplantation—single and double
- Non-cardiac surgical procedures.

Resection of highly vascular tumors and tumors invading large blood vessels.

- In pulmonary embolectomy
- Severe hypothermia—during rewarming
- In severe respiratory failure—resuscitation.

Q. Outline briefly the steps of cardiopulmonary bypass.

Figure 26.1 shows the cardiopulmonary bypass circuit.

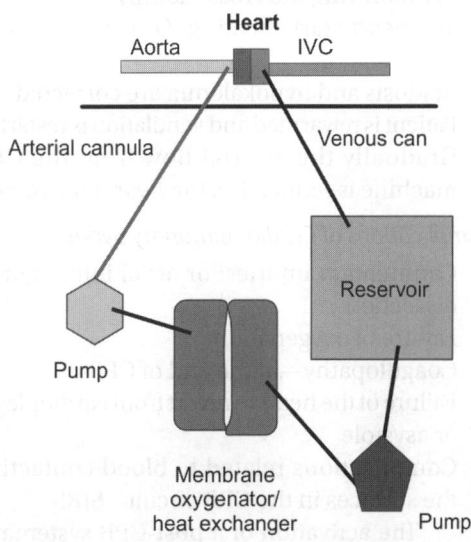

Fig. 26.1: Cardiopulmonary bypass circuit.

Steps

1. The Cardiopulmonary Bypass Circuit (The CPB Circuit)

The CPB circuit is made of:
- A venous cannula—(right atrium or separate superior and inferior vena caval cannulation.
- A venous reservoir to store blood.
- A heat exchanger to regulate temperature of blood.
- A membrane oxygenator for gas exchange.
- An arterial pump to return the oxygenated and warmed blood back to the circulation via the arterial cannula (through ascending Aorta or femoral/brachial artery).

2. Myocardial Protection and Cardioplegia

CPB and then aortic cross clamping deprives the heart of coronary flow and causes permanent myocardial damage within 15 to 20 minutes.

This requires myocardial protection by intracoronary infusion of a cardioplegic solution or total circulatory arrest and hypothermia to reduce metabolic rates.

Cardioplegic solutions: Contain potassium to stop the heart from beating.

3. Discontinuation of CP Bypass

- Perfusion is restored to the coronary arteries (by removing the cross-clamp)
- The heart starts beating. Or else may need defibrillation
- Acidosis and hypokalemia are corrected
- Patient is rewarmed and ventilation is restarted
- Gradually the arterial flow from the CPB machine is reduced as the heart takes over.

Complications of Cardiopulmonary Bypass

- Cannulation injuries: or atrial injury aortic dissection
- Failure of oxygenation
- Coagulopathy—at the end of CPB
- Failure of the heart to revert from cardioplegia or asystole
- Complications related to blood contacting the surfaces in the CPB circuit—SIRS
  - The activation of a post-CPB systematic inflammatory response syndrome (SIRS)
  - Leading to multiple organ failure.

Minimizing CPB Complications
- Mini CPB
- Beating heart surgery—for coronary bypass only.

Q. Pericardial effusion and tamponade.

It is caused by imbalance in the process of production and resorption of pericardial fluid.

Etiology
- **Acute effusion**
  Hemopericardium
  - Penetrating trauma
  - Postoperative
  - Coronary angiography
- **Chronic effusion**—causing chronic tamponade
- Tuberculosis
- Malignant infiltration of pericardium—bronchus or breast carcinomas.
- Uremia
- Connective tissue disease

Clinical Features
- Pulsus paradoxus
- Low blood pressure and a raised jugular venous pressure
- Kussmaul's sign—the jugular venous pressure rises with inspiration.

Emergency Treatment
- Pericardiocentesis—aspiration of the pericardial fluid
- Through a wide-bore needle inserted into pericardial space to left of xiphisternum.

Open Surgery: Median sternotomy or emergency room thoracotomy: (1) if pericardiocentesis fails or (2) penetrating wounds of the heart.

Treatment of Cause
- Tuberculosis ATT with steroids.
- Collagen diseases—require immunosuppressives (azathioprine) with steroid.

Constrictive Pericarditis
- Progressive thickening of pericardium which gets adherent to heart and restricts its movements leading to low input failure.
- Tuberculosis, collagen diseases and chronic renal failure are common causes.
- Treatment—pericardiectomy.

Thoracic Aortic Aneurysms (TAAs): Mostly Affects Elderly Persons

Five main types of TAA	Etiology
1. Ascending aortic aneurysm	Secondary to medial degeneration
2. Transverse aortic aneurysm	Atherosclerosis and hypertension
3. Descending aortic aneurysm	- Do -
4. Thoracoabdominal aneurysms	- Do -
5. Traumatic aneurysm	Blunt trauma to chest

Complications: Progression
- Dissection (commonly ascending aorta)
- Rupture, aortic regurgitation and congestive failure
- Distal embolization
- Pressure—esophagus, recurrent laryngeal nerve or superior vena cava
- Erosion into bronchus or esophagus, rib.

Clinical Manifestations
- Incidental finding at radiography or imaging
- Chest discomfort or pain
- Other features depending upon the complications.

Investigations
- **Chest X-ray**
  - A widened mediastinum or an enlarged calcific aortic shadow
  - Skeletal fractures seen in traumatic aneurysms.
- **MRI or CT scan**—size and extent of aneurysms. to plan for surgical or endovascular repair. **Echocardiography** with transesophageal imaging—for aneurysms involving the aortic arch.
- **Aortography**—to mark extent of the aneurysm and its relationship with aortic branches.

Treatment
- Endovascular repair
- Surgical repair—interposition grafts or complete restoration of arterial anatomy.

Indication for Surgery
- Aneurysm larger than 6 cm, aortic dissections, mycotic aneurysms, and asymptomatic
- Aneurysms larger than 5 cm in Marfan syndrome.

Traumatic aortic aneurysms: Urgent repair required—generally endovascular repair.

Surgical management varies by underlying etiology and location.

Postoperative complications: High mortality, high risk of stroke and paraplegia.

SURGERY FOR CORONARY ARTERY DISEASE

Coronary Anatomy
The left and right coronary arteries arise from the sinuses of Valsalva just above the left and right coronary cusps of the aortic valve respectively.

The left coronary artery branches into two—the left anterior descending artery (LAD) and the left circumflex artery (LCx) which gives off its obtuse marginal branches (OM1,2,3,).

Anatomical Dominance
- **The artery supplying the posterior descending artery:** Right coronary artery (90%) or left circumflex (10%)—determines the side of dominance of the circulation—right dominant or left dominant.
- **A balanced pattern circulation:** Two posterior descending arteries—one each from RCA and LCx.
- Dominance of the right or left is important in planning the CABG (coronary artery bypass grafting) by identifying the location of diseased vessels responsible for ischemia.
- The LAD is the most frequently diseased and the most bypassed during CABG surgery.

Preoperative Considerations for CABG
- History and physical examination
- Chest X-ray—state of lungs and shadows of heart and great vessels
- CT scan—for evaluation of calcification of vessels and valves.

ECHOCARDIOGRAPHY
Assessment of structure of heart walls and valves and detailed cardiac function.

Cardiac catheterisation: To evaluate and identify vessels and state of myocardial circulation.

Stress Echocardiography

Real time 3-dimensional echocardiography (RT3DE)—in planning surgery for valvular defects.

Transthoracic or transesophageal echocardiogram (TTE, TEE)—for assessment of ventricular function and valvular pathology.

Stress test: Exercise tolerance testing (ETT) or treadmill test (TMT).

Radionuclide studies (thallium-201)—to assess myocardial perfusion.

Cardiac Magnetic Resonance Imaging (MRI)

Invasive Methods of Diagnosis

Coronary angiography: The gold standard of diagnosis.

Selective coronary angiography—to diagnose and quantify the extent of coronary artery occlusion.

Q. Write a short note on indications for coronary bypass surgery.

Guidelines from the European Society of Cardiology (ESC) and the European Association for Cardiothoracic Surgery (EACTS).
- Chronic stable angina
- Acute coronary syndromes: In patients stabilised after an episode of ACS
- For complications of myocardial Infarction—ventricular septal rupture—usually 3rd–7th day.
- After infarction, with pulmonary edema and hemodynamic instability
- **Papillary muscle necrosis**—causes acute mitral regurgitation
- Mitral valve replacement with CABG
- Ventricular aneurysm occurs following partial—thickness necrosis of the ventricular wall
- **Acute failure of percutaneous coronary angioplasty**

Preparation for surgery
- Clinical assessment—coagulopathy, carotid artery disease, respiratory status, peripheral vascular disease, diabetic complications and control of diabetes, renal dysfunction drugs, such as diuretics and angiotensin-converting enzyme (ACE) inhibitors.

Risk assessment, e.g., H/o major adverse cardiac events (MACEs).

Arterial grafts—taken from
- The left internal mammary artery (LIMA), or internal thoracic artery—for the LAD.
- LIMA-LAD anastomosis avoids the late complication of vein graft atherosclerosis.
- Also tried are the bilateral internal mammary artery (BIMA) grafts.

Venous grafts—from great saphenous veins.

The operation
- Harvesting of the conduits—long saphenous vein from the leg.
- Median sternotomy dissection of LIMA.
- CPB after heparinization.
- Aortic cross clamping and arrest.
- Anastomosis carried out—aortic base to LAD, LCx or RCA, OM 1 or 2 as the case be.

Postoperative complications
- Bleeding
- Postoperative arrhythmias.
- Atrial fibrillation (AF).

Off-pump coronary artery surgery—CABG without the use of CPB.
- Can be used with a minimally invasive approach. Or through sternotomy.

Minimally invasive direct coronary artery bypass (MIDCAB)
- Anterior submammary incision—for port and dissection of LIMA with a thoracoscope.
- LIMA grafted to LAD.
- Lateral MIDCAB incisions—to access other coronary vessels. (LCx, OM1 OM2)

'Hybrid' coronary revascularization
Combined MIDCAB (typically LIMA to LAD with PCI to less accessible coronary vessels.

SURGERY FOR VALVULAR HEART DISEASE
- Early surgeries—valvular repair.
- Valve stenosis—'blind' commissurotomies.
- Later—open procedures—repair or replace under vision.
- Valves ensure unidirectional flow of blood without reflux through the heart.

Repair or Replace?

The selection of procedure (repair or replacement) or the type of prosthesis for replacement, depends upon:
- The patient's age, the need for anticoagulation
- Existing comorbidities like bleeding diathesis
- The patient's choice.

Types of Prosthetic Valves

Mechanical Valves

Any age group, for any valve
- High durability
- But thrombogenic and need lifelong anticoagulation with warfarin
- Complications—hemorrhage (intracerebral or GI tract or thromboembolism (cerebral infarct).

Biological Valves

- **Homograft (or allograft)** valves from cadavers
- **Autografts**, a patient's own valve
- **Heterografts (or xenografts)** prepared from animal tissues.

Prosthetic Valve Dysfunction and Complications

- Structural valve failure
- Paravalvular leak
- Thrombosis and thromboembolism
- **Prosthetic valve endocarditis (PVE)**
  - High risk with mechanical and bioprosthetic valves and lowest risk with homograft and autograft valves.
  - **Organisms causing PVE:** Staphylococcal and streptococcal species.

Postoperative Management

Antibiotic Prophylaxis

Antithrombotic therapy: All patients with mechanical valves require warfarin.

Causes of Mitral Valve Disease

Stenosis
- Rheumatic heart disease (common)
- Calcification of valve or chordae
- Congenital (rare)

Regurgitation
- Rheumatic heart disease
- Valve prolapse
- Left ventricular dilatation or hypertrophy

Ischemia
Bacterial endocarditis.

Mitral Regurgitation (MR)

Indications for Surgery
1. Primary mitral regurgitation—with severe symptoms or left ventricular dysfunction.
2. MR secondary to ischemic heart disease—may need repair with CABG.
3. Failed percutaneous mitral balloon valvuloplasty (PMBV).

Mitral stenosis—due to rheumatic fever.

Preoperative evaluation includes—ECG, chest X-ray, Doppler imaging and echocardiography, transesophageal echocardiogram (TEE), coronary angiography and MRI.

Medical management includes use of anticoagulation in patients with AF or left atrial enlargement. Tachy arrhythmias and cardiac failure are treated.

Approach
- A median sternotomy
- A right thoracotomy—unusually
- The mitral valve can be accessed
  - Through the left atrium in the interatrial groove,
  - Through the right atrium and then the interatrial septum or
  - Through the left atrial appendage.

Aortic Valve Disease

Aortic Stenosis (AS)

Causes
- A congenital bicuspid aortic valve
- Damage by rheumatic disease
- Senile degeneration and calcification of a normal valve.

Severity: Stenosis is graded as being mild to severe—by echocardiographic study.

Pathology: Pressure overload on the left ventricle causes left ventricular hypertrophy.

Clinical Correlation
- Symptoms—syncope, chest pain or angina, shortness of breath or congestive failure.
- Loud systolic murmur over the precordium and a murmur in the carotid arteries.
- Hypotension (low systolic pressure and low pulse pressure).

Treatment
Aortic valve replacement (AVR)—provides relief of symptoms and survival benefit.

Indications
- Severely symptomatic patients (aortic valve diameter < 1 cm)
- Patients with severe AS who have and systolic dysfunction—LVEF below 50% or those undergoing CABG or other cardiac surgery.

Aortic Insufficiency (AI) Syn: Aortic Regurgitation (AR)

Causes
- Rheumatic disease combined with AS.
- Infective endocarditis.
- Leaflet redundancy or destruction (myxomatous degeneration)
- Aortic root dilatation—Marfan syndrome
- Aortic dissection—syphilis
- Inflammatory disease (ankylosing spondylitis, SLE, ulcerative colitis).

Pathology
- Valve leaflet thickened calcified and fixed.
- Chronic AI—left ventricular volume overload.
- Echocardiographic grading—mild to severe.
- Acute AI causes severe pulmonary edema, myocardial ischemia and cardiovascular collapse.

Clinical Features
- Wide pulse pressure, visible carotid pulsation
- Early diastolic murmer over chest
- Signs of LVH.

Investigations
- Chest X-ray
- ECG
- Echocardiography with Doppler flow study
- Coronary angiography to assess coronary anatomy and state.

Treatment
Surgery: Aortic valve replacement (AVR) offers the definitive treatment.

Medical therapy—Vasodilator drugs and diuretics are used for controlling heart failure.

Indication for Surgery
Severe symptoms and progressive left ventricular dysfunction. Also in asymptomatic patients along with CABG or correction of congenital defects.

Transcatheter Interventional Aortic Valve Implantation (TAVI)
- For patients too old or too frail for AVR
- Patients with associated comorbidities
- 'Porcelain' aorta–heavily calcified ascending aorta.

ROLE OF SURGERY FOR CONGENITAL HEART DISEASES

Congenital heart diseases start in the third to eighth week of gestation.

Physiology
Fetal circulation: The right and left ventricles pump blood in parallel (adults: it is in series) hence more of oxygenated blood reaches the heart in the fetus through the right to left shunts, **(1) ductus venosus, (2) ductus arteriosus and (3) foramen ovale.**

After birth, pulmonary vascular resistance falls due to:
- Breathing
- Pulmonary vasodilatation
- Cessation of blood flow from placenta (umbilical cord is divided).

Result of fall in pulmonary vascular resistance is closure of the three fetal circulatory shunts.
- **Constriction of ductus arteriosus** within 30 minutes due to increase in blood oxygen levels.
  This causes reversal of pulmonary systemic pressure gradient and stoppage of blood flow from pulmonary artery into the aorta.
- **Closure of ductus venosus**
- **Closure of foramen ovale.**

The cutting of umbilical cord leads to:
- Fall in pressure in inferior vena cava
- Fall in right atrial pressure.

The functional closure of the shunts happens immediately after birth, and structural closure over the next 6 months. The same may fail partly or fully causing congenital heart diseases.
- Patent foramen ovale
- Patent ductus arteriosus
- Failure of septation—atrial septal defect (ASD) or ventricular septal defect (VSD).

Congenital stenosis
- Extracardiac—coarctation of aorta
- Intracardiac—supravalvular, infravalvular or valvular stenosis.

Abnormal connections of vessels and stenoses
- Tetralogy of Fallot—VSD, overriding aorta, pulmonary stenosis, right ventricular hypertrophy.
- Transposition of great vessels.
- Total anomalous venous drainage.

Diagnosis: Antenatal diagnosis is possible—detected in utero at 16-18 weeks.

Clinical presentation: Variable presentation may be with cardiac arrhythmias, or with polycythemia, cyanosis and/or hypertension thromboembolic event.

Investigations: Fetal echocardiography is preferred to cardiac catheterization (avoided).

CYANOTIC HEART DISEASES

- **Tetralogy of Fallot:** Most common cyanotic heart disease—5-10%
  Surgery—carried out early at 4-6 months of age, if possible or at the earliest.
  - A patch to close the VSD
  - Resection of the obstructing section of the infundibular septum.
    The survival rate after surgical correction is 90-95%.
- **Transposition of great vessels (TGV)—2nd most common CHD.**
  - The aorta arises from the right ventricle and the pulmonary artery from the left ventricle. It is incompatible unless there is a shunt like VSD.
  - Severe central cyanosis at birth—is the presenting feature.

Treatment:
1st stage: Creating a life saving right to left shunt and oxygenate the aortic lood.
- Percutaneous balloon septostomy
- Intravenous prostaglandins can be administered to keep the PDA open and increase systemic-pulmonary shunting.

Surgery: Arterial switch repair within the first few weeks of birth. Long-term results are good.

- **Total anomalous pulmonary venous drainage (TAPVD)**
  - Pulmonary veins drain into systemic venous circulation at coronary sinus or right atrium, superior or inferior vena cava. Associated ASD allows the child to survive neonatal period.
  - Cyanosis at one week, failure to thrive, chest infections and cardiac failure—those with pulmonary blood flow.

Surgery aims to re-establish the pulmonary venous drainage into the left atrium.

ACYANOTIC HEART DISEASES

Q. Short note on patent ductus arteriosus.

Patent ductus arteriosus (PDA)

Ductus arteriosus closes functionally through a prostaglandin inhibition mechanism within hours after birth. Following onset of respiration expansion of lungs and increase in arterial oxygen saturation and a drop in the pulmonary arterial resistance. Physical closure happens within 6 months.

Complications: PD is left-to-right shunt of blood, resulting in a high pulmonary blood flow
- Larger ductus can cause cardiac failure and can lead to shunt reversal (Eisenmenger syndrome) with cyanosis and clubbing.
- Infective endocarditis
- Left ventricular failure.

Treatment
- A cyclo-oxygenase inhibitor (e.g. indomethacin): Used to close the ductus
- Interventional cardiology: Coil ductal closure or umbrella.

Surgery for small children with wide and larger ductus— left thoracotomy. Division and suturing or ligation.

Coarctation of the aorta: 6-7% of congenital heart disease.

It is hemodynamically significant narrowing of the aorta (commonest site—descending aorta) Mostly affects male sex, in girls, associated with Turner syndrome.

Pathophysiology

- Preductal—usually in infants
- Postductal—older children or adults

1. **Differential perfusion:** The coarctation results in over perfusion of upper parts of body and poor perfusion of lower body—kidney, excess renin secretion and acidosis.
   - Left ventricular overload and failure.
2. **Differential hypertension**—upper body hypertension.
3. **Cardiac failure.**

Clinical Features

- High blood pressure in upper body
- Prominent vessels in neck
- Claudication of lower extremities and exhaustion.
  Peripheral pulsation—radio-femoral delay
  Machinery murmur—continuous—over thoracic spine or infra clavicular.
- Cardiac failure—mainly in infants

Complications

- Heart failure
- Infective endocarditis
- Rupture of the aorta
- Hemorrhagic stroke.

Chest X-ray—rib notching due to dilated posterior intercostal vessels.

Aortic knuckle shadow.

"Three sign"

1. Upper dilated left subclavian,
2. The middle—stenotic coarctation part
3. The lower poststenotic dilatation of the descending aorta.

Echocardiography is diagnostic. Infant coarctation typically presents congestive heart failure after closure of ductus arteriosus and often requires early surgical correction.

Treatment

- Infants—vigorous medical treatment—Prostaglandin (PGE-1) to reopen the ductus and general resuscitation followed by surgical correction.
- Percutaneous stenting—preferred method for adults
- Surgery—surgical repair via a left thoracotomy—childhood or young adults.
- Death—usually by the age of 40 years due to complications.

Atrial Septal Defects

Atrial septal defect causes a left to right shunt. If large, it causes pulmonary hypertension and congestive heart failure. Later leads to right to left reversal of shunt (Eisenmenger effect) and left ventricular failure.

Types of ASD

- Ostium secundum ASD—ostium primum fails to fuse.
- Ostium primum ASD—associated trisomy 21, failed development of endocardial cushion, associated mitral regurgitation.
- A sinus venosus ASD—associated anomalous pulmonary venous drainage.
- Patent foramen ovale.

Complications: Right ventricular failure, endocarditis and paradoxical emboli.

Treatment

Interventional cardiology: Transcatheter deployment of devices to close small defects especially os. secundum defects.

- Open-heart surgery with CPB and closure of the defect, either sutured or with pericardial or synthetic patch.
- Primum atrioventricular defect repaired along with mitral valve replacement, if needed.

Ventricular Septal Defects (20-25% of CHDs) (Refer Table 26.1)

Defect in the interventricular septum with left to right shunting VSDs account for 20-30%. May be isolated or with tetralogy of Fallot or complete atrioventricular defect.

Table 26.1: Types of VSD.

Type of VSD	Synonym
Perimembranous defect (75%)—defect in the membranous septum	Conoventricular VSD
Muscular defect (10%)	Trabecular VSD
Atrioventricular canal defect	Inlet defect
Subarterial defect (VSD)	Outlet or subarterial VSD

Complications

- Progressive pulmonary edema and congestive cardiac failure.
- Eisenmenger syndrome (reversal of shunt to right to left)—2nd decade.

Diagnosis: Echocardiography.

Treatment

30–50% of smaller VSDs close spontaneously in the first 5 years.

Indications for surgical closure of VSD
- For large defects
- For left-to-right shunts of >2:1
- Increasing pulmonary arterial resistance
- Failure of medical therapy.

SU26.2: Chest wall and pleural diseases.

Write short notes on the following:
1. Surgical aspects of lung abscess
2. Pleural effusion
3. Empyema thoracis
4. Empyema necessitans
5. Mesothelioma of the pleura
6. Tumors of chest wall:

Hemothorax, pneumothorax, flail chest and stove in chest are considered under chapter on thoracic trauma.

PLEURAL EFFUSION

Exudative effusions: Protein content more than 30 g/L.

Transudative effusions: Protein content—less than 30 g/L.

Analysis

- Protein
- Glucose content
- pH
- LDH.

Pathophysiology

- High pulmonary capillary pressure due to elevated left atrial pressure—heart failure or circulatory overload.
- Low intravascular oncotic pressure—low levels of the plasma proteins, e.g., malnutrition diseased liver or kidney.
- Obstructive accumulation of pleural protein—secondary to lymphatic obstruction—cancers lymphoma or metastatic.
- Increased capillary permeability—causing leak of fluid and protein—pneumonia, tuberculosis, collagen diseases.

Infected pleural infection (empyema)

And malignant effusions.

Malignant pleural effusion

- Lung cancer—most common
- Direct spread to the pleura—both parietal and/or visceral layers.
- Secondary involvement in other malignancies, i.e., breast cancer.
- Primary pleural malignancies—mesothelioma.
- Cancers obstructing the mediastinal lymphatics—as in carcinoma breast.

Diagnosis

- Biopsy—pleural biopsy—needle, CT guided, video-assisted thoracoscopic surgery (VATS) or open surgery.

Palliation
- **Drainage:** Intercostal drainage tube insertion along with chemotherapy and pain relief
- **Pleurodesis:** Instillation of chemotherapeutic drugs like cyclophosphamide.

EMPYEMA THORACIS
Suppurative collection in the pleural cavity.

Etiology
- Infection of the lungs:
  - Postpneumoneic
  - Lung abscess—rupture
  - Bronchiectasis
  - Tuberculosis
  - Fungal infections.
- Rupture of esophagus (Boerhaave's syndrome or perforating esophageal foreign bodies).
- Post-traumatic—blunt/penetrating.
- Bony infection—ribs or vertebral (TB).
- **Extrathoracic causes:** Subphrenic abscess.
- **Iatrogenic**: Post pleural aspiration, tube drainage or post-thoracotomy.

Pathology: Thick pus with a thick cortex of fibrin and coagulum over the lung.

A typical empyema after pneumonia undergoes three phases:
1. Exudative phase—thin infected content: Antibiotics + aspiration or drainage
2. Fibrino-purulent phase—drainage—a must; some may require by early decorticaton
3. The organizing phase—thick "cortex" like sheet causes trapping of lung making it unable to expand—surgery is the only remedy.

Sites of empyema
- Apical
- Basal
- Lateral diaphragmatic recess
- Mediastinal
- Interlobar.

Clinical Features
- Fever, pain and dyspnea
- Tender chest wall, dullness,
- Features of contributing illness.

Investigations
- Chest X-ray
- CT scan.

Tretment
- **Antibiotics as per the causative organism.**
- Symptomatic care—pain relief, physiotherapy to chest and help oxygenation
- Early aspiration of pus and bacterial culture (before starting antibiotic)
- Drainage of pus—intercostal drainage connected to an underwater seal
- Specific treatment—like anti tuberculous treatment
- Surgical intervention (refer below).

Surgery for Empyema
Aim
Complete drainage of pus and cause full expansion of lungs for normal air exchange.

Methods
- Intercostal drainage—for early and thin empyema
- Rib resection and open drainage—thick pus and localised empyema and in patient unfit for a major thoracotomy during the build up for thoracotomy.
- Decortication—"peeling the thick cortex" of the thickened membrane over pleura to allow complete lung expansion.
- Thoracoscopy and video-assisted thoracoscopic procedures
  - Thoracoscopic biopsy, drainage of empyema, talk pleurodesis, debridement and drainage and decortication.

EMPYEMA NECESSITANS
It is an empyema thoracis penetrating the chest wall and presenting subcutaneously.

There is an underlying empyema with a track communicating with the subcutaneous bulge.
- **Cause:** Tuberculous or non tubercujlous empyema.
- **Iatrogenic:** Following aspiration or incomplete drainage of empyema.

- **Clinical features:** A tender and fluctuant swelling over chest wall with a cough impulse. Management is similar to that of empyema thoracis.

SURGERY FOR MEDICAL CONDITIONS
- **Lung abscess**
  Surgery: Only for drainage of the pus after aspiration fails to control; or to treat an empyema.
- **Bronchiectasis:** Chronic irreversible dilatation of the medium-sized bronchi.
  - Unilateral or bilateral
  - Generalised—in lung or confined to lobe/s or segments.

Causes
- Suppurative pneumonia or bronchial obstruction
- Tuberculosis.

Treatment
Lobectomy or pneumonectomy for localized disease like segmental or lobar bronchiectasis. Surgery is avoided for generalized or bilateral disease except to control recurrent infection or bleeding.

Role of Surgery in Tuberculosis
1. Residual cavity after adequate ATT
2. Aspergilloma
3. **Hemoptysis:** Recurrent or uncontrolled, severe bleed from a cavity
4. Chronic abscess of empyema
5. Lesion in a tuberculous lung with suspicion of cancer on X-ray or scan.

Treatment
- **Lobectomy:** Resection of the diseased lobe
- Pneumonectomy
- **Empyema:** Decortication.

LUNG CYSTS
Symptomatic cysts or infected cysts are treated by resection—open or VATS.

Hydatid cysts: Resection of lobe after adequate medical treatment of the parasite.
- Albendazole high dose 400 mg 3 times a day for 6 weeks or praziquantel.

MESOTHELIOMA OF PLEURA
Etiology
- Mostly due to inhaled asbestos fibers.
- 80–90% are malignant mesotheliomas.

Clinical Features
Dyspnea, dry cough, chest pain. Rarely hemoptysis.

Diagnosis
- Thoracoscopic biopsy
- Biomarkers.

Treatment: Multimodal—Surgery, Chemotherapy and Radiation
- **Palliative surgery:** Pleurectomy or decortications.
- **Radical surgery for early tumor:** Extrapleural pneumonectomy (EPP) resection of the lung, pleura—both visceral and parietal layers, adjoining pericardium and part of the diaphragm.
- Hyperthermic chemotherapeutic pleural lavage (post resection).
- **Prognosis:** Very poor—22 months for an early tumor, 12 months for an advanced tumor.

TUMORS OF THE CHEST WALL (REFER TABLE 26.2)
- **Can arise from:** Bone—sarcoma
- **Cartilage:** Chondroma and chondrosarcoma
- **Soft tissue:** Benign—lipomas
  - Fibrous histiocytomas, fibrosarcoma
- **Chest wall mass:** Consider malignancy until proved otherwise
- Complete resection offers the best prognosis
- **Clinical features:** Swelling, pain in chest wall or both.

Table 26.2: Chest wall mass—management algorithm.

Chest wall mass (CT/MRI) small 2 cm lesion

Clear diagnosis—resection done		Unclear diagnosis—needle or incisional biopsy	
Benign: No further treatment	**Malignant:** Wide resection of tumor	Synovial cell sarcoma Liposarcoma Fibrosarcoma Desmoid' Malignant fibrous Histiocytoma (pleomorphic undifferentiated sarcoma)	Osteosarcoma Rhabdomyosarcoma **Non-rhabdomyosarcoma** Ewing's PNET (primitive neuroendocrinal tumor)
↓	↓		
Chondroma and osteochondroma	Chondrosarcoma Wide resection done	Proceed for surgery	Neoadjuvant chemotherapy followed by surgery
Esosinophilic, granuloma, fibrous, dysplasia		Wide surgical resection	

Plasmacytoma: Solitary myeloma—serum electrophoresis

Needle biopsy

Radiation with doses of 4000 to 5000 cGy

Multiple myeloma: Chemotherapy, monoclonal antibody.

Ewings' tumor: ESR elevated, young patients. Needle biopsy for diagnosis.

Treatment: Preoperative chemotherapy—radiologic imaging—residual disease—treated by surgical resection and reconstruction—followed by maintenance chemotherapy.

Primitive neuroectodermal tumors (PNETs)—neuroblastomas, ganglioneuroblastomas and ganglioneuromas—arise primitive neural crest cells that migrate from the mantle layer of the developing spinal cord.

SU26.4: Describe the etiology, pathogenesis, clinical features of tumors of lung and the principles of management.

LUNG TUMORS

Anatomy of the Bronchi Lungs

Refer **Figure 26.2** for lung segments.
- The bronchi and lungs develop from the endoderm of the primitive foregut as a bud in 4th week of intrauterine life. The stroma and vessels develop from the mesenchyme
- The right lung has three lobes—upper and middle lobes separated by the transverse fissure and the lower lobe separated by the oblique fissure from the other two.
- The left lobe has two lobes—the upper and lower separated by the oblique fissure.
- The upper lobes have three segments—on each side—apical, anterior and posterior.
- The lower lobes have four basal segments—on each side—apical, posterior, lateral, anterior
- The right middle lobe is divided into a lateral and medial segment.
- The left side has a smaller "lingula" replacing the middle lobe, with two sub segments—superior lingular and inferior lingular.

Blood supply: Each segment has a unit of a branch from pulmonary artery (deoxygenated blood), systemic supply (oxygenated blood) from the segmental branches of bronchial arteries from thoracic aorta. Segmental pulmonary vein draining oxygenated blood into pulmonary veins (two each side) and thereby into the right atrium.

The lymphatic drainage is into respective bronchial branches and divided into zones. Refer **Table 26.3**.

Types of Benign Lung Tumors
- **Mass:** A tumor larger than 3 cm in size.
- **Nodule:** A tumor less than 3 cm in size.

Hamartomas: 55% of benign lung nodules.

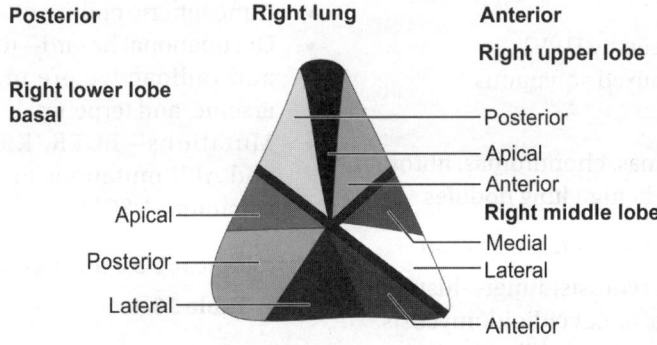
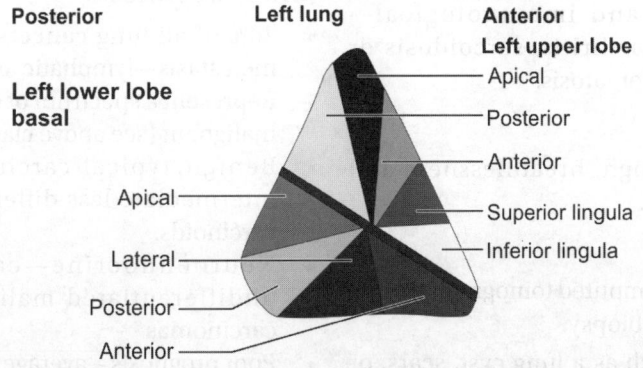

Fig. 26.2: Lung segments.

Table 26.3: Lymphatic drainage zones of bronchi and lungs (14 stations).

Supraclavicular zone	Hilar/interlobular zone
Station 1: Low cervical, supraclavicular sternal notch	Station 10: Hilar
	Station 11: Interlobar
Upper zone: (around trachea)	
Station 2: Upper paratracheal	**Lower zone (lower lobe level)**
Station 3: Prevascular/retrotracheal	Station 8: Paraesophageal
Station 4: Lower paratracheal	Station 9: Pulmonary ligament, peripheral zone (parenchymal level)
AP zone (aortic—para-aortic)	Station 12: Lobar
Station 5: Subaortic	Station 13: Segmental
Station 6: Para-aortic, subcarinal zone (tracheobronchial)	Station 14: Subsegmental
Station 7: Subcarinal	

They have "normal" tissues in " abnormal" amounts—cartilage, connective tissue, muscle and fat.

Age group—50 to 70—usually < 4 cm chest X-rays show as a coin-like round growth.

Bronchial adenomas: Adenomas are common.

Papillomas are less common.

Types of papilloma:

- Squamous (caused by HPV)
- Glandular and mixed squamous
- Glandular.

Rare tumors: Lipomas, chondromas, fibromas, neurofibromas and benign lung nodules.

Pulmonary nodules are fairly common

Granulomas: Tuberculosis; fungi—histoplasmosis, aspergillosis, or coccidioidomycosis.
- Infection from human papilloma virus.
- A lung abscess (usually caused by bacteria).
- Inflammatory and immunological—as rheumatoid arthritis, sarcoidosis or Wegener's granulomatosis.

Clinical features

Mild persistent cough, breathlessness and Wheeze, hemoptysis.

Diagnosis

Chest X-ray or CT (computed tomography) scan, a bronchoscopy and biopsy.

Birth defects such as a lung cyst, scars, or other lung malformation.

LUNG CANCERS

Etiology

Known Factors

- Cigarette smoking—about 15% of heavy smokers develop lung cancer and accounts for 88–85% of all cases.
- Passive smoking increases the risk of lung cancer by 30%.
- Atmospheric pollution.
- Occupational hazard—mining of chromium and radioactive ore uranium, cadmium, arsenic, and terpenes.
- Mutations—EGFR, KRAS, BRAF, ROS-1 and ALK mutations are recorded in non-squamous NSCLC.

Histological Classification of Lung Cancers

Refer **Table 26.4**.

SMALL CELL LUNG CANCER (SCLC) (OAT CELL CANCER)

- 20% of all lung cancers aggressive, early metastasis—lymphatic and hematogenous.
- Represent a spectrum of disease—benign to malignant (see above classification).
- Benign/typical carcinoid tumor—the intermediate less differentiated atypical carcinoids.
- Neuroendocrine—carcinomas—the undifferentiated malignant small cell carcinomas.
- Poor prognosis—average survival is less than a year despite a chemotherapeutic response.

Table 26.4: Histological classification of lung cancers	
Small cell lung cancer—SCLC-25%	**Non-small cell lung cancer (NSCLC) 75%**
• Small cell carcinoma 20% • Neuroendocrine tumors (NET)—1% • Carcinoid—4–5%	• Adenocarcinoma—**40%** • Bronchoalveolar cell carcinoma—**lepidic growth** • Squamous carcinoma—25% • Large cell undifferentiated

Treatment

- **Chemotherapy:** Various regimes with combination of cyclophosphamide, cisplatin, etoposide, doxorubicin, and vincristine.
- **Radiotherapy:**
  - Thoracic radiation therapy to improve local control of the primary tumor
  - Prophylactic cranial irradiation—because brain metastases are noted in 80%.
- **Surgery:** Infrequent role—only for early disease (rarely diagnosed at this stage)
  - Lobectomy (very infrequent chance) for T1 N0 T2 N0—for resection
  - Solitary peripheral pulmonary nodules with no evidence of metastatic disease.

NON-SMALL CELL LUNG CANCER (NSCLC)

Epithelial NSCLC

- **Adenocarcinoma**—40% the most common type, peripherally located early metastases. Women and non-smokers are also affected in high numbers.
- **Squamous carcinoma**—25% appears as a cavitating tumor.
  - Localized or locally spreading in the lobe, nodes, chest wall and mediastinum.
- **Large cell undifferentiated** is a discrete type of NET.
  - Aggressive behavior, early nodal and cerebral metastases.
- **'Lepidic' neoplastic lesions** (formerly—bronchoalveolar carcinoma (BAC))
  - Often multifocal primary tumors.
  - Four subtypes—precursor lesions, minimally invasive; lepidic adenocarcinomas and frankly malignant variety.

X-ray: Shows a patchy diffuse shadow ('ground glass').

Neuroendocrine tumors

- Small cell cancer
- Large cell undifferentiated lung cancer and
- Carcinoid—less aggressive.

Carcinoids

Typical carcinoids—central tumors—arise from major bronchi. Metastases are rare.
- Clinically—present with cough or hemoptysis.
- Immunohistochemistry: Carcinoids express neuron-specific enolase(NSE), chromogranin, and synaptophysin.
- Surgery is frequently curative.

Neuroendocrine carcinomas or atypical carcinoids:
Arise in lung periphery and aggressive.

Diagnosis: Sites—80% in bronchi, 20% in alveoli.
- Slow growing and highly vascular
- 20%—risk of metastases
- Treated by surgery and systemic therapy.

Staging of lung cancers TNM to, Tis, T1-4, N0–3 M0–M1-a,b,c
Stages of non-small cell lung cancer (simplified)
• **Stage I:** Tumor confined to lungs, no lymphatic spread • **Stage II:** Tumor in lung and limited spread to peripheral lymph node—bronchial and beyond • **Stage III:** Tumor—upto main bronchus and hilar nodes and mediastinal lymph nodes disease • **Stage IV:** Disseminated—contralateral, extrathoracic, disseminated to other systems or organs

Clinical Presentation of Lung Cancers

Depend on the site of the tumor the spread to adjacent structures; the extent of metastases.

Symptoms

A persistent cough, weight loss, dyspnea, and non-specific chest pain hemoptysis, recurrent pneumonia or clubbing. Carcinoid syndrome indicates pulmonary or hepatic metastases.

Paraneoplastic symptoms: Muscle weakness, myasthenic syndrome nausea, vomiting, fluid retention, high blood pressure, high blood sugar, confusion, seizures, coma.

Investigation

- Chest X-ray
- High resolution CT (contrast enhanced)—tumor, lung, bronchi, pleura and nodes assessed) and CT guided FNAC from tumor
- Biopsy for histological subtyping and genomic mutations in tumor
- FDG (PET scan)—micro nodules are picked
- **Bronchoscopy:** Biopsy, brush cytology, segmental bronchial lavage and transbronchial needle aspiration (TBNA)
- Endobronchial ultrasound (EBUS) and EUS FNAC of the tumor or TBNA.

Surgical Approaches for Diagnosis

Mediastinotomy or VATS through 2nd space are used for biopsy of lesions.

Video-assisted Thoracoscopic Surgery (VATS)—Short Notes

- Thoracoscopic technique to gain access to the chest cavity.
- **Application:** VATS alone or VATS with limited (mini) thoracotomy.
  - Most lung resections are performed through two or three port incisons and completed.
  - Advantage—speedy post operative recovery
  - Pain is far less as the ribs are not spread or divided (unlike in an open thoracotomy).
  - The technique avoids rib-spreading.

Treatment of Lung Cancers

Prognosis depends on—histological type of the tumor, stage of the tumor, and the general condition of the patient. Fitness to undergo resection of lung.

Best chance of cure is with—early detection and surgical resection.

Prognosis—5 year survival for early tumors—without nodes is 35 to 55-60% (as per T stage) and with significant nodal disease—it drops to below 15%.

Surgical Management of Lung Cancer

Aim of Surgery

- To remove the tumor and lymph nodes completely.
- To conserve as much lung as possible.

Selection: Early stage lung cancer (T1-3, N0-1), 90% of NSCLC survive for ten years.

Types of Surgical Resection

- Wedge resection or segmentectomy—for small peripheral tumors.
- Resection of the lobe (lobectomy)—lobar central tumors
- Pneumonectomy—for recurrent tumors and central tumors near main bronchus.
- Lung-sparing bronchoplastic or sleeve resection—for proximal endobronchial tumors to preserve normal parenchyma.
- Mediastinal lymph node dissection—for staging and locoregional control.

Complications of Lung Resection

- Bleeding
- Respiratory infection—basal collapse and hypoxemia
- Persistent air leak—and postoperative pneumothorax.
- Failure of lung to expand (collapse of lung)—required rethoracotomy.
- Bronchopleural fistula—more after pneumonectomy

Non-surgical Local Ablative Therapy

- **Radiofrequency ablation:** For small lesions <2 cm and metastases.
- **Targeted radiation therapy:** Stereotactic body radiation therapy (SBRT)—Syn: Stereotactic ablative body radiation (SABR).
  - As the first-line therapy for patients with resectable NSCLC
  - In nonoperable patients.

- **Chemotherapy:**
  - *Adjuvant chemotherapy:* After resection of early tumor larger than 4 cm (stage Ib) or higher-stage molecular profiling.
- **Targeted therapy**
  - Sotorasib—NSCLC—(non small cell lung cancers) with KRAS G12C mutations.
  - Erlotinib or crizotinib—for tumors with elevated levels—epidermal growth factor receptor (EGFR).
- **Immunotherapy**
  Immune modulation:
  - Monoclonal antibody against the programmed death ligand 1 (PD-L1) on cell surface membrane.
- Nivolumab—tumors with high expression of PD-L1, responded better to nivolumab.
- Pembrolizumab—against metastatic lung carcinoma expressing PD-L1 > 50%.

METASTATIC LUNG CANCERS

Pathology

- The biology of primary malignancy determines the behavior of its metastases.
- Metastases may be hematogenous, lymphatic or including direct extension to the chest.

Diagnosis

- 95% of pulmonary metastases remain asymptomatic as they are located in peripheral part.
- Diagnosis is usually made at follow up after treating primary cancer.

CT scan—helps detect nodules but subject to missing small nodule and false positives.

PET CT may detect smaller lesions; a new solitary nodule may be new primary lesions.

Staging

Parameters of prognostic significance: Resectability, disease-free interval, and number of metastases and site of primary tumor.

Long-term survival after metastasectomy

- Favorable tumors—sarcoma and breast, colon, and genitourinary metastases.
- Unfavorable tumors—melanomas and esophageal, pancreatic, and gastric cancers.

Note:
But the outcome is changing with newer modalities with chemotherapy, hormonal and targeted therapy, and immunotherapy.

Criteria for metastasectomy

- Should be completely resectable technically.
- Primary tumor should be controlled.
- Adequate lung reserve should be available after resection.
- Absence of extrathoracic metastases.

Treatment

Surgery

Parenchyma conserving procedures (wedge resection, laser, or cautery excision (to meet future risk of recurrent metastases and need for resurgeries).

Surgical Approaches

They include, median sternotomy, thoracotomy —posterolateral or anterolateral (as required) and VATS.

Procedures

- Wedge resections with a 1 cm margin.
- **LASER or cautery resections:** Lumpectomy—for multiple nodules in the lung.
- Anatomical resection—for central lesions attempting to conserve lung parenchyma.

Adjuvant chemotherapy and radiation for pulmonary metastases

Radiation therapy for pulmonary metastases:
- For palliation of symptoms due to extensive pleural, bony, or neural involvement.
- SBRT (Stereotactic Body Radiation Therapy) —for metastases from colon cancer.

Neoadjuvant or adjuvant chemotherapy—cis -platinum-based chemotherapy.

Surveillance

The follow-up protocols are as per primary tumors, need CT scans.

SU26.3: Describe the clinical features of mediastinal diseases and the principles of management.

MEDIASTINAL DISEASES AND PRINCIPLES OF MANAGEMENT

Anatomy of Mediastinum (Refer Figure 26.3)

Mediastinum is the central space in the chest—between the thoracic inlet(first rib) and the diaphragm below. Between the right and left pleural cavities, stretching between sternum in front and vertebral column behind.

It harbours the heart with the great vessels, trachea and esophagus, along with lymph nodes draining the chest. Also the thoracic duct, sympathetic chain run in the space.

Arbitrary Divisions

Depicted in the **Figure 26.3** and explained in **Table 26.5**.
- **Superior mediastinum:** Above a plane from sternal angle to vertebral column posteriorly T1 to T4.
- **Anterior mediastinum:** Lies behind sternum and to left of midline between sternum and pericardium between pleural membranes.
- **Middle mediastinum:** Pericardium.
- **Posterior mediastinum:** The space behind the pericardium, in front of the vertebral level T5-T12, below the plane of superior mediastinum and above the diaphragm.
- **Inferior mediastinum:** Mostly the lower recess of anterior mediastinum and its surgical importance is in respect of tumors and herniae.

A more practical and pragmatic division is division into three compartments:
1. Anterosuperior—anterior plus superior (inferior is also a part of anterior)
2. Middle—or the visceral (pericardium with heart and great vessels)
3. Posterior (posterior space)—includes para-esophageal area and paravertebral sulci.

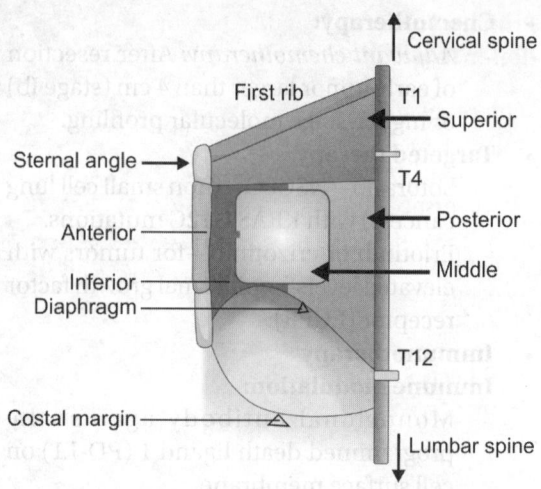

Fig. 26.3: Anatomy of mediastinum.

Table 26.5: Contents of (compartment wise) of mediastinum.

Compartment of mediastinum	Anatomical structures
Superior	Thymus, trachea, esophagus, great vessels, thoracic duct Both vagus nerves, recurrent laryngeal nerve, phrenic nerves
Anterior	Thymus, internal thoracic arteries and veins, parasternal lymph nodes Nerves—none
Middle	The heart and its great vessel roots, trachea and main bronchi ascending aorta, pulmonary trunk, pericardiacophrenic arteries vena cava, pulmonary veins, pericardiacophrenic vein Nerves—phrenic, vagus, sympathetic
Posterior	Esophagus, descending aorta, azygos hemiazygos veins, thoracic duct Nerves—vagus, splanchnic, sympathetic chain
Inferior	No major structures normally but hernia and tumors occupy this space

Primary Tumors of the Mediastinum
(Refer Table 26.6)

Clinical symptoms of mediastinal mass/tumors
Pain—chest
Compressive symptoms
Breathlessness—tracheal compression or displacement
Venous congestion (superior vena caval syndrome)—congested veins in neck, chest wall and upper limbs.
Hoarseness of voice—recurrent laryngeal nerve
Dysphagia—esophagus
Horner's syndrome—sympathetic chain
Late stage—diaphragmatic paralysis.
Pleural effusion
Haemorrhage, due to erosion of major vessels by malignant lesions
Specific to the respective pathology—like myasthenia gravis in thymoma or hypoglycemia in insulinoma

Diagnosis: Image guided biopsy or mediastinoscopic biopsy.

Imaging:
- CT Scan and MRI—for visualization of soft tissue and vascular lesions.
- FDG -PET scan.

Nuclear imaging in mediastinl pathology: Relevant to the mediastinum
- Fluorodeoxyglucose 18F (FDG -18 F) breast and colon cancer, melanoma
- Metaiodobenzylguanidine MIBG tagged iodine 123-I,131-I,- in pheochromocytoma, neuroblastoma
- Iodine 131-I, 123-I for retrosternal goiter, thyroid cancer
- Octreotide (iridium 111 tagged)—for neuroendocrine tumors (APUD)—medullary thyroid carcinoma carcinoid, pheochromocytoma, gastrinoma, insulinoma, glucagonoma, small cell lung cancer.
- **Monoclonal antibodies** 111In, 99mTc NSCLC, colon and breast cancer, prostate cancer metastases.
- Gallium 67Ga- Lymphoma, NSCLC, melanoma.
- Sestamibi 99mTc and Thallium 201T—differentiation of thyroid cancers and parathyroid tumors.

TREATMENT OF MEDIASTINAL MASS LESIONS (REFER TABLE 26.7)
Surgery
- Generally surgical excision or decompression.
- Radiotherapy or/and chemotherapy for lymphomas.
- Medical treatment to contain endocrine or paraneoplastic symptoms.

Q. Write a short notes on thymoma.

THYMOMA (REFER TABLE 26.8)
- Arises from the thymus gland—being the most common mediastinal tumor, (25%) in adults.
- **Pathology:** Variable—benign to aggressively invasive.
- Masaoka classification system to stage thymomas.
- Indicator of malignancy is capsular invasion.

Table 26. 6: Primary tumors of the mediastinum.

Primary tumors of the mediastinum (common tumors only)
Common: Thymoma lymphoma, neurogenic tumors and germ cell tumors

Tumor pathology	Adults incidence %	Children–incidence in %	Mediastinal compartment
Neurogenic tumors	20	40	Posterior
Cysts	20	18–20	All
Thymomas	20–25	06	Anterior
Lymphomas	13–15	20	Anterior/middle
Germ cell tumors	11–12	11–12	Anterior
Mesenchymal tumors	7–8	9–10	All
Endocrine tumors	06	-rare	Anterior/middle

Table 26.7: The surgical approach to mediastinal pathology.

Surgical approach to mediastinal pathology: Depends on the anatomical location of the pathology

Superior mediastinum	Transcervical (neck incisions) or combined with sternotomy
Anterior mediastinum	Median sternotomy
Posterior mediastinum	Posterolateral thoracotomy or VATS
Middle mediastinum	Through anterolateral thoracotomy or VATS

Table 26.8: Staging system for thymoma.

Masaoka staging system for thymoma

Stage I	Encapsulated tumor with no capsular invasion
Stage II	Capsular invasion or invasion into the mediastinal fat or pleura
Stage III	Gross invasion into the pericardium, great vessels, or lung
Stage IVA	Pleural or pericardial dissemination
Stage IVB	Lymphogenous or hematogenous metastasis

Clinical presentation

- (1) Myasthenia gravis, (2) mediastinal mass—compressive symptoms or obstruction (less common) of airway and esophagus.
- A myasthenic crisis may be the first manifestation.

Investigations: CT or MRI—chest mediastinum.

Diagnostic test for myasthenia: Acetylcholine receptor (AChR) antibodies in serum.

Treatment: Thymectomy—resection of thymus gland relieves Myasthenia gravis (MG) even when the thymoma is not demonstrated.

Transcervical approach or minimal access surgical approach through mediastinoscopy.
- Management of myasthenic crisis:
  - Emergency plasmapheresis.
  - Immunoglobulin to neutralize Anti Acetylcholine Receptor Antibody (AChR Ab).
  - Supportive ventilation and nutrition.
- Long-term control of myasthenic symptoms:
  - Pyridostigmine 600 mg /day or neostigmine tablets 15–30 mg every 6–8 hours.
- Immunosuppression to block formaton of AChR antibodies:
  - Azathioprine 50 mg/day or
  - Mycophenolate mofetil (MMF) 500 mg/day (anti T and B cells)

Germ Cell Tumor

- 12–14% of all mediastinal masses. Anterior mediastinal tumor.
- Most common site of extragonadal germ cell tumor.
- Contain elements from all three cell types (mesoderm, endoderm and ectoderm).
- Most (75%) are benign. Include dermoid cysts (teratomatous).

Clinical presentation

Young males with compressive symptoms—high levels of serum alpha-fetoprotein, human chorionic gonadotrophin and carcinoembryonic antigen suggest malignancy.

Treatment

- Chemotherapy
- Persistent mass on CT—needs resection
- If tumor markers fail to come to normal levels, chemotherapy is continued.

Lymphoma and mesenchymal tumors like lipoma are common in anterior mediastinum.

Thyroid

Retrosternal goiter is an extension from neck into anterior mediastinum.

Ectopic thyroid (and parathyroid) tissue—may be in anterior or/and posterior compartment.

Mass effect—airway compression and obstruction—stridor.

Treatment
- Cervical incision and excision.
- Larger ones require a median sternotomy.
- Neurogenic tumors arise from peripheral nerves or from sympathetic chain. They may be asymptomatic or with compressive symptoms, neurological deficit or due to catecholamines from pheochromocytoma or neuroblastomas.

Metastatic lymph nodes: Mimicking a primary mediastinal lesion.

Management includes management of primary lesion (as the case may be) and palliation of mediastinal compressive symptoms.

Arteries, Veins and Lymphatics

Chapter 27

Arterial System	
SU27.1	Describe the etiopathogenesis, clinical features, investigations and principles of treatment of occlusive arterial disease.
SU27.2	Demonstrate the correct examination of the vascular system and enumerate and describe the investigation of vascular disease.
SU27.3	Describe clinical features, investigations and principles of management of vasospastic disorders.
SU27.4	Describe the types of gangrene and principles of amputation.
Veins	
SU27.5	Describe the applied anatomy of venous system of lower limb.
SU27.6	Describe pathophysiology, clinical features, investigations and principles of management of DVT and varicose veins.
Lymphatic System	
SU27.7	Describe pathophysiology, clinical features, investigations and principles of management of lymph edema, lymphangitis and lymphomas.
SU27.8	Demonstrate the correct examination of the lymphatic system. Bedside clinics.

Arterial Diseases

Competencies SU27.1, 27.2 and 27.4 are considered together.
SU27.3 is discussed after SU 27.4.

OCCLUSIVE ARTERIAL DISEASE OF THE EXTREMITIES

This chapter deals with peripheral arterial occlusive diseases affecting the extremities.

Causes of Arterial Occlusion in Upper and Lower Limbs

Enlisted below in **Table 27.1**.

Etiopathogenesis

Arterial occlusion leads to ischemia of the part/organ supplied by the artery. The effects vary from organ dysfunction to infarction when the supply is totally cut off.

The impact of occlusion is related to the rapidity, extent and degree of occlusion and availability of a collateral/alternate source of arterial supply. The affected body parts/organs show pathological and clinical effects ranging between ischemia and infarction.

Table 27.1: Etiology of arterial occlusion.

Acute (sudden) occlusion	Chronic (slow and progressive) occlusion
Embolism (cardiac)—thrombus from MI, valve, atrial fibrillation Arterial—aneurysm, ulcerated plaque Paradoxical (venoarterial) embolism **Thrombosis**—arterial, dissecting aneurysm **Trauma** Blunt/crush/penetrating injuries, ruptured intima, vessel wall hematoma, external pressure by fracture or muscle hematoma Arterial lacerations/division Iatrogenic—angiography, plaster casts Acute compartment syndrome Vibration—mechanical/sonic Thermal Frost bites **Acute infective thrombosis** **Acute ergot poisoning**	**Atherosclerosis** **Arteritis** Thromboangiitis obliterans Polyarteritis nodosa (collagen diseases) SLE, Wegener's granulomatosis. Temporal arteritis (Takayasu) **Chronic vasospastic diseases** Industrial—hazard of vibrating tools) **Upper limb**—thoracic outlet syndromes Cervical rib Raynaud's disease Etiological factors contributing: Smoking Diabetes mellitus

Table 27.2: Rutherford's classification of acute ischemic limb.

Grade	Impact	Sensation	Doppler signal wave Artery	Doppler signal wave Venous	Need for revascularization to save the limb
I	Viable	Normal	Present (weak)	Normal	Can be done in 24 hours
II	Threatened	Paresthesia			
IIA	Marginally	Mild	Absent	Present	Prompt— 6–12 hours
IIB	Immediately	Severely	Absent	Present	Immediate needed within 6 hours
III	Irreversible	No sensation	Absent	Absent	Major amputation/resections needed

Clinical Features of Ischemia in Limbs

Summarised in **Table 27.2** above.

> Q. Discuss clinical features of ischemia of limb—acute and chronic.

> Q. Define acute ischemia and classify acute ischemic limb.

Acute occlusion:
Ischemic symptoms of less than 2 weeks.

Pain, pulseless, pallor, poikilothermia (cold), paresthesia, paralysis.

Gangrene of the limb (wet gangrene)—due to sudden occlusion, cell death and tissue edema and failed venous return.

Pain is sudden, severe and persistent. The limb is pulseless, pale, paralysed (nerve ischemia) and held down hanging by patient. **Rutherford's classification of acute ischemic limb—relevant for urgent treatment.**

Chronic Occlusion
- **Pain:** Intermittent claudication leading progressing to rest pain.
- Pain reduced by; dependency of limb: Dusky foot (sunset foot).
- **Skin:** Superficial painful ulcers. Skin turgor lost, nails brittle, hair loss.
- **Hyperesthesia**—indicates severe ischemia.
- **Temperature** changes—cold to feel.
- **Wasting of muscles** is an important feature ischemia (mainly gluteal, thigh and calf muscles)

- **Arterial pulsation**: Weak/absent pulsation.
- Bruit over arteries.
- Capillary circulation—delayed or absent
- Venous filling delayed
- **Dry gangrene**
- **Pre-gangrene:** Severe rest pain with color changes and edema.
- Raynaud's syndrome: Due to vasospasm in the arterioles (discussed in next section)
- In scleroderma, SLE, TAO, uncommonly in atherosclerosis.

Claudication

> **Q. Define and grade claudication. (Short note)**
>
> **Ischemic pain** (in the muscle)—due to metabolites including the p-substance and prostaglandins that irritate the nerve endings ("crying of dying nerves"). It is crampy burning and deep, worsened by activity and elevation of limb, relieved by rest. The limb held in dependent position to facilitate gravitational flow of blood. In lower limbs it is called claudication (claudicare – to limp). It is of burning type in skin.
>
> Claudication is classified as per severity of occlusion and degree of ischemia.
>
> **Boyd's classification**
> - Grade I: Pain on walking, disappears on continued walking
> - Grade II: Pain on walking but can walk with pain
> - Grade III: Pain on walking which compels the patient to take rest for relief.
>
> **Fontaine classification of chronic ischemia (clinical stages)**
> - Stage 1: Asymptomatic
> - Stage 2: Intermittent claudication affecting normal life
> - Stage 3: Rest pain
> - Stage 4: Ulceration or gangrene

GANGRENE

Macroscopic death of tissue with superadded putrefaction (due to saprophytes)

Causes of gangrene: Atherosclerosis, thrombosis and embolism, arteritis including TAO collagen disorders, drugs, trauma.

Contributors: Diabetes, smoking (Old mnemonic - RESTED—Raynaud's, Ergot, Syphilis, Thrombosis, Embolism, Diabetes)

Types of Gangrene

Dry gangrene— due to slow arterial occlusion (chronic ischemia) - ischemic part gets separated off the live part of the limb by the body's healing granulation tissue (blood vessels and fibroblasts) seen **typically as a line of demarcation.**

Signs of Gangrene

Loss of—pulsation, sensation, color (original) and function (limb).

The gangrenous part looks—black (iron sulfide), shrunken, sunken, shriveled, mummified with odor of hydrogen sulfide (due to saprophytic action on the heme molecule).

Line of demarcation—red line (of hyperemia) between the gangrene and live parts—separates the dead from live—made of live granulation tissue—capillaries and fibroblasts.

It is not seen in wet gangrene due to infection and microthrombi in the marginal vessels.

Wet gangrene

Usually follows sudden occlusion of artery and vein or death of tissue with infection.
- Seen in acute ischemia, traumatic gangrene, diabetic limbs
- Line of demarcation is absent
- There are skip areas of gangrene proximally and the definite levels are unpredictable
- Prognosis is worse due to risk of spreading proximally.

Gas gangrene: Due to gas forming clostridium group of gram positive anaerobic bacilli—*Clostridium perfringens Cl. oedematiens* and *Cl. septicum* and saccharolytic clostridia.

Tissue crepitus is typical—seen post-traumatic limbs (not a part of ischemia).

SIGNS ELICITED ON EXAMINATION OF ISCHEMIC LIMB

- Appearance—wasting, dry skin, gangrene if present
- Gait—painful, bearing weight on normal side
- Circulation—capillary filing delayed
- Absence of arterial pulsations
- From foot arteries to external iliac arteries palpated to localize occlusive site/s.
- Muscle wasting.

Buerger's Test and angle of ischemia:
- In a supine patient, elevate the leg until the patient complains of pain and measure the angle between leg and bed (normal upto 90 degree—reduced to less than 60 in ischemic limbs). The ischemic **feet will be pale** after holding in elevation for 2–3 minutes.
- Hypertension and thickened arteries in atherosclerosis
- **Cardiovascular system:** Arrhythmia, ischemic disease, valvular disease.

Short notes:

Ankle-brachial pressure index (ABPI)—ratio of BP at Ankle to BP at arm
- Calculated by dividing the systolic blood pressure at the ankle by the systolic blood pressure in the arm.

Lower blood pressure in the leg suggests occlusive peripheral artery disease (PAD).

Ankle Brachial Index:
- ABPI: 1–1.2—normal
- Below 0.9—warning of ischemia
- Below 0.7—significant ischemia
- Below 0.5—severe ischemia (0.4 and below—critical ischemia)
- Below 0.3—may be seen in gangrenous limbs.

Q. Define and discuss critical limb ischemia (CLI). (Short notes)

Criteria
- Rest pain with chronic claudication.
- Skin (mainly foot) ulcerations—non-healing and edema of foot
- Ankle Systolic pressure below 40 MM Hg
- ABPI—0.4 or less (<0.3 is usually in gangrenous limb).

Clinical features: Vary according to cause of ischemia and duration.

Treatment varies—from non-interventional treatment and revascularization to amputation for intractable cases.

Importance: Critical limb ischemia mandates urgent evaluation and revascularization of limb.

Levels of arterial obstruction and clinical presentation: In lower limb ischemia. Summarised below in **Table 27.3**.

Table 27.3: Level of arterial obstruction and clinical presentation.

Obstruction level	Claudication
Aortoiliac	Gluteal and upper thigh, with impotence
Iliofemoral	Thigh and leg, gluteal may be seen in some
Femoropopliteal	Thigh leg, foot

Clinical Features (Related to Degree of Occlusion and Morbid Anatomy of Limb)

These are detailed in **Table 27.4**.

DIAGNOSIS AND MANAGEMENT

Type and site (level) and degree of occlusive arterial disease, if possible etiology and clinical grade of ischemia. These provide the way to investigate and plan appropriate treatment.

Investigations
- **Blood:** Hemoglobin, cell counts, platelets, coagulation profile
- Blood sugar, HbA1c, renal function tests, lipid profile
- Specific tests for immunological diseases (ANA, pANCA)
- Urine analysis
- ABPI: Ankle brachial pressure index.

Colour Doppler study—allows visualization of flow—direction and arterial tree

Duplex scan: It is combination of B mode ultrasound and Doppler study

Doppler principle helps detect velocity of blood flow through arteries and assess sites and degree of occlusion (higher velocity indicates more severe narrowing).

Normal arterial flow wave is triphasic: A positive (systolic) wave, a second negative wave (early diastolic back flow) and a third positive wave (elastic recoil of arterial wall).

In occlusion, it is biphasic, then a monophasic in severe occlusion and flat in total occlusion.

Information obtained: Site, degree and number of occlusions in arteries and the state of collateral circulation.

Table 27.4: Clinical features vis a vis degree of occlusion.

Degree of occlusion	Pathology	Symptoms	For example, lower limb claudication Boyd's grade
Mild/partial	Compensated ischemia through collaterals or/and reduced function	None or mild	Pain on walking and disappears on walking. (Grade I)
Moderate and progressive	Failing compensation—inadequate collateral and progressive ischemia	Mild but persistent and may be progressive	Walks with pain and limps (Grade II)
		Persistent and severe	Compelled to take rest for relief of pain (Grade III)
Severe	Decompensated occlusion and ischemia minimal collateral supply	Critical ischemia threatens limb	Rest pain-persistent (Grade IV)
	With failed collaterals	Non-salvageable state Pre-gangrene	Pain, edema, hyperesthesia, blue black color
Total	Cell death with putrefaction	Gangrene	Loss of pulsation, circulation, sensation, color, function Black color by ferrous sulfide

Q. Write a short note on arteriography.

- Radio contrast imaging of arterial tree by injecting a radioopaque dye into artery.
- Dye used: Iodine containing—sodium diatrizoate.
- Indications:
  - Indicated only when a direct arterial revascularization procedure is planned.
  - Non-invasive Doppler duplex scan and CT angiography have replaced arteriography for diagnostic purposes.
- Contraindications (relative): Hypersensitivity to the contrst dye. Uncorrected coagulopathies and bleeding disorders, renal failure.
- Arteriography is classified as per the route of access to the artery and injection of dye.
- For example, for lower limb ischemia:
  - Direct puncture arteriography—ipsilateral femoral artery is punctured for a popliteal aneurysm or injury of femoropopliteal tree. Dye flows distally to depict artery.
  - Retrograde arteriography- (seldinger technique) Opposite (normal) femoral artery is punctured with a specially designed Seldinger needle and a catheter is passed proximally into abdominal Aorta. the dye is injected which flows into distal arterial tree (iliofemoral) on both sides. This is used to depict the occluded arterial tree on side.
  Also both sides can be studied.
  - Transbrachial femoral arteriography—brachial artery is cannulated and cather passed into descending aorta to inject the dye (used when the femorals are blocked or to study abdominal Aortic aneurysm.)
  - Trans lumbar Aortography—direct puncture of abdominal aorta through paravartenbral space.

Use: Depiction and recording of arterial tree with details of obstruction - number, site/s, and degree of blocks in artery/arteries. State of collaterals. Distal "run off" (see below).

Complications of arteriography: (Invasive procedure)
- **Dye:** Hypersensitivity and anaphylaxis.
- Acute renal failure.
- Paraplegia—due to spasm of spinal arteries due to entry of dye into the arteries following injection of dye into aorta.

Needle: Hemorrhage and periarterial hematoma—late pseudoaneurysm.
- Dislodged atheromatous plaque and distal embolism
- Thrombosis at site of puncture
- Dissection of artery and obstruction. Aortic dissection at lumbar site of puncture.

Q. Short note on distal run off.

It is the flow of dye in the arterial tree distal to the site of main (usually the first) occlusion. It shows state of the distal arterial tree which allows flow of blood to the ischemic part. A poor distal run off predicts a poor outcome of a an arterial reconstruction, bypass or stenting as the blood can't reach the distal ischemic tissue. But a good distal run off is due to patency of distal arterial tree and results of reconstruction are good.

Digital Subtraction Angiography (DSA)

This allows computerized subtraction of images of soft and bony tissues allowing clarity in delineating arterial image after injection of contrast and following the same to the limb vessels.

A catheter is placed in an artery by seldinger technique and dye injected. Computerised images with digital subtraction record the clear images. DSA is almost replacing direct angiography.

MRI and MR Angiography and CT Angiography

Help in depicting the arterial tree. Useful in aneurysms, angio malformations and tumors. Intravenous contrast is injected after a plain CT/MR imaging is done. Also these are complementary to an arteriography.

Q. Management of acute limb ischemia. (Long answer question)

TREATMENT OF ACUTE LIMB ISCHEMIA (ALI)—MUST BE STARTED IMMEDIATELY

Principles: Total arterial occlusion beyond 6 hours causes irreversible ischemia.
- Diagnosis and stratify (Rutherford grading I/II/III)
- Any fall in ABPI of 10 to 20% calls for immediate revascularization in lower limbs.
- Post-traumatic ischemia needs swift dealing with the injuries along with revascularization of limb and arterial repair.
- Non-traumatic acute ischemic limbs usually have a cardiac or large vessel source of emboli which need to be treated.

Treatment
- **Heparinization:** Intravenous heparin bolus 80 units. kg body weight (about 5000 IU) followed by and a continuous infusion at 16–18 units/kg monitoring of APTT (maintain between 60 and 80).
- Pain relief—analgesics are a must—preferably opioids—morphine.
- Emergency Doppler study—to evaluate—arterial injury/state of occlusion and stratify.
- Immediate—CT angiography—in Grade II and III.
- Intervention—act as per diagnosis.

Non-traumatic ALI
- **Embolism:** Fogarty catheter and balloon embolectomy (with distal thrombectomy
- **Thrombosis:** Thrombolysis and pharmaco mechanical thrombectomy.

Thrombolysis with streptokinase/urokinase. Followed by trans-arterial catheterization and thrombectomy/thromboembolectomy.
Intraoperative arteriography (for documentation of patency)
Intra-arterial nitroglycerine 100 micrograms to prevent vasospasm.

Post-traumatic ALI: Explore and act as per the cause:
- Relieve vasospasm—intra-arterial papaverine
- Evacuation of hematoma
- Arterial repairs/ arterial bypass (emergency grafting).
 Concurrent treatment of fractures and soft tissue injuries.
- Urgent fasciotomy in acute compartment syndrome—causing ALI.
- Transesophageal endoscopic ultrasonography (EUS) to study the heart and the aorta for possible sources of emboli.

TREATMENT OF CHRONIC LIMB ISCHEMIA

Principles: About three fourth of the patients can be managed by non-interventional methods
- **Diagnosis:** Stratification and cause of ischemia.
- Non-interventional management.
- Interventional management—radiological/surgical.

Treatment

General and Non-interventional Treatment
- **Lifestyle modification:** Total stooping of smoking in smokers.
- Modification of diet, exercise and yoga.
- Care of diabetes, mellitus, obesity, hyperlipidemia.
- Graded limb exercises to increase blood supply to limbs, e.g., Buerger's exercises.
- Coronary angiography and treatment—to improve cardiac output and mitigate limb ischemia.

Medications
- Peripharal Vasodilators (cAMP)—phosphodiesterase inhibitor: Cilastazole.
  - Nitroglycerin, xanthinol nicotinate.
- Antithrombotics—antiplatelet drugs—clopidogrel 70 mg/day or aspirin 75 mg/day.
- Statins, antidiabetic therapy and antihypertensive therapy as needed.

Interventional Treatment

> **Q. Endovascular interventional revascularization procedures.**

PTA: Percutaneous Transluminal Angioplasty and Stenting of the Occluded Artery
- Done under local anesthesia.
- Arterial puncture to pass a balloon catheter over a guidewire balloon dilatation of the occluded arterial segment and placing of a suitable stent (titanium/drug eluting/bio stent). Antithrombotic therapy is continued.
- Useful in patients with claudication, ulcers, critical ischemia and in reducing levels of amputation in gangrene.

Percutaneous angioscopic LASER atherectomy and stenting.

SURGICAL TREATMENT

Procedures: Depend on site and type of arterial block.
- **Localized and short blocks (less than 10 cm)—preferably single or few**
  - Endarterectomy—removal of intimal plaque with inner layer of media.
  - Thromboendarterectomy—removal of thrombus with endarterectomy.
  - Arterioplasty (e.g., profundaplasty)—after endarterectomy the arteriotomy is closed by a patch of vein or graft to widen the lumen of narrowed artery.
- **Diffuse, long segment or multiple blocks**
  Bypass grafting: A synthetic graft (generally PTFE) connects a patent proximal vessel to distal patent vessel and ensures flow, bypassing the blocked segment.

For example, aortofemoral bypass—for an iliac occlusion.

A good distal run off is crucial for success of all arterial reconstructions and bypass procedures.

Results: (Generally)

Good
- In those with Rich distal run off
- In proximal blocks, single blocks, short blocks
- In atherosclerosis.

Poor
- In those with multiple blocks
- In immune arteritis
- Poor results in blocks in lower leg and foot.

Amputations
- For gangrene—level of amputation varies according to level of cut off of arterial supply.
- Incapacitating rest pain in critically ischemic limb, where revascularization is not feasible or possible.
- **Sympathectomy:**
  - Temporary relief of vasospasm in arterioles of skin. No effect on rest pain
  - To overcome vasospasm in the skin and help healing of the ulcers
  - To save a flap viability in an amputation and thereby limit the amputation to a lower level.

Recent advances
- **Gene therapy and stem cell therapy:** Intra-arterial injection of stem cells has been used with success in stimulating vascularity in the muscles of the affected limb.

Same principles are applicable to upper and lower limbs—with respective regional anatomy of vessels and functions under consideration.

Q. Short notes on reperfusion injury.

Following revascularization, circulation is restored. This results in the formation of oxygen-free radicals, which damage the tissue, and accumulation and sequestration of WBCs in the microcirculation. This prolongs the ischemia and prevents flow of nutrients into tissues, causes tissue necrosis. Also releases intracellular byproducts of ischemia into circulation endangering life. More often seen in lower limbs than in upper.

Fasciotomies are performed during the arterial intervention to prevent reperfusion injury and compartment syndrome. If not done, fasciotomy should be immediately done post-operatively.

Q. Acute compartment syndrome. (Short notes)

It happens in the fascial compartments of the limbs—when the intracompartmental pressure exceeds capillary perfusion pressure (30 mm Hg)
- Post-traumatic tissue edema/muscle hematoma
- Post revascularization procedure.

This is the result from prolonged ischemia and delayed reperfusion causing cell membrane damage and the interstitial fluid accumulation in the necrotic muscles and nerve tissue.

Treatment: Fasciotomy.

Preventive: Should be done in all patients with acute limb ischemia of longer than 6 hours or combined arterial and venous injuries.

Therapeutic: Emergency four-compartment fasciotomy should be performed for lower leg compartment syndrome. Thigh compartment fasciotomies—indicated in ACS of thigh.

In the upper extremity, fasciotomies of the forearm and hand may be needed to prevent compartment syndrome after emergency revascularization.

Delay leads to tissue death and needs amputation.

AINHUM (Short Notes)
- Gangrene of a toe (usually 5th) or a finger due to progressive constricting ring at the root occluding the digital arteries.
- Etiology unknown.
- Treatment—usually amputation of the toe or finger.

Early recognition and division of the constricting band may save the digit.

VASOSPASTIC CONDITIONS AND ARTERITIS

Q. Short note on thromboangiitis obliterans.

Syn: Buerger's disease

Definition: Inflammatory thrombotic condition of arteries and superficial veins—characterized by: (1) Obliterative—arteritis of medium and small arteries, (2) Superficial thrombophlebitis and (3) Raynaud's phenomena.

Etiology: Believed to be of an immune mechanism against toxin in the beedie/cigar leaves.

Pathology: Panarteritis (all layers), periarteritis, phlebitis, arteriolar ischemia, thrombosis. Raynaud's phenomena are due to arteriolar spasm due to ischemia of vaso vasora of arterioles of fingers/toes with resultant loss of vasomotor tone.

Clinical Features
- Beedie smokers, mostly males of 25 to 45 years.
- Intermittent claudication—with progressive increase in claudication distance.
- Later stage—rest pain and gangrene.
- All four limbs can be affected but mostly lower limbs.
- Systolic pressure is mostly normal or lower.
- Absence of peripheral arterial pulsation—without thickening of vessel walls differentiates it from atherosclerosis.
- Associated phlebitis is less common and so are Raynaud's phenomena.
- Buerger's test is positive. The patient prefers to keep the leg hanging and dependent.
- Doppler study reveals multiple occlusions in any or many of the arteries. TAO commonly affects arteries of lower limb—femoral or its

distal branches. It affects arteries distal to axillary artery in upper limb.
- The large vessels like iliacs and carotids are spared (unlike atherosclerosis). The visceral arteries are also not affected (unlike in SLE and autoimmune arteritis).
- Arteriography shows a corkscrew pattern with occlusions, collaterals with a poor distal run off (but rarely done now after Doppler as there is no scope for arterial surgery).

Treatment

Strict advice to stop smoking, Buerger's exercise, vasodilators and aspirin.
- Sympathectomy has a limited role in temporary reprieve from skin ulceration.
- Placental extracts were used for the same.
- Omental pedicle transposition—to revascularize the limb to relieve rest pain (omentoplasty)
- **Amputations:** For gangrene and incapacitating rest pain—at various levels depending on the individual case.

Q. Short note on Raynaud's disease.

RAYNAUD'S DISEASE AND SYNDROME

- **Raynaud's phenomena**—cause the syndrome of Three features in digits:
- **Pallor (local syncope)** sudden vasospasm in arterioles—cuts off arterial supply
- **Cyanosis—local cyanosis**—capillary flow with deoxygenated stagnated blood
- **Redness with throb—hyperemia**—arterioles dilate and fresh oxygenated blood flows.

Due to vasospasm of digital arterioles following exposure to trivial stimuli—exercise, heat cold, vibration, climatic changes etc.

Raynaud's disease is a vasospastic disorder of unknown origin and sensitivity of digital vessels and arterioles of hands to trivial stimuli that trigger Raynaud's phenomena.

Clinical Features

Refer **Table 27.5**.

Differential Diagnosis of Raynaud's Disease

Collagen diseases (SLE, polyarteritis), acrocyanosis, TAO, occupation involving exposure to vibrating tools, Exposure to cold weather; atherosclerosis.

Table 27.5: Comparison of Raynaud's disease with Buerger's disease.

Raynaud's disease	Buerger's disease (TAO)
• Females in age group 25–45 years • Smoking is not a factor • Upper limb • No major vessels involved • No phlebitis • Gangrene is less common than in TAO.	• Males in age group 25–45 years • Beedie smoking is integral to TAO • Lower limb preferred (upper less often) • Medium and small arteries occluded • Phlebitis may be seen • Gangrene usual culmination

Treatment Raynaud's Disease

Main objective is to avert an episode of spasm by avoiding triggering factors and agents. Avoid exposure to cold.

Medications

- Vasodilators—Nifedipine, (calcium channel blockers), nitroglycerine and isosorbide.
- Angiotensin II—receptor blockers-losartan.
- Phentolamine—(alpha 1 blockers), prostacyclin.

Surgery (indicated for threatened gangrene). Thoracic sympathectomy T2/3 (sympathetic denervation of upper limb)—thoracoscopic route.

Collagen disorders frequently present with Raynaud's syndrome; Digital gangrene is common. Steroids and immunosuppressants are used for treatment.

Acrocyanosis: May be confused with Raynaud's disease but it is painless and not episodic.

Occupational vasospastic disorders—need change in working atmosphere in addition to therapeutic measures.

Q. Thoracic outlet syndrome (TOS). (Long or short question).

A clinical syndrome involving the upper limb due to compression of neurovascular structures to the upper limb at the thoracic outlet, made of the first rib and its osteomuscular attachments.

Features

- Neurological—85%
- Vascular—Arterial or venous
- Combined neurovascular.

Etiology and pathology: Essentially three syndromes (Refer **Figure 27.1**).

1. **Scalenus anticus syndrome**
   - Sclene triangle—boundaries: The floor is made by first rib, and sides by the scalenus anticus and scalenus medius muscles.
   - Contents—trunks of brachial plexus and 2nd part of subclavian artery.
   - Compression due to pressure by the scelenus anticus or a cervical rib which narrows the space.
2. **Costoclavicular syndrome**
   - Space between clavicle and first rib.
   - Compression due to clavicle—sagging shoulder in females. Bony callus after fracture of clavicle, hypertrophic subclavius muscle, any other swelling. Compresses cords of plexus and 3rd part of artery and subclavian vein (less common).
3. **Hyperabduction syndrome**
   - Hyperabduction syndrome (pectoralis minor syndrome) compression in the space between pectoralis minor and first rib.
   - Hypertrophied muscle, bony swelling.

Q. Short notes on cervical rib syndrome.

Cervical rib (extra rib)—from C-7 transverse process to the first rib—through the scalene triangle causes elevation of the floor of the triangle, narrowing the latter.
Females more commonly affected.

Types of cervical rib: Unilateral or bilateral; (more common)

- Complete from C7 transverse process to first rib.
- **Incomplete:** Partly grown into a bony lump—blind end
- Partly bone and fibrous—ending with a band
- A complete fibrous band replacing the rib. (common)

The trunks of brachial plexus and subclavian artery or/and veins- get compressed at their exit from the scalene triangle by the scalene muscles—first rib.

Subclavian artery—is compressed and it also rubs against the rib causing thrombosis, stenosis, and poststenotic aneurysmal dilatation. Thrombus forms in the dilated part of artery, releasing emboli into distal arteries.

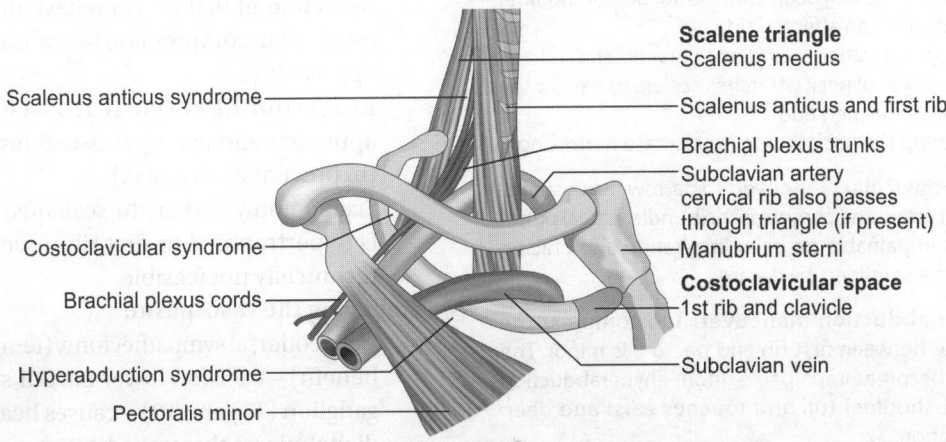

Fig. 27.1: Thoracic outlet syndrome pictorial display only-not actual.

Venous congestion or thrombosis may occur in subclavian or axillary veins.

The above may remain asymptomatic or cause thoracic outlet syndrome.

Diagnosis—X-ray/MRI neck for TOS (given below).

Clinical features of TOS (including cervical rib)

Neurological—more common.

Neuralgia along inner side of arm and forearm.

Later—weakness or wasting of small muscles of hands and hypothenar muscles.

Digital gangrene of little and ring fingers.

Arterial: Ischemic pain, vasospasm with Raynaud's syndrome

Pulsation: Adson's test positive if artery is patent or absence of pulsation (due to embolism and digital gangrene.

Venous: Arm edema and axillary vein thrombosis (uncommon feature).

Q. Clinical tests to diagnose thoracic outlet syndromes (TOS).

Adson's test: The patient's palpable radial pulsation on affected side, disappears upon performing the Adson's maneuver—diagnostic of scelenus anticus syndrome.

Adson's maneuver: Aims to narrow scalene triangle and compress neurovascular structures.
- Wide stretching of arm and abduction of shoulder abduction on affected side.
- Deep inspiration—to elevate first rib and
- Extension of neck (stretches sceleni to narrow the triangle further) and
- Turning the neck to side (to increase narrowing)

Costoclavicular maneuver: To narrow the costoclavicular angle and compress the bundle. Radial pulsation is impalpable on deep inspiration and bracing both the shoulders backwards.

Hyper abduction maneuver: Top compress the bundle between first rib and pectoralis minor. The pulse becomes impalpable upon—hyperabduction of the shoulder (till arm touches ears) and deep inspiration.

Differential diagnosis
- **Neurological** disorders like syringomyelia, peripheral neuropathy
- Vascular—occlusive arterial diseases
- SLE, Raynaud's, Ergot poisoning, occupational
- Embolism form heart, great vessels, aneurysms

Investigations
- Neurological evaluation of brachial plexus—including nerve conduction tests
- Doppler evaluation with duplex scan of great vessels and upper limb vessels.
- CT angiography/MR angiography—to study arterial occlusion.
- **Cervical rib:** X-ray neck, MRI neck.
- Blood tests—for anemia, diabetes, collagen disorders, systemic disorders.

Treatment
- Exercise to those with sagging shoulders.
- Advise to lose weight in case of hyperabduction and costoclavicular syndromes.
- Analgesics and neuroanalgesics (gabapentin).
- Vasodilators—nitroglycerin and cilostazol.
- Antiplatelets—aspirin.
- Surgery.

Surgery
Aims
- **Decompression of the neurovascular bundle**
  - Resection of first rib (to relieve the neurovascular compression)—transaxillary approach.
  - Resection of cervical rib—cervical approach and extra periosteal resection (to prevent recurrence.)
  - Scalenotomy—when the scalenus muscle is hypertrophied or first rib resection is technically not feasible.
- **Relieving the vasospasm:**
  - Cervicodorsal sympathectomy (temporary benefit)—excision lower part of stellate ganglion (T1) and T2)—causes healing of digital ulcers threatened gangrene. Thoracoscopic or supraclavicular approach.

- **Revascularization of limb:**
  - Arterial bypass
- **Surgery for complications**
  - Aneurysmal repair after resection of cervical rib
  - Amputation—for gangrene.
  - Fasciotomy—for acute compartment syndrome.

SU27.4: Gangrene and principles of amputation.

Note: Gangrene has already been discussed in previous section of this chapter.

Q. Define gangrene, types of gangrene and enumerate indications for amputation.

Amputation: It is a surgical operation to dismember an extremity or a part thereof.

General indications: As told classically in Bailey and Love's short practice of surgery.

- **Limb is dead:** Death of tissues due to Irreversible cessation of blood circulation.
  - Gangrene—arterial occlusion, venous gangrene.
- **Limb is deadly**: A threat to life—
  - Life threatening infections threatening septicemia, gas gangrene.
  - Wet gangrene with spread of infection, necrtising fascitis, severe cellulitis.
  - Malignancies—osteosarcoma, melanoma, some squamous cell carcinoma.
  - Arterio venous fistulas - causing cardiac failure.
- **Limb is a dead loss:** An encumbrance; better life can be given without the limb.
  - Post-traumatic—with irreparable tissue necrosis or sepsis.
  - Disasters with entrapped limb—(life saving on site amputations)
  - Severe rest pain with critical limb ischemia—uncorrectable or failed vascularization.
  - Severe elephantiasis of distal limb where a prosthesis is only hope to rehabilitation
  - Paralysis with severe contractures (e.g, polio) and fused joints due to any cause.

Accordingly amputations may be emergency or elective.

Level of amputation—is decided buy the indication viz., the disease, local anatomy of the limb (upper or lower) and the quality of rehabilitation and life after each type of amputation.

Philosophy of amputation:
- The amputation should serve the indication well.
- Length of residual limb should allow the best possible prosthesis and rehabilitation.
- Level of amputation should allow least possible dismemberment to allow the amputee to return to as normal a lifestyle physically and mentally as possible.

General technical considerations in limb amputations:

Types: Emergency or elective

Guillotine amputation: Done in emergency situation where the gangrenous part is removed (e.g., gas gangrene or post-traumatic gangrene). Line of division is through the skin, muscle and bone at the same level and stump is left open with the flaps to be closed later.

Flap closure: Primary or delayed (in infected cases like diabetic infective gangrene).

Flaps: Equal or unequal—usually long posterior flap. Ratio of anterior: posterior 1:2 with total length of flaps from level of amputation should be equal to circumference of the limb.

Types of Amputation stump

End bearing: Prosthesis is fitted on to the end.
Side bearing (non end bearing): Prosthesis fits to the sides of the stump and weight is not directly transmitted through end of stump to the prosthesis.

Ideal stump: It should
- Be cone shaped, rounded and non end nearing.
- Have a scar soft, supple and healed by primary intention.
- Not adherent to underlying tissues, bone or nerves, away from end bearing part.
- Have a mobile and functional joint above with normal joint sensation and normally functioning muscle action on the joint.

- Have normal blood supply and normal sensation.

  Have adequate length to allow a proper fitting of a prosthesis, e.g., minimum length recommended in lower limb amputations: Above knee: 7-8 inches—(20 cm from greater trochanter). Below knee—3-4 inches (7.5-10 cm) from tibial tuberosity. However current day prostheses are tailor made to the individual needs and lengths.

Types of amputations in practice

Lower limb: Toe amputations
- Metatarsophalangeal, tarsometatarsal or midtarsal amputations.
- Syme's amputation—calcaneum bears the weight after the fore foot s divided talonavicular joint.
- Below knee and above knee amputations.
- Disarticulation of hip and hind quarter amputation.

Upper limb:
- Fingers, forearm, above elbow, below elbow.
- Disarticulation of shoulder.

Principle steps of amputation:
- Marking line of bony division
- Marking skin flaps, incisions and raising flaps
- Division of muscles
- Division of nerves 5 cm above stump and ligation of vessels—artery is ligated first and then the vein.
- Suturing of muscles covering the stump—to make a cushion for skin.
- Skin closure with or without a drain (must in infected cases and optional in clean cases).

Complications:
Immediate: Hematoma, stump infection, flap necrosis, osteomyelitis and necrosis of bone.

Late: Scar adhesion to bony stump, cut end of nerve causing an adherent neuroma and pain. Contracture of the joint.

Phantom limb: Patient feels the existence of a limb after amputation and some feel a painful limb (painful phantom). Exact mechanism is not established but may be due to sensory stimuli from stump neuromas or inadequate analgesia during perioperative period. Setting a psychological cycle.

Difficult to treat, reassurance with psychotherapy needed. Carbamazepine is used.

Postoperative rehabilitation
- Stump care and dressing
- Physiotherapy to joint
- Crutches to walk
- Temporary prosthesis followed by regular prosthesis after healing of the stump wound.

Veins

> SU27.5: Describe the applied anatomy of venous system of lower limb.
>
> SU27.6: Describe pathophysiology, clinical features, investigations and principles of management of DVT and varicose veins.

APPLIED ANATOMY OF VENOUS SYSTEM OF LOWER LIMBS

Anatomy

Venous system of the lower limb—divided into the **superficial venous** system and the **deep venous system,** which accompanies the arterial branches, deep to deep fascia of the leg, connected by perforating veins.

The superficial veins of the lower limb: Anatomical variations are very common.

Two main venous trunks—the great (long) saphenous and the short saphenous veins arise from the dorsal venous arch on the foot.

Great saphenous vein (GSV) arises from medial end of the arch.

Runs anterior to medial malleolus and up the leg medial to tibia, along with saphenous nerve to curve behind medial condyle of femur before continuing in the medial thigh.

The GSV pierces the cribriform fascia in femoral triangle to join the common femoral vein (CFV)—at the saphenofemoral junction (SFJ), a point 3-4 cm below and lateral to the pubic tubercle.

Tributaries of GSV in thigh are variable before it joins CFV.
- Accessory (anterior) saphenous vein (ASV) is the major tributary—it arises at lateral side of knee and joins the GSV near the SFJ after ascending anteromedial to the GSV upto the thigh. It is often mistaken as a duplication of GSV.

The short (small) saphenous vein (SSV)—arises from the lateral side of the dorsal venous arch and runs posterior to the lateral malleolus and upwards in the leg accompanied by sural nerve. It runs in the posterior midline of leg, to join popliteal vein after piercing the fascia at the saphenopopliteal junction (SPJ)—in the popliteal fossa.

The position of SPJ is variable—the SSV runs under the deep fascia for a variable length in most cases to join at the level of knee or higher. It may continue beyond popliteal vein proximally to pierce the fascia of thigh to terminate in the deep veins of thigh; or the SSV may continue into thigh as the vein of Giacomini, which may terminate in the GSV (a few).

The deep veins of the lower limb:

Leg veins: Three pairs of venae comitantes, (six) accompany the three leg arteries (anterior and posterior tibial and peroneal arteries).

Popliteal vein—formed by the six leg veins in the popliteal fossa, also joined by the soleal and gastrocnemius veins.

The femoral vein starts as continuation of popliteal vein at the adductor canal and runs in the thigh—joined by deep femoral vein that joins about 4 cm below the inguinal ligament to form the common femoral vein, passes under inguinal canal to become external iliac vein after receiving the great saphenous vein in femoral triangle

Perforator veins (perforate the deep fascia of leg or thigh)

They are valved veins that allow unidirectional blood flow from the superficial to the deep venous system.

Perforator sites—not constant.

Calf—medial and lateral sets, around the knee and mid thigh.

Venous valves: They are in superficial and deep veins and allow unidirectional cephalad flow. Their failure causes stasis and congestion.

VENOUS PATHOPHYSIOLOGY

Importance of venous return: Venous system contains 60% of the total blood volume with an average pressure of around 5-10 mm Hg. The venous return impacts cardiac output by influencing myocardial contraction.

Venous return is influenced by mainly mechanical factors, stimuli from autonomic nerves and endocrine factors.

Intravascular Pressure gradient across the arteries to veins in lower limbs.

Arterial pressure at arteriolar end: 30 mm Hg, capillaries—about 12 mm at the venous end vein—10 mm at venules and falling gradually to 5 mm at the vena caval entry to right heart.

Standing Position

Effective venous return to the right atrium is ensured against a pressure of 100 mm Hg in erect posture, by a gradient of 200–300 mm Hg due to the following:
- Decrease in intrathoracic pressure during inspiration.
- Calf muscle pump—contraction of calf muscles containing deep veins during ambulation.
- **Filling of deep veins:** The venous pressure falls during the muscle relaxation and this sucks in the blood from the superficial veins into deep veins.

Finally the venous inflow is maintained normally at around 30 mm Hg.

VENOUS HYPERTENSION AND CHRONIC VENOUS INSUFFICIENCY (CVI)

Failure of mechanism of venous return and anti reflux— leads to stagnation and increase in venous pressure. This sets in a vicious cycle—through further structural damage to vein—dysfunction and destruction of valves, thickening and dilatation of vein with resultant loss of compliance and worsening of venous hypertension, and its ill effects—increase in capillary pressure, edema and irreversible damage to the soft tissues of the leg and foot.

CHRONIC VENOUS INSUFFICIENCY (CVI)

Q. Etiology of chronic venous Insufficiency.

Etiology

A. Congenital
- Absence or defective, incompetent valves.
- Defective venous wall.

B. Primary (i.e., cause undetermined), venous system dysfunction—valve or wall:
- Varicose veins—dilatation and tortuosity with elongation of the veins.
- Loss of venous tone and thickened wall.

C. Secondary (e.g., post-thrombotic, post-traumatic).
- Venous occlusion and compression
  - DVT—thrombus
  - Post DVT incompetence of valves
  - Traumatic
  - Iatrogenic
  - Arteriovenous fistula
- Deficient calf muscle pump function
  - Immobility, paralysis of muscles
- Other factors worsening the CVI:
  - Increased intrathoracic pressure: COPD, CCF
  - Increased intra-abdominal pressure
  - Tumors, ascites, pregnancy, constipation
  - Pelvic/abdominal radiotherapy

Q. Describe the pathology and soft tissue complications of varicose veins.

Pathology

Over 80% of chronic venous disease is due to reflux from incompetent venous valves.

Changes in the vein wall: Increased matrix metalloproteinases, inflammatory cell infiltration, decreased elastin content, collagen deposition smooth muscle cell proliferation.

Result: Rigid, non-compliant veins with dilatation and elongation and tortuosity.

Secondary valvular dysfunction: Due to vein wall changes.

Soft tissue complications:
- Skin changes—pigmentation, (hemosiderosis) and ulceration.
- Subcutaneous—lipodermatosclerosis (LDS)
- Telangiectasia—over malleoli.
- Eczema—an erythematous dermatitis.
- Chronic inflammation and fibrosis causing a 'woody' leg.

Soft tissue—edema
- This is 'pitting edema' in early stage
- Muscle hypertrophy and fibrosis
- Contractures of the Achilles tendon

Venous ulcer: Painful ulcer—due to periostitis—usually over malleoli ankle with features of venous hypertension and CVI.

CVI—includes the following pathologies:
- Telangiectasias
- Varicose veins
- Venous ulceration
- Venous claudication—bursting pain on walking.

> **Q. Describe the CEAP classification for chronic venous disorders.**

CEAP (Clinical-Etiology-Anatomy-Pathophysiology) classification for CVD (for chronic venous disorders)

C—Clinical classification - C0–6
C0: No visible or palpable signs of venous disease
C1: Telangiectasias or reticular veins
C2: Varicose veins; distinguished from reticular veins by a diameter of 3 mm or more
C3: Edema
C4: Changes in skin and subcutaneous tissue secondary to CVD
C4a: Pigmentation or eczema
C4b: Lipodermatosclerosis or atrophie blanche
C5: Healed venous ulcer
C6: Active venous ulcer

Symptoms: Aching, pain, tightness, skin irritation, heaviness, muscle cramps. Some are asymptomatic.

E—Etiological classification c, p, s, n
Ec: Congenital
Ep: Primary
Es: Secondary (i.e., post-thrombotic)
En: No venous cause identified

A—Anatomic distribution—s, d, p, n
As: Superficial veins involved
Ad: Deep veins involved
Ap: Perforator veins involved
An: No venous location identified

P—Pathophysiologic dysfunction—r, o, r o, n
Pr: Reflux
Po: Obstruction
Pr,o: Reflux and obstruction
Pn: No venous pathophysiology identified

Differential Diagnosis of Venous Disease
- **Lymphedema** presents with pitting edema without pigmentation and ulceration.
- **Arterial disease:** Painful ulcers generally at the tips of the toes with discrete edges and limb pallor on elevation. Patient has history of claudication and absent pulses.
- **Squamous cell carcinoma**—venous ulcers can mimick or turn into SCC.
- **Others:** Trauma, arteriovenous malformation (AVM), orthostatic edema.

Clinical Features
Varicose veins with involvement of only superficial system or perforators or deep venous system or in combination.

Factors influencing prevalence:
- Age—prevelance increases with age
- Gender—more women than men
- Familial susceptibility
- High intra abdominal pressure—pregnancy
- Occupation with prolonged standing—surgeons, nurses, barbers, policemen
- Smoking and obesity are associated with higher incidence.

Symptoms
- Vague heaviness and aching, in legs and thighs—worse in the evening upon lying down.
- Later—throbbing, burning or bursting over affected limb—worse on prolonged standing, and relieved by elevation.
- Itching and ankle swelling.
- **Skin changes:** Telangiectasia (not associated with malleolar flare and
- Reticular veins
- Venous ulcers.

Signs
- Tortuous dilated subcutaneous veins GSV in 70%, SSV in <25%.
- Trendelenberg test and tourniquet tests are performed to localize the incompetent valves— (SFJ/valves). The same principles are applied to test the Short Saphenous system too.

> **Q. Short notes on clinical signs of deep vein thrombosis.**

Signs of Deep Vein Thrombosis (DVT)
- Perthes test—bursting pain when patient walks with a tourniquet tied round the upper thigh
- Inverted beer bottle appearance—in a long standing post DVT limb with CVI.

- Calf tenderness and Homan's test (pain on stretching tendo Achilles) are features of acute DVT.
- Abdomen—mass, ascites, portal hypertension.
- Chest—COPD, cardiac failure.

Saphena varix: A soft reducible swelling due to large dilated veins around the SFJ.

Disappears in recumbent position and a thrill is palpable while coughing.

Diff diagnosis: Femoral hernia.

> **Short note:**
> **Complications of varicose veins**—CEAP classification considers these features.
> Bleeding, infection, skin changes, ulceration.
> Periostitis, equines deformity, squamous cell carcinoma in chronic ulcer.

Investigations

> **Duplex ultrasound scanning**—most accurate way—venous anatomy, valves, perforators reflux, obstruction
> **MR venography**—for secondary varicose veins, deep veins or variations in venous anatomy
> **Invasive**—(rarely done): Contrast venography
> Ascending venogram and descending venography
> **Intravenous ultrasonography (IVUS)**

Details of the investigations are given below.

> **Q. Short note on role of duplex ultrasound scan in evaluation of venous disease.**

Duplex ultrasound scanning—most accurate way to assess anatomy and complications.

The B-mode—gives a pulsed wave

Colour Doppler—shows blue for venous flow towards heart and red for reflux.

Doppler study is done to look for: Venous reflux in the superficial and deep venous systems, distribution of varicosities, state of venous junctions and perforators. Venous valvular competence, presence of acute or chronic DVT.

MR venography—for secondary varicose veins, deep veins or variations in venous anatomy.

Invasive (rarely done)

Contrast venography

Ascending venogram—superficial veins are occluded by a bandage to the limb and dye is injected into into dorsal vein of foot and bandage is released to locate the incompetence perforator. (Duplex scan has replaced it)

Descending venography—to record the dysfunctional valves in deep system by injecting dye into femoral vein asking the patient to do valsava maneuver.

Intravenous ultrasound (IVUS).

Management

Progress of varicose veins is unpredictable with reference to development of complications.

> **Treatment modalities**—many available with different outcomes in different patients: Selection varies on individual patient and choice of surgeons.

> **Compression treatment:** To reduce reflux and venous pressure.
> - Use of compressive elastic stockings during standing—desirable pressure 15–35 mm hg
> - Can cause skin necrosis, tourniquet effect and distal edema by improper application
> - Advocated only as an adjunct to interventional treatment or on temporary basis.

> **Endovenous ablation:**
> - Endothermal—LASER/RFA
> - Non-endothermal non-tumescent—USGFS (foam sclerotherapy)
> - Catheter-directed sclerotherapy and mechanicochemical ablation
> - Catheter directed endovenous glue (cyanoacrylate).

> **Surgery:**
> - Phlebectomy
> - Stripping
> - Trendelenberg operation
> - Subfascial ligation of perforatots (Cocket and Dodd)
>   **Minimally invasive surgery—SEPS** (subfascial endoscopic perforator vein surgery)

Details of treatment:

> **Q. Short note on endovenous thermal ablation (endothermal ablation) of varicose veins.**

This is replacing the surgical stripping of the veins in a large proportion of cases.

- Endovenous laser ablation (EVLA)—uses LASER as the thermal source.
- Radiofrequency ablation (RFA)—uses electromagnetic energy as thermal source.

Concept: A Thermal device is inserted percutaneously inside the incompetent vein to produce thermal energy causing permanent occlusion of vein.

Advantage over surgery: High efficacy, marginally safer, rapid recovery superior quality of life post-procedure, mostly an outpatient procedure under local anesthetic.
EVLA has lower recanalisation rates than RFA.

Disadvantage: EVLA can only ablate main veins but not minor varicosities and bunches.

Complications: Deep venous thrombosis.

Non-endothermal, non-tumescent ablation
Note: No heat used to ablate, hence no need for tumescent anesthetic injection.
- Sclerotherapy—injection of a sclerosing agent directly into the superficial veins, e.g., sodium tetradecyl sulphate causes—inflammatory sclerosis.

Q. Short notes on ultrasound-guided foam sclerotherapy (UGFS).

- **Ultrasound-guided foam sclerotherapy (UGFS):** The use of foam increases the effective volume of the detergent agent and improves endothelial contact of the foam. The foam is prepared with 1:4 sclerosant: Air (Tessari's method). This foam should be injected within 2 minutes.
  Application: Popular for recurrences and localized varicosities.
  Used also for main truncal varicose veins.
  Complications: Phlebitis, high recurrence, pigmentation.
  Advantage, less painful, no need for anesthesia, minor varicosities can be treated, can be done in ulcerated skin too, low cost
- **Catheter-directed sclerotherapy and mechanochemical ablation:**
  - *Concept:* Mechanical and chemical damage to venous endothelium
  - *Procedure:* It involves a device that deploys an angled wire from the end, connected to a motorized handle.
  - The catheter is placed within the lumen of affected vein lumen and liquid sclerosant is infiltrated via the catheter: The catheter is withdrawn while spinning the wire mechanically by triggering the switch.
  - *Indication:* This is done for main veins and combined with surgery for tributaries. (removed by phlebectomy).
- **Endovenous glue:** Endoluminal application of cyanoacrylate adhesive through an endovenous catheter and sealing the lumen by compression of vein.

Q. Principles of surgery for varicose veins.

Surgery for Varicose Veins (Refer Figure 27.2 for Varicose Vein Stripping)
- **Trendelenburg operation** (ligation of saphenofemoral junction and tributaries at the SFJ and great saphenous venous stripping.
- **Saphenopopliteal junction ligation and small saphenous stripping** is done to treat SSV incompetence.

Complications:
- Hemorrhage and, hematoma, infection.
- Damage to nerve during venous stripping to saphenous nerve (GSV) or sural nerve (in SSV).
- Damage to deep veins (common femoral or popliteal vein)
- Recurrence.
- Thromboembolism.
- **Phlebectomy**—removal of small veins.

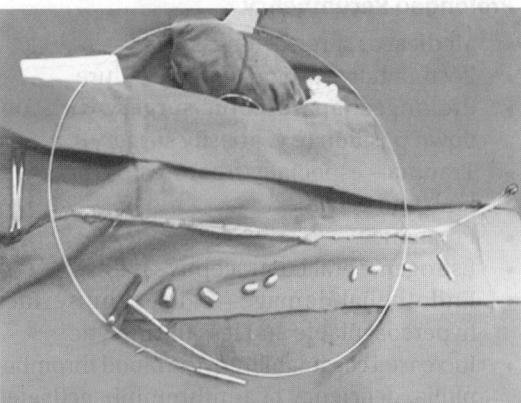

Fig. 27.2: Great saphenous vein stripped.

Indications: To treat localised varicosities and recurrent varicosities and as an adjunct to stripping of man trunks (GSV/SSV) and to endovenous mechanochemical ablation.

- **Perforator Ligation**
  - In patients with skin changes and ulcers
  - Subfascial ligation (Cocket and Dod operation)
  - Subfascial endoscopic perforator ligation surgery (SEPS)

Recurrent varicose veins: Very common and detected clinically in over 20% of the operated patients and by duplex scan in 50–70% more common in surgery for SSV.

Causes of recurrence:
- Neovascularization
- Reflux in residual main trunk of vein
- Failure of initial surgery.
- Reflux in a new site of venous junctions.

DEEP VENOUS THROMBOSIS (DVT)

> **Q. Etiopathogenesis, clinical features and management of acute deep vein thrombosis.**

- Acute DVT
- Chronic DVT—persistent etiological factors or undiagnosed/untreated acute DVT.

Etiological Factors

Virchow's triad of venous thrombosis:
- Abnormal surface (e.g. endothelial damage) blood in contact with the surface).
- Abnormal flow (e.g. stasis of blood);
- Abnormal blood (e.g. high platelet count)

Prolonged Recumbency
- Medical or surgical illness
- Postoperative period, cardiac failure
- Prolonged laparoscopic surgery with foot down position (e.g. obesity surgery)
- Trauma—especially fractures of the lower limb and pelvis
- Pregnancy
- Estrogen—oral contraceptive pill
- Endothelial damage—causes the surface hypercoagulable and less fibrinolytic
- Increased coagulability of the blood thrombophilia, deficiency of antithrombin, activated protein C.

Clinical Diagnosis of Acute DVT
Risk factors assessment including h/o previous DVT. Family h/o coagulatory disorders.

Clinical Presentation and Examination Findings

- Pain in calf or full extremity, swollen calf (increased circumference)
- Dilatation of superficial veins (of short duration)
- Pain on dorsiflexion of the ankle (Homan's sign)
- Tenderness over calf (Moses' sign).

Phlegmasia alba dolens represents a more severe form of DVT.
Most of the deep venous channels of the extremity are occluded sparing only collateral veins and some degree of venous return is maintained.
Patients present with edema, pain, and white appearance (alba).
Typically—seen in pregnancy or postpartum—due to compression of left common iliac vein.

Phlegmasia cerulea dolens—occurs with extension of thrombus into the collateral venous system, resulting in limb pain and swelling, cyanosis, a sign of arterial ischemia and finally leading to venous gangrene.

Chronic DVT presents with a post-thrombotic limb—turgid, pigmented with venous ulceration and considerable incapacitation. The leg has an inverted beer bottle appearance.

Investigation: Duplex scanning of limb (B-mode ultrasound with color Doppler imaging) Blood—coagulation profile, antithrombin, activated protein C and S.

Treatment of deep vein thrombosis
Aim:
- To reduce the risk of pulmonary embolus.
- To avert or minimize problems of post-thrombotic syndrome (PTS) limb.

1. **Anticoagulation**
   - Rapid anticoagulation under APTT monitoring
     - Therapeutic dose of low-molecular-weight heparin (LMWH) (e.g enoxaparin 7500–10000 or dalteparin

or unfractionated (plain) heparin intravenously (10000 units) followed by a contiuous infusion.
- Fondaparinux 7.5 mg subcutaneous—for patients sensitive to heparin.
- Bivalirudin (a direct thrombin inhibitor).
– Warfarin—started for long term anticoagulation with monitong of prothrombin time/INR
- Continued for 6 months or more if needed.
- NOACs—NOvel anticoagulants: Factor Xa inhibitors—rivaroxaban and apixaban; thrombin inhibitors—dabigatran.
2. **Inferior vena cava filter** on temporary basis—in patients who can't be anticoagulated to prevent embolism.
3. **Prevention of Post-thrombotic syndrome** (limb):
   – Thrombolysis (tissue plasminogen activator is injected into the thrombus through the vein.
   – Endovenous thrombectomy and stenting.
   – Venovenous bypass procedures. The results are unpredictable.

Venous Ulcers

Ulcers secondary to venous hypertension and its complications.

Etiology

They include—"the varicose ulcers" (superficial varicosities with ulceration) and "post-thrombotic ulcers"—secondary to the recanalized deep veins or and perforators.

Site: Varicose ulcers—usually at or around the malleoli—medial in GSV or lateral SSV. Post-thrombotic ulcers—lower leg, posterior or in front, usually multiple and small.

Complications

Infection

Painful walking—incapacitation, equinus deformity, periostitis.

Malignancy—squamous cell carcinoma on long-standing.

Differential Diagnosis

Arterial ulcers, malignant ulcers. Ulcers of collagen disorders, sickle cell disease.

Evaluation

- Duplex scanning of limb to study the system.
- Blood investigations for immunological and metabolic parameters.
- Cardiovascular system.

Treatment

> **Q. Short notes on Bisgaard's method of treatment.**
>
> - Rest and elevation, compression therapy—wake up to bed time- compression bandage
> - Dressing the ulcer—treatment of infection with systemic antibiotics and local dressing with topical antiseptics—povidone iodine, zinc oxide
> - Massage the muscles of calf
> - Exercise—active and passive

Intervention

- Sclerotherapy—foam sclerotherapy under US guidance is currently followed.
- Endovenous ablation for axial veins = Laser or RFA.
- Phlebectomy—incision and avulsion of dilated venous radicals from around the ulcer especially in post-thrombotic ulcers.
- ligation and stripping—for primary varicosity of main GSV /SSV or surgical.
- Subfascial ligation.
- Skin grafting for ulcer—split thickness graft.

Lymphatic System

> **SU27.7:** Pathophysiology, clinical features, investigations and principles of management of lymphedema, lymphangitis and lymphomas.
>
> **SU27.8:** Demonstrate the correct examination of the lymphatic system.

LYMPHEDEMA

Definition

Lymphoedema is swelling of a body part (limb) caused by the accumulation of high protein interstitial fluid secondary to inadequate lymphatic drainage (capillary filtration being normal).

Incidence—approx 1 in 5000 at birth.

Pathogenesis of Lymphedema

- Normally interstitial pressure is negative and lymphatic pressure is positive at rest.
- A transient rise in interstitial pressure above the lymphatic pressure causes a prograde lymphatic flow. A failure of this mechanism results in lymphedema.
- Retrograde increase in lymphatic pressure due to lymphatic obstruction or high abdominal pressure.

Pathology (Refer Table 27.6)

Note:
Lymphedema is exclusively extrafascial spares subfascial space.

Contrast: All other types of oedema may involve both epifascial and subfascial space—viz., cardiac, renal, hypoproteinemic or any inflammatory edema.

Venous edema—both capillary filtration and lymphatic drainage are defective.

Complications

Eczema, fungal infection, of skin and nails, fissuring, and warts lymphangiosarcoma.

Lymphangioma—due to dilated dermal lymphatics forming "blister'on the skin. They contain clear or blood stained fluid. They undergo thrombosis and fibrosis forming hard nodules and fibrose, forming hard nodules

CLASSIFICATION OF LYMPHEDEMA (REFER TABLE 27.7)

> **Q. Define and classify lymphedema.**

Clinical Features of Lymphedema

> **Q. Describe clinical features and grading of lymphedema.**

Making an early diagnosis is important because early measures can be highly effective at this stage to prevent the disabling late disease.

Stages

Reversible stage: Pitting and resolution on recumbency (morning).

Irreversible stage: Fibrosis, dermal thickening and hyperkeratosis.

Table 27.6: Pathology of lymphedema.	
Effects of lymphedema	*Result*
Lymphostasis and lymphotension	Stasis of growth factors and other active peptides, glycosaminoglycans and bacteria.
Accumulation of:	
1. Inflammatory cells (macrophages and lymphocytes)	Increase in protein-rich interstitial fluid edema fluid) deposition of ground substance
2. Fibroblasts	Fibroplasia due to collagen production with subdermal fibrosis
3. Activation of keratinocytes	Dermal thickening

Table 27.7: Classification of lymphedema.

Two main types of lymphedema:
1. Primary—cause undetectable clinically
2. Secondary

Based on severity: Lymphedema may be:
- Mild: <20% excess limb volume
- Moderate: 20–40% excess limb volume
- Severe: >40% excess limb volume.

1. Primary lymphedema: Three types—congenital, praecox and tarda
The cause is unknown or unproven—thought to be caused by 'congenital lymphatic dysplasia'. Congenital aplasia, hypoplasia, or hyperplasia of lymphatic vessels and nodes.

Based on lymphangiographic (or lypmphoscintigraphic) abnormality
- Aplasia (about 15%)
- Hypoplasia (65–70%)
- Hyperplasia-dilated lymphatics (10–15)

Types: Based on family history, age of onset and lymphangiographic abnormality:
- **Congenital primary lymphedema** (present at birth) 10 to 15% of all cases
  - Hereditary (Milroy disease) or nonhereditary.
- **Praecox** (early in life) or Meige disease—about 75%
  - Females mostly affected (80-90%).
  - Unilateral (70%) or bilateral.
  - Presents in teenage or 20s—swelling of the foot and ankle - worse on prolonged standing.
- **Tarda** (late in life)—10–15%
  - Both men and women affected
  - Age of onset—25 to 40 years.

2. Secondary lymphedema
- Caused by obstruction to lymphatic drainage by known factors. Infection—recurrent and chronic
- Infestation: Parasites—filarial lymphangitis and lymphadenitis (*Wuchereria bancrofti*)
- Infiltration: Malignancies—primary- lymphoma; metastatic carcinoma in lymph nodes
- Irradiation: Post-irradiation state
- Interruption: By injury to of lymphatics—post-traumatic
- Intervention: (Surgical), e.g., radical mastectomy, axillary or groin lymph node dissection

Clinical Classification: (Brunner)—Grading
- **Subclinical (latent):** Only pathological changes but no clinically visible lymphedema.
- **Clinical grade**
  - *Grade I:* Pitting edema, reducing or disappearing on elevation of limb. At rest.
  - *Grade II:* Non-pitting edema, no reduction on elevation
    - Stemmer sign positive (skin over the toe can't be pinched)
  - *Grade III:* Edema with irreversible skin changes, i.e., fibrosis, papillae.

Symptoms
- Heaviness of limb
- Tightening of clothes
- Visible thickening pain—mild to severe
- Generalized debility.

Signs
- Skin and subcutaneous changes—edema, thickening, nodules, ulceration
- Lymphorrhea
- Ulceration (rare but occurs when there is venous hypertension)
- **Malignant change (lymphangiosarcoma):**
  - Severely dilated lymphatics with lymphorrhea
  - Non healing ulcerated nodules and purple or red discoloration of nodules are suspicious of lymphangiosarcoma.

Differential Diagnosis of Lymphedema

Other local and systemic causes of limb swelling should be excluded.

Primary v/s Secondary

History and clinical examination.
Progress of lymphedema—slower in primary lymphoedema than in secondary lymphedema.

Investigations

- Evaluation for other causes of edema—heart, kidney, thyroid, liver, hypoproteinemia.
- Imaging studies—to evaluate lymphedema—cause and grade.

Lymphangiography (old practice)—injection of a radiopaque dye directly into lymphatic channels through a small catheter and recording by radiography.

Lymphoscintigraphy (has replaced lymphangiography)

- Radiolabeled (technetium- 99m) colloid injected into the second web space between the patient's toes. The patient exercises his limb and images are taken of the limb and whole body. Abnormal accumulation of tracer is seen in lymphedema.

CT scan and MR: To find any mass obstructing the lymphatic system.

MR scan: Also to differentiate lymphedema from

- Lipedema(excessive subcutaneous fat and fluid) and
- Chronic venous edema.

TREATMENT OF LYMPHEDEMA

Conservative Treatment

Objectives

Control edema, maintain health of the skin. Avoid infection—cellulitis and lymphangitis.

- **Medical treatment:**
  - Limited by the physiologic and anatomical nature of the condition.
  - Diuretics are ineffective—due to high interstitial protein content and fibrosis.
  - **Analgesia:** Non-opioids—paracetamol NSAIDs or Opioids: Codeine.

- **Combination of physical therapies (CPT)**
  Two-stage treatment: Skin care followed by the application of compression bandages
  Skin care and good hygiene.
- **Treating complications:**
  - **Eczema:** Topical hydrocortisone cream, fungal infections—topical fluconazole
  - Cellulitis and lymphangitis
    - I/V antibiotics to cover staphylococci and beta-hemolytic streptococci
    - Limb elevation and immobilization.
- **Surgical treatment**
  - **Aim**
    - To reduce limb size and restore limb function.
    - Restoration of lymphatic drainage when possible.
  - **Indications**
    - For functional impairment.
    - Intractable lymphorrhea with recurrent infections.
    - Risk of lymphangiosarcoma.

  Less than 10% qualify for surgical treatment and results are generally poor.

Procedures for Restoration of Lymphatic Drainage

Lymphatic Transposition

- **Direct**—lymphovenous bypass, (anastomosing the dilated lymphatics to veins)
  - Nodovenous anastomosis (lymph node to vein)
  - Lymphatic grafting
- **Indirect**—mesenteric bridge—omental pedicle transposition procedures.

Limb Reductive Procedures

Resection of hypertrophied subcutaneous tissue and thickened skin to reduce limb size to facilitate limb function.

- **Homan's procedure:** Staged resection of strips of subcutaneous tissue and dermal part by raising skin flaps and primary closure (high skin necrosis rates)
- **Sistrunk operation:** Wedge resection of skin and subcutaneous tissue and primary closure.

- **Charle's procedure:** Subcutaneous and skin removed down to deep fascia and split skin graft done.
- **Swiss roll cake procedure:** After resection the dermal skin flap is rolled in layers.

> **Q. Short note on acute lymphangitis.**

ACUTE LYMPHANGITIS

- Acute infection of lymphatic vessels
- **Common causative organisms:** *Streptococcus pyogenes, Staph. aureus.*
- The infection from an area spreads to the respective draining local lymphatics and further to the nodes with potential for systemic sepsis (septicemia).
- **Predisposing conditions:** Injury-trivial or severe, diabetes mellitus, filariasis.

Clinical Features
- H/o injury or infection of respective part.
- Pain and fever with chills.

Local Signs
Local warmth, tenderness, red streaks along line of inflamed lymphatic vessels.

Complications
- Immediate—septicemia.
- Intermittent and long-term—recurrent lymphangitis.
- Lymphedema, fibrosis and hypetrophy of the part.

Differential Diagnosis
Acute cellulitis (often coexist): Red streaks along the skin are absent in cellulitis and distal edema favour lymphangitis.

Investigations
- **Blood:** Polymorphonuclear leukocytosis.
- Blood sugars may be elevated.
- Ultrasonography of the part—to look for any underlying collection or cellulitis.

Treatment
- Intravenous antibiotics—penicillin and aminoglycoside or piperacillin.
- Rest and elevation of the part:
- Pain relief—analgesics— NSAIDs and antipyretic
- Drainage of abscess—if there is any.

Lymphomas

- A group of heterogenous malignancies of the lymphoreticular system with about 70 subvarieties.
- **The cell of origin:** Arising from stem cells leading to proliferation of the respective cell clones - from B-cell, T-cell or NK cells (natural killer cells).
- Lymphomas arise from lymphoid tissue anywhere in the body where is found.

The Major Sites

- **Lymph nodes:** Lymph nodes—including inside the chest, abdomen, and pelvis.
- **Spleen:** The spleen makes lymphocytes and other immune system cells.
- **Bone marrow:** Commonly affected.
- **Thymus:** It is important in the development of T lymphocytes.
- **Adenoids and tonsils:** More often affected in NHL.
- **Digestive tract:** The stomach, intestines, and many other organs.

They account for about 15% of all cancers in children.

Etiological Factors

- Genetic factors.
- Racial predisposition, e.g., Burkitt's Lymphoma in African.
- Infection:
  - *Viral:* HIV, Epstein-Barr virus, infectious mononucleosis.
  - *Bacteria: H. pylori*—claimed as having association with MALT lymp
- Familial syndromes, e.g., Sjogren's syndrome-30 fold increase of NHL.
- Ionising radiation, radiotherapy.
- Celiac disease and association with intestinal T-cell lymphoma
- Occupation hazards: Industrial chemicals—aniline dye workers;
- Smoking—higher incidence found.

Classification of Lymphomas (Refer Table 27.8)

> Q. Classify lymphomas. Describe clinical features and management of Hodgkin's disease.

WHO modified REAL (Revised European American Lymphoma) classification
(Simplified for easy reference) Must Know

Hodgkin's lymphoma (HL)

Predominant HL (HL)
- Nodular lymphocytic type

Classical HL (CHL)
- Nodular sclerosis CHL—most common
- Lymphocyte rich CHL
- Mixed cellularity CHL
- Lymphocyte depletion CHL

Non Hodgkin's lymphoma (NHL)
- **Immature (precursor) cell neoplasms**
  - **B-cell:** Acute lymphoblastic leukemia (B-ALL), lymphoblastic lymphoma (B-LBL)
  - **T-cell:** Acute lymphoblastic leukemia (T-ALL), lymphoblastic lymphoma (T-LBL)
- **Mature (peripheral) cell neoplasms**
  - **B-cell** origin: All B cell related non-Hodgkin's lymphomas
  - **T-cell and NK cell origin:** All T cell related non-Hodgkin's lymphomas

Precursor lymphoid neoplasms.
Immunodeficiency: Associated lymphoproliferative disorders.

Table 27.8: Classification of lymphoma.

Hodgkin's lymphoma (HL)	Non-Hodgkin's Lymphoma (NHL)			
	Behaviorally	**Microscopically**	**Lymphocyte cell type**	
	Indolent	Low grade	B-cell	T-cell
	Aggressive	Intermediate grade	Small cell	Low grade T-cell
		High grade	Large cell	Anaplastic T-cell

Non Hodgkin's Lymphoma

Two types—based on clinical behavior:
1. **Indolent**—slow spread and better prognosis
2. **Aggressive**—rapid spread and end.

Three grades—based on microscopic features—**low grade, intermediate and high grade.**

Q. Short notes on Burkitt's lymphoma.

BURKITT'S LYMPHOMA

Cell Type
- Medium-sized cells. Mainly affects children and more males than females.
- **Burkitt-like lymphoma**, has slightly larger cells but different chromosome changes.

Different Varieties of Burkitt's Lymphoma
- **African endemic variety:** Most are linked to infection with the Epstein-Barr virus (EBV) and Infectious mononucleosis: Tumor of the jaw or other facial bones.
- **Non-endemic or sporadic:** Some of these are linked to EBV infection. Usually present as a large tumor in the abdomen or also in the ovaries, testicles, or other organs. They can spread to the brain and spinal fluid.
- **Immunodeficiency-associated type of Burkitt lymphoma**—is associated with HIV or AIDS or who have had an organ transplant.
  Rapid growth and progress. But curable in over half the cases with intensive chemotherapy.

HODGKIN'S LYMPHOMA

It is of B-cell origin.
Age—bimodal—young and old (teenage and over sixty years of age.

Q. Short note on pathology of Hodgkin's lymphoma.

Affects lymph nodes—mainly neck, axillae, groin, mediastinum and peripheral, spleen, and later extra lymphatic spread and distant spread to liver, lungs, bone, brain, other organs.

Gross: Lymph nodes are fleshy, pinkish grey, and rubbery in consistency.

Microscopy: Lymphocytic infiltration, histiocytes, reticulum cells, and fibrous tissue

Dorothy-Reed-Sternberg cells: Diagnostic of HL
Giant cells with two large mirror image nuclei-**giving an "Owl eye" appearance,**
It is said to be modified germinal centre of B cells without normal surface antigens.

Q. Describe clinical features of Hodgkin's disease.

CLINICAL FEATURES OF LYMPHOMAS

Varies with stage and type of lymphomas.

General symptoms: Weakness, weight loss, loss of appetite, anemia.
- Lymph nodal mass in neck—node or nodes—discrete, soft and rubbery
- Mediastinal mass.
- Splenomegaly.
- Constitutional symptoms of prognostic importance—the B-symptoms—indicating poorer outlook.

B-Symptoms: Fever, Night Sweats, Loss of Weight (>10%)

Differential diagnosis of cervical nodes in lymphomas:
- Tuberculous lymphadenitis (matted nodes often, and abscess formation)
- Infectious mono nucleosis—tender and discrete nodes of recent origin
- Secondaries—head/neck malignancies—stony hard and non-tender, fixity to vessels (late stages)
- From papillary thyroid carcinoma—discrete, soft.

Q. Ann - Arbor staging for lymphoma. (Important)

Rationale of Ann Arbor staging: (Refer Table 27.9)
- HL starts in lymph nodes and spreads serially contiguously to other nodes/ nodal groups.
- Then the disease also involves spleen, the main centre of B- cells, the cell of origin of HL.
- Late spread is to other organs—liver, bone, brain, other organs like genitalia, thyroid, bowel.

Table 27.9: Ann Arbor staging for lymphoma.

Stage	Nodes and spread	B symptoms	E	S	SE
I	A node or nodes of single group	A-absent B- present	IE—limited contiguous extra-nodal spread	IS—node plus spleen	I–S + E = I–SE
II	Two or more nodes or groups of nodes on same side of diaphragm	A-absent B- present	IIE—nodes and extralymphatic spread on same side of diaphragm	IIS—nodes plus spleen	
III	Two or more node/groups—on either sides of diaphragm	A-absent B- present	IIIE—node and non contiguous extra-lymphatic site on either sides of diaphragm	IIIS—nodes plus spleen	
IV	Systemic spread or extensive no contiguous extranodal spread	A- absent B- present	Diffuse disease in liver, spleen, bone, brain, viscera, skin, etc		

Table 27.10: Comparison between Hodgkin's and Non-Hodgkin's lymphoma.

	HL	NHL
Incidence	More common	Less common
Age	Young and elderly (bimodal) Teens /20s and plus 60 (mean 35)	Generally 50 plus (mean 55 years)
Lymph nodes	Cervical nodes mainly Central and axial nodes, e.g., mediastinal, para-aortic, inguinal	Any node Generally more peripheral and diffuse nodal involvement Mesenteric nodes, often involved
	Discrete soft rubbery	Matting may happen
Nodal spread	Sequential and contiguous	Scattered and unpredictable
Peripheral nodes	Rare (e.g. epitrochlear)	common
Waldeyer's ring	Less commonly affected	Commonly affected
Splenomegaly	Very common	Less common
Reed Sternberg cells	Diagnostic	Absent
Treatment	Radiotherapy Chemotherapy	Mainly chemotherapy
Prognosis	Predictable and good for early stage	Variable with different varieties

- The prognosis is commensurate with spread of disease and hence the staging helps in therapy.

Four stages are described focusing on lymph nodes and extralymphatic spread and spleen.
- Each stage may be A **without B symptoms or B with B-symptoms.**
- Further suffixes indicate involvement extralymphatic sites(E) and spleen(S).

Q. Differences between Hodgkin's and non-Hodgkin's lymphoma (Refer Table 27.10).

Comparison between Hodgkin's and Non-Hodgkin's Lymphoma

INVESTIGATIONS AND DIAGNOSIS
Blood
- Blood counts, ESR, smear study (ALL, CLL, anemia)
- LDH—prognostic pointer
- Renal and liver functions.

Imaging
- Chest X-ray—to study mediastinal mass and lungs
- Ultrasonography
  - Neck to study nodes and thyroid
  - Abdomen—to study liver, spleen, abdominal nodes and pelvis
- CECT—abdomen and chest, neck
- MRI and PET scan—to study extranodal spread
- **Invasive investigations for diagnosis and staging:**
  - FNAC—node-not recommended—a complete node is needed to study structure for diagnosis of lymphoma and further for subtyping by immunohistochemistry.
  - **Node biopsy**—full node biopsy recommended.
  - **Immuno histochemistry**—for complete sub typing of lymphoma. IHC (Immuno Histo Chemistry) Markers in Lymphoma : CD 3 - for all T/NK cell lymphomas; CD 20 is a pan B cell marker. Ki-67 indicates cells in growth phase. CD 56 -NK cell lymphomas; Further details not covered .
  - **Bone marrow biopsy**—for staging and assessing response to treatment.

Staging laparotomy: (Short notes)

Indicated in Hodgkin's for staging before planning treatment.
Rarely done currently because the imaging studies (read above) have minimized the need for a staging laparotomy. **Laparoscopic exploration** provides a better option when needed.

Procedure
- Midline laparotomy, inspection
- Splenectomy
- Biopsies from—liver, ovaries, mesentery, omentum
- Lymph nodes—para aortic, celiac, mesenteric, iliac and bone biopsy from iliac crest.

TREATMENT OF LYMPHOMA

> **Q. Describe the treatment of lymphoma.**

Treatment of Hodgkin's Lymphoma
Modalities
- Radiotherapy (RT)
- Chemotherapy(CT)—ABVD regime
- Immunotherapy/targeted therapy—monoclonal antibodies
- Stem cell transplantation.
- Surgery: Splenectomy, bleeding organs.

Stage IA and IIA
- **Radiotherapy:** Mantle field or extended field radiotherapy:
- **Supradiaphragmatic disease**—Y field—mediastinum, neck both sides and axillae.
- Subdiaphragmatic disease: Inverted Y field—para-aortic, mesenteric, bilateral iliac nodes.

Stage IB and IIB - RT + CT
Chemotherapy recommended in addition in case of large mediastinal mass, High LDH, presence of "B " symptoms and severe anemia.

Stage III and IV
Chemotherapy or CT with immunotherapy (monoclonal antibodies).

Chemotherapy Regimens
- **ABVD regimen**—most common.
- Adriamycin (doxorubicin)—30 mg/sq mtr surface
- Bleomycin—10 mg/sq. meter
- Vinblastine—6 mg/sq meter
- Dacarbazine—(DTIC) 350 mg/sq. meter

AVD regimen: Without Bleomycin given with immunotherapy (Brentuximab - for CD 30 +ve)

BEACOPP regimen. Bleomycin, etoposide, adriamycin (doxorubicin) cyclophosphamide, oncovin (vincristine), procarbazine, prednisolone.

Other regimens—(less in use) Stanford V regimen: Adriamycin , bleomycin, vincristine, vinblastine, mechlorethamine, etoposide and prednisolone.

MOPP regimen (given up) mustine hydrochloride, oncovin (vincrisitne), procarbazine, prednisolone.

Treatment of relapsing HL: High dose CT with stem cell transplantation.

Immunotherapy and gene therapy—using retuximab or brentuximab with AVD.

Prognosis: 5 year survival St I and II: 80–85%, St IIIA: About 65%, St IIIB and IV: Approx 35–40%

Treatment of Non-Hodgkin's Lymphoma (NHL)

Treatment options in NHL
Depending on the type and stage of the lymphoma and other factors.
- Chemotherapy—CHOP or CVP regime
- Immunotherapy - monoclonal antibodies (anti CD 19, anti CD 20, anti CD 52), anti - CD79b antibodies); and immunomodulators
- Targeted therapy: Monoclonal antibodies or specific tumor cell enzyme inhibitors
- Radiation therapy is useful in the following conditions:
  - Prior to stem cell transplantation
  - For skeletal spread- spine and cranial
  - For stage I and II (selected cases)
  - Palliation of pain in skeletal spread
- High-dose chemotherapy and stem cell transplant
- Surgery—for localized NHL—splenectomy, thyroidectomy, gastrectomy
- Palliative and supportive care for non-Hodgkin lymphoma
  - Against infection: Antiviral and antibiotics, intravenous immunoglobulin (IVIG)
  - Against neutropenia, thrombocytopenia and anemia
  - Palliative care

Chemotherapy: CHOP or CVP regime

CHOP: Cyclophosphamide, doxorubicin (**H**ydroxydaunorubicin), vincristine (**O**ncovin) and **P**rednisone Or CVP - (CHOP less H—leaves out daunorubicin.
Chemotherapy may be combined with an immunotherapy drug, rituximab (rituxan).

Immunotherapy: Monoclonal antibodies—Retuximab/brentuximab—MAbs against cell proteins.
The MAbs target the surface proteins on the tumor cells (e.g.Retuximab)and kill them. Or they are given as carriers of a chemotherapeutic drug to deliver chemotherapy into the cell they target the cell.

High dose chemotherapy and stem cell transplantation
Used for aggressive and relapsing lymphomas.
- Prognosis: Over all 50% 5 year survival—generally worse than in Hodgkin's lymphoma
- High grade lymphomas like diffuse large B-cell lymphoma (DLBCL) and Burkitt's respond well to early therapy, but have a relapsing rates.
- The advances have led to better prognosis, with the immunotherapy and stem cell transplantation.

TIPS FOR EXAMINATION OF LYMPHATIC SYSTEM

Have a reasonably good knowledge of:
- Anatomy of the lymphatic system. General and with reference to a specific region/body system.
- Pathological conditions—affecting the region and general diseases with a local or focal presentation, e.g. TB—lymphadenitis in neck.
- History taking
  - General symptoms—fever, weakness, loss of weight and appetite
  - Specific symptoms—region or system—in the draining organs of the lymph nodal region.
    - Pain, swelllng, draingn areas (groin nodes are enlarged in pathologies of leg or urinary system and history should include both).
    - Other history—contributing to the diagnosis—family history of cancer
    - Treatment history
    - Endemicity—in filariasis, malaria.
- Examination
  - General examination—anemia, built, skin conditions
  - Lymph nodes—draining the area of the presenting part—consistency of nodes is important
  - Other nodal areas examination.

- Systemic examiniation—spleen, lever, genitals, chest and mediastinum, skeletal system including the spine and neurological examination.

Always Remember
- Lymphatics drain from deeper plane to superficial plane
- Veins drain from superficial to deep plane
- Red streaks are typical of lymphangitis
- A thickened vein is felt and seen in superficial phlebitis
- Lymphedema is superficial—hence distal and pitting
- Venous edema (deep vein obstruction) is more proximal, more over the muscular parts of limb and skin surface is turgid and brawny
- If there is any lesion, examine the nodes draining that region or organ and one nodal group more proximally. Also examine corresponding nodes on other side in case of extremities
- If there is a lymph nodal swelling, examine all areas/organs draining into that lymph node group.

Section 6

Hernia, Peritoneum and the Digestive Tract

- 28: Abdominal Cavity, Hernia and Digestive Tract
- 28.1: Hernia, Peritoneum and Retroperitoneum
- 28.2: Esophagus and Stomach
- 28.3: Spleen, Liver and Biliary Tract
- 28.4: The Intestines
- 28.5: The Vermiform Appendix
- 28.6: Tumors of Colon, Rectum and Anal Canal

Abdominal Cavity, Hernia and Digestive Tract

Chapter 28

28.1: HERNIA, PERITONEUM AND RETROPERITONEUM

SU28.1	Describe pathophysiology, clinical features, investigations and principles of management of hernias.
SU28.2	Demonstrate the correct technique to examine the patient with hernia and identify different types of hernias.
SU28.3	Describe causes, clinical features, complications and principles of management of peritonitis.
SU28.4	Describe pathophysiology, clinical features, investigations and principles of management of intra-abdominal abscess, mesenteric cyst, and retroperitoneal tumors.

HERNIOLOGY

HERNIA

This section mainly deals with hernia of groin and abdominal wall.

Definition

- Abnormal protrusion of contents of a container through a normal or abnormal opening.
- Abdominal hernia: Abnormal protrusion of any intra-abdominal structure through a normal or abnormal opening (or a gap) in the abdominal wall.

Types

- **Internal hernia:** Contents within the cavity entrapped in a gap within the abdomen. For example, diaphragmatic hernia or intra-abdominal-paraduodenal hernia.
- **External hernia:** Protrusion outside the abdominal cavity.

Sites of Abdominal Wall Hernia
(Refer Figure 28.1)

- Groin—inguinal hernia, femoral hernia, pre-vesical hernia
- Anterior abdominal wall (ventral hernia):
  - Umbilical hernia and paraumbilical hernia. Epigastric hernia.
  - Spigelian hernia (along the line of spiegel).
- **Incisional hernias:** Any part of abdominal wall after failed healing of a surgical wound.
- Others: Lumbar hernia—superior and inferior—through the lumbar triangles of Grynfeltt and Petit respectively, obturator hernia, gluteal hernia, perineal hernia.

ETIOLOGY AND PATHOGENESIS OF HERNIA

Hernia is the outward protrusion of the abdominal contents through an anatomical point of weakness in the abdominal wall effected

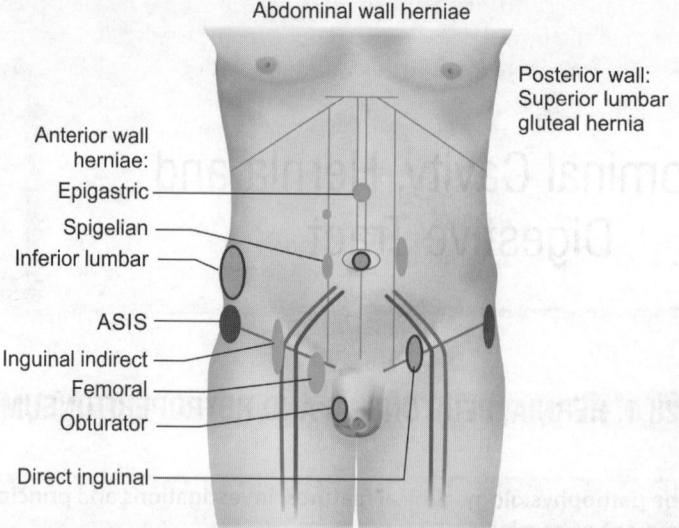

Fig. 28.1: Abdominal wall hernia sites

by the intraabdominal pressure. The abdominal wall is made of the three layers of muscle and a layer of fascia transversalis.

> **Q. Etiological factors contributing to the herniogenesis.**

Etiological Factors Contributing to the Pathogenesis of Hernia

- Weak fascial layers, particularly the fascia transversalis, due to inherited defective synthesis of collagen (there is a reversal of ratio of type I to/type III collagen, normal being 3:1).
- **Anatomical factors:** Structures passing through natural defects, e.g., vas deferens and gonadal vessels through inguinal ring femoral canal, obturator nerve. These gaps can be the site of herniation.
- **Developmental failure:** For example, umbilical defects due to failure of closure of umbilical scar.
- **Pathological factors:** Hematoma, injury, neurological disorders, myopathies, causing muscle loss or weakness.
- Surgical trauma—to abdominal muscles and fascia.
- Weakening of fascia and muscles—ageing and pregnancy.
- High intra-abdominal pressure—pregnancy, ascites, tumors, chronic cough, constipation, prostatic enlargement with BOO (bladder outlet obstruction), gymnastics and sports.
- **Metastatic emphysema:** Smoking causes weakness of musculofascial structure by altering the collagen characteristics (similar to inherited defective collagen).

Overall, hernia is a disorder of collagen and less a localized disease, initiated by various factors enumerated above.

Parts of an Abdominal Wall Hernia

- **Hernial sac**—made of peritoneum—has a mouth, a neck, a body and a fundus.
- **Coverings of sac**—abdominal wall layers.
- **Hernial contents**—bowel (enterecele), omentum (omentocele).
- **Extra peritoneal contents**—e.g., fat in a epigastric hernia, bladder or cecum in a sliding hernia.

Reducible hernia (uncomplicated hernia) is one where contents protrude and get reduced freely back into the peritoneal cavity.

Complications of Hernia and Nomenclature

- Irreducible hernia—contents can't be reduced and they stay outside.

- Obstructed hernia—irreducibility and occlusion of lumen of the bowel.
- Incarcerated hernia—an obstructed hernia with large bowel.
- Inflamed hernia—irreducible hernia with an inflamed peritoneal structure (e.g., inflamed appendix in a hernial sac or an inflamed fallopian tube).
- Strangulated hernia—irreducibility PLUS compromised vascularity of contents (leads to ischemia and infarction of the content).

Diagnosis of hernia involves knowledge of:
- Anatomy of the area concerned.
- Pathology of swellings from any structure in the area.
- Clinical signs—to diagnoses hernia and differentiate the same from other swellings.
- Look for complications in a hernia.

Diagnostic Feature of Any Hernia
- A swelling which appears upon causing a rise in intra-abdominal pressure—when the patient coughs, the swelling shows "an expansile impulse on coughing".
- Reducibility (in uncomplicated hernia).

PRINCIPLES OF TREATMENT OF HERNIA

Surgical repair of hernia is the only cure.

Aim—is to prevent complication of strangulation.

Goal
- Returning herniated contents back into the abdominal cavity.
- Prevent them from herniating again—by repairing the weakened area of the wall.

The abdominal wall is made of the three layers of muscle and an endoabdominal fascia (fascia transversalis). All hernia repairs aim at strengthening the weakened fascia transversalis and the transversus abdominis muscle, **with or without** a reinforcement with a synthetic mesh.

Those repairs without a mesh are called "tissue repairs" (suturing or darning techniques).

The reinforcement of the layers is done by placing a synthetic mesh, generally of polypropylene.
- Superficial to the fascia transversalis (ONLAY)
- Within the defect—"plug and patch mesh " (inlay)
- Deep to the fascia transversalis (SUBLAY), but superficial to peritoneum Or
- Intraperitoneally—intraperitoneal Onlay Mesh -(IPOM) repair.

The fibrous tissue grows through the pores of the mesh to help form a strong scar and prevent hernial recurrence.

Types of Mesh
Synthetic mesh: Non-absorbable
- Polypropylene knitted—most popular
- Polytetrafluoroethylene (PTFE)—woven
- **Synthetic absorbable mesh** (polyglycolic acid or polyglactin)—used only for temporary closure of abdominal wounds but not for hernia repairs.

Composite mesh for intraperitoneal use: To prevent adhesion between the bowel and mesh.

The surface facing the peritoneum is covered by a layer of absorbable material like cellulose or polyglactin and the muscle facing surface is polypropylene.

Biological mesh: Fibrous tissue without cellulose and non-immunogenic.

It provides a 'scaffold' for neovascular ingrowth and new collagen deposition. As the fibrous tissue matures, the host enzymes break down the biological implant to replace it with naturally formed remodeled fibrous tissue of the host.

GROIN HERNIAS (HERNIAE)

Groin refers to the area where the lower limbs join the main part of the body, including the area around the genitals.

Covers an area of anterior abdominal wall just above Inguinal ligament and the upper thigh just below (covering the femoral triangle) and the area covering the pubic crest, suprapubic area and root of the scrotum.

Anatomy of Inguinal Canal

Each of the inguinal canals, (right and left) is about 4-5 cm long, running obliquely from the internal inguinal ring, an aperture about 1.25 to 1.5 cm in size, just lateral to the inferior epigastric vessels, to the external ring, a triangular opening made of the pubic crest and the two crura of the external oblique aponeurosis.

Boundaries of the Canal

- Anterior wall—the external oblique aponeurosis, whose fibres run obliquely and medially.
- Floor—reflected fibres of the inguinal ligament.
- Roof—arching fleshy fibers of internal oblique and transversus abdominis which join medially to form the conjoint tendon, to be inserted to the pubic crest.
- **Posterior wall:** Fascia transversalis and partly by the arching fibers of conjoint tendon (medial part).

The deep (internal) inguinal ring is at the mid-inguinal point and lies lateral to the inferior epigastric artery and vein, which run upwards and medially to the rectus.

Hesselbach's Triangle

- Medial: Lateral border of rectus
- Lateral: Inferior epigastric vessels
- Base: Inguinal ligament.

SURGICAL ANATOMY OF FEMORAL HERNIA

> Q. Describe surgical anatomy of femoral hernia.

Femoral Ring
Boundaries

- Anterior: Inguinal ligament (Poupart's).
- Posterior: Iliopectineal ligament (Cooper's).
- Medial: Lacunar ligament (Gimbernat's)—sharp and often strangulates the hernial sac.
- Lateral: Femoral vein separated by a thin fibrous septum.

Surgical femoral ring: Lies about 1.25 cm above the anatomical femoral ring as a defect in the fascia transversalis.

Femoral canal—occupies the medial part of the femoral canal separated from the femoral vein by thin fibrous septum and opens at a about 2–2.5 cm lateral to pubis. This space contains fat and lymph node of cloquet. The femoral hernia occupies this space and projects through the opening, which the femoral hernia protrudes.

Femoral ring is large in a wider female pelvis and in elderly females with loss of fat.

> Q. How do you classify groin hernias?

> Q. What is European hernia society (EHS) classification?

CLASSIFICATION OF GROIN HERNIAS

Inguinal Hernia

- Congenital hernia:
  - Patent Processus Vaginalis (forming a congenital hydrocele in chidren)
  - Congenital hernia due to a preformed sac, vestige of the processus—young adults.
- Acquired hernia
  It is due to:
  - Herniation through the defective fascia transversalis.
  - **Indirect:** Through the deep (internal) inguinal ring.
  - **Direct:** Through Hesselbach's triangle.
  - **Combined:** Indirect and direct (Pantaloon hernia).
  - **Sliding:** An intra-abdominal organ (colon or bladder) forms part of a wall of the sac.

Femoral Hernia

NYHUS' CLASSIFICATION OF GROIN HERNIA

(Basis: Defect in fascia transversalis and its strength)

- Type I: Indirect hernia with a normal internal ring
- Type II: Indirect hernia with an enlarged internal ring
- Type IIIA: Direct inguinal hernia
- Type IIIB: Indirect hernia with posterior wall weakness (pantaloon hernia)
- Type IIIC: Femoral hernia;
- Type IV: Represents all recurrent hernias.

European Hernia Society (EHS) Classification

Nomenclature

- P - primary hernia, R - recurrent hernia.
- L - lateral/indirect, M - medial/direct,
  F - Femoral hernia
- Size: Assumed finger breadth = 1.5 cm
- X = not investigated
- 0 = no hernia detectable.
- 1 = smaller than 1.5 cm (one finger)

- 2 = less than 3 cm (two fingers)
- 3 = >3 cm (more than two fingers).

E.g: PF1 is primary femoral hernia 1.5 cm sac, RM2 is recurrent direct hernia 1.5–3 cm sac.

Special Types of Hernia

Depending upon the state of contents (**Refer Figure 28.2**).

(Each is a short question)

- **Littre's hernia:** Meckel's diverticulum in a hernia sac.
- **Richter's hernia:** A strangulated hernia with only a part of the circumference of the bowel stuck and strangulated. Here, there is no obstruction of the bowel. The patient passes loose stool and later, altered blood due to strangulation.
- **Amyand's hernia:** Inguinal hernia with acute appendicitis in the hernia sac.
  Amyand's triad: Acute appendicitis in an inguinal hernia and undescended testis.
- **Narath's hernia:** Femoral hernia with posterior dislocation of hip.
- **Maydl's hernia ("W loop" strangulation):** A strangulated hernia, where the bowel loop gets strangulated in the sac like a "W" shaped loop, the intraperitoneal component of the "W" undergoing gangrene.

> **Q. Short notes on Fruchaud's Myopectineal orifice.**

FRUCHAUD'S MYOPECTINEAL ORIFICE (REFER FIGURE 28.3)

Myopectineal orifice (MPO) is an area of lower anterior abdominal wall, covered by weakened fascia transversalis. It is the potential area for groin hernias.

Margins of this orifice:

- Lateral boundary—the iliopsoas muscle
- Medial boundary—rectus sheath and rectus abdominis muscle
- Superiorly—the arching fibers of transversus abdominis and internal oblique muscle and tendons.
- Inferior boundary—the ilio-pectineal line and cooper's ligament and pecten pubis.
- The MPO is overlies the preperitoneal space between fascia transversalis and peritoneum. (Bogros' space).

Application

- **Focus of hernia repair today is to repair the whole area of weakness and not just the hole in the weakened area, the site of herniation.**
- The MPO is dissected and reinforced in a preperitoneal repair—open or laparoscopic.

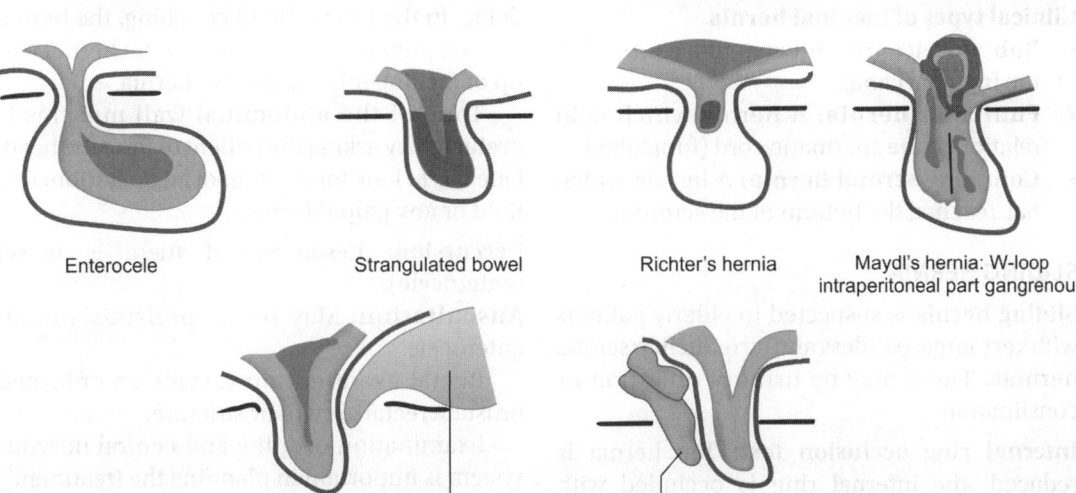

Enterocele   Strangulated bowel   Richter's hernia   Maydl's hernia: W-loop intraperitoneal part gangrenous

Sliding hernia bladder   Cecum

Fig. 28.2: Types of of hernia depending upon the state of contents

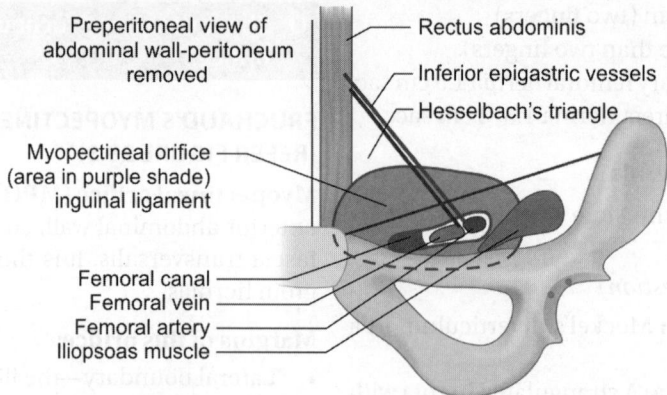

Fig 28.3: Fruchaud's myopectineal orifice.

INGUINAL HERNIA

Clinical Features

History: Swelling in the groin disappearing on lying down or history of the patient reducing the same, pain indicates adhesions or incarceration; severe and continuous pain along with persistence of the swelling is suspicious of strangulation.

Chronic cough, constipation and dysuria indicate straining. Details of strenuous work or sport may add to the assessment.

Signs: A reducible swelling with expansile impulse on coughing.

Clinical types of inguinal hernia
- **Bubonocele:** An indirect hernia confined to the inguinal canal.
- **Funicular hernia:** A hernia which is in relation to the spermatic cord (funiculus)
- **Complete scrotal hernia:** A hernia which has reached the bottom of the scrotum.

SLIDING HERNIA

Sliding hernia is suspected in elderly patients with very large, painless and, irreducible scrotal hernias. There may be urinary retention or constipation.

Internal ring occlusion test: The hernia is reduced; the internal ring is occluded with thumb. Patient coughs and is observed for appearance of hernia through the Hesselbach triangle (direct hernia). An indirect hernia won't appear on coughing.

Flaws: Wrong marking of the internal ring and overocclusion of the ring with thumb to cover lateral part of the Hesselbach's triangle where a small direct hernia may be missed and a pantaloon hernia will be misdiagnosed as a direct hernia, missing the indirect component.

Finger invagination test: The scrotal skin is invaginated gently with the little finger, which is pushed into the external ring, the ring just admits the little finger but is wider after the hernia has passed through the same, the finger is passed upwards and laterally - either it will feel the posterior wall made by fascia transversalis or will go backwards through the defect in the fascia. Upon coughing, the hernia hits the pulp of the finger in a direct hernia and tip of the finger in an indirect hernia.

Tone of the abdominal wall muscles is evaluated by asking the patient to raise the head. One has to look for any scar of an operation, free fluid or any palpable mass.

Percussion: Resonance if there is bowel (enterocele).

Auscultation: May reveal peristalsis in an enterocele.

Rectal examination reveals an enlarged prostate rectal growth or stricture.

Examination of spine and central nervous system is important in planning the treatment.

Respiratory system and cardiovascular stem are examined.

Femoral hernia: Easy to miss; narrow neck, cough impulse may not be present.

Seen below and lateral to pubic tubercle while inguinal hernia is seen above and medial.

Signs of strangulation of a hernia: Irreducibility, absence of cough impulse, redness and edema, tenderness, associated abdominal distension.

Q. Differential diagnosis of groin hernia.

Differential diagnosis of groin hernia

Inguinal hernia: Can be mistaken for:
- Femoral hernia
- Hydrocele in the scrotum
  - One can get above the scrotal swelling
  - Hernia is reducible and expands on coughing
- Varicocele, lipoma of the cord.

Femoral hernia: Mistaken for:
- Inguinal hernia, saphena varix, lymph node, lipoma, aneurysm, psoas abscess, rupture of adductor longus.

Investigations in Hernia: Diagnosis is Largely Clinical

- CT scan to find occult hernias, interparietal and abdominal wall hernias.
- MRI may show a hidden entrapped sac of hernia in cases with persistent pain.
- Evaluation of other systems, e.g. Marfan syndrome—hernia with aortic regurgitation.
- Ultrasound—abdominal mass, fluid, liver and kidney diseases, renal pathology.
- Post operative - ultra sound—collections in hernia wound.
- X-ray chest—to assess respiratory system.

General Investigations

- Blood—hemoglobin, sugar, renal parameters, liver function test, coagulopathies.
- ECG and echo cardiogram—before surgery.

Surgical Philosophy

- What is the treatment for hernia? Surgical repair.
- Why surgery? to avoid complications (strangulation) or to treat existing complication.
- Surgery for all hernias? Wherever the risk of developing strangulation is high.

- Which hernias have the high risk of developing strangulation?
  - Indirect hernia—have a narrow neck, run obliquely through the inguinal canal.
  - Direct hernia which protrudes through the external ring
  - Irreducibility of hernia—indicates adhesions or incarceration.
  - History of pain in hernia—indicates adhesions or obstruction.
  - Patients with high physical activity—sportspersons, laborers, any profession involving high physical activity.
  - Young patients.

"Must Surgery" when?
- Strangulation and any complication—immediate
- Reducible hernias with pain and difficulty in reducing the hernia.
- Sliding hernia with bladder (cystocele); colonic incarceration.

Observation "wait and watch policy"
- Hernias with wide neck (direct hernia), and those self reducing, pain free, hernias.
- Elderly patients with sedentary life style.
- Co-morbidities—cardio vascular of respiratory that increase morbidity of surgery.

Treatment

Inguinal Hernia

Principle

- Herniotomy—dissection of a the sac, reduction of contents and ligation of sac at its neck and excision of the distal part of the sac.
- Reinforcement of the posterior wall of inguinal canal (of fascia transversalis) to prevent recurrence with sutures (herniorrhaphy) or (generally) a synthetic mesh (hernioplasty).

Herniorrhaphy
- Repair of the posterior with the tissue available locally within the inguinal canal.
- Fascia transversalis, conjoint tendon and inguinal ligament or the iliopectineal ligament. These repairs are called the **Tissue repairs**, using sutures to approximate the structures to close the gap in front of the weak posterior wall so as to strengthen the

latter. Bassini's and Shouldice's repair are two classical examples.

Hernioplasty

Here the reinforcement is done using any material foreign to the inguinal canal.
Fascia lata, skin, or a synthetic mesh.
- Bassini repair-multiple interrupted sutures with non absorbable material (polypropylene or polyamide) appose inguinal ligament with conjoint tendon (with fascia transversalis as per Bassini).
- Shouldice's repair: Continuous polypropylene sutures are used in 4 layers incorporating (1) Repair of fascia transversalis—in two layers of—double breasting (overlapping) and (2) repair of muscle—in two layers—of approximating the conjoint tendon with the inguinal ligament—a deep and a superficial layer.

> Q. What is tension free repair? Explain with example.

TENSION REPAIRS

(Syn: Tissue repairs/suture repairs)
Here the approximation of local structures by sutures leads to fibrosis over 12 to 20 weeks. But the region is subject to abdominal pressure, constant movement and distraction of the muscles resulting in tension along the line of healing of the wounds. Hence these are called Tension repairs. This leads to wound failure and high risk of recurrence of hernia.

Tension Free Repair

Reinforcement of the defective wall is done by placing a synthetic mesh over the gap overlapping the edges of the gap by atleast 2.5 cm, to allow for shrinkage of scar. The mesh helps growth of fibrous tissue through its pores while holding on the healing edges "without tension".

> Q. What are the methods to deploy a mesh in a groin hernia repair?

Methods of Deployment of Mesh

Lichtenstein Mesh Onlay Tension Free Repair
- Polypropylene mesh is cut to size and deployed to cover and overlap margins of the defective fascial posterior wall of the inguinal hernia. Mesh is fixed to inguinal ligament below, rectus medially and conjoint tendon above, it is split laterally to encircle the spermatic cord and rejoined to sutured to the internal oblique laterally.

This procedure is **Considered gold standard**—has low recurrence rate, easy to learn and has a short learning curve.

Disadvantages:
- Risk of inguinodynia (groin pain) due to nerve entrapment —ilio inguinal. Ilio hypogastric or genitofemoral nerve in the mesh or fibrous tissue.
- Infertility due to ischemia of testis due to the entrapment of testicular vessels.
- Medial recurrences.

Preperitoneal Mesh Inlay (Sublay)

The myopectineal orifice (MPO) is dissected and a large mesh is deployed to cover the entire MPO, reinforcing the whole of weakened fascia transversalis and not merely the hole, thereby preventing any recurrence or occurrence of a new hernia—inguinal or femoral.

Methods to Deploy the Pre-peritoneal Mesh: Laparoscopic or Open

Laparoscopic
- TEP: Totally extra-peritoneal—pre-peritoneal mesh inlay repair— most popular.
- TAPP: Transabdominal (peritoneal) pre-peritoneal inlay procedure.
- IPOM: **Intraperitoneal** "Onlay"
The mesh is placed over the MPO with in the peritoneal cavity—done for recurrences after both laparoscopic ad open methods have failed.

Open
- Nyhus' Repair—supra inguinal approach—transverse incision
- Stoppa repair—for bilateral hernia—supra pubic transverse incision—Pfannenstiel incision—use of a single giant sized mesh
  - (30 × 20 cm) to cover MPOs on both sides.
  - Also called (Giant Prosthetic Repair of Visceral Sac- "GPRVS").

Q. Enumerte the complications of inguinal hernia surgery.

Complications of Inguinal Hernia Surgery

- Hemorrhage—at operation or reactionary due to slipped ligature.
- Infection—of mesh or wound.
- Recurrence—failed wound healing, failure of surgical technique in open mesh onlay.
- Nerve entrapment and groin pain—inguinodynia.
- Infertility—due to entrapment of testicular vessels and ischemic atrophy of testis.
- In laparoscopic repair—injury to bowel, bladder or iliac vessels.

Q. Diagnosis and treatment of femoral hernia (refer clinical features).

SURGERY FOR FEMORAL HERNIA

- Femoral hernias make about 8–10% of all abdominal wall hernias.
- Female—male ratio is about 8:1.
- Diagnosis is often made at laparotomy for intestinal obstruction.
- High degree of suspicion is needed.
- Surgery is advised early owing to the strangulation due to narrow neck of hernia.

Surgical Approach: Open or Laparoscopic

- **Laparoscopic approach** is preferred wherever possible.
- **TEP or TAP** and the MPO is reinforced with a large polypropylene mesh.
- Associated inguinal hernia can also be tackled.

Open approach:

- **Low (Lockwood approach):** Incision in the thigh just below inguinal ligament, dissection of the sac and reduction of contents with closure of sac.
  Repair by approximating the inguinal ligament to the Cooper's ligament.
  Modification: Currently, a mesh plug is inserted into the femoral ring.
- **Inguinal approach (Lotheissen approach):** Inguinal incision(similar to incision for inguinal hernia repair) is deepened through the fascia transversalis to dissect the femoral ring and the hernia.
  Repair of femoral ring by suture approximation of conjoint tendon to the Cooper's ligament.
  Modification: Currently, preperitoneal mesh is placed instead of the tissue approximation. The overlying fascia transversalis is sutured.
- **High (suprainguinal) approach (McEvedy's approach):** Open preperitoneal approach—oblique pararectus incision to enter preperitoneal space and dissection.
  Femoral ring is repaired by suturing inguinal to Cooper's ligament.
  Modification: A preperitoneal mesh is preferred to a suture repair.
- **Nyhus approach:** Supra-inguinal transverse incision and a preperitoneal mesh reinforcement of the MPO is done as for the inguinal hernia.

Q. What are the principles of operation for a strangulated groin hernia.

Strangulated Groin Hernia

- Emergency operation is required
- Incision over the inguinal area just 2 cm above and parallel to line of inguinal ligament which is extended upto the root of scrotum.

Inguinal hernia: The sac is dissected, opened and collected toxic/infected fluid is let out the constriction at external ring or internal ring is now released and contents of the sac inspected for gangrenous contents **(Fig. 28.4)**.

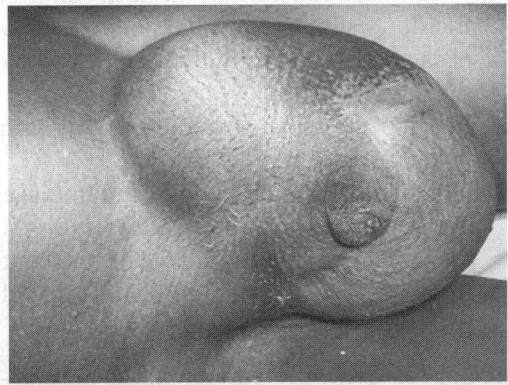

Fig. 28.4: Strangulated inguinal hernia.

Any gangrene of intestines requires resection and anastomosis, preferably through a laparotomy. Mesh repair is usually deferred and a simple suture repair is done to avoid wound infection and failure. A mesh is deployed only if there is no significant contamination or infection.

Strangulated Femoral Hernia

Inguinofemoral approach: Incision from above the inguinal ligament downwards to the upper thigh over the line of femoral canal. Dissection of sac from below and reduction by pulling inward from above the inguinal side (Resection of the strangulated bowel if needed).

VENTRAL HERNIAS

Umbilical hernia, epigastric hernia, lumbar hernia, Spigelian hernia and incisional hernia are included. Post-traumatic hernia also a type of ventral hernia.

> **Q. Short notes on umbilical hernia.**

Umbilical Hernia

Congenital—failure of umbilical scar to close.
- Most hernias subside with the closure of umbilicus by 1 year in 80% and another 15% by two years of age.
- Only the symptomatic, irreducible and strangulated hernias need to be repaired before 2 years of age. Persistent hernias after the age of 2 years are repaired surgically.

Mayo's repair: General anesthesia in children.
- Incision—subumbilical incision, dissection of sac, reduction of contents and closure of the sac.
- Repair of the defect—by simple sutures using polypropylene or
- By Mayo's operation in older children aged 5–10 years. It involves "double breasting" of the upper and lower lips of the rectus sheath in transverse axis using non-absorbable (polypropylene) sutures.

Acquired: Generally paraumbilical hernias—defects juxtaposed to the umbilicus.

- More common in females.
- Common association with—obese, post pregnancy, associated with hypothyroidism, cirrhosis, ascites.
- May present with as reducible hernia or with pain and irreducibility.
- Acute strangulation is often a complication.

Diagnosis
- Clinical diagnosis of hernia
- **Ultrasound:** To evaluate for intra abdominal mass or fluid, liver and kidneys, uterus and adnexa in females.
- Evaluation of the liver function and renal function, thyroid status, diabetes.

Treatment
Surgery is planned electively after optimizing comorbidities.

Surgical repair
- Mayo repair is not preferred due to very high rate of recurrences.
- Mesh repair is preferred
- Options:
  - Onlay patch
  - Retro rectus sublay of a large mesh
  - Laparoscopic—intraperitoneal onlay mesh (IPOM).

> **Q. Short notes on epigastric hernia.**

EPIGASTRIC HERNIA (SYN: FATTY HERNIA OF LINEA ALBA)

Small vessels in deep layer of the abdominal wall pierce the linea alba to reach the subcutaneous plane. These openings enlarge due to pressure and also obesity. The extra-peritoneal fat herniates through these openings to present as small and painful swelling in the supra umbilical linea alba. Usually there are multiple gaps. Uncommonly the sac may be large and containing omentum.

Clinical presentation—includes
Pain, swelling or only dyspepsia—more often postprandial discomfort or fullness with negative endoscopic evaluation reports and no pathology found at ultrasonography.

Treatment: Surgery involves reduction of the contents, closure of sac and repair of midline defect with polypropylene sutures and reinforcement by a mesh placed (by retrorectus sublay method).

Laparoscopic repair: The defect is identified by taking the falciform ligament down and then the extra peritoneal herniated contents are reduced; often multiple defects can be visualized, A repair is effected by placing a mesh—IPOM or a retrorectus sublay.

> Q. Long or short note on incisional hernia.

INCISIONAL HERNIA

They are very common (10-30%) after abdominal operations—emergency operations have a higher risk.

Etiology and Predisposing Factors

- Patient: Illness-poor nutrition or obesity, sepsis, immunosuppression-steroids, diabetes, post operative cough.
- Surgery and surgeon: Defective technique, wrong choice of suture material or its length.
- Wound: Unhealthy tissue, infection.

All incisional hernias begin to form early in the postoperative period. The musculofascial layers disrupt as the skin heals.

Even though the hernia may present in one site there may be multiple defects along the previous wound. The skin over the hernia becomes thin and atrophic. Dermatitis or sinuses of due to infected suture material may be seen.

Clinical presentation includes pain and partial obstruction—post prandial bloating, constipation. Some may develop acute obstruction or strangulation of bowel.

Investigation: CT and sonography help in recognition of the defect and associated unsuspected defects, contents of the sac, plane of the sac (interparietal) and state of intra abdominal contents.

Surgical Repair

Principles of Surgery

- Release of obstructing adhesions and freeing the abdominal wall.
- Identifying all the defects in previous wound.
- Creating plane for repair—through suturing and/or mesh placement.
- Repairing and reinforcement of entire length of wound.

Challenges

- Dense adhesions—damage to the bowel during dissection and the risk forming of readhesions.
- Loss of tissue planes and destroyed tissue resulting from previous surgery.
- Contents of a large hernia can cause high intra abdominal pressure and abdominal compartment syndrome (ACS). This can compromise respiratory movements, compress vena cava reducing the cardiac input and result in poor renal perfusion and oliguria.

Surgical Repair of the Hernia

Open surgery: Excision of old scar, release of adhesions and adherent bowel or omentum. Repair of incisional hernia by suturing the entire length of wound and placing the mesh.

Placing the Mesh - Options

- **Onlay:** Superficial to the sutured rectus sheath.
- **Retrorectus sublay:** A larger mesh is placed in a plane behind the rectus sheath—underlapping the length of previous wound by 3-5 cm all round.
- **Abdominal wall reconstruction (AWR) and component separation**—for a large and recurrent ventral hernia or one with multiple defects.

  Tissue planes are re dissected and recreated by dissection between the muscle and the fascia (endoabdominal fascia) far into the lateral side and giant sized mesh is placed in the pre-peritoneal plane. The anterior or posterior component of the rectus sheath is sutured to close the wound with non-absorbable sutures.
- **Laparoscopic methods:**
  - Adhesiolysis and returning herniated contents

- IPOM repair - a dual layer tissue separating mesh is fixed under the entire wound length covering all the defects and with adequate overlap.

Or

Component separation—incising the posterior rectus sheath and relaxing incision over the transversus abdominis to facilitate closure by suturing the edges of the rectus.

In presence of gross peritoneal contamination—a simple closure of the wound is recommended and no mesh is used.

RARE HERNIAS

> **Q. Short notes on spigelian hernia, lumbar hernia and obturator hernia.**

Spigelian Hernia

Herniation through small defects in the spigelian fascia (aponeurosis of transversus abdominis)—a line along the lateral border of rectus called the Spigel's line. The hernia protrudes and stays deep to the external oblique. There may be no palpable swelling at times.

Differential Diagnosis

- When there is swelling, a lipoma or a neurofibroma.
- Ultrasonography or CT scan—can assess the defect and plane of the swelling.
- Repair involves preferably a laparoscopic release and an IPOM or TAPP. For an extraperitoneal mesh fixation.

Lumbar Hernia

Herniation through the lumbar triangle—superior or inferior (more common).

Superior lumbar triangle (Grynfeltt-Lesshaft): twelfth rib above, medial border—the erector spinae (sacrospinalis) and lateral border—the posterior margin of internal oblique muscle.

Inferior lumbar triangle (Petit's): Boundaries: Iliac crest below, medial border—latissimus dorsi, lateral border—the external oblique muscle.

Primary hernia—less common.

Secondary—postoperative incisional hernias (renal operation or drainage of cold abscess).

Differential diagnosis
- Cold abscess from spine.
- Pseudohernia: Phantom hernias—post polio muscle paralysis.
- Lipoma.

CT scan—to evaluate the hernia, the spine and the abdominal wall.

Treatment: Surgical repair
- Open or laparoscopic repairs—with mesh fixation.
- TAPP: Laparoscopic mesh placement in extraperitoneal plane or open preperitoneal mesh repair.
- Open fixation.

Obturator Hernia

- Passes through the obturator canal.
- Often diagnosed for obstruction at laparotomy for intestinal obstruction.

Perineal hernia: Through the pelvic floor.

Gluteal and Sciatic hernia: Through greater and lesser sciatic foramina respectively.

PARASTOMAL HERNIA

- Herniation by the side of colostomy or ileostomy.
- It is due to widening of the muscle defect through which the bowel has been brought out. Weakness of musculo fascial layer.
- The hernia can develop obstruction.
- It poses difficulty in applying the ostomy bags.

Treatment: Surgical Options
- **Re-siting of colostomy:** Dissection of hernia, closure of stoma hole and shifting the stoma to another site.
- Suturing of the edges of the widened stoma defect and narrowing it with mesh reinforcement.
- Laparoscopic repair by deploying a mesh around the stoma with a central hole to accommodate the stoma loop.

THE PERITONEUM

> SU28.3: Describe causes, clinical features, complications and principles of management of peritonitis.

PERITONEAL CAVITY

This is the largest cavity in the body, with a surface area of 2 square meter. The peritoneum is lined by a single layer of mesothelium made of flattened polyhedral cells, resting on a thin layer of fibroelastic tissue with a rich network of vascular and lymphatic capillaries, nerve endings, and immune-competent cells, particularly lymphocytes and macrophages.

Normally, peritoneal fluid present is < 50 mL.

Two parts:
1. Parietal—lining inner aspect of abdominal wall.
2. Visceral peritoneum—covers the viscera.

Parietal peritoneum is supplied by somatic nerve endings and sensitive to pain, with accurate localization. Visceral layer is poorly innervated and pain is felt in umbilical area without localization.

Functions of the Peritoneum

- Pain perception—parietal layer
- Visceral lubrication—both layers
- Fluid and particulate absorption—(property made use of useful in peritoneal dialysis.
- Inflammatory and immune response
- Fibrinolytic activity.

Peritoneal Exudates
- Bacterial—appendix, TB
- Traumatic
- Chemical—bile
- Ischemia—vascular occlusion/strangulation
- Allergy.

PERITONITIS

Defined as inflammation of the peritoneum. The peritoneum, otherwise sterile environment, reacts to various pathologic stimuli with a fairly uniform inflammatory response.

Peritonitis may be—infectious/sterile (e.g., chemical/mechanical).

> Q. Describe etiology, clinical features and management of acute peritonitis.

ACUTE PERITONITIS

Localized or generalized.

Etiology (Refer Figure 28.5)

Primary Peritonitis: Spontaneous bacterial peritonitis **(SBP)**.

Secondary peritonitis—a septic focus is known.
- Bacteria—acute bacterial peritonitis—gastrointestinal or non-gastrointestinal.

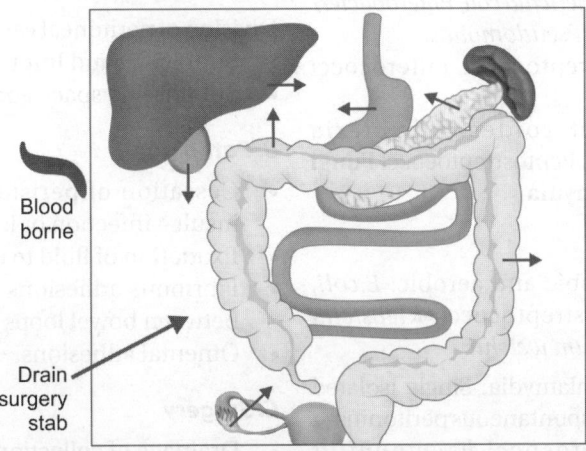

Fig. 28.5: Etiology of acute peritonitis.

- Traumatic—surgical or blunt trauma
- Bacterial translocations (transmural spread)
  - Acute pancreatitis
  - Inflammatory bowel, intestinal obstruction
  - Ischemia, e.g. strangulated bowel, vascular occlusion
- Allergic, e.g. starch particles.

Tertiary peritonitis—in immunocompromised patients with previous co-morbidities; in ICU patients.
- Chemical peritonitis—bile (without infection), barium.

Most cases, irrespective of the etiology, get infected by bacteria due to bacterial translocation from the intestinal flora.

Source of Infection
- Hollow viscus perforations: Perforated appendix, duodenal ulcer of gallbladder intestinal strangulation, ischemic bowel.
- Female genital tract—fallopian tube and vagina, pelvic inflammatory disease.
- Exogenous infection—surgery, trauma, dialysis, drains, catheters.
- Hematogenous infection.

Primary Peritonitis (spontaneous bacterial peritonitis)—generally due to a single organism. Mostly spreading from fallopian tubes or hematogenously from the lungs.

Microbiology of Acute Peritonitis

Bacteria Commonly Found
- Gram-negative: *Escherichia coli, Enterobacter/Klebsiella, Proteus, Pseudomonas.*
- Gram-positive: Streptococci, enterococci staphylococci
- **Anaerobic** -Bacteroides Eubacteria *Clostridium welchii*, Peptostreptococci **Fungi** Candida 2%, **chlamydia**.

Usually Polymicrobial
From GI tract, anaerobic and aerobic: *E.coli*, bacteroids, anerobic streptococci, *Klebsiella pneumoniae, Clostridium welchii*.

Non GIT-gonococci/Chlamydia: Single isolated strains seen in primary spontaneous peritonitis—pneumococci/streptococci, *haemophilus influenzae*.

Others: TB, secondary fungal colonization—in HIV and immunocompromised.

Pathogenesis
Bacterial numbers are more in distal bowel. When there is stasis and obstruction, proximal bowel also gets affected by more bacteria favoring the infection.

Gram negative bacteria secrete endotoxins (lipopolysaccharides) which act on the host causing the release of tumour necrosis factor (TNF) from leukocytes and its systemic absorption leading to endotoxic shock. Gram positive organisms produce exotoxins.

> **Q. Describe factors favoring spreading or localization of peritonitis.**

FACTORS SPREADING/DECIDING SEVERITY
- Speed, degree and duration of contamination, e.g, perforation and vigorous peristalsis and anything that stimulates peristalsis, enema, oral feeding.
- Age of patient—children and elderly
- General health—debility
- Virulence of organisms
- Nature of underlying cause
- Immunosuppressed states—HIV/diabetes/old age/steroids
- Disruption of localization.

Factors Favoring Localisation of Peritonitis

A. Anatomy
Division of peritoneal cavity into compartments:
- Supracolic and Infracolic
- Subphrenic space and pelvic

B. Pathology
- Cessation of peristalsis as a response to insult—infection or inflammation
- Exudation of fluid to dilute
- Fibrinous adhesions to contain infection—between bowel loops and to the parieties.
- Omental adhesions.

C. Surgery
- Drainage of collections
- Placing drains—to prevent spread.

Complications

Systemic
- Septic shock
- Pneumonia
- ARDS, renal failure
- Marrow suppression
- **Multiple organ system failure**.

Abdominal
- Paralytic ileus
- Bowel adhesions—obstruction
- Residual/recurrent abscess—pelvic abscess, subphrenic, paracolic
- Portal pyemia—liver abscess.

PERITONITIS: CLINICAL FEATURES

Localized Peritonitis (Refer Figure 28.6)
- Clinical features of the etiological factor (e.g., appendicitis)
- General features—fever/tachycardia
- Local: Guarding—rigidity-absent in pelvic or retroperitoneal and posterior sepsis
- Silent collection—localizing signs may be absent until too late in the course.

Generalized Peritonitis

Early: May resolve or localize
- Severe pain worsened by movement
- Tachycardia—progressive
- Tachypnea
- Temperature high

Abdomen
- "Still"
- "Rigid" and tender
- "Board"—like feel
- "Silent"—paralytic ileus.

Late Signs

> **Q. Short note on facies hippocratica.**

- "Silent" and progressive distension of abdomen.
- Circulatory failure
- Cold clammy extremities
- **Hippocratic facies**—"anxious look"
- Dry tongue, sunken eyes, hollow temple
- Circulatory collapse and death.

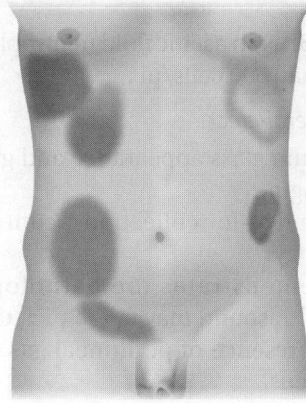

Intraperitoneal localised collections in peritonitis e.g., right and left subphrenic, right and left paracolic, pelvic, inter bowel collection

Fig. 28.6: Localised peritonitis

History and Examination

The diagnosis of peritonitis is usually clinical.
- 30% of patients are completely asymptomatic
- Fever and chills (80% of patients)
- Abdominal pain or discomfort—acute or insidious is the chief complaint in 70% of patients
  - Initially, the pain—dull and poorly localized (visceral peritoneum)
  - Later—steady, severe, and more localized pain (parietal peritoneum)

History should include recent abdominal surgery, previous episodes of peritonitis, travel history, use of immunosuppressive agents.
- Distension discomfort diarrhea
- Anorexia and nausea. Vomiting due to underlying visceral organ pathology (i.e., obstruction) or secondary to peritoneal irritation.
- Worsening or unexplained encephalopathy.
- Renal failure.

Assessment and Monitoring

Diagnostic Tests

Blood—leukocytosis
- Leukocytosis (>11,000 cells/µL),
- Coagulation parameters like prothrombin (PT) and partial thromboplastin time (APTT) along with liver function are assessed. Amylase may be elevated.
- Blood culture.

Peritoneal fluid

The predictor of SBP is an ascitic fluid neutrophil count of greater than 500 cells/μL.

X-ray abdomen-lateral/erect

For example, ground glass appearance and gas under the diaphragm.
- Ultrasound study—for collections, contributory pathology.
- CT- scan—demonstrates the pathology better as the ultrasound may fail to pick the pathology in presence of peritoneal gas or bowel gas in ileus.

Evaluation of Diabetes

Peritoneal aspiration—for culture, nature of collections.

TREATMENT OF ACUTE PERITONITIS

General Care
- Assessment—charts of vital parameters, input and out put, organ function.
- Access lines and circulation.
- Alimentation—fluid replacement and balance of electrolyte.
  Nutrition—intravenous until peristalsis returns and toxicity settles.
- Aspiration—nasogastric tube—to decompress the bowel and to take out toxic collections.
- Antimicrobials—broad spectrum—cephalosporin or piperacillin and metronidazole.
- Analgesia:
  - Additional support—against complications—ARDS—ventilator support or organ dysfunction, (e.g., dialysis).

Specific Care

Intervention in Peritonitis
- Diagnostic aspiration under image guidance. For bacteriology/assess contents/malignancy.
- Guided peritoneal aspiration of abscesses and lavage for general peritonitis
- Image (sonographic or CT) guided drainage of collections and tube drainage.
- Laparoscopic exploration, lavage and drainage.
- Open surgery.

Surgery

The goals of surgery
- To eliminate the source of contamination.
- To reduce the bacterial inoculum.
- To prevent recurrent or persistent sepsis.

Role of surgery
- Damage control—wash and drain.
- Definitive surgery—same stage/delayed.
- Re- look laparotomy.
- Repeated peritoneal lavage (laparostomy).
- Surgery for late obstruction/residual abscesses.

Details
- Laparotomy or laparoscopic exploration
- Drainage of collections, peritoneal lavage, removal of all exudates, leaving drains
- Definitive surgery for the cause—e.g., appendectomy, closure of perforation, release of intestinal obstruction, resection of gangrenous bowel or cholecystectomy.

Nonoperative Treatment

Treatment for primary pathology by non operative measures -
Pancreatitis, pneumococcal, streptococcal peritonitis.

Peritoneal Lavage
- Crucial in managing peritonitis to remove the toxins and pool of infection.
- Can be done with saline and antibiotic solutions and drains leaf behind.

Treatment of complications of peritonitis—as necessary (discussed in next section).

SPECIAL TYPES OF PERITONITIS

> Q. Short note on post-operative peritonitis.

Post-operative Peritonitis

Most cases follow surgery for intra-abdominal sepsis (e.g., perforations); but can occur after any laparotomy.

High morbidity and mortality can deteriorate rapidly to develop septic shock and multiple organ failure.

Early diagnosis and treatment are crucial to patient's survival.

Clinical Features

A post-operative state, where the patient "looks and feels "ILL".
Signs of failing peripheral circulation are seen: High pulse rate and gradually falling pulse volume until collapse.

Abdominal Signs

- **"Silent abdomen"** peristaltic sounds absent.
- "Delay" in return of peristaltic sounds.
- Important: In most of the cases show, there is **no localization of pain, and no guarding.**
- Tachycardia and failing circulation only raise the suspicion.

Investigation

- Leukocytosis.
- Elevated CRP.
- Sonography—fluid collections in peritoneal cavit or between bowel loops.
- Distended edematous and aperistaltic bowel loops.

Treatment

- Aggressive antibiotics, fluid and electrolyte replacement.
- Early surgery alone can save.
- Re-exploration, peritoneal lavage, and drainage of purulent collections. In addition, the pathology like a disrupted suture line may be tacked or a life-saving fecal diversion done.

BILE PERITONITIS

Cause

- Following biliary surgery, bile duct injury or leakage from T-tube.
- Leakage from GI anastomoses duodenal, gastric/pancreatic or jejunal.
- **ERCP complication:** Endoscopic perforations of duodenum or bile duct.
- Perforation of gall bladder, duodenum (ulcer or trauma) or jejunum.
- It has a high mortality due to infectivity and also to the loss of potassium ions.
- Signs of sepsis and biliary leak in the post operative period should warn the surgeon.

Treatment

- Immediate surgery—lavage, drain, look for biliary obstruction.
- Endoscopic or open—endo-stenting of biliary tree.
- Heavy antibiotic cover and maintaining the fluid/electrolyte balance.

Q. Short notes on Meconium peritonitis.

MECONIUM PERITONITIS
(REFER FIGURE 28.7)

(Also refer neonatal intestinal obstruction)

- Associated with muco viscidosis and meconium plug syndrome.
- In intrauterine life, the exudate calcifies in the peritoneal cavity.

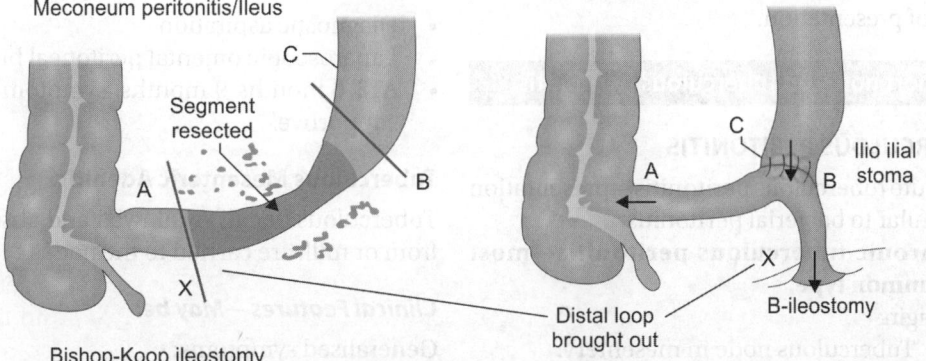

Fig. 28.7: Meconeum peritonitis

Pathology
- Usually due to perforation secondary to neonatal obstruction.
- Sterile to start with, later leads to bacterial peritonitis (3-4 hours).

Clinical Features
A new born baby with a tense abdomen, failure to pass meconium.

Diff. Diagnosis
- Intestinal obstruction due to other reasons in the new born.
- X-ray—calcification, gas and fluid shadows.
- Prognosis—bad due to associated sepsis, obstruction, bad lungs.

Treatment
Immediate laparotomy, resection of the obstructed long loop of ileum and a Bishop Koop ileostomy.

ABDOMINAL TUBERCULOSIS
- Mesenteric lymphadenitis
- Peritonitis
- Ileocecal, jejunoileal, gastroduodenal
- Pelvic
- Urogenital.

General Pathology of Tuberculosis
- Granulomatous infection—caseation
- Inflammatory response—exudation from peritoneal surface
- Fibroblastic response—adhesions
Combination of the above leads to various types of presentation.

> Q. Short notes on tuberculous peritonitis.

TUBERCULOUS PERITONITIS
- Acute tuberculous peritonitis—presentation similar to bacterial peritonitis.
- **Chronic tuberculous peritonitis—most common type.**
  Origin:
  - Tuberculous node in mesentery.
  - Tuberculous lesion—mesentery, ileocecal, pyosalpinx.
  - Blood borne from lungs—miliary or cavitatory.

Varieties of presentation:
- Ascitic—general ascites—distension
- Encysted—localized collection, with or without obstructive features.
- Fibrous—plastered loops generally causing intestinal obstruction.
- Purulent—presents like bacterial peritonitis, may be secondarily infected with bacteria.

Diagnosis
- High ESR
- Ascitic fluid tap—biochemical and microscopic analysis of ascitic fluid—exudates, lymphocytes
- AFB-Ziel Nielsen staining of ascitic fluid
- NAAT test - of ascitic fluid for TB
- Peritoneal biopsy—laparoscopic.

Treatment
- Antituberculous therapy and surgery—to relieve obstruction or to drain.
- Risk of surgery—adhesion, internal/external fistula.

Acute Type—Tuberculous Peritonitis
- Acute pain/fever/guarding.
- Serous fluid.
- Peritoneal/omental nodules/granulomas
  D/D: Acute bacteria peritonitis, pancreatitis.

Investigation
- Diagnostic aspiration
- Laparoscopic omental peritoneal biopsy
- ATT 6 months-9 months, symptomatic and supportive.

Tuberculous Mesenteric Adenitis
Tuberculous bacilli swallowed and absorbed—from or milk are carried to the nodes.

Clinical Features—May be:
Generalised symptoms:
- Abdominal pain-vague or "appendicitis" like pain RIF

- Intestinal obstruction—due to adherent loop
- Ileo-cecal lymph node mass
- Pseudomesenteric cyst (caseous nodes between mesenteric leaves)
- Asymptomatic but demonstrated radiologically.

Treatment: ATT; Surgery: to drain pus/relief of obstruction.

> SU28.4: Describe pathophysiology, clinical features, investigations and principles of management of intra-abdominal abscess, mesenteric cyst, and retroperitoneal tumors.

COMPLICATIONS OF ACUTE PERITONITIS AND INTRA PERITONEAL ABSCESS

Usually follows an attack of localised or diffuse peritonitis.

Preferred sites: (Refer Figure 28.8)
- Sub-phrenic
- Pelvic
- Paracolic—right or left side
- RIF/interloop.

> Q. Discuss sites and clinical signs of intraperitoneal abscesses after acute peritonitis

LOCALISED INTRA-ABDOMINAL ABSCESS

Signs vary according to the site and location of abscess **(Refer Figure 28.9)**.

Clinical Features
Symptoms
- Vague pain
- Fever
- Lassitude, anorexia, "unwell"
- Local features depending on location
- For example, shoulder pain in subphrenic abscess or mucus diarrhea in pelvic abscess.

Signs
- Tachycardia
- Distension
- Ileus
- P/R—bulge into anterior wall of rectum/vagina in pelvic abscess.

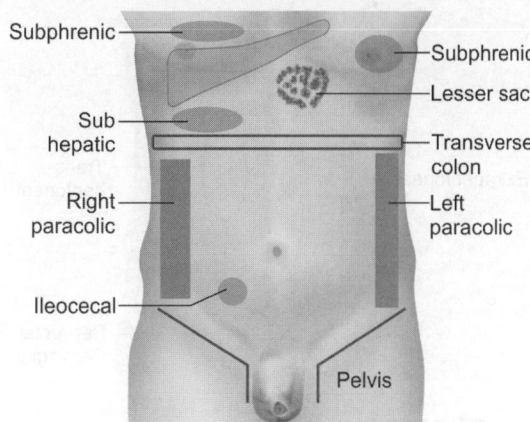

Fig. 28.8: Sites of intraperitoneal abscesses post peritonitis

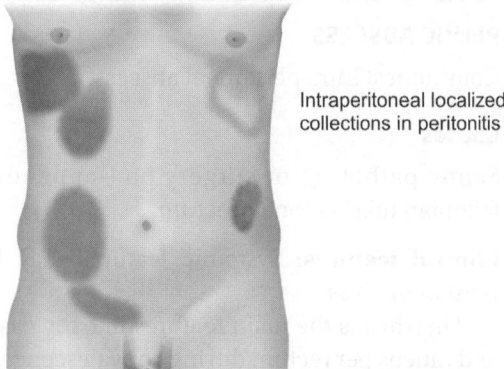

Fig. 28.9: Intraperitoneal abscesses.

Investigations
- Leukocytosis and elevated CRP levels
- X-ray
  - Erect posture (lateral decubitus (for an ill patient) shows free air and ground glass opacity
- USG/CT—diagnosis and serial monitoring.

Treatment—Peritoneal Abscess (Refer Figure 28.10)
- Antibiotic—to contain infection.
- Monitor—wait for localisation near abdominal wall.
- Aspiration—CT/USG guided.
- Open drainage
  - Extraperitoneal drainage
  - Transperitoneal drainage.

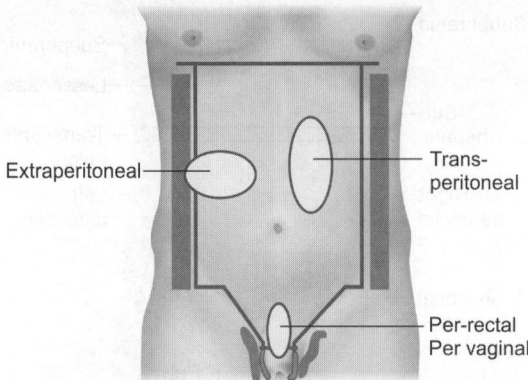

Fig. 28.10: Drainage of peritoneal abscesses.

Q. Discuss etiopathology, clinical features and management of pelvic abscess.

PELVIC ABSCESS

Commonest Intra peritoneal abscess.

Causes

Septic pathology or surgery on—appendix, fallopian tube, colon or rectum.

Clinical features: Systemic features may be present or absent

Diarrhea is the main features in early cases and mucus per rectum during convalescence.

Pathology and Consequences

- Abscess may rupture per rectally and resolve
- May worsen and rupture into general peritoneal cavity to cause septic shock.

Clinical features: Refer intra-peritoneal abscess.
- Fever, abdominal pain, difficulty to pass stools or urine may be there.
- Per rectal examination: Bulge and tenderness in the rectal wall.
- Laboratory: leukocytosis.
- USG: To detect and localize.

Treatment

- Antibiotics.
- **Drainage:** Per rectal drainage/vaginal drainage.
- Rarely laparotomy.

Q. Describe subphrenic spaces, etiology, pathology, clinical features and management of subphrenic abscess. (important)

SUBPHRENIC SPACES AND ABSCESS

- **Anatomy of subphrenic spaces:** (Refer Figure 28.11)
- **Subphrenic space** is the area between the diaphragm above and the transverse colon below.

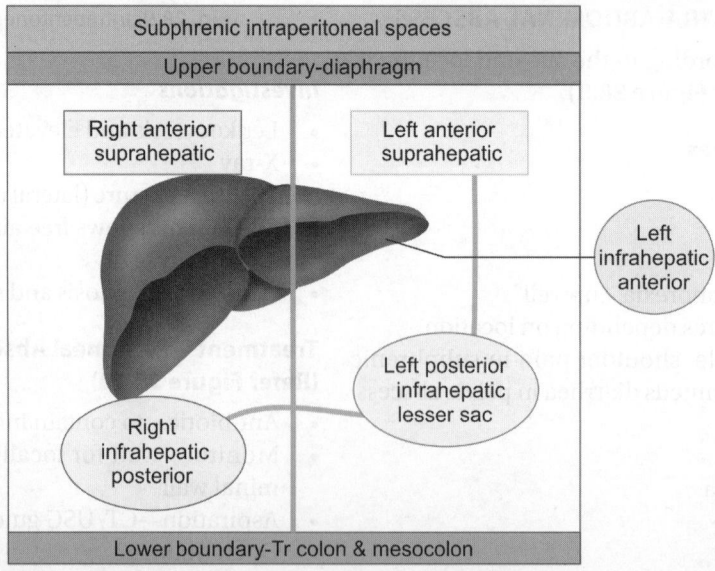

Fig. 28.11: Subphrenic spaces.

- **Subdivided into seven spaces: Refer Table 28.1**
- **Extraperitoneal—3 spaces**: Right and left perinephric spaces and the bare area of the liver.
- **Intraperitoneal—4 spaces**: As shown below.
- The falciform ligament divides it into left and right and liver into supra and infrahepatic.
- Left suprahepatic and infrahepatic spaces are generally inter communicating.
- Lesser omentum divides this space into anterior and posterior (lesser sac) infrahepatic.

SUBDIAPHRAGMATIC ABSCESS (REFER FIGURE 28.12)

Etiology of subphrenic abscess—usually follows peritonitis **(Refer Table 28.2)**.

Table: 28.1 Anatomy of subphrenic spaces.

Intraperitoneal spaces	
Falciform ligament divides into right and left	
Right	**Left**
Right lobe of liver divides into	**Left lobe of liver divides into**
Anterior (supra hepatic) and **Posterior** (subhepatic)	**Anterior**—anterior to lesser omentum Supra hepatic and subhepatic and **Posterior** (lesser sac)
Extraperitoneal spaces		
Right perinephric	Bare area of liver	Left perinephric

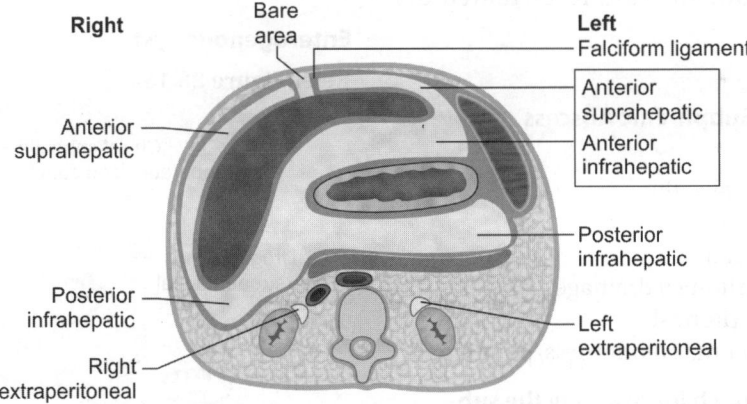

Fig. 28.12: Subphrenic abscesses.

Table 28.2: Etiology of subphrenic abscesses.

Right side	Left side
Liver abscess	Gastric perforation
Duodenal ulcer perforation	Splenic abscess
Gall bladder perforation or gangrene	Colonic perforation
Appendix—abscess, gangrene, perforation	Pancreatic abscess
Laparotomy for peritonitis	Post-trauma
Post-trauma	

Clinical Features

"Pus somewhere, pus nowhere, pus under diaphragm".

Symptoms
- Follow an infective focus in abdominal cavity days/weeks after temporary improvement.
- Fever—swinging, anorexia, weight loss, hiccup

Signs
- Tachycardia
- Epigastric, fullness, rigidity +/-, mass
- Pleural effusion.

Diff. Diagnosis
Pyelonephritis, liver abscess, empyema thoracis.

Investigations
- To prove pus
- To localize pus
- To exclude differential diagnosis
- To remove pus.

WBC counts; leukocytosis.
X-ray—effusion, air/fluid level/tented diaphragm.
USG/CT.

Treatment of Subphrenic Abscess
- Antibiotic
- Accurate localization
- Aspirate under guidance
- Adequate drainage
    - Extraperitoneal drainage
    - Transperitoneal
    Incision over max tenderness/pointing.

Surgical Approach for draining the subphrenic abscess:
- Anterior subcostal
- Posterior trans costal (bed of 12 th rib)
- Midline laparotomy—for left subphrenic abscess or lesser sac abscess.

MESENTERIC CYSTS
Refer **Figure 28.13**.

> Q. Classify the mesenteric cysts.

Types
- Chylolymphatic
- Enterogenous
- Urogenital remnant
- Teratogenic and dermoid.

> Q. Short notes on: 1. Types and pathology of mesenteric cysts. 2. Clinical diagnosis and differential diagnosis of mesenteric cysts. 3. Treatment of mesenteric cysts.

Pathology of Mesenteric Cysts
Refer **Table 28.3**.

Chylolymphatic Cyst
Refer **Figure 28.14**.

Enterogenous Cyst
Refer **Figure 28.15**.

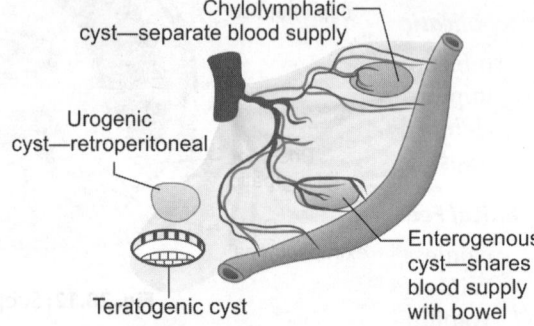

Fig. 28.13: Mesenteric cysts—types.

Table 28.3: Differentiation of mesenteric cysts.

Chylolymphatic cyst	Enterogenous cyst
Commonest	It occurs on mesenteric border of intestine
• Congenitally segregated lymphatic tissue	• Essentially a duplication of bowel
• Thin wall/lined by flat epithelium	• Thick wall, has mucosa, mucinous content
• Has a separate blood supply	• Shares the blood supply with the respective bowel segment
• Can be enucleated.	• Removed with intestinal segment

Chapter 28: Abdominal Cavity, Hernia and Digestive Tract

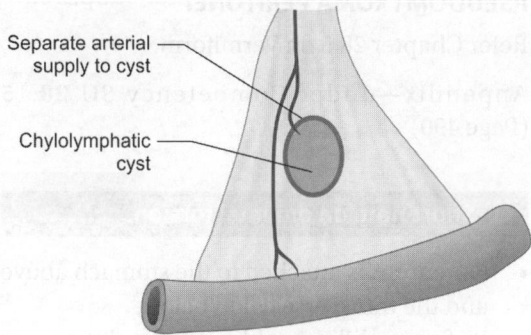

Fig. 28.14: Chylolymphatic cyst.

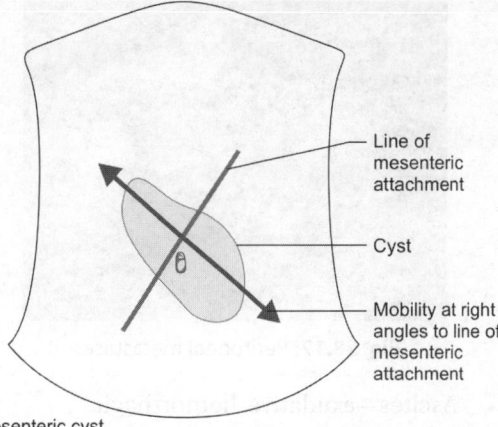

Fig. 28.16: Clinical features of mesenteric cyst.

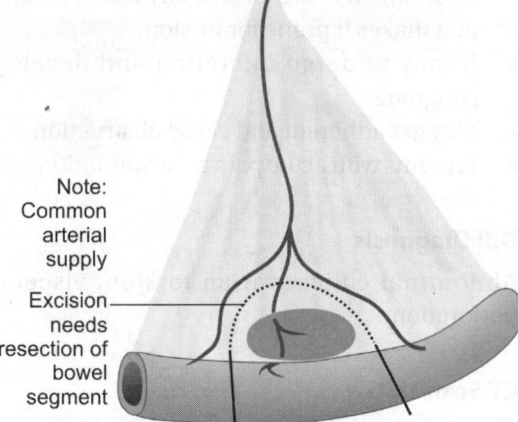

Fig. 28.15: Enterogenous cyst.

Complications
- Infection
- Rupture
- Hemorrhage
- Intestinal obstruction.

Clinical Features (Refer Figure 28.16)
- Painless abdominal swelling
- Pain—recurrent abdominal pain
- Vomiting
- Cystic—a fluid thrill is felt
- Mobile—at right angle to line of mesenteric attachment
- Dull in centre and resonant around
- **Acute abdomen**—due to hemorrhage or infection. Rarely rupture.

Differential Diagnosis
- Tuberculous abscess of the mesentery
- Hydatid cyst of the mesentery

- Peritoneal inclusion cyst
- Post-traumatic—hemorrhagic cyst (serosanguineous cyst).

USG/CT Scan

Treatment
- Excision of the cystic swelling
- The enterogenic cyst is resected with the adjoining bowel loop.

Acute Mesenteric Adenitis

Etiology
- Suspected to be due to viral infection or to *Yersinia*. Follows respiratory infection.
- Usually seen in childhood and teenage.

Clinical Features
- Central pain abdomen.
- Vomiting; fever.

Diff. Diagnosis: Acute appendicitis.

Usually self limiting.
If in doubt diagnostic laparoscopy and appendectomy is done.

> Q. Short note on carcinomatosis peritonei.

CARCINOMATOSIS PERITONEI (FIG. 28.17)
- Infiltration of peritoneal cavity by carcinoma
- Pancreas, stomach, ovary, breast
- Studded with nodules, omental nodules

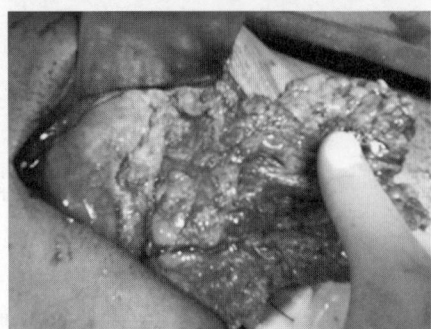

Fig. 28.17: Peritoneal metastases.

- Ascites—exudative/hemorrhagic
- DD: TB peritonitis
  - Pseudomyxoma peritonei.

Investigations
X-ray
- Ascites
- Obstructive signs

CT—mimics TB—fat stranding, omental nodules.

Treatment
Palliative-repeated paracentesis and intra peritoneal hyperthermic mitomycin/fluorouracil.

Prognosis is poor.

PSEUDOMYXOMA PERITONEI
Refer Chapter 28.5 on Vermiform.

Appendix—under Competency SU 28.15 (Page 490)

Q. Short note on omental torsion.

- Omentum is attached to the stomach above and the transverse colon below.
- Its free mobility enables it to reach any part of abdomen.
- Attachment to any part or any tumor arising in it makes it prone for torsion.
- It may undergo infarction and develop gangrene.
- May get adherent and cause obstruction.
- Presents with acute pain as "acute abdomen".

Diff Diagnosis
Abdominal colic; ovarian torsion, visceral perforation.

CT Scan/USG
Treatment—laparoscopic/open resection.

RETROPERITONEUM

RETROPERITONEAL PATHOLOGY

Q. Short notes on psoas abscess.

Psoas Abscess

- Psoas abscess is generally due to tuberculosis of spine or TB lymphadenitis of the paravertebral lymph nodes.
- Secondary to infections of kidney and upper urinary tract—ruptured perinephric abscess.
- Gastrointestinal perforations (uncommon)—complications of IBD
- Infected retroperitoneal hematoma
- Hematogenous—in patients who are immunocompromised or elderly with debility
   - Then abscess tracks underneath the psoas sheath and points to the groin. Sometimes as a dual swelling above and below the inguinal ligament.
   - It may track under iliacus and point in the iliac fossa.

Clinical Features

- Back pain, lassitude and fever.
- Swelling in the groin or iliac fossa.
- Fixed flexion deformity of the hip evident on inspection
- Pain is felt upon passive extension of hip (psoas spasm.)

Diagnosis and Treatment

- CT scan—guided diagnostic aspiration of pus and therapeutic drainage.
- Antibiotics as per the report.
- Antituberculous treatment—as per the protocol.
- Unusually, open drainage may be required.

Q. Classify and enumerate the retroperitoneal tumors.

RETROPERITONEAL TUMORS

Primary tumors (Refer Table 28.4)

- **Secondary tumors**—spread from other organs—renal, adrenal, pancreatic.
- **Primary tumors of retroperitoneum:** Sarcomas—fat, muscles, fibrous tissue and nerves. And lymphomas—lymph nodes.

Q. Short notes on retroperitoneal lipoma.

RETROPERITONEAL LIPOMA

- More commonly seen in women.
- Macroscopically—commonly grow very large.

Complications

- Retroperitoneal lipoma undergoes myxomatous degeneration.
- Sarcomatous change.
- Compression of ureter or nerves.

Clinical Presentation

- A large lump inside the abdomen or pain.
- Or as vague abdominal pain.

Diagnosis

Ultrasonography and CT scanning.

RETROPERITONEAL SARCOMA

They make about 2% of all solid malignancies and about 15–20% of all sarcomas.
Mostly seen in the 40–50 year age group. No age is exempt.

Table 28.4: Retroperitoneal tumors.

Benign-retroperitoneal tumors—20%	Primary retroperitoneal malignancies—80%
Lipoma	Retroperitoneal liposarcoma, leiomyosarcoma—50%
Neurofibroma, neurilemmoma	
Leiomyoma	Myxoid sarcoma, synovioma (rare)
Extra-adrenal chromaffinoma	Retroperitoneal lymphoma—mostly NHL
Paraganglioma	Teratomas
Benign teratomas	

Common Types: Adults

- Liposarcoma
- Leiomyosarcoma
- Undifferentiated pleomorphic sarcoma (malignant fibrous histiocytoma.
- **Histological grading:** Low, intermediate and high (Gr I, II and III).

Clinical Presentation

- Very large rapidly growing tumor.
- Often asymptomatic.
- Non-specific symptoms—such vague abdominal pain and fullness.
- May cause pressure or obstructive uropathy or neural deficit due to compression or infiltration of retroperitoneal nerves.
- Later, they metastasize to lungs and bone.

Investigation

- Imaging—MRI and CT—complement each other in detection and staging of the tumor.
- Image guided core biopsy.

Treatment

Surgery

Wide surgical resection is the definitive treatment and only chance of a cure.

Most of the times, this involves complete resection of the tumor an adjoining viscus like kidney, adrenal, intestinal loop, etc.

Chemotherapy and radiotherapy (CT, RT) are used as adjuvant to surgical debulking for inoperable or non-accessible tumors. or residual tumors owing to involvement of vital structures, e.g., the proximal superior mesenteric vessels or bilateral renal vessels.

Drugs used are—doxorubicin, ifosfamide, dacarbazine (DTIC) methotrexate.

Radiotherapy: External beam (EBRT) or intra-operative (IORT).

Neoadjuvant therapies (chemotherapy, EBRT or combination RT and CT)—to downstage the tumor and achieve higher resection rates and also to reduce local recurrence.

Chemosensitive tumors: High grade (Gr 3) liposarcoma, leiomyosarcoma, and undifferentiated pleomorphic sarcoma.

Monoclonal antibodies are used for metastatic tumors.

Targeted therapy, e.g., anti angiogenetic agent, tyrosine kinase inhibitors, and mammalian target of rapamycin inhibitors (mTOR inhibitors), e.g., Trabectedin-used in synovial sarcoma, myxoid sarcoma and, leiomyosarcoma.

Prognosis

5 year survival rates are poor—35-50%, irrespective of tumor cell type and even after complete resection. However the low-grade liposarcomas are curable.

28.2: Esophagus and Stomach

SU28.5	Describe the applied anatomy and physiology of esophagus.
SU28.6	Describe the clinical features, investigations and principles of management of benign and malignant disorders of esophagus.
SU28.7	Describe the applied anatomy and physiology of stomach.
SU28.8	Describe and discuss the etiology, clinical features, investigations and principles of management of congenital hypertrophic pyloric stenosis, peptic ulcer disease, carcinoma stomach.
SU28.9	Demonstrate the technique of examination of a patient with disorders of the stomach.

ESOPHAGUS

SU28.5 Describe the applied anatomy and physiology of esophagus.

APPLIED ANATOMY OF ESOPHAGUS

Embryology

Esophagus develops from foregut endoderm—beginning 4th week. The caudal foregut gives off the ventral diverticulum. Then the laryngo-esophageal fold fuses as a septum thus dividing the diverticulum into ventral laryngo-tracheal tube and a dorsal esophagus.
Incomplete separation of the ventral from the dorsal tube causes a tracheo-esophageal fistula. The mesoderm contributes to the muscle layer.

Anatomy (Refer Figure 28E-1)

The adult esophagus is a tubular structure 25 cm long starting from cricopharyngeal sphincter (at C 6 level, which is 15 cm from upper incisor tooth and made of cricopharyngeus and thyro-pharyngeus) and extending through the posterior mediastinum upto the gastro-esophageal junction (approximately T12 level), which is about 39–40 cm from upper incisor.

Q. Describe the anatomical division and surgical division of esophagus.

It is divided into three parts—cervical, thoracic and abdominal (refer **Fig. 28E-1**).

The cervical esophagus: From cricopharynx to the thoracic inlet (suprasternal notch) 15–18 cm.

Thoracic esophagus: From suprasternal notch 18 cm—to the level of diaphragmatic hiatus (T10).
- Upper thoracic 18 cm to level of crossing of aortic arch 25 cm (T5)
- Mid thoracic—25–32 cm level of inferior pulmonary vein.
- Lower thoracic—upto diaphragmatic hiatus—approx 37 cm.

Intra-abdominal—diaphragmatic hiatus to gastro-esophageal junction—40 cm

Surgical division:
- Upper third—cricopharynx to aortic arch.
- Middle third—aortic arch to inferior pulmonary vein.
- Lower third—inferior pulmonary vein to gastro-esophageal junction.

Esophageal mucosa is lined by squamous epithelium and columnar epithelium in the lowest 2–3 cm. Submucosa is thick and the toughest layer. Muscularis is made of skeletal muscle in proximal part and smooth muscle. distally. There is no serosal cover.

Arterial supply is segmental from multiple branches of thoracic aorta. Veins form a plexus around the esophagus and drain mainly into Azygos vein (and also into hemiazygos and posterior intercostal veins) and inferior thyroid vein in neck.

Lymphatics: Intercommunicating network. Lymph node groups: Cervical, mediastinal and subdiaphragmatic—paracardiac (three fields).

Nerve supply: Vagus nerve—carries fibers of sympathetic and parasympathetic.

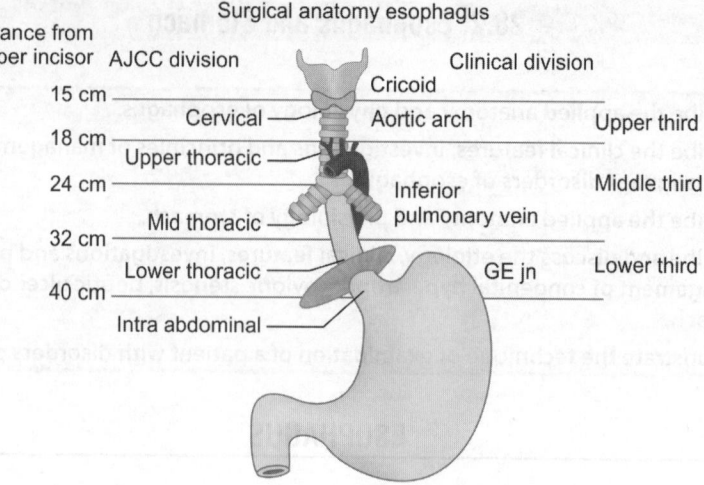

Fig. 28E-1: Surgical anatomy of esophagus.

Q. Enumerate esophageal constrictions.

Esophageal Constrictions

- Cricopharynx—15 cm
- Aortic arch crossing—20 cm
- Left bronchus—22–23 cm
- Diaphragmatic aperture—37–38 cm

Functional Divisions of Esophagus

- Proximal sphincter—cricopharyngeal sphincter.
- Body of esophagus
- Lower esophageal sphincter

Q. Describe the physiology of swallowing and the esophageal peristalsis.

Physiology of swallowing

Initial part of swallowing is voluntary—from mouth upto the cricopharynx—the synchronous movements happen between the oropharyngeal structures to allow the food past the cricopharyngeal sphincter to enter esophagus.

Past cricopharynx: It is involuntary.

- **Primary peristalsis**: Esophageal movement follows the cricopharyngeal relaxation to drive the swallowed food down to the abdomen.
- **Secondary peristalsis**: Reflex peristalsis that follows irritation or distention, generally following the primary peristalsis—more of emptying the esophageal contents.
- **Tertiary contractions** (peristalsis): Non-propulsive segmental contractions of the esophagus-happen without stimulation.

Long answer question: Describe the lower esophageal sphincter (LES), the anti-reflux barrier mechanism and factors influencing LES function

Short question: Describe lower esophageal sphincter and transient lower esophageal sphincter relaxation (TLESR/TLOSR).

LOWER ESOPHAGEAL SPHINCTER (LES)

" A" 3 cm long zone of increased pressure in the lower esophagus" that allows:

- Synchronous relaxation to allow esophageal emptying into the stomach.
- Maintain the tone to prevent the gastro-esophageal reflux.

Anti-reflux Barriers

This is achieved by anatomical and physiological parts.

Anatomical Barriers

- Diaphragmatic aperture—the crura act like a pinch cock when diaphragm contracts.
- Intra—abdominal part of esophagus (2.5 to 3 cm)—compressed by intra-abdominal pressure.
- Angle of His at the junction of the esophagus with fundus like a flap valve.
- Rosette like folds of the mucosa at the lower esophageal end.

Physiological Barriers

- Tone of the LES.
- Ensured by the myenteric smooth muscle plexus, mainly the Auerbach's plexus (between circular and longitudinal muscle layers) and Meissner's plexus in submucosa.
- Normal resting LES pressure: 10 to 30 mm Hg.
- During complete relaxation: Below 10 upto 7 mm Hg (not zero).
- In reflux, the pressure falls and allows reflux of gastric contents.

Causes of Fall in LES Pressure

- Smoking, fatty food, citrus fruits, full stomach.
- Hypothyroidism, gastrointestinal hormones—glucagon(anti-gastrin effect), secretin.
- Drugs; nifedipine, statins, antidepressants, anatomical barriers against.

Elevated LES Pressure

Abnormally high gastrin (Zollinger-Ellison syndrome)

Transient lower esophageal sphincter relaxation (TLESR)

Episodes of transient relaxation of LES which happen postprandially and at times during sleep. These are meant to let off the intragastric gaseous pressures, but they allow reflux.

The reflux is reversed by a corrective esophageal contraction to clear the contents.

Abnormalities and Disorders of LES

- Failure to relax—high pressure—achalasia.
- Low pressure—gastroesophageal reflux disease (GERD).
- Esophageal motility disorders.
- Presbyesophagus—generally lower esophageal tone.
- Failure of Auerbach' plexus in entire esophagus by diseases.

> **SU28.6:** Describe the clinical features, investigations and principles of management of benign and malignant disorders of esophagus.

Q. Enumerate the clinical features of esophageal disease.

Clinical Features of Esophageal Disease

- **Dysphagia**—difficulty in swallowing.
  - Patient being aware of the swallowing.
  - The patient feels the food takes longer to reach the lower end
  - Feels food sticking inside.
  (Normally one is unaware of the food moving past the cricopharynx during normal swallowing)
- **Pain on swallowing (odynophagia)**—seen in conditions of inflammation and ulceration.
  - Aphagia—inability to swallow.
  - Drooling usually follows dysphagia.
  - Aspiration—of esophageal content into respiratory tree.
- **Chest pain due to esophageal spasm**—difficult to distinguish from cardiac pain.
- **Heartburn: Reflux or regurgitation**—seen in gastro esophageal reflux disease.

Q. Enumerate the investigations for esophageal disorder.

- **Endoscopy**—the primary investigation to study the esophageal pathology—luminal or wall structural. Biopsy or cytology is also done.
- **Endoscopic therapeutics**—for resection of superficial lesions, control of bleeding (varices or tumors), LASERs, stenting and for endosonography.
- **Endosonography:** Ultrasound transducer loaded to the tip of the endoscope allows study the layers of the esophageal wall to the evaluate early lesions and the mediastinal nodes.
- **Endomicroscopy** to study dysplastic changes in GERD and detect adenocarcinoma.
- **Oral contrast CT** study the luminal and wall abnormalities and IV contrast to study the wall and extra-esophageal pathology—tumors, nodes abnormal vessels, bony masses.
- **MRI**—to study the wall.
- **Barium swallow study:** Now obsolete and replaced by endoscopy and CT scan study.
- **Esophageal manometry:** Used to diagnose esophageal motility disorders. It provides for complete study of esophageal body function and behaviour of the LES.
- **24 hour pH monitoring** and recording of combined pH impedance.
  - Most accurate method for the diagnosis of gastroesophageal reflux.

- Useful in patients with atypical reflux symptoms and normal endoscopic findings.
- Those who fail to respond to medical therapy.
- **Third space endoscopy:** Submucous or intermuscular space is entered at endoscopy and therapeutic procedures are done.

Q. Etiology of dysphagia, evaluation (Refer Table 28E-1).

EVALUATION OF DYSPHAGIA

History and Examination

- Duration and progress
- Initiation of swallowing or terminal
- Painful or painless
- For liquids or for solids
- Partial or progressive
- Past history of ingestion of drugs, corrosives, hot liquids, radiation
- Neurological history and clinical status
- Family history.

Investigations

- Medical and neurological evaluation and ENT evaluation for oro pharyngeal dysphagia: ENT evaluation, oral evaluation.
- Specific causes for esophageal dysphagia: Like systemic diseases and neurological disease.
- Chest X-ray—for mass in the mediastinum and bony abnormality.
- Endoscopy, biopsy, endoscopic staining (iodine) for detection of cancers.
- Endomicroscopy for Barrett's esophagus.
- Esophageal manometry.
- 24 hour pH monitoring.
- CT—contrast enhanced—for esophageal and extra-esophageal disease.
- Endosonography (endoscopic USG)
- Ultrasonography of abdomen and neck.
- MRI—for wall lesions and mediastinal nodes.

ESOPHAGEAL PERFORATIONS

Spontaneous

Q. Spontaneous rupture of esophagus (Boerhaave's syndrome).

Boerhaave's syndrome (Baro-trauma due to luminal high pressure caused by wretching or vomiting against a closed glottis after a heavy drink or meal)
- Full thickness rupture the lower esophagus and leak into pleural cavity, usually left side causing empyema and into the mediastinum causing mediastinitis.
- Pain in chest and breathlessness with features of mediastinitis.
- Surgical emphysema—in neck and mediastinum.
- X-ray or CT- show mediastinal air.
- Contrast CT shows leak.

Emergency surgical exploration, suturing of esophagus, drainage of mediastinum and pleural cavity and aggressive antibiotic therapy are needed. Delay increases the mortality steeply.

Table 28E-1: Etiology of dysphagia.

Summary: Causes of dysphagia

Oropharyngeal
- Oral and pharyngeal painful, obstructive lesions, candidiasis, iron deficiency anemia causing sideropenic dysphagia (Plummer-Vinson syndrome)
- Extrinsic pressure in neck—large thyroid, lymph node mass, tumor, bony mass neurological—myasthenia gravis, post polio, motor neurone disease polyneuropathy.

Esophageal
- Luminal and mural—foreign body, esophageal web, Schatzki's ring, strictures—peptic, malignant, corrosive, post radiation, candidiasis.
- Extrinsic compression—mediastinal masses, dysphagia lusoria (double aortic arch).
- Neuromuscular dysfunction—achalasia, scleroderma.

Traumatic
- Penetrating—injury—bullet or stabs.
- Iatrogenic—endoscopy—mainly rigid or during therapeutic endoscopy—balloon dilatation.
- Instrumentation—dilatation of stricture. Insertion of nasogastric tube, accidental esophageal intubation during endotracheal intubation
- Foreign body—eroding through the wall when stuck for many days.

Diseases
Peri-esophageal abscess or diverticulum, growth.

Management (Refer Table 28E-2)
- CT scan to locate sit of leak and assess the fluid collections—neck, chest or abdomen.

Treatment
Conservative: Small (endoscopy) perforations—pass a nasogastric past the perforation, antibiotic and monitor for signs of sepsis.

Surgery: Primary repair in early cases with no sepsis, to drain collections—cervical drainage, chest drains, peritoneal drains, diversions—esophagostomy, gastrostomy.

Endoscopic stents to cover the growths or strictures causing perforations.

Q. Mallory-Weiss syndrome.

Mallory-Weiss Syndrome

Spontaneous **linear and vertical tear of the mucosa at cardia** (on the gastric mucosa in 90% distal to squamo-columnar junction and on esophageal side in 10%) caused by a violent bout of retching or vomiting (usually but not always, following a intake of alcohol or heavy meal).
Some cases may have a deeper tear short of a complete tear causing intramural hematoma causing pain and dysphagia.

Clinical features of Mallory-Weiss tear: Hematemesis—mild or severe.

Treatment
Emergency control of bleeding by endoscopic injection of sclerosant or glue (cyano acrylate) or laser therapy or surgical suturing (rarely).

Table 28E-2: Treatment of esophageal perforations.

Conservative treatment	Emergency surgical treatment
• Early minimal leak and small perforation • No signs of sepsis • No foreign body • No signs of obstruction • CT—shows minimal leak into mediastinum	• CT-gross contamination of peritoneum pleural cavity with large collections • Signs of sepsis • Obstructive signs, foreign body inside Boerhaave syndrome

Corrosive Injury
Acids—cause coagulation necrosis of lining—limit the injury deeper layers, but can cause stasis at pylorus and severe fibrosis.

Alkalis—cause liquefaction necrosis and penetrate deeper and through the entire wall to cause long and tough strictures.

Treatment
Emergency jejunostomy—for feeding and free drainage of the esophageal contents through a nasogastric tube if possible.
- Nutrition; initially intravenous and then through jejunostomy.
- Endoscopic surveillance and
- Oral contrast CT scan to assess the scarring of esophagus and stomach.

Definitive surgery: Delayed—12 weeks after inflammation settles.

Choice of procedure in surgery depends on the site and extent of scarring:
- Esophageal strictures—are usually left alone and a colonic conduit is taken sub-sternally to connect stomach with cervical esophagus.
- Resection of the scarred esophagus and part of the stomach and replace with a colonic conduit (a more hazardous operation).
- Scarred Stomach: A total gastrectomy and a jejunal pouch for reconstruction and esophagojejunostomy.
- Gastric outlet obstruction is managed by an antrectomy or a gastrojejunal bypass.

Q. Etiology and principles of management of esophageal strictures.

Esophageal Strictures: Causes

Congenital: Failure of recanalization—part of atresia with/without Tracheo esophageal fistula

Acquired
- Traumatic—chemical
- Peptic—early—Schatzki's ring, later a Frank stricture at lower end of esophagus
- Thermal—accidental hot liquid swallowed—may be short or long
- Radiation-induced
- Chemical-induced (corrosive -acid/alkaline)— usually long.
- Medication-induced—localized scarring following ulceration due to a tablet medication getting stuck, e.g., vitamin C, analgesics doxycycline.

Iatrogenic: Prolonged nasogastric tube feeding.
- Instrument induced
- Malignant -strictures

Diagnosis: Endoscopy, MRI and CT are complementary—assess the tissue.

Treatment

Malignancy—as per protocol for the respective cancer.

Benign strictures: Treatment depends upon short or long strictures.

Short strictures
- Upper esophagus; LASER coring and self dilatation. SEMS—unsuitable. Near the cricopharynx.
- Mid esophagus: SEMS—self expanding metallic stent.
- Lower esophagus again—a LASER coring of the stricture preferred—SEMS may slip and migrate.

Surgery: Esophagectomy for long strictures with colonic conduit replacement.

Indications: Long strictures, undilatable strictures, technical difficulty in stentng or LASER coring. And Malignancy.

ESOPHAGEAL DIVERTICULA

Outpouching of the wall of esophagus.

Types

- Pulsion diverticula—luminal high pressure pushes the mucosa through the wall.
- Traction diverticula—adhesion of the wall of esophagus to a granuloma of histoplasmosis or TB. Lymphadenitis: This causes a mid-esophageal pouching.

Sites
- Cricopharyngeal diverticulum: Zenker's diverticulum—pulsion diverticulum—through the Killian's dehiscence.
- Mid-esophageal—mostly traction diverticula.
- Epiphrenic divertiula—pulsion diverticula just above diaphragm.

Traction diverticulum causes obstructive symptoms and sometimes fistula with bronchus.

The pulsion diverticula are mostly associated with some neurological disorders that cause incordination in esophageal motility.

Clinical Features

Mainly due to the underlying disorder and less due to diverticula.

These diverticula are asymptomatic unless they enlarge and accumulate food.

They cause extrinsic pressure and dysphagia. Infection due to the stagnant food, which aspiration and halitosis.

Treatment

- Treat the underlying neurological disorder if any.
- Surgery:
  - Zenker's diverticulum—posterior pharyngeal myotomy.
  - Diverticulopexy—obliteration of diverticulum to prevent food from getting there.
  - Diverticulectomy—removing the pouch.
  - Diverticulo-esophageal anastomosis (for large epiphrenic diverticula).

CLASSIFICATION OF ESOPHAGEAL MOTILITY DISORDERS

- **Of pharyngoesophageal junction**
  - Pharyngoesophageal (Zenker's) diverticulum
  - Myogenic—myasthenia, muscular dystrophy
  - Neurological—stroke, motor neuron disease, multiple sclerosis, Parkinson's disease

- **Of the body of the esophagus**
  - Diffuse esophageal spasm (corkscrew esophagus)
  - Reflux associated
  - Nutcracker esophagus
  - Eosinophilic esophagitis and allergic
  - Autoimmune disorders, e.g., especially systemic sclerosis
  - Idiopathic
- **Of the lower esophageal sphincter**
  - Achalasia
  - Incompetent lower sphincter (i.e. GERD)

> **Q. Causes of dysphagia, pathogenesis, diagnosis and treatment of achalasia cardia (long answer).**

ACHALASIA CARDIA

A state of failure of lower esophageal sphincter (LES) to relax resulting in spasm of the LES.

Cause

- Loss or absence of Auerbach's plexus.
- Congenital absence or deficiency of Auerbach's plexus.
- Acquired: Progressive loss of the myenteric plexus at LES causing functional obstruction—trypanosomiasis, viral infections and immunological mechanisms postulated.

Pathogenesis

- Failure of the LES to relax synchronously in response to esophageal peristalsis.
- Resulting in functional obstruction at the lower end of esophagus.
- In some, there is associated hypomotility of the esophageal muscle also.

Types of Achalasia

Three distinct **types** based on manometric findings:
1. **Type I (classic)**—with minimal contractility in the esophageal body,
2. **Type II (intermitent)**—achalasia with intermittent panesophageal pressurization and
3. **Type III (spastic)**—with premature or spastic distal esophageal contractions (vigorous achalasia).

Consequences

- Stasis in proximal esophagus,
- Progressive dilatation and hypertrophy of the esophagus—mega esophagus.
- Subsequent to hypomotility and stasis, there is infection in the stagnant pool.
- Esophagitis in the wall.
- Aspiration of contents.
- Malignancy in a small number (about 0.4%), They have an increased risk of cancer 25–30 years (squamous cell carcinoma—11 times the risk in normal and less commonly adenocarcinoma).

Pseudoachalasia is an achalasia like disorder caused by obstruction due to submucous carcinoma or , benign tumors of GE junction, paraneoplastic feature of lung cancer, LES failure in amyloidosis or sarcoidosis.

Clinical Features of Achalasia

Age: Mostly between 20 and 40 years.
Sex: More in females.

Symptoms

- **Early symptoms:** Chest pain due to esophageal spasm.
- Progressive dysphagia, more for liquids.
- Heartburn due to esophagitis.
- Aspiration of stagnant esophageal contents causing pneumonitis and lung abscess. .
- **Late feature:** Painful swallowing, nutritional deficiency, and weight loss.
- Recurrent chest in infection with nocturnal cough, laryngospasm. Halitosis and candidiasis of esophagus.

Differential Diagnosis

- Carcinoma—dysphagia is progressive and is for solids.
- Scleroderma and diffuse spasm.
- Stricture of esophagus.
- Pseudoachalasia.

Investigations

- Esophageal manometry—is diagnostic.
  - Classically, the LES does not relax completely on swallowing, no peristalsis

and there is a zone of raised resting pressure in the esophagus.
- X-ray—absence of fundal gas shadow.
- Contrast CT (or barium swallow): Advanced cases may show typical signs:
  - Mega esophagus: Massively dilated and aperistaltic and with a smooth pencil like lower end—the "sigmoid esophagus" whose lower end looks like a "bird's beak" (Fig. 28E-2).
- Endoscopy—recumbent, esophagus with stagnant "cesspool", mucosal ulcerations.
  - Resolution esophageal manometry.

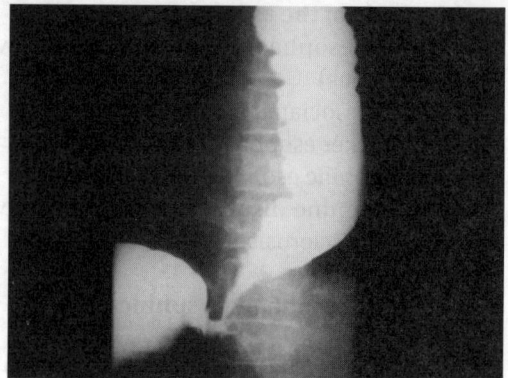

Fig. 28E-2: Achalasia cardia.

Treatment

Mild cases—calcium channel blocker—nifedipine, nitroglycerine.

Botulinum injection—endoscopic botulinum injection into muscle—last for 3 months.

Definitive Treatment

Early treatment recommended to reduce risk of carcinogenesis and respiratory complications
- **Endoscopic pneumatic dilatation**—rupture of circular muscle.
  Disadvantage
  - Uncontrolled dilatation (due to variability between patients)
  - May require repeat dilatation
  - Risk of rupture and peritonitis
- **POEM—per oral endoscopic myotomy**—endoscopic incision and division of circular muscle. It has evolved as an alternative to surgery.
- **Surgery:** Heller's cardiomyotomy with partial fundoplication (refer **Figure 28E-3**)—open or laparoscopic approach.

Surgical division of serosa and circular muscle at the lower end of esophagus—incision from the junction upwards to the level of crus of diaphragm, deepening through muscle layer until the submucosa bulges and downwards for at least 2.5 cm. The post myotomy reflux is minimized by adding an anti reflux procedure like a Toupet or Dorr's partial fundoplication.

Esophagectomy

Uncommonly indicated for cases with high risk of carcinoma (endoscopic biopsy) or in cases

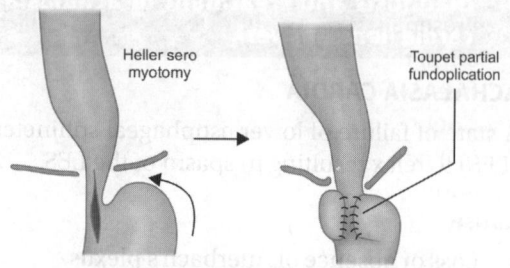

Fig. 28E-3: Heller's cardiomyotomy.

with a giant esophagus and recurrent and severe respiratory complications.
Secondary achalasia—Chagas' disease.

> Q. Write a short answer on tracheoesophageal fistula.

ESOPHAGEAL ATRESIA AND TRACHEOESOPHAGEAL FISTULA

Failure of laryngobronchial tube to separate from the esophagus
Often associated with other anomalies—VACTERL:
- V - Vertebral defects
- A - Anal atresia
- C - Cardiac anomalies (defects)
- TE - Tracheoesophageal fistula
- R - Renal agenesis, Radial hypoplasia
- L - Limb abnormalities.

Types of Tracheoesophageal Fistula (Refer Figure 28E-4)

- In **85% cases, the upper end is blind and lower end communicating with trachea.**

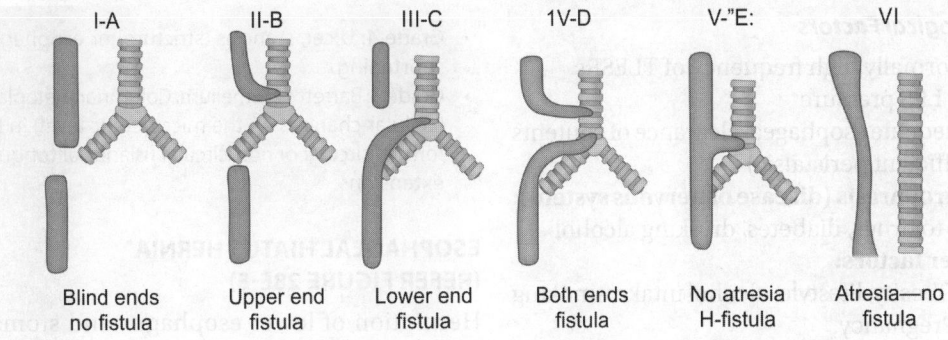

Types of esophageal atresia and tracheoesophageal fistula

Fig. 28E-4: Types of tracheoesophageal fistula.

- Presentation in newborn as soon as the baby cries, the gastric contents enter respiratory tree and cause chemical pneumonitis.
- Cough and cyanosis—are pathognomonic in a newborn.
- Should be recognized within 24 hours for saving the life.
- A catheter passed per orally fails to pass down the esophagus
- Radiography with water soluble contrast, if possible, is done to identify the fistula.

Treatment

- **Immediate surgery** to prevent aspiration of gastric contents into lungs.
  - a gastrostomy is done for feeding
- **Definitive repair**—done when the child improves.
  - Thoracotomy, division of fistula and restoration of esophageal continuity by anastomosing the two ends.
  - Or if the gap is large, a colonic or jejunal loop transposition may be needed.

Complications

- Associated anomalies often add to the morbidity and mortality.
- Anastomotic leak leading to mediastinal and pleural infections.

> **Q.** Describe pathophysiology of gastro esophageal reflux disease and surgical principles of anti-reflux surgery. Write note on surgical treatment for esophageal hiatus hernia.

GASTROESOPHAGEAL REFLUX DISEASE (GERD/GORD)

- This is a clinic-pathological entity denoting the esophageal damage and symptoms due to abnormal gastroesophageal reflux across the lower esophageal sphincter.
- The resting LES pressure is around 10-25 mm Hg, falling upto 1 to 3 mm Hg during act of swallowing when it relaxes to allow passage of esophageal contents into stomach.
- The LES also undergoes short physiological spells of transient relaxation postprandially (TLESRs) and at other times like during sleep, to clear the esophageal contents.
- During these TLESRs, reflux can occur, especially during sleep.

In early GERD, the frequency of TLESRs increases and reflux events take place beginning the acid damage to the esophageal mucosa.

Later stages: Persistent lowering of LES pressure sets in—below 7 mm Hg allowing free reflux.

Other Factors Causing GE Reflux

Anatomical Factors

- **Loss of the length** of intra-abdominal of esophagus: Here the LES can't contract (sphincteric failure) e.g., in hiatus hernia. But, All those with GERD do not have a hernia and all those with a hernia need not have GERD.
- Weak diaphragmatic pinch.
- Altered obliquity of angle of HIS
- Weakened gastric mucosal rosette.

Physiological Factors
- Abnormally high frequency of TLESRs
- Low LES pressure
- Inadequate esophageal clearance of contents (inefficient peristalsis)
- **Gastroparesis (disease of nervous system):** Due to drugs, diabetes, drinking alcohol
- **Other factors:**
  - Obesity, lifestyle, alcohol intake, smoking
  - Pregnancy.

Pathogenesis
The abnormal reflux is caused by—
- High gastric pressure causing fundal stretching and
- A relaxed LES.

The esophageal squamous epithelium is exposed to acid reflux causing inflammation, erosion, ulceration and in the long run, metaplasia of the squamous into columnar epithelium (intestinal metaplasia) called Barrett's epithelium, the seat of a future adenocarcinoma.

Pathology
The acid reflux damaging the mucosa and subsequent changes are graded and classified under various systems:

> **Q. Classify and grade the severity of gastro-esophageal reflux disease.**
>
> **Los Angeles Classification of GERD**
> - Grade A: Isolated mucosal erosion/s (one or more) < 5mm.
> - Grade B: Isolated mucosal erosion/s (one or more) > 5mm.
> - Grade C: > 1 mucosal breaches bridging the tops of mucosal folds—involving < 75% of circumference of esophagus.
> - Grade D: > 1 mucosal breaches bridging the tops of mucosal folds—involving > 75% of circumference of esophagus.
>
> **Savory - Miller Classification Reflux Esophagitis**
> - Grade 1: Single or multiple erosions on a single fold.
> - Grade 2: Multiple erosions affecting multiple folds. Erosions may be confluent.
> - Grade 3: Multiple circumferential or rounded erosions.
> - Grade 4: Ulcer, stenosis (stricture) or esophageal shortening.
> - Grade 5: Barrett's epithelium. Columnar metaplasia (cellular changes on the microscopic level) in the form of circular or non-circular (islands or tongues) extensions.

ESOPHAGEAL HIATUS HERNIA (REFER FIGURE 28E-5)
Herniation of lower esophagus and stomach through the diaphragm.
- **Type I:** Sliding (most common)—esophagus and stomach herniated through hiatus. sq -col jn is high cardia herniates.
- **Type II:** Para-esophageal hernia "rolling" hernia—herniation of gastric; fundus through a defect adjacent to esophageal hiatus. G-E junction is in normal position.
- **Type III:** Mixed type-sliding and rolling both gastric cardia (S-C Jn) fundus herniate.
- **Type IV:** Mixed type with additional herniation of other viscera like colon or spleen.

Clinical Features of GERD
Cardinal Features
- Heart burn.
- **Acid reflux** or regurgitation in the mouth and **"bitter" taste due to acid.**
- **Difficulty** in swallowing. Less commonly odynophagia—due to severe esophagitis.

Atypical Symptoms
- Recurrent pharyngitis, cough, hoarseness, wheezing
- Non-cardiac chest pain
- Secondary anemia—due to micro-bleeding form ulceration.

Diagnosis: Most often empirical.

Differential diagnosis:
- Acid peptic disease and peptic ulcers
- Angina pectoris and ischemic heart disease
- Achalasia cardia
- Carcinoma esophagus
- Gallstones and pancreatic diseases.

Clinical Features of Hiatus Hernia
- **Sliding hernia:** Features are those of GERD; secondary anemia, hematemesis.

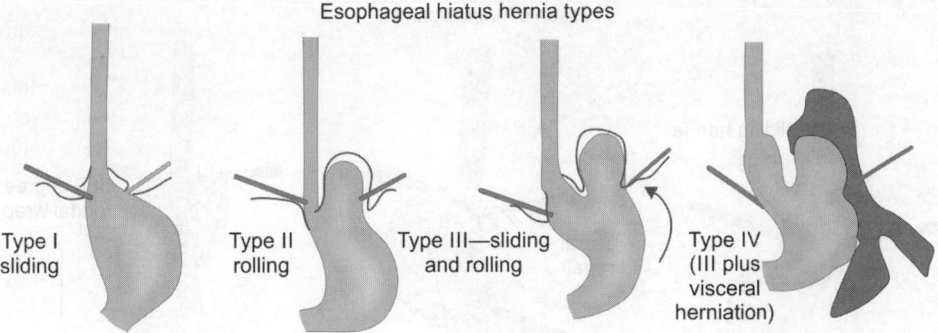

Fig. 28E-5: Types of esophageal hiatus hernia.

- **Rolling hernia:** Chest pain, pressure on heart, gastric obstruction due to gastric volvulus.

Confirmatory Tests and Evaluation of GERD

- 24-hour pH monitoring and recording is the 'gold standard' for diagnosis of GERD; all PPI or H2 blockers are stopped 2 weeks prior to pH metry.
- Esophageal manometry; length and pressure of the LES are important in planning the antireflux procedure.
- Endoscopic grading (see above) and biopsy from areas of Barrett's mucosa.
- Endomicroscopy—where the endoscope provides for a magnification view of the mucosa for selecting areas for biopsy.
- CT scan—for assessment of gastroesophageal anatomy (before planning a surgery).
- Blood—anemia, diabetes.
- Cardiovascular disease.
- Chest X-ray for pneumonitis.

Treatment of GERD

After evaluation, the treatment strategy is decided.
- Medical treatment—first line
- Endoscopic treatment
- Surgery

Medical treatment of GERD

- Proton pump inhibitors—are the cornerstone to keep gastric pH above 5.
- Omeprazole 20 mg or esomeprazole 40 mg. Pantoprazole 40 mg, twice daily for about 8–10 weeks followed by once daily for maintenance.
- Prokinetics: Domperidone 10–30 mg Itopride 50 mg 3 times daily or Levosulpiride 25–75 mg per day. These will add to esophageal clearance and also increase LES pressure.
- Those who fail to respond to above must be investigated for an alternative diagnosis.
- Diet and lifestyle modification—avoid fat rich food.

Endoscopic treatment of GERD

Indication: With a confirmed diagnosis of GERD, if symptoms are not controlled or endoscopic findings show progression or worsening of the grade or Barrett's epithelium is suspicious.
Aim: To augment a failing **LES (LOS)**.
Goal—to narrow LES and to increase the pressure to help reduce the GE reflux.
- Radiofrequency ablation (RFA) of mucosa upto the level of sphincter and induce scarring—most effective of all endoscopic procedures in on long term follow up (5-10 year)
- Endoscopic suturing devices - endoluminal plication of gastric mucosa just below the cardia—this is believed to augment the Angle of His.
- Injection of submucosal polymers into the lower esophagus just above and at LES.
- "Gatekeeper reflux repair" system. Endoscopic placement of preformed radiopaque hydrogel into submucosa and augment the LES.
- **Barrett's esophagus**: Endoscopic evaluation and RFA or submucous resection of suspected dysplastic areas.

Surgery for GERD

Aim—to prevent reflux by restoration or creation of a new anti-reflux barrier.
Goals:
- Ensuring a length of 2.5 to 3 cm of intra-abdominal esophagus.

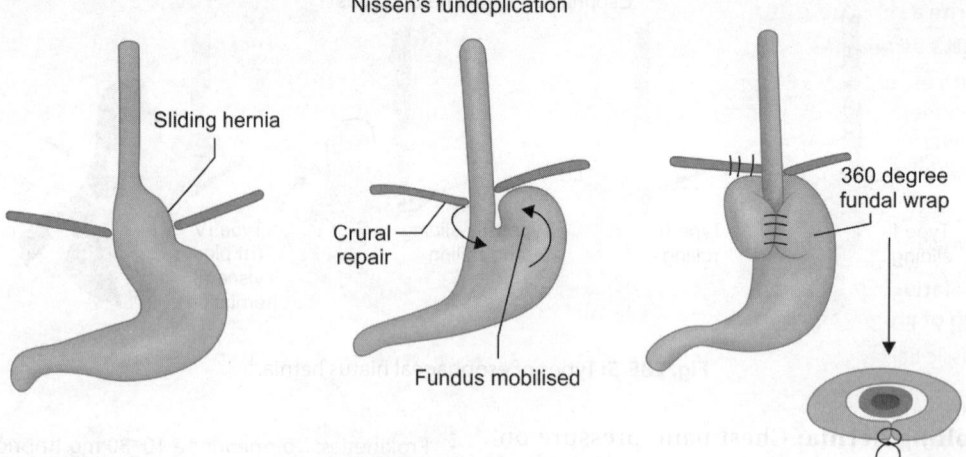

Fig. 28E-6: Nissen's fundoplacation.

- Tightening the diaphragmatic crura to prevent herniation of esophagus.
- Fundal wrapping of the intra-abdominal esophagus to boost LES and prevent herniation.

Surgical Procedures

For GERD and hiatus hernia. These are performed by open laparotomy, laparoscopically (or robotic-assisted laparoscopic technique) or less commonly by thoracic approach.

Transabdominal Procedures

Nissen's Fundoplication
- 360° fundal wrap (Refer **Figure 28E-6**).
- Most widely practiced and accepted.
- Here a 2.5 cm wide wrap of gastric fundus is swung around the mobilized lower esophagus and sutured creating a 360 degree wrap- to buttress the lower sphincter and also to prevent the reherniation of the esophagus into the chest. Also the diaphragmatic crura are tightened around the esophagus.

Complications
- The tight wrap may prevent free belching and cause a "Gas Bloat" sensation in stomach.
- Also a slipped wrap may cause recurrence of reflux as well as obstruction to esophagus.

Partial Fundoplication **(Refer Figure 28E-7)**
- Only a part the circumference is wrapped;
- Toupet—posterior partial fundoplication: Unlike Nissen's, here the wrap covers 270°

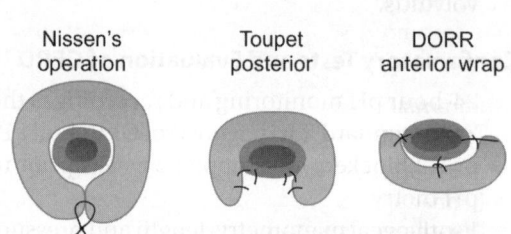

Fig. 28E-7: Types of fundoplications:

around the esophagus leaving the anterior wall open, without a wrap providing for a free air movement—avoiding the "gas bloat".
- **Dorr's—anterior partial fundoplication—** the fundus is wrapped 180° from the front —just to boost the Angle of His and to prevent reherniation.

Transthoracic Procedures
- **Belsey mark IV:** The herniated stomach is pushed back into abdomen. The fundus is wrapped around the esophagus like a collar (hood) and sutured to the diaphragmatic hiatus, which is plicated and narrowed around the esophagus as an extra buttress. Now this procedure is reserved only for recurrent large hernias with short esophagus.
- **Reconstruction of short esophagus—Collis' gastroplasty:** Making a gastric tube and wrapping the fundus around the new tube along with plication of the diaphragmatic hiatus.

Q. Write a short note on Barrett's esophagus.

Barrett's esophagus

Barrett's esophagus is characterised by metaplastic replacement of normal squamous epithelium of the lower esophageal mucosa by gastric mucosal epithelium.

Barrett's esophagus may be diagnosed if there is any intestinal metaplasia in the esophagus.

The relative risk of cancer rises with increasing length of abnormal mucosa.

- Classic Barrett's (≥3 cm columnar epithelium)
- Short-segment Barrett's (<3 cm of columnar epithelium);
- Cardia metaplasia (intestinal metaplasia at the esophagogastric junction without any macroscopic change at endoscopy.

The squamo-columnar junction moves proximally with time as the reflux continues.

Differential diagnosis at endoscopy—sliding hiatus hernia. Both may coexist.

Microscopy: Intestinal metaplasia—presence of columnar epithelium with mucus secreting goblet cells in the esophageal mucosa.

Clinical features—Barrett's may be asymptomatic (contrasting with esophagitis).

pH monitoring will show abnormal pH profiles despite asymptomatic state.

Complications
- Barrett's ulcer—ulceration in the columnar metaplastic mucosa.
- Stricture—at squamocolumnar junction.
- **Adenocarcinoma**: 0.5% per year; 25 times higer risk than in general population.

Surveillance
- Repeat endoscopy and multiple biopsies at 2 year intervals.
- Any dysplasia—may be subjected to active treatment.

Treatment
Aim—prevent development of adenocarcinoma.
- Endoscopic mucosal resection (EMR)
- LASER ablation
- Radiofrequency ablation (RFA)
- Photodynamic therapy, argon-beam plasma coagulation (APC).

Note: An antireflux surgery will not reverse metaplasia and cannot prevent carcinoma.

CARCINOMA OF ESOPHAGUS

Sixth most common cancer in India, squamous cell carcinoma is most common in Asian countries but adenocarcinoma makes almost 55–60% of esophageal cancers in the west.

Age: Usually after 50 years of age, but sometimes in very young age too.

Etiology
- Tobacco
- Indians: Areca (betel nut) and pan beeda.
- Alcohol
- Barrett's esophagus: Adenocarcinoma.
- Achalasia cardia
- Plummer-Vinson's syndrome: Corrosive strictures, human papilloma virus (HPV 16, 18).
- Esophageal candidiasis
- Diet, deficiencies (Vitamin B2, A, C)
- Mycotoxin.

Pathology
Gross pathology (Refer **Table 28E-3**).

Distribution of Tumor
Refer **Table 28E-3**.

Macroscopic Types
- Fungating growth (60%)
- Polypoidal growth
- Ulcerative growth (20%)
- Stricture—annular
- Diffuse infiltrative.

Spread
Esophageal cancers are aggressive and spread early—locally, through lymphatics, blood.

Local Spread
- Around the lumen.
- Transmural—along the wall.
- Extraesophageal—to trachea, bronchus, aorta, veins, left recurrent laryngeal nerve.

Complications
- Tracheo/bronchoesophageal fistula
- Mediastinitis due to perforation growth
- Fatal hemorrhage from aorta due to aortic infiltration.

Table 28E-3: Distribution of esophageal cancer.

Site of tumor	Asian countries (India) (90% SCC)	Western countries 30–35% SCC, 60% adenocarcinoma
Upper third	17%	15%
Middle third	50–55%—squamous cell carcinoma	25%
Lower third	30–34%	60%—adenocarcinoma

Lymph Nodes

- Spread through periesophageal lymphatic network
- Cervical nodes—cervical level 5—lower jugular and supra clavicular
- Mediastinal—periesophageal nodes, nodes in tracheoesophageal groove
- Inferior mediastinum—above diaphragm
- Subdiaphragmatic nodes and paracardiac nodes and then to the celiac nodes.

Blood spread—to liver, lungs, brain and bones.

Microscopy

- Upper 35 cm—squamous cell carcinoma
- Lower 3-5 cm—adenocarcinoma.

Uncommon tumors

- Melanoma
- Leiomyoma (rarely sarcoma)
- Gastrointestinal stromal tumor.

Clinical Features of Carcinoma Esophagus

Men are affected more than females (M:F ratio 3:1 for SCC and 12:1 for adenocarcinoma).

Classical Features

- Dysphagia—for solids (manifests when over 60% of lumen is occluded. An intelligent patient will notice an increase in the time taken by the swallowed bolus reach the stomach
- Regurgitation
- Weight loss and cachexia
- Aspiration pneumonitis, loss of voice
- Supraclavicular nodes
- Anemia
- Backache.

Features of metastases: Pleural effusion, ascites, lung metastases.

STAGING ESOPHAGEAL CARCINOMA

Refer **Table 28E-4**.

Stage

Stage	T	N	M
Stage 0:	Tis	N0	M0
Stage I:	T1 or 2	N0	M0
Stage II:	T3	N0	M0
	T1-2,	N1	M0
Stage III:	T1-2	N2	M0
	T3	N1	M0
Stage IV:	Any T	Any N,	M1
	T4	N1-3	M0

Investigations

- **Endoscopy and biopsy**
  - Histological type and confirmation.
  - Chromoendoscopy: Different stains are instilled locally through endoscope for improved localization of tumors.
  - NBI narrow band imaging: Spectral splitting and viewing under green and blue light facilitates better recognition of tumor.
  - Endomicroscopy—endoscopic evaluation under magnification better identification of dysplasia in Barrett's. The same can be biopsied at endoscopy.
- **Ultrasonography of abdomen** to assess hiatal and peritoneal spread and metastases in liver.
  - Sonography of neck nodes and FNAC.
- **Radiology**
  - Chest X-ray—shows aspiration pneumonia.
  - Contrast enhanced CT scan—is the best to stage the tumor and nodes, local extension, to trachea, aorta, bone, mediastinal fat, pericardial infiltration.

Table 28E-4: Staging of esophageal carcinoma.

Tumor		Node	Number of nodes	Metastases
Tis	High grade dysplasia			
T1	Invading mucosa and submucosa, lamina propria	N0	No nodes	M0—no mets
T2	Invading muscularis propria	N1	1-2 nodes	pM1—micromets
T3	Extra-esophageal spread	N2	3-6 nodes	
T4a	Spread to lung, pleura, azygos vein, diaphragm, pericardium	N3	7 or more nodes	cM1—clinical metastases
T4b	Spread to trachea, aorta, bone			

- **Bronchoscopy**—identifies the invasion of trachea (fistula) and also widening of carina due to subcarinal nodal spread.
- **Laryngoscopy** to evaluate vocal cords (recurrent nerve).
- **Transesophageal endosonography**
  - Useful for evaluating the invasion of esophageal layers, periesophageal nodes, cardia and left lobe of the liver also.
  - It can identify nodes smaller than 5 mm.
  - EUS guided transesophageal nodal needle aspiration cytology is also done.
- **Blood tests**: Hematocrit; ESR; liver function tests. Other investigations in management.
- **Laparoscopy:** Undertaken before deciding on proceeding with a total esophagectomy, to look for and take biopsies from any peritoneal and liver metastases.
- **PET scan** using 18 F-fluorodeoxyglucose (FDG) with CT (PET-CT) SCAN to evaluate the tumor response to radiotherapy.
- Flow cytometry, p53 gene study, immunohistochemistry.

TREATMENT OF ESOPHAGEAL CARCINOMA

Rationale

- Esophageal cancer is aggressive and has poor prognosis. Only 10% of the patients live for 5 years if treated.
- Two prognostic factors are: 1. Depth of invasion of tumor and 2. Nodal spread.
- Best chance of a cure is for a node negative early stage tumor (T1, 2 N0, M0,—both squamous or adenocarcinoma). A total nodal clearance is a must to exclude any nodal metastases.

Modalities and Aim of Treatment

- Surgery—curative or palliative.
- Radiotherapy and chemotherapy—adjuvant or neoadjuvant.
- Endoscopic treatment—preventive, curative, palliative and adjunct to other modalities.

Philosophy

- Curative approach v/s palliative approach.
- **Curative therapy** is radical esophagectomy.

Indications for Radical Surgery

Early stage tumor confined to esophagus (T1, T2 N0, M0) in a patient who is assessed fit for the major surgery.

Multimodal Therapy

For node positive disease (T1,2 N1)—adjuvant or neoadjuvant (RT CT).

Palliative Therapy

- Hematogenous metastases.
- Contiguous organ invasion.
- Peritoneal spread.
- Advanced lymph node spread.

Chemotherapy and Radiotherapy Combined as a Curative Modality

- For proximal squamous cell carcinoma (selective set of patients)
- Early low grade tumors small in size
- Disadvantage: High rate of recurrence.

Endoscopic curative therapy: Only for T1 N0 M0 tumors, low grade (unsuitable for any tumor T1b and beyond, high grade).

- **Endoscopic mucosal resection (EMR):** Entire lesion is sucked into a double lumen endoscope and resection is completed.
  Indications:
  - Tumors-stage: Tis (high grade dyplasia); T1a, N0 M0 curative therapy.
- **Endoscopic submucosal resection (ESMR):** Involves a submucosal dissection and resection of T1a—tumors with normal margins of 1 cm.

Curative Surgery
- Surgery alone: T1 a/b and T2a N0 Mo
- Surgery and RT +CT - for N1 disease,

Palliative surgery T3+, N1+, M1 disease. Palliative surgery or multimodal.

Note: Post-cricoid tumor (squamous cell carcinoma):
- Primary radiotherapy is the mainstay of this carcinoma—5000–6000 cGy.
- Pharyngolaryngectomy with colonic transposition is also done (it has a higher morbidity).

SURGERY FOR ESOPHAGEAL CARCINOMA

It is done as appropriate to the site of the esophageal tumor.

Carcinoma of upper third of esophagus—these are squamous carcinomas:

Radical surgery: Three phase esophagectomy (McKeown):
- **Total esophagectomy with three field lymphadenectomy**—cervical, mediastinal and infradiaphragmatic field (para cardiac, and subdiaphragmatic nodes).

McKeown's operation: The operation has three phases:
1. Abdominal—to mobilize the stomach
2. Thoracic—for mobilizing the esophagus
3. Cervical—for delivery of the specimen and anastomosing the stomach to the pharynx, the anastomosis is in the neck.

Carcinoma of Middle Third of Esophagus
- **Two phase esophagogastrectomy** (Ivor Lewis operation or Lewis -Tanner operation) with two field lymphadenectomy (abdominal and thoracic fields).

Operation:
- Abdominal phase—mobilisation of stomach and lower esophagus, division of esophageal hiatus
- Right thoracotomy, mobilization of esophagus, delivery of the specimen through thorax and anastomosis between proximal esophagus and stomach- in the thorax.

- **McKeown's total esophagectomy with two field lymphadenectomy:** This is also practiced by some—for upper middle third (more proximal growths closer to the aortic arch) for better clearance.

Carcinoma of Lower Third of Esophagus
- **Ivor Lewis two phase** esophagogastrectomy is preferred. Generally:
  1. Resection of lower third of esophagus and proximal stomach with two field lymphadenectomy (thoracic and abdominal) with an intra-thoracic anasotomosis.
  2. Resection of lower esophagus and stomach through through a thoraco-abdominal incision with a limited approach to lymph nodes—for growths of the intra-abdominal esophagus.
- **Trans-hiatal total esophagectomy T.H.E. (Orringer) with lymphadenectomy:**
  - The abdominal phase—involves dissection of stomach and esophagus, lymphadenectomy, resection of the growth and creation of a gastric tube along the greater curvature, widening of the esophageal hiatus and trans hiatal mobilization of the lower middle and lower esophagus along with lymphadenectomy.
  - Cervical phase to dissect the cervical esophagus, blunt and blind dissection of the upper esophagus with finger in the mediastinum and "Pull up" of gastric tube into the neck for anastomosis between gastric tube and proximal esophageal stump.

Advantage: Avoids thoracotomy and risk of an intra thoracic anastomotic leak.

Technique: All these operations are performed by any of the contemporary techniques viz.

Open surgery: Laparotomy, thoracotomy and neck exploration.

Minimal access: Laparoscopic mobilization. Thoracoscopic and open neck.

Robotic assisted: The same can be done by robotic-assisted laparoscopy.

Palliative Surgery

- Feeding jejunostomy for facilitating radiotherapy.
- Placement of tubes through the growth: Celestin, Soutter, Mousseau Barbin tube.

RADIOTHERAPY AND CHEMOTHERAPY (COMBINATION)

- Curative role a selected set of patients with early (T1 N0 M)—well differentiated tumors
- As part of multimodality treatment:
  - Adjuvant chemo radiation—for node positive tumors after radical surgery.
  - Neoadjuvant therapy to facilitate a radical surgery in a T1-2 N1 or T3 disease.
- Palliative: For squamous cell carcinomas—stage I and IV—to palliate dysphagia and for esophago-bronchial fistulae after stenting.

Radiotherapy:
External beam radiation therapy (EBRT)—usually 5000 cGy to mediastinal and cervical fields.

Chemotherapy—combination of:
- Cisplatin; methotrexate; mitomycin C; 5 FU for adenocarcinoma.
- Paclitaxel, bleomycin and etopaside for squamous cell carcinoma.

PALLIATION IN CARCINOMA ESOPHAGUS

Palliation of dysphagia, bleeding, drooling, aspiration and pain.

Surgery

- **Soutter tube or Mousseau-Barbin tube:** Placed through the growth. These have been replaced by endoscopic stenting.
- **Feeding jejunostomy:** For nutrition.

Endoscopic Maneuvers

- Endoscopic stents: Self-expandable metallic stent (SEMS) passed over a guidewire.
  - For palliation of dysphagia and to shut a fistula due to tracheobronchial infiltration.
- Endoscopic LASER coring of the growth: Nd:YAG laser may cause perforation or need repetition. Radio frequency ablation and photodynamic therapy are less effective procedures.

Cause of Death in Esophageal Cancer

- Drooling and aspiration
- Cancer cachexia.
- Sepsis
- Perforation of growth and mediastinitis
- Malignant tracheoesophageal fistula
- Respiratory infection and death.

STOMACH

SU28.7: Describe the applied anatomy and physiology of stomach.

SU28.8: Describe and discuss the aetiology, the clinical features, investigations and principles of management of congenital hypertrophic pyloric stenosis, peptic ulcer disease, carcinoma stomach.

SU28.9: Demonstrate the correct technique of examination of a patient with disorders of the stomach.

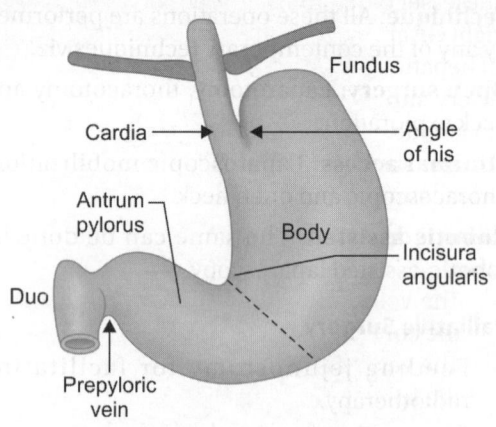

Fig. 28G-1: Anatomy of stomach

APPLIED ANATOMY AND PHYSIOLOGY OF STOMACH

(Refer **Figure 28G-1**)

The stomach develops from the endoderm of the foregut, with the dorsal mesogastrium forming the greater omentum and the ventral mesogastrium forming the lesser omentum. Parts of stomach: Cardia, fundus, body, antrum and pylorus.

Arterial Supply of the Stomach

(Refer **Figures 28G-2 and 28G-3**)

The branches of the celiac artery (the foregut trunk) form a network to supply the stomach. The arteries are: 1. Left gastric artery and 2. Right

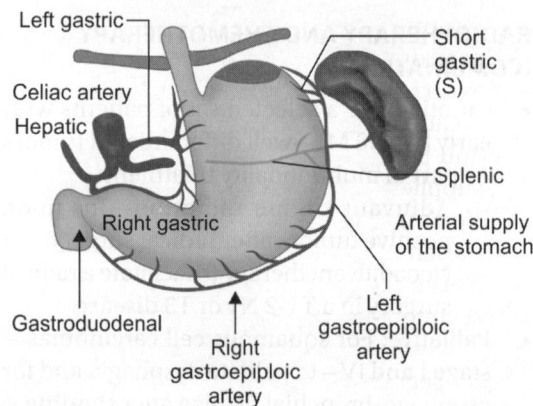

Fig. 28G-2: Arterial supply of stomach—anterior view.

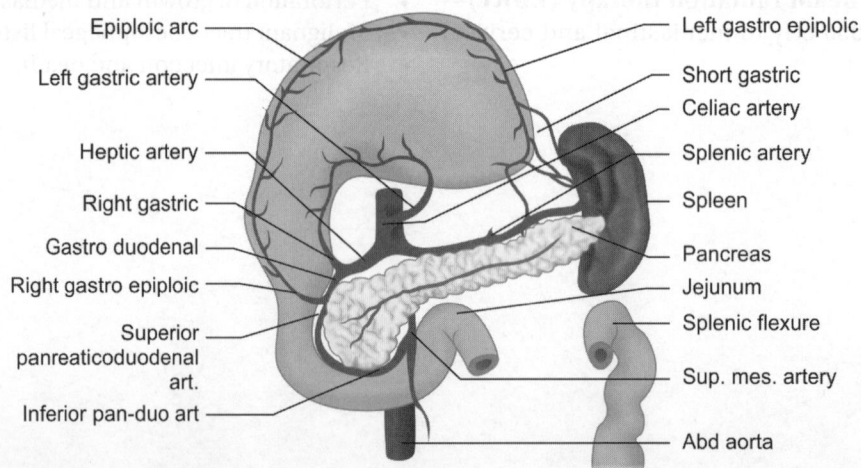

Fig. 28G-3: Posterior view of blood supply to the stomach

gastric artery (from the hepatic artery), run along the lesser curvature to anastomose and supply the lesser curvature; 3. The epiploic arteries: The right GE artery, from the gastroduodenal division of hepatic and the left GE artery from the splenic artery supply the greater curvature by forming an arcade.

The short gastric branches from the splenic artery supply the fundus.

Venous drainage of stomach—is into the portal vein.
- The veins along the lesser curve, including the coronary vein, drain into the portal vein.
- The veins along the greater curve drain into the splenic vein, which joins the portal vein.

Duodenum
- **Arterial supply**: The superior and inferior pancreaticoduodenal arteries, from the gastroduodenal and superior mesenteric arteries respectively form the arterial arcade to supply the C- loop of duodenum and pancreas. The right gastric artery also supplies the first part of duodenum.
- **Venous drainage**—into the superior mesenteric and portal veins.
- **Nerve supply: Vagus nerve**—supplies the secretomotor fibers.
    - Sympathetic supply is from spinal segments T8 and T10.

NERVE SUPPLY TO THE STOMACH
Refer **Figure 28G-4**.

Extrinsic supply: Vagus nerve—is both afferent and efferent.
The two vagi—anterior (left) and posterior (right)—enter through diaphragmatic hiatus.

This gives off the hepatic branch and the posterior—the celiac branch to the splanchnic plexus,

Both the anterior and posterior vagi supply the stomach along the lesser curvature, respectively as anterior and posterior nerves of Latarjet, with the twigs supplying the antrum and pylorus like a "crow's foot".

The vagus has a secreto-motor function (parasympathetic).
- Secretory function—stimulates the parietal cells to produce acid.
- Motor—stimulates peristalsis (fundus has the "pace maker' of stomach).
  Induces adaptive relaxation of pyloric sphincter.

Sympathetic supply: From celiac plexus—gets afferent impulses and inhibits peristalsis.

Intrinsic innervations: Meissner's submucous plexus (not very prominent in stomach).

Myenteric (Auerbach's) plexus: Significant all through the stomach except fundus.

Structure of Stomach
- Mucosa—thick folds in fundus, but thin and relatively adherent in antrum; lined by columnar epithelium.
- Submucosa—with laminal propria, vessels, lymphatics and Meissner's nerve plexus.
- Muscle: Three layers—inner circular, middle oblique and outer longitudinal, and Auerbach's myenteric plexus.
- Serosa.

MICROSCOPY OF GASTRODUODENAL MUCOSA

Gastric mucosa has—1. mucus secreting cells, 2. specialized cells—parietal (oxyntic) cells, chief cells and 3. the endocrine cells.

Gastric epithelium—single layer of columnar epithelium. It is flat with mostly mucus secreting cells in body and antrum.

The mucosal folds in the fundus and body have crypts, which contain parietal and chief cells.
- Parietal cells—mainly in the crypts of "acid producing" **distal body** and produce

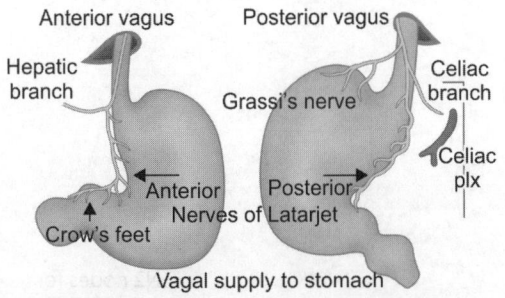

Fig. 28G-4: Nerve supply to the stomach.

hydrogen ions for gastric hydrochloric acid.
- Chief cells: Mostly in crypts of the **proximal body** producing pepsinogen (proteolytic).
- Neuroendocrine cells:
  - G cells—mainly antrum—secrete gastrin.
  - D cells—seen all over the stomach—somatostatin (antisecretory).
  - Enterochromaffin-like (ECL) cells—all over the stomach—secrete histamine to stimulate the H_2 receptors on parietal cells for acid production.

Duodenum

- The duodenum is lined by columnar epithelium, secreting mucus.
- It has endocrine cells that produce secretin and cholecystokinin.

Q. Describe the lymphatic drainage and levels of lymph node stations of stomach.

Lymphatic Drainage of Stomach (Refer Table 28G-1)

The lymphatic drainage of stomach is complex:

The submucous lymphatic network deep to the lamina propria is intercommunicating.

Generally three zones are:

1. **The primary drainage is into the peri gastric nodes**—the para cardiac, chains along the lesser and greater curvature and the supra and sub pyloric groups, numbered (refer **Table 28G-1**) as stations 1 to 6.
2. **The second level of drainage is to the distant nodes**: Left gastric, hepatic and celiac

Table 28G-1: Gastric lymph node stations (Japanese Research Society for Gastric Cancer).

Station number	Node stations	Oncological importance
1	Right para cardiac nodes	St 1, (2) D1 Gastrectomy
2	Left para cardiac nodes	
3	Nodes along lesser curvature	St 3-6 removed at D1 gastrectomy
4	Nodes along greater curvature	
5	Supra pyloric nodes	
6	Infra pyloric nodes	
7	Left gastric nodes	Stations 1, 2, 3–6 and 7–12 removed in D2 gastrectomy
8	Common hepatic nodes	
9	Celiac nodes	
10	Splenic hilar nodes	
11	Nodes along splenic artery (superior pancreatic)	
12a, p, b	Nodes along hepatoduodenal ligament a—artery, p—portal vein, b—bile duct	
13	Nodes at posterior pancreatic head	Distant node stations
14	Nodes at superior mesenteric vein.	
15	Nodes at middle colic vein	
16	Para-aortic nodes	
17	Anterior surface of pancreas	
18	Inferior surface of pancreatic body	
19	Infra diaphragmatic	
20	In the diaphragmatic hiatus	
110	Lower esophageal	N2 nodes for cancer cardia
111	Supra diaphragmatic	

on the right side (stations 7-9) and nodes at splenic helium(station 10) along splenic (station 11) and hepatoduodenal (12-a, p, b) ligament (relation to artery, portal vein and bile duct).

3. **Third level drainage is to the extra-regional nodes** and these are further classified as the extra-stations, in the superior mesenteric or para-aortic and even the thoracic level.

Application

The gastric resections for carcinoma are based on the knowledge of the drainage.

Gastric Lymph Node Stations (Japanese Research Society for Gastric Cancer)

Refer **Table 28G-1, Fig. 28G-5 and Fig. 28G-6**.

Gastric lymph node stations—stations 1 to 6. Refer **Figure 28G-5**.

Gastric lymph node stations—stations 7–12. Refer **Figure 28G-6**.

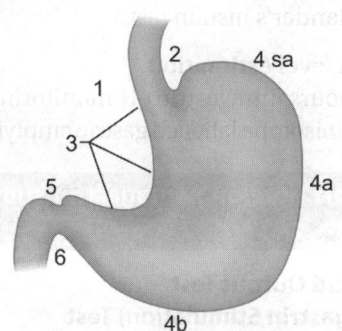

Fig. 28G-5: Gastric lymphnode stations—stations 1 to 6

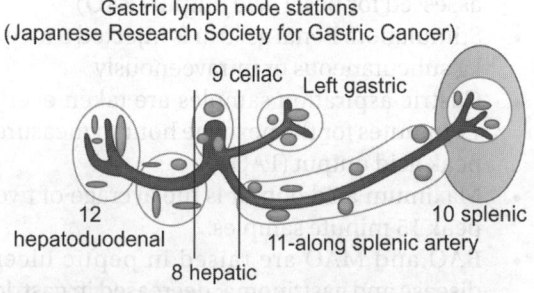

Fig. 28G-6: Gastric lymph node stations—stations 7 to 12.

SURGICAL PHYSIOLOGY OF STOMACH AND DUODENUM

> Q. Describe the gastroduodenal secretory functions.

Stomach Contents

Food, saliva, gastric acid, mucus and regurgitated duodenal bicarbonate and bile.

The stomach prepares an acidic chyme by breaking food and mixing with acid and empties the same into duodenum for further digestion.

Duodenum Secretes

- Mucus
- **Secretin,** which inhibits acids and stimulates pancreatic bicarbonate secretion.
- **Cholecystokinin** stimulates—a. contraction of gallbladder and b. the bile flow into duodenum to alkalinize the acid chime.

Gastric Acid Secretion

The parietal and chief cells produce **acid and pepsin** respectively. Factors regulating the acid production:
- Neurotransmitters - acetylcholine
- Neuropeptides
- Peptide hormones.

The proton pump in the parietal cell produces hydrogen ions.
- Histamine: ECL cells of stomach produce histamine, which acts on H_2 receptor on parietal cell to stimulate the proton pump.
- Vagus and gastrin stimulate the ECL cells to stimulate histamine release.
- Food in antrum stimulates G cells.

Acid inhibits gastrin production by negative feedback.

Inhibitors of Acid Production

- Secretin
- Somatostatin—the peptide inhibits the G cell, the ECL cell and the parietal cell.

Three Phases of Acid Production

1. The cephalic phase—mediated by vagus. Secondary to sensory arousal.
2. The gastric phase is stimulated by food in stomach, by releasing Gastrin (G-cells).

3. The intestinal phase—the duodenal chyme releases secretin to inhibit acid; the chyme and small bowel contents inhibit gastric emptying.

Proton pump produces the hydrogen ions (by a hydrogen–potassium-ATP ase pump).
- In exchange for intraluminal potassium, which enter the crypts. as the hydrogen ions are pumped against high concentration gradient.

Gastric Mucus and the Gastric Mucosal Barrier

Gastric Mucus

A viscid layer of mucopolysaccharides produced by the glands of stomach and pylorus. It is a protective barrier against mechanical and acid peptic damage of the gastric mucosa.

Factors Causing of Breaking of the Mucous Barrier

Hypovolemia and ischemia, shock, bile, non-steroidal anti-inflammatory drugs (NSAIDs), alcohol and trauma.

Peptides and Neuropeptides

Produced by the special neuroectodermal cells in lining.

Their action:
- Endocrine—cell to blood circulation and to the target.
- Paracrine—cell to intercellular space and thence to the target.
- Neurocrine—neural cells secrete them which act across the synapse on the target.

> **Summary of Gastric Acid Secretion**
> - Gastric distention—stimulates muscarinic (M-1)—release of acetyl choline.
> - Acetylcholine—stimulates muscarine receptor (M3)—on parietal cell.
> - Acetylcholine—stimulates ECL cells—release of histamine.
> - Histamine stimulates H1 receptor on parietal cell.
> - Food stimulates G cells to release gastrin.
> - Gastrin stimulates G-cell receptor on parietal cell.
> - Stimulated parietal cell—makes the proton pump to pump hydrogen ions into the lumen—in exchange for potassium ions in the lumen, which combine with chloride to form **hydrochloric acid**.

Gastroduodenal Motility

> **MMC—migrating motor complex—90 minute cycle.**
> - **I phase**: Fasting phase of quiescency—40 minutes
> - **II phase**: Phase lasts for 40 minutes).
>   The gastric pacemaker in fundus generates waves passed upto the pylorus (3 per minute). Then duodenal waves are generated. They are 10/minute and passed) onto the small intestine.
> - **III phase**; 10 minute—vigorous contraction in intestine.
>
> Stimulation of secretion and motility
> - Gastrin, acetylcholine, histamine, 5- HT, CCK.
>
> Inhibition of secretion and motility
> - Secretin, enteroglucagon, somatostatin prostaglandin.

INVESTIGATION OF STOMACH AND DUODENUM: GASTRIC FUNCTION STUDY

Acid stimulation tests:
- Pentagastrin test (# see below)
- Kay's augmented histamine test:
- Hollander's insulin test.

Gastrin level estimation
- 24 hours intragastric pH monitoring
- Radioisotope labelled gastric emptying study.

> **Q. Short note on pentagastrin stimulation test.**

Peak Acid Output Test (Pentagastrin Stimulation) Test

- Patient fasts overnight
- A naso gastric tube is placed and stomach emptied
- Next hour aspiration of gastric secretion is assessed for basal acid output (BAO)
- Stimulation: Penta gastrin is injected 6 mcg/kg subcutaneous or intraveenously
- Gastric aspiration samples are taken every 15 minutes for the next one hour to measure peak acid output (PAO)
- Maximum acid output is the average of two peak 15 minute samples.
- BAO and MAO are raised in peptic ulcer disease and gastrinoma; decreased in gastric cancer, pernicious anemia or atrophic gastritis.

Augmentin Histamine Test of Kay
Same principle but less preferred for better safety of pentagastrin.

Hollander's insulin test—This test is to detect a failed vagotomy. If vagus is intact, insulin induced hypoglycemia stimulates acid secretion through vagus.

> **Q. Short note on gastrin and hypergastrinemia.**

GASTRIN

It is a pentapeptide—secreted by G cells of the gastric antrum.
Normal fasting plasma levels: 50 ng/L.

Three types (of different molecular weight):
1. G-34: Big gastrin (G 34) little gastrin
2. G-17: Little gastrin (0% is in this form)
3. G-14: Mini gastrin (Gu) most common 90%; mini gastrin (G14).

Gastrin stimulates acid production
- It has trophic effect in the parietal cells and also the ECL cells producing histamine.
- It maintains mucosal defence.
- G cell population increases in antral G cell hyperplasia, duodenal ulcer, G-cell.

HYPERGASTRINEMIA

Ulcerogenic Disorders
- Gastrinoma of pancreas
- Antral G cell hyperplasia
- Short gut syndrome, gastric outlet obstruction.

Hypergastrinemia due to low acidity (negative feedback)
- Long-standing treatment with proton pump inhibitors (omeprazole).
- Pernicious anemia
- Vagotomy, atrophic gastritis (hypochlorhydria)
- *H. pylori*, chronic renal failure.

Gastric Motility Studies
- **Gastric dysmotility problems:** Particularly for postoperative gastroparesis.
- Radioisotope-labelled liquid and solid meals are ingested by the patient.
- Gastric emptying is observed on a gamma camera.
- It helps separate study of emptying of solids and liquids.

Endoscopy
Gastro-duodenoscopy: With biopsy, narrow band imaging (NBI) or chromo endoscopy.

Forward viewing scope for routine diagnosis and therapeutics—control of bleeders, polypectomy, submucous resection of early tumors.

Side viewing endoscope: To view the blind areas of stomach (fundus, angle of His), pyloric channel, juxta-pyloric duodenum, duodenal papilla, third part of duodenum.
- **Endoscopic ultrasound**: Best to assess the T-stage of early gastric cancer by evaluating the depth of invasion and also the perigastric nodes and hepatoduodenal nodes. To assess duodenum and head of pancreas.
- Ultrasonography of abdomen and pelvis—as adjunct to evaluation of stomach.
To evaluate liver in cancer or varices, pancreas in pancreatitis, spleen in portal hypertension.

Contrast Enhanced CT Scan
- Best to stage gastric cancers—lymph nodes and hepatic metastases.
- But less sensitive to detect small and superficial lesions. (false negative rate).
- **MRI**—better than CT to detect liver lesions otherwise no advantage over CT.

PET—functional imaging based on a tracer being taken up by metabolically active tumor cells (actively dividing cells). Fluorodeoxyglucose (FDG) is the usual tracer. The PET is combined with CT for a combined structural (anatomy) and functional scan information (PET-CT study).

It is increasingly being used in the pre-operative staging of gastroesophageal cancer.

Diagnostic Laparoscopy
Detection of peritoneal disease—undetected by imaging (smaller than 3-4 mm).

Laparoscopy is combined with peritoneal cytology.

> **Q. Short notes on *Helicobacter pylori*.**

HELICOBACTER PYLORI
- Gram-ve—flagellated organism looks like a spiral.

- Infection with *H. pylori* is believed as the most common human infection.
- *H. pylori* is now classified by the World Health Organisation as a class 1 carcinogen.
- *H. pylori* infection is a prime etiological factor for chronic gastritis, duodenal and gastric ulcers, gastric cancer and gastric MALTomas.
- The organism is a urea splitter—hydrolyzes urea to produce of ammonia, a strong alkali.
- The ammonia acts on antral G cells and releases gastrin leading to gastric acid hypersecretion.
- The negative feedback mechanism to reduce gastrin release may be defunct.

Diagnosis
- Urea breath test or rapid urease test at endoscopic biopsy is done.
- Ig G—also done by ELISA method.
- PCR—for the urease gene.
- Infection with *H. pylori* produces enzymes and disrupts the gastric mucous barrier.
- *H. pylori* infection results in chronic gastritis and may progress to gastric ulceration.

Eradication Therapy
- Triple therapy—for 2 weeks.
- Amoxycillin—500 mg thrice daily.
- Clarithromycin—500 mg twice daily.
- Esomeprazole—40 mg twice daily.
  Triple therapy is given to all with duodenal ulcers or symptomatic infection.

> **SU28.8:** The etiology, the clinical features, investigations and principles of management of congenital hypertrophic pyloric stenosis (CHPS), peptic ulcer disease, carcinoma stomach.

> **Q. Congenital hypertrophic pyloric stenosis (CHPS).**

CONGENITAL HYPERTROPHIC PYLORIC STENOSIS (CHPS)

A congenital condition with hypertrophy of circular layer of pyloric muscle due to defective neuromuscular plexus, (Auerbach's plexus), resulting a thickened pyloric sphincter and gastric outlet obstruction.
- Incidence: 3-4 in 1000 new births.
- Sex: Male: female = 4: 1; first born male child is the preference

Pathology of CHPS
- Hypertrophied pyloric ring—hypertrophy of circular layer of muscle.
- Excess of acetylcholine seen in the nerve endings
- The myenteric (Auerbach's) plexus does not innervate the muscle.

Clinical Features
- Usually first born male child
- Presents between 3 and 6 weeks after birth.

Complaints
- Vomiting—projectile and non-bilious.
- Failure to thrive.
- Child is hungry.

Signs
- Abdomen; visible gastric peristalsis; moving from left to right.
- Pyloric mass palpable in right hypochondrium (pyloric tumor)
- Dehydration
- Hypokalemia
- Alkalosis.

Differential Diagnosis
- Duodenal atresia—bilious vomiting, no mass palpable.
- Intracranial hemorrhage—consciousness level altered.
- High intestinal obstruction (jejunum) due to neonatal volvulus or malrotation of midgut.
- Acute gastroenteritis.

Diagnosis is essentially clinical.
- Ultrasound study—shows a typical pyloric mass of thickened muscle and a longer than average pyloric canal (15 m or longer) and in coronal view a target sign.
- Gastrografin study is rarely performed now.
- Electrolytes—hypokalemia, high hematocrit.

Treatment

Ramstedt's Pyloromyotomy

Prepoperative

Correction of dehydration, hypokalemia and alkalosis by infusion of glucose, potassium and half normal saline.

Operation: Under general anesthesia.
- Small laparotomy—transverse incision right hypochondrium
- Deliver the pyloric mass
- Longitudinal incision over the pylorus only through serosa and muscle fibres till the mucosa bulges.

Endoscopic Treatment
- Endoscopic pyloromyotomy is under trial and is being tried.
- Endoscopic balloon dilatation—results are inconsistent and generally not preferred.

Prognosis: Very good after surgery.

Q. Classify gastritis.

GASTRITIS

Refer **Table 28G-2**.

Gastritis refers to inflammation of the gastric mucosa, microscopically proved.

Classification: Based on cause, quantum of inflammatory infiltrate and degree of gastric atrophy.

Q. Write note on auto immune gastritis.

Autoimmune Gastritis (Previously called Type A Gastritis)

- Autoimmune condition
- Anti parietal cell antibodies—cause atrophy of parietal cell mass and

Table 28G-2: Types of gasrtitis

• Autoimmune (type A) gastritis	• Menetrier's disease
• H. pylori (type B) gastritis	• HIV gastritis
• Reflux	• Granulomatous gastritis
• Erosive gastritis	• Eosinophilic gastritis
• Stress gastritis	• Lymphocytic gastritis
	• Acute bacterial (phlegmonous) gastritis

- Hypochlorhydria and achlorhydria
- Deficiency of intrinsic factor (from parietal cells) and malabsorption of vit B12m lead to pernicious anemia.
  The atrophy does not affect antrum (no parietal cells there)
- Chronic hypergastrinemia—due to hypochlorhydria led negative feedback. Gastrin causes hypertrophy of ECL cells producing high level of histamine.
- ECL cells develop a microadenomas which can turn malignant (carcinoids)

These patients are predisposed to the development of gastric cancer, and benefit from endoscopic surveillance.

Q. Write a short note on *H. pylori* gastritis.

H. pylori Gastritis
- Previously called type B gastritis.
- Antral gastritis or pan gastritis (proximal gastritis without distal inflammation is not included).
- These lead to peptic ulcer disease.

Reflux Gastritis (Alkaline Gastritis)

Due to the bile reflux.

Etiology; previous gastric surgery—gastro jejunostomy or gastrectomy with GJ.
- Biliary dyskinesia—after cholecystectomy.
- Bile breaks the mucosal barrier and leads to nitrosamine formation and in the long run can be carcinogenic.

Treatment
- Sucralfate—mucosal protective; bismuth salts were used earlier.
- Bile chelating agents and prokinetic agents (domperidoen, itopride, cinitapride, levosulpiride) are useful in the treatment.
- Revisional surgery for diverting bile to distal ileum (Roux-en-Y).

Q. Short note on erosive gastritis and stress related gastritis.

Erosive gastritis
- Due to the damage to the gastric mucosal barrier;
- Cause: NSAIDs and alcohol.

- Mechanism: Inhibition of COX-1 (cyclooxygenase-type 1) receptor enzyme, blocking the production of cytoprotective prostaglandins in the stomach. This leads to mucosal damage and ulceration.

Stress gastritis
- The stress of illness—trauma, infection or surgery or otherwise, can cause reduced arterial supply and hypoxia to mucosa of the stomach. This causes ulceration and bleeding.
- Preventive measures in stressful situation: PPI or H2 blockers.
- Treatment in stress bleed:
  - Intravenous Ranitidine or omeprazole/esomeprazole/pantoprazole to push the astric pH levels to 4.5 from below 2.
  - Use of sucralfate to cover and protect it from acid pepsin digestion (sucralfate gets deactivated at a pH above 5).
  - **Surgical resection of the stomach (blind sub total gastrectomy)—rarely required.**

Menetrier's disease
Giant rugal hypertrophy of proximal stomach—with achlorhydria.

Premalignant disease
- Overexpression of transforming growth factor alfa (TGF - alfa) which binds to EGF receptor.
- When found with dyspepsia and diagnosed, **Treatment is**—a subtotal gastrectomy and lifelong supplementation of iron and vitamin B12.

Other Types (Rare)

- **Lymphocytic gastritis**—associated with *H. pylori*: T cell infiltration of gastric mucosa and submucosa.
- **HIV gastritis**—due to cryptosporidiosis.
- **Granulomatous gastritis**—Crohn's and tuberculosis.
- **Eosinophilic gastritis**—responds to steroids and chromoglycate.
- **Phlegmonous gastritis**—infective—often anaerobic bacteria which invade intermuscular planes leading to infective thrombosis and gastric gangrene.

PEPTIC ULCER
- "Ulceration due to the digestion of gastroduodenal lining by pepsin activated in presence of acid. And hence called "acid peptic digestion" of gastroduodenal lining.
- The golden phrase "No Acid No Ulcer ' Still Holds Good, irrespective of etiology.
- It is the net result of acid peptic attack against the mucosal defence.

ETIOLOGY AND PATHOGENESIS
Refer **Table 28G-3**.

PATHOLOGY OF PEPTIC ULCERS
All ulcers tend to occur in alkaline mucosa. Refer **Figure 28G-7**.

Duodenal Ulcers
Most in the first part—rarely 2nd part (ZES, hypersecretion).

Gastric Ulcers
- Lesser curvature—most common 70%
- Prepyloric antrum and pyloric channel
- Junction of alkaline with acidic mucosa of stomach
- Uncommon sites—greater curvature, fundus.

Progression: All ulcers penetrate muscle layers, there is inflammation and fibrosis.
- They heal by fibrosis causing scarring.
- Superficial ulcers (acute ulcers—involve mucosa and submucosa).

Complications: Perforation or bleed.
- Caused by NSAIDs, steroids, alcohol, stress of trauma, surgery or burns.
- Present with massive bleed.

Duodenal ulcers
Site: Anterior wall or posterior wall or double "kiss ulcers", 2nd part less common.

Multiple ulcers seen in hypergastrinemia or Zollinger-Ellison syndrome.

Jejunal ulcers: Follow gastrojejunal anastomosis, e.g., biliary or bariatric surgery.

> **Q. Complications of peptic ulcer.**

Complications of Peptic Ulcers
Acute complications:
- Perforation
  - Duodenal ulcers—usually anterior duodenal ulcers.

- Gastric ulcers:
   Anterior—into peritoneal cavity
   Posterior—into lesser sac.
- Bleeding: Posterior duodenal ulcers replace by gastric ulcers.
  - Hematemesis   30%   60%
  - Melena   70%   40%

Chronic complications:
- Penetration: Posterior ulcers penetrate through the wall—into the neighboring organ.
  - Into pancreas
  - Into colon and cause a fistula (gastrocolic)
- Stenosis: Duodenal/pyloric stenosis
  - Hour glass stomach
  - Teapot stomach (progressive fibrosis and shortening of a lesser curvature)
- Malignant change—duodenal ulcers—unlikely
  - Gastric ulcers—2–3% (different from ulcerative gastric cancer de novo)
    Risk of malignant change—if ulcer is larger than 2 cm.
    Greater curvature ulcers.
    Ulcers in pyloric channel or prepyloric antrum.

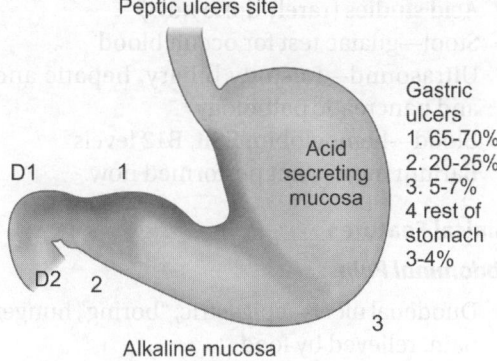

Fig. 28G-7: Distribution of peptic ulcers.

Gastric ulcers
1. 65-70%
2. 20-25%
3. 5-7%
4 rest of stomach 3-4%

Investigations

- **Upper GI endoscopy and biopsy** (10 biopsies of a gastric ulcer is mandatory)
- ***H. Pylori***—urea breath test or endoscopic biopsy of pre-pyloric mucosa for rapid urease test (RUT)
- Serum gastrin assay—in multiple ulcers in duodenum

Table 28G-3: Acid peptic attack versus mucosal defence.

Mechanism of acid peptic attack		
• Stress acts through higher stimuli from CNS on vagus to release **acetylcholine**. • Smoking, spirit, spices stimulate G cells of antrum to release **gastrin** which activates H_2 receptor.	ACh stimulates gastrin receptor to release gastrin. Also, Ach and gastrin both stimulate histamine 2 receptor to release histamine	Histamine activates parietal cell ATPase - hydrogen potassium pump (proton pump) resulting in-
Endocrine • Hyperparathyroidism (HPT), ZES gastrinoma— all stimulate ECL cells to release histamine		Exchange of hydrogen (H^+) ion for potassium ion (K^+) from gastric lumen to produce HCl (hydrochloric acid)
Gastric lumen • Pepsinogen is activated by hydrochloric acid (released from parietal cell) into pepsin. • Active pepsin, *Helicobacter pylori*, luminal bile luminal irritants, aspirin, steroids, NSAID, alcohol. **All the above damage mucus barrier and the mucosal cell barrier breaking the mucosal defence**		
Mucus barrier—defective mucus		
Mucosal cell barrier		

Submucosa
• Vascularity—hypovascularity: Ischemia—acute stress, burns, head injury, shock, chronic ischemia
• Cytoprotective
  – Prostaglandin
  – Somatostatin		

- Acid studies (rarely done now)
- Stool—guaiac test for occult blood
- Ultrasound—to study biliary, hepatic and and pancreatic pathology
- Blood—hemoglobin, ESR, B12 levels
- Barium meal is not performed now.

Clinical Features

Abdominal Pain

- Duodenal ulcer—epigastric, "boring", hunger pain, relieved by food
- Periodicity—periodic attacks of pain of 2-6 weeks alternating with pain free periods of 2-6 weeks
- Gastric ulcer—no periodicity observed
- Pain is not relieved (sometimes worsened) by food intake, not a typical hunger pain
- Vomiting; unusual in the absence of stenosis—in duodenal ulcer
- Vomiting may be seen in 50% of gastric ulcer patients
- Hematemesis and melena ratio
- Duodenal ulcer; 30%: 70 %; gastric ulcer it is 60%: 40% respectively
- Weight—gain in duodenal ulcer, loss in gastric ulcer.

Treatment of Peptic Ulcers

> **Q. Short note on medical treatment of peptic ulcers.**

- *H. pylori* eradication; anti-*H. pylori* regime: For 14 days (upto 21 days recommended by some)
    - Amoxicillin 500 mg thrice a day Clarithromycin 500 mg twice a day
    - Esomeprazole 40 mg twice daily (or pantaprazole 40 mg bid omeprazole 20 mg bid) Metronidazole 400 mg Q8H is also used in place of amoxicillin.
- Followed by maintenance with a Proton Pump inhibitor (esomeprazole 40,mg/day or omeprazole 20 mg/day) for 4 weeks
- Check endoscopy for confirming ulcer healing
- **Acute ulcers**: Intravenous PPI and oral sucralfate as a mucosal protective initially, until gastric pH goes above 5 (sucralfate gets inactivated at pH above 5).

Ulcers not responding to *H. pylori* eradication and PPIs are investigated for gastrinoma and immnological disorders (IgG 4).

> **Q. Short note on principles of surgical treatment peptic ulcers.**

Surgery

- Has a limited role in treatment of uncomplicated peptic ulcers today.
- The surgical operations are more often reserved for the peptic ulcer complications and complications of earlier surgeries done for peptic ulcers.

Rationale of surgery for peptic ulcers

- Acid reduction—vagotomy or
- Diversion of food away from ulcer bearing mucosa—gastrojejunostomy.
- Resection of ulcer bearing part of stomach—partial distal gastrectomy.

Vagotomy

Vagus is secretomotor nerve.

- **Truncal vagotomy**: Anterior (left) and posterior (right)vagus are divided below diaphragmatic hiatus. It causes gastroparesis. Therefore a drainage operation is done by anastomosing stomach to jejunum (gastrojejunostomy)
- **Selective vagotomy**: Anterior vagus divided below the hepatic branch near left gastric artery and posterior below the celiac branch. This will preserve the innervations of hepatobiliary tree and the celiac plexus. But the motor ablation requires a gastrojejunostomy.

Highly selective vagotomy (proximal gastric vagotomy—HSV or PGV): (Refer **Figure 28G-8**)

The terminal branches of both the vagi supplying the lesser curvature are divided close to the stomach from the cardia to the proximal antrum, preserving the branches of the "crow's foot" supplying the antrum and pylorus, retaining the antral and pyloric motility and gastric emptying. Hence there is no need for a drainage procedure.

Gastrojejunostomy (Refer Figure 28G-9): Vagotomy induces gastroparesis. Pyloric stenosis causes gastric outlet obstruction. Both are relieved by gastrojejunostomy; it helps gastric drainage. If done without vagotomy, it allows healing of duodenal ulcer, but causes jejunal ulcers due to acid flooding the jejunal mucosa.

Pyloroplasty (Refer Figure 28G-10): Here the stenotic pylorus is opened in longitudinal axis and sutured in transverse axis to effect a patent pylorus to drain the stomach after vagotomy.

Partial gastrectomy (Refer Figure 28G-11): Distal two thirds of stomach is removed—to remove ulcer bearing area of stomach that includes lesser curve, prepyloric zone and junction of acidic and alkaline mucosa of stomach. The acid levels in gastric ulcer are normal or lower. The proximal gastric stump secretes less acid than normal after resection of antrum (antrum secretes gastrin and stimulated acid secretion).

The gastric resection is followed by restoration of gastrointestinal continuity—by anastomosing the gastric stump to the first part of duodenum as in Billroth I operation or to a loop of jejunum as in Billroth II operation—(after closing duodenal stump).

Complications of Surgery for Peptic Ulcers

- Recurrent ulcers—due to incomplete vagotomy or hypergastrinemia (gastrinoma).
- Postvagotomy diarrhea—variable from mild to severe
- Bilious vomiting—jejunogastric reflux
- **Dumping syndrome:** The rapid passage of food into jejunum causes shifting of fluid from intravascular compartment into jejunal lumen (sequestration of fluid) and hence low intravascular volume, vasomotor symptoms (resulting in epigastric fullness, flush, sweating and high packed cell volume)
- **Late dumping**—due to hypoglycemia.

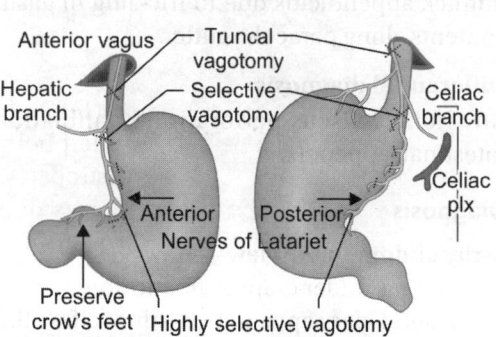

Fig. 28G-8: Highly selective vagotomy.

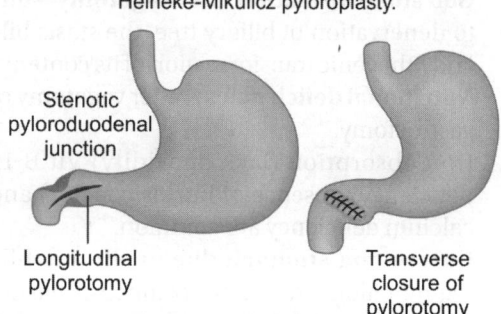

Fig. 28G-10: Pyloroplasty

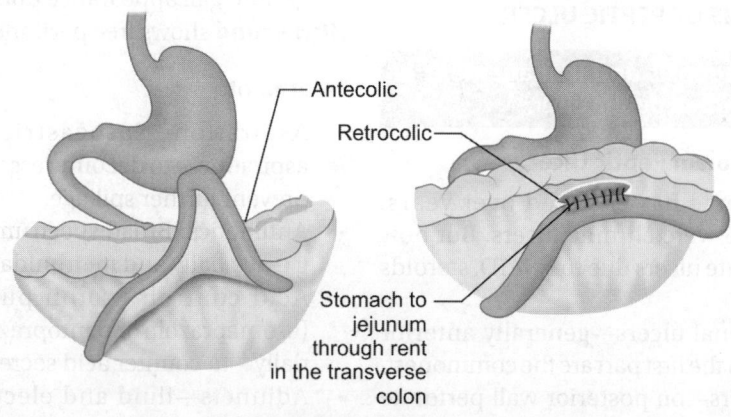

Fig. 28G-9: Gastrojejunostomy

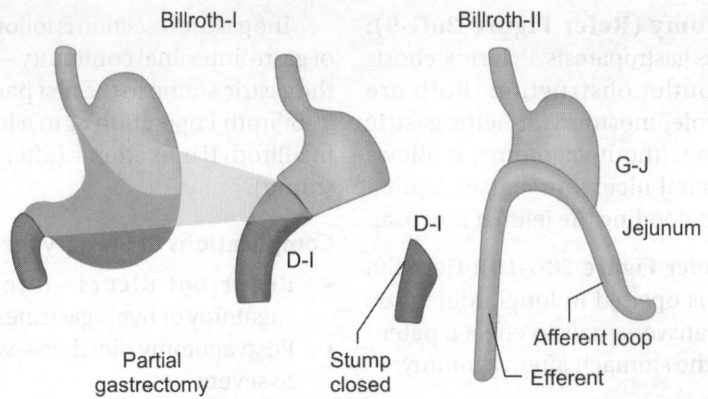

Fig. 28G-11: Partial gastrectomy: Billroth types

- **Jejunal ulcers**—in incomplete vagotomy and/or hyper secretors of acid.
- **Afferent loop obstruction (early post op period)**—causes bilious vomiting
- **Efferent loop obstruction**— late due to fibrosis or adhesions
- **Retrograde jejunogastric intussusception**
- **Gall stone formation after vagotomy**—due to denervation of biliary tree, the stasis bile and lithogenic transformation of its contents.
- **Nutritional deficiencies**—after vagotomy or gastrectomy.
  Iron absorption (lack of acidity) Vit B 12 deficiency (absence of intrinsic factor) and calcium deficiency are common.
- **Carcinoma stomach** due to chronic bile regurgitation, breakdown of mucosal barrier and formation of nitrosamines in the stomach (average 15-20 years after GJ).

COMPLICATIONS OF PEPTIC ULCER

> Q. Clinical diagnosis and management of acute perforated peptic ulcer.

Acute Perforation of Peptic Ulcer

- The incidence has changed over years. Earlier, 80 % were chronic ulcers. But now most are acute ulcers due to NSAID, steroids or stress.
- Site: Duodenal ulcers—generally anterior wall ulcers in the first part are the commonest. Gastric ulcers—on posterior wall perforate into the lesser sac.
- Sex: Male: female ratio about 8:1.
- Age: No age is exempt but mostly seen between 30 and 40.
- **Pathology and clinical presentation**: Refer Table 28G-4.

Valentino's appendix: Slow perforations—may mimick appendicitis due to trickling of gastric contents along paracolic gutter.

Differential diagnosis:
Any hollow viscus perforation—gallbladder, intestinal, appendix.

Diagnosis

X-ray abdomen: AP view—shows
- Free gas under diaphragmatic dome
- Ground glass appearance—due to free fluid in peritoneal cavity
- Localized dilated loops of ileum amidst ground gall appearance due to septic ileus

Ultrasound shows free peritoneal gas.

Treatment

- Aspiration: Nasogastric (Ryle's) tube aspiration—to decompress the stomach and prevent further spillage.
- Antibiotics: Broad spectrum—ceftriaxone 2 g twice daily and metronidazole.
- Acid control: Proton pump inhibitors (esomeprazole or pantoprazole) 40 mg twice daily—to counter acid secretion.
- Adjuncts—fluid and electrolyte supplementation.

Table 28G-4: Pathology and clinical features of acute perforated peptic ulcer.

Pathology	Clinical Features
I stage of peritonism (peritoneal reaction to sudden spillage of irritating gastric contents)	Sudden acute pain in epigastrium—patient rolls up and screams. Signs may not be obvious except for mild guarding
II stage of reaction (3–6 hours) Reactive secretion of peritoneal fluids to dilute the gastric spillage	Clinical stage of illusion (patient feels better) • No pain, quiet look • But abdomen tense, distended and silent (absence of peristalsis) • Pulse rate high, and volume low.
III stage of peritonitis Bacterial proliferation is established	• Signs of peritonitis and septic shock • On examination: Silent, board like abdomen. Tender and rigid, scanty naso gastric aspirate • Area of liver dullness is obliterated by resonance • Flanks are dull • High pulse rate, tachycardia, • Rectal tenderness in recto-vesical pouch

- Assessment: Monitoring
- Action: Early surgery
  - Laparoscopy or laparotomy
  - Exploration and mopping of all peritoneal free contents
  - Closure of perforation and omental patch on the suture site
  - Biopsies from gastric ulcer edges in a gastric perforation
  - Peritoneal toilet with saline and drainage.

Prognosis is poor in patients with
- Late presentation or delay in diagnosis (>24 hours)
- Shock
- Elderly age increasing age (>75)
- Medical comorbidities.

Q. Non-operative treatment of perforated peptic ulcer.

Nonoperative treatment (Hermann Taylor Regimen)
- This is to allow the perforation to close by natural healing while supporting the patient.
- All non-operative measures are started.

Indications:
- Patient is unfit medically for surgery
- A small perforation with minimal peritoneal soiling is expected
- Patient reports late (after many days) when the healing would have already happened (healing underway), provided there are no signs of peritonitis.

Postoperative Follow Up
- Aggressive anti *H. pylori* regimen—amoxicillin, clarithromycin and PPI (e.g., omeprazole)—2 weeks (or 3 weeks—as per the local protocol)
- Continue with PPI for 6 weeks.
- Gastroscopic evaluation: For ulcer healing and sequelae—pyloric or duodenal stenosis.

Majority of patients recover as they have an acute ulcer perforation. They are advised lifestyle modification including abstinence from alcohol, smoking, spicy food.

Elective Surgery required only for:
- Benign ulcers—not healing or duodenal ulcers with stenosis
- Persistent pain and incapacitation (usually posterior penetrating ulcers).

Gastric ulcer: If biopsy proves malignancy—oncological protocol is followed.

Q. Etiology of hematemesis and melena; management of acute bleeding peptic ulcer.

HEMATEMESIS AND MELENA

- Bleeding—a common complication of peptic ulcers, as chronic and occult or overt.
- Hematemesis and melena are the manifestation of overt bleed while a guaiac test of stools detects occult blood in stool.

- The incidence of hematemesis v/s melena in peptic ulcers is 30:70 in duodenal ulcer and 60:40 in gastric ulcer.

Differential Diagnosis of Upper Gastrointestinal Bleeding

- Chronic peptic ulcer
- Acute gastroduodenal ulcers/erosions
- Esophageal varices
- Carcinoma stomach
- Mallory-Weiss syndrome
- Peptic ulcer in Meckel's diverticulum
- Medical causes—purpura, hemophilia.

BLEEDING PEPTIC ULCER: MASSIVE BLEED

- Acute erosive gastritis or *H. pylori* gastritis—alcohol or NSAID gastritis
- Stress induced gastritis, aspirin or clopidogrel, anticoagulants.
- Peptic ulcers:
  - Usually elderly men, atherosclerotics
  - Eroded artery at the base of the ulcer crater.

Diagnosis and management—an emergency:
- Resuscitation and monitor: Transfusion
- Fluid and electrolyte replenishment
- Nasogastric tube aspiration with saline wash out to clear the stomach of blood
- Catharsis—to clear the bowel of decomposing blood (to prevent encephalopathy due to absorption of nitrogenous products formed in the gut).
- Empirical intravenous (IV) proton-pump inhibitors (omeprazole or pantoprazole)—40 mg bolus and repeated every 12 hours.
- Diagnostic upper gastro intestinal endoscopy.
- Investigation—to exclude coagulopathy or other medical causes.
- If variceal bleed and medical causes are excluded and an ulcer bleed is established—endoscopic control of bleeding is performed for an active bleed or for endoscopic stigmata of recent bleed.

High-risk stigmata of recent ulcer bleed:
- Active bleeding vessel at the base of ulcer—90% will rebleed
- Clot on the vessel at the ulcer base—50% will rebleed

- White patch and slough over the bleeding vessel in ulcer base—30% rebleed risk.
- Ulcer crater with clear floor and base—no risk of rebleed.

Methods of endotherapy:
- Laser coagulation of vessel.
- Endoclip application to the vessel.
- Injection of sclerosant into ulcer base or vessel base—adrenaline or sodium tetra decyl sulfate.

Emergency transcatheter arterial embolization (TAE) for duodenal ulcer.
An arterial catheter placed into the gastroduodenal artery detects the bleeder and the same is embolized with gelatin foam or metal coils. But risk of rebleed is more than in surgery and a rebleed makes surgery more morbid.

Surgery

Emergency

- Surgery for patients who continue to bleed
- Failure of endotherapy
- Those requiring more than six units of transfusions.

Emergency control of bleeder—laparotomy, duodenotomy, **under running** of the bleeding vessel at the ulcer base (usually the gastro epiploic) and **ligation of a feeding artery** (gastroduodenal artery) is performed. The pylorotomy is closed transversely as a **pyloroplasty.**

Acid controlling—Highly selective or truncal vagotomy is done if the patient is in stable state.

Distal gastrectomy for large gastric ulcers with massive bleeds.

Blind subtotal (80%) gastrectomy for uncontrolled diffuse erosive bleeds: This procedure is rarely done except as a desparate need today.
- Concomitant *H. pylori* eradication—started in immediate postoperative period.
- Endoscopic review after 6 weeks of PPI.

Prognosis: Overall less favorable.
- High risk of rebleeds (overall 25%), with mortality steeply increasing in rebleeds

- Delay in diagnosis and delay in decision before surgery
- Elderly age and atherosclerosis add to morbidity.

Other Causes

Stress ulcers; Medical management; sucralfate locally through naso gastric tube and PPI. Endotherapy for any major bleeds.

Emergency surgery—uncommonly needed—blind subtotal gastrectomy.

Dieulafoy's lesion: Gastric arteriovenous malformations, may cause severe bleeding.

Treatment

- If detected at endoscopy-endoscopic clips, injection of cyanoacrylate glue or sclerosant are the options.
- If found at surgery, excision of the lesion with part of gastric wall is performed.

Mallory-Weiss syndrome: Linear tear found at endoscopy can be treated by laser or sealant injections. Most of the cases are successfully treated by endotherapy. Rarely surgery is required where a gastrotomy just below cardia and under running of the tear is done.

Tumors: Small bleeding tumors and benign angiomas are controlled by LASER or sclerotherapy/glue followed by elective or emergency surgical resections.

Gastrointestinal stromal tumors (GIST) or leiomyoma:
- They present commonly with massive bleeds and are treated by Emergency gastric sleeve resections.
- Endoscopy may reveal an ulcerated bleeding tumor and CT or MRI may help in a fit patient.

PYLORIC STENOSIS IN DUODENAL ULCER

Pathology

- A misnomer: Chronic duodenal ulcer leads to scarring in first part of duodenum.
- Pyloric channel ulcers (uncommon) cause pyloric stenosis.
- There may be partial or total obstruction of pyloric outlet causing massive dilatation of stomach.

Physiological Consequences of Pyloric Stenosis

Loss of hydrogen and chloride ions from vomiting gastric contents—results in metabolic **alkalosis** with hypochloremia and hypokalemia. Later kidney compensates by absorbing potassium in exchange for hydrogen, to excrete hydrogen ions, thereby causing a paradoxical aciduria.

Clinical Features

- Epigastric pain—pattern changes—persistent and worse after meals. Loss of periodicity
- Vomiting—more towards evening, regurgitant, copious, foul smelling
- Vomitus—non-bilious, often contains undigested food of previous day/s.
- Loss of appetite and weight.

Examination Reveals

- A dilated stomach with visible gastric peristalsis (VGP)—induced by a large glass of water given to the patient.
- In fasting state, the stomach can be seen with stagnant fluid by sign of succession splash by auscultation (normal gastric emptying time is between 120 and 180 minutes).

Scratch test: A dilated stomach may be demonstrated by the scratch test to mark the greater curve of the stomach—which is at or below the umbilicus.

Differential diagnosis—pyloric carcinoma with gastric outlet obstruction.

Investigation

Diagnosis

- Gastroscopy and biopsy of pyloric scar.
- CT scan—dilated stomach with thickened gastric walls and stagnant fluid.
- Blood examination:
  - Serum electrolytes—low levels of potassium, sodium, (also often magnesium and calcium)
- Metabolic slkalosis:
  - Urine: Acidic with low pH (aciduria).

High hematocrit due to loss of fluid.

Treatment: Surgery for relief of obstruction and correcting high acid secretion.

Preoperative:
- Hydration and correction of hypokalemia and alkalosis.
- Daily infusion of fluids with potassium, sodium and calcium.
- Reducing gastric wall edema for overcoming the atony and regaining the peristaltic activity: Allowing only liquid diet, daily gastric wash outs with normal saline till clear aspirate is obtained (takes many days).
- After the patient is evaluated for medical comorbidities, surgery is undertaken.

Surgery—laparoscopic or open route.
- Relief of gastric outlet obstruction—gastrojejunostomy.

Correction of hypersecretion of acidity -
- Truncal vagotomy is generally preferred.
- Proton pump inhibitors—in the immediate postoperative period.
- *H. Pylori* eradication after the patient starts taking oral feeds regularly.

Endotherapy: Endoscopic balloon dilatation of mild pyloric stenosis is practiced with risk of recurrence and disruptive rupture of pylorus. Self-expanding stents have not found favor.

GASTRIC VOLVULUS

Axial rotation of stomach by more than 180°, causing a closed-loop obstruction.

Types
- Organo-axial 70%
- Mesentero-axial or 25%
- Combined 5%.

Presentation: Acute abdominal emergency or as a chronic intermittent problem.

Borchardt's Diagnostic triad of gastric volvulus.
- Severe epigastric pain
- Retching with inability to vomiting
- Inability to pass a nasogastric tube.

Types:
- Organo-axial—most common.
  - The stomach twists on its longitudinal axis (the line joining the cardia with pylorus) as acute condition. This is usually associated with a large paraesophageal hernia or defects in diaphragm. The stomach gets trapped in the gaps or strangulated.
- Mesentero-axial: less common. The greater and lesser curvatures are bisected
  - Antrum twists on the fundus and posterior wall is seen anteriorly. The stomach twists on a more horizontal axis around line of the left gastric artery.
  - Presentation—intermittent and incomplete obstruction, strangulation is uncommon.

Etiology
- Laxity of ligament (30–35%)—gastrosplenic, gastroduodenal, gastrophrenic and gastrohepatic
- Diaphragmatic defects (45%)
- Secondary to operations—fundoplication, esophagectomy, vagotomy,
- Neurological disorders; poliomyelitis
- Increased intra-abdominal pressure—tumors

Diagnosis: CT scan is diagnostic and helps plan surgical approach.

Treatment
Acute Stage
- Endoscopic reduction and elective surgery later to prevent recurrence
- Emergency surgery—if gangrene is suspected or if endoscopic reduction fails.

Elective Surgery
- Decompression
- Derotation of stomach
- Deterrents against (prevention of) recurrence
- Defective anatomy corrected.

Surgical approach can be open or laparoscopic the procedures may be as below:
- Simple gastropexy—fixing gastric wall to anterior abdominal wall by suturing or performing a tube gastrostomy.
- Gastrojejunopexy with division of the gastrocolic omentum. The greater curvature is sutured to the jejunum by taking seromuscular sutures

- Partial gastrectomy—for strangulation gangrene, if any
- Diaphragmatic hernia repair
- Repair of eventration of the diaphragm.

ACUTE DILATATION OF STOMACH

Sudden massive dilatation of stomach following disruption of neuromuscular transmission.

Etiology
- Major trauma—spinal, abdominal, limbs
- post anesthesia (epidural anesthesia)
- Postoperative—Nissen's fundoplication, following repair of large ventral hernias
- Acute gastric volvulus
- Psychiatric illness with polyphagia
- Hypokalemic alkalosis
- Sepsis—including peritonitis.
- Reflex—spinal jackets.

Complications
- Respiratory distress and hypoxia
- Ischemia and necrosis/gangrene of stomach
- Perforation or rupture of stomach
- Septic shock
- acute abdominal compartment syndrome and renal/respiratory failure.
- Death—unrecognized gangrene—mortality is upward of 80%.

Clinical Features
- Acute pain and severe distension of epigastrium
- Difficulty in breathing
- Associated electrolyte abnormality
- Naso gastric tube aspirate—copious, non-bilious and often brownish (mucosal ischemia).

Diagnosis
- X-ray
- CT scan.

Treatment
- Nasogastric tube aspiration
- Intravenous fluids and correction of potassium and other electrolyte abnormalities
- Antibiotic coverage in sepsis
- Supportive—ventilator support if need be
- Monitoring.

Acute gastric dilatation is a serious condition which can be rapidly fatal.

Surgery
- Suspected gangrene or perforative peritonitis.
- Failure of decompression and nonoperative measures.
- Resection of infarcts and necrotic tissue, gastrostomy and a feeding jejunostomy.
- Peritoneal drainage.

GASTRIC CANCER

Epidemiology and Risk Factors in Pathogenesis of Gastric Cancer
- Ethnicity
- Atrophic gastritis and achlorhydria
- Pernicious anemia
- Watery diarrhea, hypokalemia, and achlorhydria (WDHA) syndrome (VIPoma)
- Menetrier's disease (giant rugal hypertrophy of mucosa with proteinuria)
- Intestinal metaplasia
- Dysplasia
- Smoking and obesity
- Pernicious anemia
- Genetic factors (3-4%)—hereditary gastric cancer syndromes
- Operations for benign peptic ulcers—risk of cancer in gastric remnant 15-20 years later
- **Hyperplastic polyps:** Large, pedunculated polyps (>1 cm) and villous adenomas show an creased risk of gastric cancer.
- Chronic atrophic gastritis.

Genetic: 95-96% are sporadic 3-4% may have a familial link.

Germline mutations
- In p53 (Li-Fraumeni syndrome) and BRCA2.
- CDH 1—encoding adhesion protein E cadherin—an autosomal dominant factor.
- Mismatch repair gene deletions (MMR deletions).

HER -2 neu over expression (15-25%).

Hereditary nonpolyposis colorectal cancer (HNPCC) syndrome and polyposis syndromes:

- Familial adenomatous polyposis, MUTYH-associated adenomatous polyposis
- Juvenile polyposis syndrome, PTEN-associated hamartoma tumor syndrome (Cowden syndrome), and Peutz-Jeghers syndrome.
- Infection with *Helicobacter pylori*
- Chronic *H. pylori* infection and antibodies to *H. pylori* are associated with higher risk of cancer in distal cancer (not the cancer of cardia). The intestinal type of gastric cancer is associated with *H. pylori* related pangastritis, achlorhydria and intestinal metaplasia of gastric epithelium.

Diet: Salt, smoked or poorly preserved foods with high content of nitrates, nitrites produce intragastric luminal carcinogens. Diet high in raw vegetables, fresh fruits, vitamin C, vitamin A, calcium, and antioxidants are believed to be protective.

Q. Pathology and staging of carcinoma of stomach.

PATHOLOGY OF GASTRIC CANCER

Gastric Cancers (Refer Table 28G-5)
- Adenocarcinoma—from mucus secreting cells
- Lymphoma
- Neuroendocrine tumors, e.g., carcinoid
- Leiomyosarcoma
- GISTs—gastro intestinal stromal tumors.
- Adenosquamous and squamous cell carcinoma.

Table 28G-5: WHO—histologic typing of gastric cancer.

• Adenocarcinoma	• Adenosquamous carcinoma
• Papillary adenocarcinoma	• Squamous cell carcinoma
• Tubular adenocarcinoma	• Small cell carcinoma
• Mucinous adenocarcinoma	• Undifferentiated carcinoma
• Signet-ring cell carcinoma	• Others

Types
- Proximal tumors (GE Junction)—not related to *H. Pylori*.
- Distal adencarcinomas—associated with *H. Pylori*.

Lauren's classification—microscopy is correlated well with prognosis.

Intestinal type: (associated with metaplasia)—polypoid or ulceration.
Acinar architecture retained and differentiated, better prognosis.

Diffuse type—deep infiltration and early spread, poorly differentiated, signet ring cells common—more of a scirrhous type—it has a poor prognosis.

Classification of Gastric Carcinoma

Q. Short note on early gastric carcinoma

Early gastric cancer (Refer Figure 28G-12)
Confined to mucosa and submucosa T1, any N.
- Type I: Elevated (protruding)
- Type II: Superficial—IIa elevated, II b flat and II c depressed
- Type III: Excavated—invades deep submucosa.

Q. Classify advanced gastric carcinoma.

Advanced gastric cancer: Borrmann's classification (Refer Figure 28G-13).
- Type I: Polypoid
- Type II: Ulcerative (ulcerated growth)
- Type III: Crateriform—deep ulceration and irregular margins
- Type IV: Diffuse infiltrating (linitis plastica).

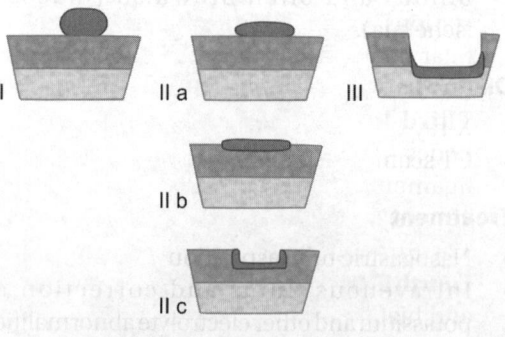

Fig. 28G-12: Early gastric cancer

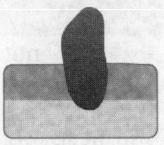 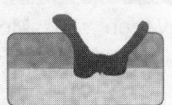 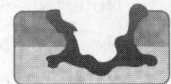 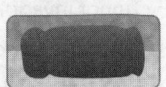

Type I: Polypoid   Type II: Ulcerative   Type III: Excavated ulcer   Type IV: Diffuse infiltrating (linitis plastica)

Fig. 28G-13: Advanced gastric cancer: Borrmann's classification.

Q. Short note on leather bottle stomach.

Linitis plastica (leather bottle stomach): Adenocarcinoma, poorly differentiated and (Lauren's) diffuse type, submucous infiltration, intact looking mucosa with loss of mucosal folds, may be localized of diffuse type.
Early metastasis and poor prognosis.
Treatment: Total gastrectomy and reconstruction with esophagojejunal anastomosis.

Spread of the Tumor

Local—with in the stomach—along the submucosa and through the muscle and then the serosa to peritoneal cavity.

(S) Serosal spread is the single most important prognostic factor.

Outside the stomach—to nearby organs or into the abdominal wall and peritoneal cavity.

(P) spread—all over the peritoneal cavity and into the pelvis.

Lymphatic spread (L)

- **First level nodes from cardia to pyloric stations 1-6:** The tumor cell can spread to any of the perigastric nodes through submucous lymphatic network.
- **The second level nodes** receive these cells—stations-left gastric, hepatic, celiac, splenic hilar nodes and those along splenic vessels (stations 7-11).
- **Third level** spread is to extra-regional nodes—associated with the hepatoduodenal ligament, head of pancreas, middle colic vessels, superior mesenteric vein, (stations 12-16).
- **Fourth level**—para-aortic, subdiaphragmatic and hiatal and supra hiatal nodes (stations 17-20, 110-112).

Supraclavicular node: Troisier's sign.
Umbilical nodule: Sister Joseph's nodule—due to spread along the ligamentum teres.

Blood spread (M)—through portal vein into the liver.

Later diffuse hematogenous spread may happen to lungs, skin, testis or ovaries (Krukenberg tumor), or even bones.

STAGING (Refer Table 28G-6)

Stages: I, II, III—considering the local tumor invasion and nodal spread.

Summary of staging of carcinoma stomach

- Stage I: Refers to the early gastric carcinoma
- Stage II: To the advanced carcinoma with resectable local and lymphatic spread (T1,2 N0/N1)
- Stage III: Locally advanced and/or extensive lymphatic spread (T3N1, T4, N2+)
- Stage IV: Denotes the hematogenous, nonregional lymphatic and peritoneal spread.

Clinical Features

- **Dyspepsia group:** Middle aged man complaining of a recent "indigestion", vague epigastric discomfort, fullness, loss of appetite, loss of weight.
- **Obstructive group:** Epigastric pain, vomiting the food, and ball rolling sensation and visible gastric peristalsis.
- **Triple "A" group:** Anemia, asthenia and anorexia
- Cachexia
- Hematemesis (15%), melena
- Mass group: Epigastric mass—with vomiting (distal growth) or dysphagia (proximal growth) or without vomiting (growth in the body).

Table 28G-6: TNM staging (Adopted from AJCC)

Tumor (T)	Tumor invasion level	Node (N)	Nodal invasion	Met (M)	
Tx	Tumor not assessed	Nx	Not assessed	Mx	Not assessed
T0	No tumor evident	N-0	No nodes	M0	No metastasis
Tis Ca- in situ	High grade dysplasia or lamina propria not invaded	N1	N1-1-3 nodes	M1	Distant spread
T1 a	Lamina propria invaded	N2	3-6		Hematogenous Non-regional nodes level 16, 17, 18 Peritoneal disease micro or macro
T1 b	Submucosa invaded	N3	7 or more		
T2	Muscularis propria	N3 a	7-15 regional nodes		
T3	Subserous plane	N3 b	16 or more regional		
T4a	Serosa breached				
T4b	Adjacent organs invaded				

- **Perforation** can perforate uncommonly.
- **Features due to metastases**:
  - Ascites
  - Nodules in the rectovesical pouch, Blumer's shelf.
  - Troisier's sign-paplable supraclavicular (Virchow's) node.
  - Hepatomegaly—hard nodules with umbilication.
    * Umbilical nodule (Sister Joseph's nodule)
    * Cutaneous secondaries, unusual sites like testic, small bones.
    * Trousseau sign-migrating thrombophlebitis, (diff diagnosis—in carcinoma pancreas).

Differential diagnosis of following features:
- Dyspepsia and pain—acid peptic disease and ulcers
- Mass—pancreatic, colonic, lymph nodes
- Ascites—ovarian or other malignancies
- Anemia—any medical cause
- Melena or hematemesis.

Q. How do you investigate a case of suspected carcinoma stomach?

Investigations for evaluation of gastric carcinoma

- **General:** Blood test for anemia, high ESR.
  - Stool guaiac test for occult blood
- **Upper** gastrointestinal endoscopy—biopsy.
- Narrow band imaging for evaluation of early lesions.
- **Ultrasound**—to evaluate peritoneal, liver and nodal metastases.
- **Endoscopic ultrasound (EUS)** is most accurate in distinguishing early gastric cancer (T1) from more advanced tumors and evaluation of depth of invasion. Nodes < 0.5 cm are detected.
- **Contrast enhanced multislice CT scan**—for evaluation of local, nodal and metastatic disease.
- **Positron emission tomography–computed tomography (PET-CT):** Using fluorodeoxyglucose (FDG) as radio tracer. Use: FDG PET CT study helps in preoperative detection of regional disease and metastases and avoid a morbid radical surgery for advanced disease. PET helps in detection of recurrences and metastases after treatment.
- Laparoscopy and peritoneal cytology for detecting metastases and avoiding a radical surgery.
- Carcinoembryonic antigen (CEA), may be elevated in some
- **Genomic evaluation: Immunohistochemistry (IHC)**—Post surgery, the specimens are tested with immunohistochemistry methods:
  - For mismatch repair genomic mutations, MMR mutations
  - For microsatellite instability (MSI); HER-2 neu receptor (15-30% test positive).

> **Q. Short note on treatment of carcinoma of stomach, also refer summary at end.**

TREATMENT OF CARCINOMA STOMACH

Surgery is the cornerstone of treatment of carcinoma of stomach.

Adjunct modalities: Chemotherapy, radiotherapy, local ablative therapy, immunotherapy and targeted therapy.

Summary of treatment is described after the details:

> **Principles and nomenclature of gastric surgery for cancer (Refer Figure 28G-14)**
>
> **Radical surgery (with or without adjunct therapy) is the only hope for cure.**
>
> Radical surgery involves complete removal of all disease with no residual cancer.
> - R0 - no residual disease after resection
> - R1 - microscopic residual disease after an apparently R0 resection, e.g., micro mets in residual - nodes, tumor cell spillage surgery, small areas of serosal breach (T4 a disease)
> - R2 - gross residual tumor tissue left behind, e.g., release of tumour adherent to abdominal wall, liver or pancreas or large lymph nodes left behind.
>
> **Extent of Gastric resection in cancers:**
> - **Total Gastrectomy:** Entire stomach including lower 3 cm of esophagus and 2 cm of post pyloric duodenum—continuity is restored by anastomosing esophagus to jejunum (loop or a pouch with a Roux-en-y)—usually reserved for proximal gastric cancers only.

- **Subtotal gastrectomy**-The G-E junction and proximal stomach (about 20–25%) is preserved and anastomosis as in total gastrectomy done for most cancers.
  This is referred to as a Distal Gastrectomy (that removes distal three fourths).
- **Esophagogastrectomy** resection of lower esophagus and proximal part of stomach (fundus and body) with anastomosis between proximal esophagus and distal gastric remnant (body or antrum)

Cancer of cardia: A gastric cancer within 2 cm of cardia is treated as lower esophageal cancer.

Radical resections: "Radical" refers to the curative intent of operation, which involves a total loco-regional clearance of the cancer.

En bloc removal of tumor bearing stomach with a tumor free margin of 5 cm proximally and duodenal cuff of 2 cm from first part of duodenum, the gastro-hepatic and gastro-colic omentum and the obvious and potential regional lymphatic field and may include removing extra-regional lymphatic area.

These surgeries are—total radical gastrectomy or radical distal subtotal gastrectomy (Refer **Fig. 28G-15**).

> **Dissections of lymph nodes are named after the extent of dissection.**
> - D1 - lymphadenectomy - N1 lymph nodes—stations 1-6
> - D2 - lymphadenectomy - N2 lymph nodes—stations 1-6; 7-11 (11s,12 a included).

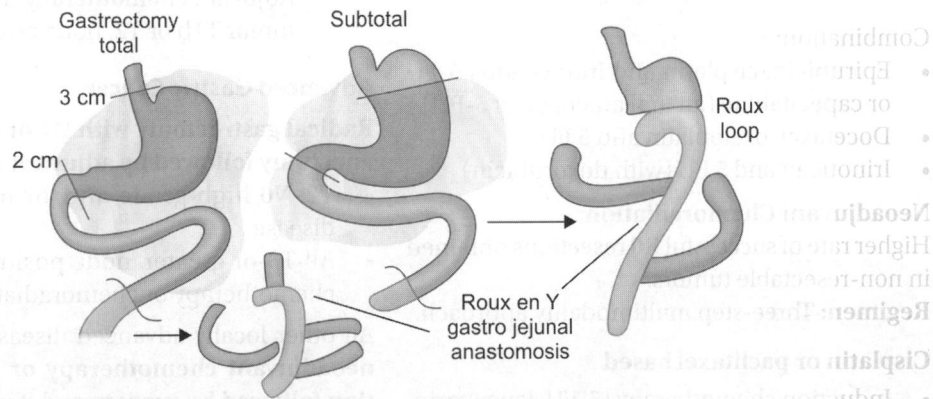

Fig. 28G-14: Gastrectomies in gastric cancer.

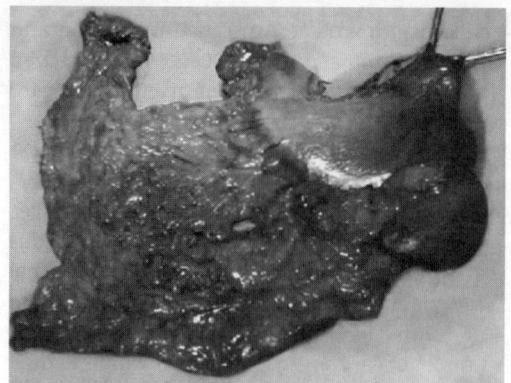

Fig. 28G-15: Radical total gastrectomy.

- **D3** - N3 lymph node dissection - 1–6 + 7–11 + 12–15 (usually not done as it is a more morbid procedure with no survival advantage over D2.
- **D4** - removal of pancreatic and paraortic nodes not practiced now—no advantage.

Palliative surgery—for locally advanced and inoperable disease.
- Local resection—for an obstructive lesion with peritoneal or/and N3 disease; also as adjunct to chemotherapy.
- Gastrojejunostomy to overcome a non-resectable obstructing growth.

Chemotherapy: Combination cytotoxic chemotherapy—adjuvant therapy after surgery for all advanced gastric cancers and selected early cancers.
- Neoadjuvant chemotherapy is advised for locally advanced disease as it improves the outcome following surgery.

Combination:
- Epirubicin, cisplatin and intravenous 5-FU or capecitabine (an oral analogue of 5-FU)
- Docetaxel, oxaloplatin and 5 FU
- Irinotican and 5 FU (with doxorubicin)

Neoadjuvant Chemoradiation
Higher rate of successful **R0** resections obtained in non-resectable tumors.
Regimen: Three-step multimodality approach.

Cisplatin or paclitaxel based
- Induction chemotherapy (5-FU, leucovorin, and cisplatin or paclitaxel)
- Chemoradiation therapy (45 Gy plus concurrent 5-FU), and followed by gastrectomy with D2 gastrectomy.

Paclitaxel based:
- Two cycles of 5-FU, cisplatin, and paclitaxel 28 days apart with concurrent radiation followed by surgery
- Gastrectomy with spleen-preserving D2 lymphadenectomy.

Immunotherapy/targeted therapy with chemotherapy: For metastatic or recurrent tumors.
- To boost T-cell-tumor immunity in patients.
- Enterectrinib injection or Larotrectenib tablets
- For high Microsatelite instability tumors- NIvolumab or pembrolizumab
- For HER 2 Neu positive tumors -Trastuzumab
- Anti -VEGF agents -Ramucirumab with Irinotican.

SUMMARY OF TREATMENT OF GASTRIC CARCINOMA

Early Gastric Cancer
- **EMR**: Endoscopic mucosal resection.
- **Indication:** T1 a N0, well differentiated < 2 cm or > 2 cm without ulceration.
- **Surgery:** Radical gastrectomy D1
- Indications:
  - Surgery alone: T1a N0—high grade, larger than 2 cm or ulcerated lesions.
  - All low grade T1b and any T2 N0
  - Adjuvant chemotherapy: For high grade tumor T1b or T2, node positive.

Advanced Gastric Cancer

Radical gastrectomy with D1 or D2 lymphadenectomy followed by adjuvant therapy for:
- T2-N0 high grade and/or node positive disease.
- All T3-or greater, node positive—adjuvant chemotherapy or chemoradiation.

All other locally advanced disease: Treated by **neoadjuvant chemotherapy or chemoradiation followed by surgery** and if needed, follow up chemotherapy.

Follow up:
Every 3 months for the first 2 years following resection.
- Clinical examination is performed, along with study of complete blood cell count, liver function tests, prealbumin, vitamin B12, and vitamin D levels).
- CT scan: Chest, abdomen and pelvis, every 6 months after surgery for 2 years, yearly for 5 year. Endoscopy—for recurrence—after 1 year and 5 years.

Recurrent and Metastatic Carcinoma
- Chemotherapy (irinotican) or chemo with immunotherapy or targeted therapy (Nivolumab/Pembrolizumab/Enterectrinib or trastuzumab (HER 2 neu positive) or anti VEGF drugs-Ramucirumab).
- Radiotherapy to reduce pain in bone metastases.

HIPEC: Hyperthermic Intraperitoneal Chemotherapy
Mitomycin C or oxaliplatin-based regimen. Laparoscopic HIPEC also practiced along with systemic chemotherapy.

Indications
- Peritoneal metastases or T4 tumor with HIPEC is given along with a cytoreductive surgery (CRS).
- **Cytoreductive surgery:** Palliative gastrectomy and addition of peritonectomy.

PALLIATION IN GASTRIC CANCER
Surgical Palliation
- **For obstruction**:
  - Gastric outlet obstruction.
    - Palliative distal gastrectomy for mobile growths.
    - Anterior gastro jejunostomy for fixed growth.
  - For obstruction of cardia—feeding jejunostomy and local chemoradiation.
- **Bleeding from growth**
  - Palliative resection of the part of stomach with the growth.
- **Perforation**—resection is the best palliation
  - Suture with a patch of omentum.

Symptomatic and Supportive
- Relief of pain, vomiting, bony pain.
- Nutritional support.

Prognosis is better with:
- Tumor early stage
- Tumor lower grade
- Tumor histo type intestinal (worse with diffuse)
- Peritoneal (serosal) invasion—negative—important factor.
- Node negative or N1.

Five year survival: T1—90%, T2—60-70%, T3—50% T4—less than 20%.

OTHER TUMORS OF STOMACH
Gastrointestinal Stromal Tumors (GISTs)
- GISTs make 1-3% of all gastrointestinal tumors, arising in any part of the GI tract.
- They are tumors of mesenchymal origin, 50% are seen arising from the stomach.
- The tumors are associated with a mutation in the tyrosine kinase c-kit oncogene. These tumors are sensitive to the tyrosine kinase antagonist imatinib.
- Seen affecting both sexes equally.
- The biological behavior of these tumors is linked to its size and mitotic index although unpredictable.
- Spread: Metastases—peritoneum and liver, lymphatic spread is late.
- The gross appearance: Ulceration of mucosa overlying the tumor, severe bleeding or noticed at endoscopy.
- Diagnosis: Endoscopic biopsy can be negative unless the tumor has ulcerated.
- Targeted biopsy by endoscopic ultrasound is more accurate.

Treatment
- Unpredictable behavior.
- Size: >5 cm—high risk for metastases.

Surgery is the best option when resectable.
- Local wedge resection for smaller tumors.
- Gastrectomy for larger tumors (without lypmhadenectomy).
- Hepatic metastasectomy.

Large tumors involving multiple viscera: Imatinib for 3–6 months prior to operation
- To reduce size and vascularity of tumor.
- Adjuvant imatinib for large resected tumours should be continued indefinitely.

Sunitinib: For Imatinib failures.

Prognosis: Improved with imatinib.

GASTRIC LYMPHOMA

Primary gastric lymphomas make 5% of all tumors of stomach, accounting for 65% of all lymphomas of the gastrointestinal tract, which is the most common site of extranodal non-Hodgkin lymphoma (NHL).

The two primary histologic types
- Low-grade marginal zone B-cell lymphomas of the mucosa-associated lymphoid tissue (MALT); MALT lymphomas are associated with *H. pylori*
- High-grade diffuse large B-cell lymphoma (DLBCL).

Symptoms
- Nonspecific and this causes delay in diagnosis.
- Clinical features: Pain (85%), loss of appetite (40%), weight loss (25%).
- Bleeding (20%), and vomiting (18%).
- Obstruction and perforation occur. Perforations often follow chemotherapy.

Investigation
Endoscopy
Multiple biopsies—from each region of the stomach, duodenum, and gastroesophageal junction (GEJ) as well as normal-appearing mucosa. Deeper biopsies, including possible endoscopic mucosal resection (EMR), if needed.
- *H. pylori* tested by RUT or urease breath test
- Translocations are evaluated.

Staging: To establish "primary" against a "systemic" lymphoma.
- CT scans of the chest and abdomen
- Bone marrow aspirate study
- Full blood count
- Lactate dehydrogenase and beta-2-microglobulin.

Treatment
No consensus on treatment.
- Surgery (gastrectomy) alone?
- Chemotherapy alone?
- Early-stage, low-grade mucosa-associated lymphoid tissue (MALT) lymphoma—antibiotics and proton pump inhibitors for the eradication of *H. pylori* and results in long-term remission.

Diffuse lymphomas: Chemotherapy is the choice. Surgery is to deal with perforation or bleeding—usually involves a gastrectomy.

> **Q. Short note on gastrinoma.**

ZOLLINGER-ELLISON SYNDROME

Hypergastrinemia and persistent, multiple peptic ulceration, ulcers in unusual sites—second part of duodenum; no esophagitis as gastrin increases the lower esophageal sphincter (LES) pressure.

Cause
- **Gastrinoma**—duodenal wall or pancreas
- Sporadic or as a part of multiple endocrine neoplasia type 1 (MEN-1) (pituitary, parathyroid and pancreatic tumors)
- G-cells: Hypersecretion of acid causing Zollinger-Ellison syndrome (ZES).
- About 25% are in association with MEN-1, 50% are multiple (most are with MEN-1).

> **Sites of primary gastrinoma—found in Passaro's triangle in 70 to 90% of patients.**
>
> **Passaro's triangle** (gastrinoma triangle)—a triangular area between three points:
> 1. At the junction of the cystic duct and common bile duct
> 2. At the junction of the second and third portion of the duodenum
> 3. At the junction of the neck and body of the pancreas
>
> The duodenal loop—from G cells of Brunner's glands. But gastrinomas can be anywhere and multiple; hence the need for whole body imaging.
>
> **Suspect ZES:** in a patient with multiple peptic ulcers in atypical locations (2nd or 3rd part of duodenum) that fail to respond to antacids.
>
> Diarrhea—seen in 20% of patients with gastrinoma.

Differential diagnosis of hypergastrinemia:
Pernicious anemia, atrophic gastritis.
G-cell hyperplasia, treatment with proton pump inhibitors, renal failure, retained or excluded antrum, and gastric outlet obstruction.

The diagnosis of ZES:
Serum gastrin level >1000 pg/mL. PPI stopped before the test.

Pentagastrin test:
The very high basal acid output but no marked response to pentagastrin, due to the maximal stimulation of parietal cell mass by the gastrin from the tumor, leaving nothing for the pentagastrin to stimulate.

Localisation test of choice: SSTR (octreotide) scintigraphy in combination with CT.
More sensitive than CT detects 85% of gastrinomas and tumors <1 cm.

Selective angiography (if octreotide scan is not done).

EUS (endo ultrasonography) assists in the preoperative localization of gastrinomas <1 cm, for tumors in the pancreatic head or duodenal wall.

Serum calcium—to rule out MEN.

Treatment and prognosis
Tumors outside the gastrinoma triangle have a worse prognosis.

Surgery for primary sporadic gastrinoma
Tumor enucleation, when possible.

Pancreaticoduodenectomy—if inevitable—when enucleation not possible total gastrectomy (earlier to the imaging modalities, this was the practice).

A highly selective vagotomy—for unresectable disease or no localization is done for the tumor.

For inoperable cases:
- Proton pump inhibitors (PPIs)—omeprazole or pantoprazole—mitigate the damage and symptoms.
- Most cases have an indolent course including malignant gastrinomas with liver secondaries.
- Gastrinomas with hepatic metastases
  - Hepatic resection for secondaries
  - Chemotherapy with streptozotocin and doxorubicin (± 5 fluorouracil),
  - Removal of all resectable disease (cytoreductive surgery)
  - Hormonal therapy with somatostatin analogues
  - Biotherapy with interferon,
  - Hepatic embolization alone or with chemotherapy (chemo-embolization).

Summary of treatment of gastrinoma: ZES

Treatment

Localized tumor:
- Enucleation—for gastrinoma in the pancreas not involving the main pancreatic duct.
- Pancreatic resection—for solitary gastrinomas with no metastases.

Inoperable or metastatis tumors:
- A highly selective vagotomy—for unresectable disease or no localization is done for the tumor
- Metastasectomy done for oligometastases
- Local ablation—radiofrequency ablation (RFA) for metastases
- Transarterial chemoembolization (TACE)—for liver metastases
- Chemotherapy; streptozotocin, doxorubicin, 5-FU.

28.3: Spleen, Liver, and Biliary Tract

SU28.10	Describe the applied anatomy of liver. Describe the clinical features, investigations and principles of management of liver abscess, hydatid disease, injuries and tumors of the liver.
SU28.11	Describe the applied anatomy of spleen. Describe the clinical features, investigations and principles of management of splenic injuries. Describe the post-splenectomy sepsis and prophylaxis.
SU28.12	Describe the applied anatomy of biliary system. Describe the clinical features, investigations and principles of management of diseases of biliary system.

SPLEEN

SU28.10: Describe the applied anatomy of liver. Describe the clinical features, investigations and principles of management of liver abscess, hydatid disease, injuries and tumors of the liver.

SU28.11: Describe the applied anatomy of spleen. Describe the clinical features, investigations and principles of management of splenic injuries. Describe the post-splenectomy sepsis—prophylaxis.

SPLEEN

Applied Anatomy of Spleen
(Refer Figure 28S-1)

Develops in dorsal mesogastrium from 6th intrauterine week, moves with rotation foregut to left side. Weight: 75-250 g in adult, measure 10 × 7 × 3 cm occupying the space below left dome of diaphragm and gastric fundus with long axis along the 10th rib and the hilum just above the pancreas.

The splenic artery from celiac trunk gives off multiple branches to pancreas along its upper border (as it runs in the gastrosplenic ligament), the left gastroepiploic artery and the vasa brevia and ends by dividing into superior and inferior branches in splenic hilum.

The splenic vein is formed at the hilum from tributaries and runs posterior to pancreatic border receiving multiple tributaries and joins the superior mesenteric vein to form the portal vein.

The splenic pulp is invested by an external serous and internal fibroelastic sheath. The lymphatic drainage: The white pulp drains

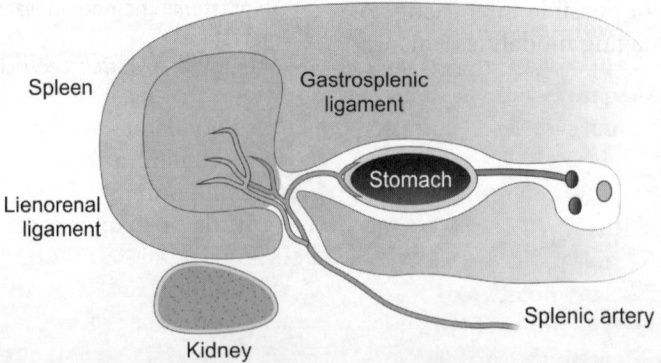

Fig. 28S-1: Splenic anatomy

through efferent vessels which run with arterioles and emerge from nodes at the hilum. These nodes and lymphatics drain into the celiac nodes via retropancreatic nodes.

Sympathetic nerve fibers from the celiac plexus innervate splenic arterial branches.

Q. What are the functions of the spleen?

Functions of the Spleen

Immune, storage, culling, repair of RBC and cytopoietic.

- **Immune function**: Maturation of lymphocytes.
  - 65% of T-lymphocytes and 15% of B lymphocytes are in the spleen.
  - Speen produces—specific immunoglobulin M (IgM) against the foreign antigens, non-specific opsonins, properdin and tuftsin. The antibodies from the B- and T-cell origin, which bind to macrophages and leukocytes to stimulate phagocytic and anti tumor functions.
- **Filter function**: RBC, platelets, Hb, iron, bacteria
  - "Culling"—the endothelial macrophages remove the effete platelets and red cells in the splenic sinuses and cords.
  - Also filtering of iron and hemoglobin.
- **Pitting**: Repair of RBCs
  - Removal of inclusions—nuclear remnants —Howell Jolly bodies
  - Precipitated hemoglobin or globin remnants—Heinz bodies
- **Reservoir function:** RBC and platelets
  - Contains approximately 8% of the red cell mass—more in a large spleen.
  - Platelet reserve—sequestration.
- **Hemocytopoiesis:** Haemopoiesis in the fetal spleen (4th week)
  - Stimulation of the white pulp
  - Proliferation of T and B cells
  - Following antigenic challenge.

This is also seen in myeloproliferative disorders, thalassemias and hemolytic anemias.

Q. Short notes on splenunculi.

SPLENUNCULI

Accessory splenic rests (small spleens) congenitally present in about 10–30% of population.

May be single or multiple.

Sites: Splenic hilum—50%-related to splenic vessels.
- Behind the tail of the pancreas—30%
- Splenic ligaments
- Greater omentum
- Mesocolon

Their importance: When a splenectomy is performed as a curative measure for hemolytic anemias like hereditary spherocytosis and ITP, the splenunculi must be carefully searched for and removed, to prevent failure of treatment due to the splenunculi continuing to contribute to the persistence of disease.

Splenosis: Due to spillage of splenic cells during surgery or following trauma to the spleen.

Splenic Cysts

- Non-parasitic **splenic cysts** are rare.
- Splenic primary cysts (true) or pseudocysts (secondary).

Splenic Infarction

Etiology

- Myeloproliferative syndrome.
- Portal hypertension
- Splenic vein thrombosis
- Sickle cell disease
- Pancreatic disease
- Iatrogenic—vascular occlusion during surgery (e.g., spleen—preserving distal pancreatectomy).

Clinical Feature

- The infarct may be asymptomatic or
- Pain- left upper quadrant and left shoulder tip pain.

CECT: Contrast-enhanced CT will show a perfusion defect in the enlarged spleen.

Treatment

Conservative—symptomatic and supportive. Splenectomy—only if there is an abscess formation in the spleen.

> **Q. Enumerate the etiology of splenic rupture and its clinical features.**

SPLENIC RUPTURE

Refer Table 28S-1.

Clinical Features of Splenic Rupture (Both Traumatic and Spontaneous)

Diseased spleen is more prone for rupture.

Grade I: Sudden Death (Due to Massive Hemorrhage)

Grade II: Shock →Recovery →Signs of Splenic Rupture

- Initial shock (internal bleeding)
- Increasing pallor
- High pulse rate sigh and restlessness.

Local signs: Abdominal distension
- Rigid abdomen, tenderness in left upper quadrant
- Shifting dullness (blood in peritoneum)

Ballance's sign: Right flank—dullness—shifting on lateral position (free blood)
- Left side: Flank dullness - but does not shift on lateral position (due to the clot and perisplenic contained collection of blood which is walled off and clotted).

Kehr's sign: Pain felt at left shoulder tip due to diaphragmatic irritation when patient is put in Trendelenburg position (foot end raised).
Blood in rectovesical pouch.

Grade III: Delayed Rupture Occurs Between 7th and 14th Day

Apparently normal patient develops sudden hypotension and signs of internal bleed and may die instantaneously if not recognized. Often the event precipitated by straining at stool or coughing.

Mechanism

- Initial blood is localization by omentum
- Subcapsular hematoma—bursts
- Because it gets digested by the pancreatic juice activated due to traumatic pancreatitis.

Complications of Splenic Rupture/Trauma

- Hemorrhagic shock due to blood loss
- Sepsis
- Pancreatitis due to associated injuries to tail of pancreas, diaphragmatic injury
- Hemothorax
- Disseminated intravascular coagulation (DIC)
- Splenic artery pseudoaneurysm
- Splenic arteriovenous fistula.

Diagnosis of Splenic Rupture

- Ultrasound examination—the safest and fastest way to assess
- CT scan—particularly in splenic trauma to assess grade and decide the line of treatment.
- X-ray—obliteration of splenic shadow and psoas shadow
    - Associated fracture ribs—9-11 as a clue
    - Fluid between intestinal loops
- Radioisotope scan— Technetium 99m labeled colloid scan.

Table 28S-1: Splenic rupture—etiology.	
Splenic traumatic rupture	*Spontaneous rupture*
Types: Blunt and penetrating Blunt injury to the abdomen Accidents—road traffic Fall form a height Blow or fall of a large weight or stone on abdomen Industrial—accidents (belt injuries)	• Inflammatory • Malarial spleen • Neoplastic • Splenic infarcts • Myeloproliferative diseases • Hematological disorders • Splenic vein thrombosis • Amyloidosis • Storage disorders—Gaucher's

> Q. Describe mechanism and classification of splenic trauma, clinical diagnosis and management of splenic trauma.

> Q. Write short notes on FAST - Focussed Assessment by Sonography in Trauma and Diagnostic peritoneal lavage in splenic trauma.

SPLENIC TRAUMA

Must know—main question.

Mechanism (refer splenic rupture above)

Focussed assessment with sonography for trauma (FAST) is done in emergency room during resuscitation. Triage is started as per ATLS recommended line of management.

Diagnostic Peritoneal Lavage (DPL)

Instillation of normal saline 1 litre into peritoneal cavity with the help of a subumbilical catheter, turning the patient to right and then to left and then aspirating the fluid. The same is analysed —culture (bacterial). It is sent for microscopy, cytology, culture, and biochemical analysis.

It is significant if the aspirate contains— gross blood >10 mL, > 1 lakh RBCs, >500 WBCs, amylase > 175 bile, bacteria or food particles.

Emergency CT scan is the standard of care in all splenic injuries to decide on management.

Classification of Splenic Trauma

Refer **Table 28S-2**.

Angiography

CT angiography is for diagnosis—of aneurysm or injury to the vascular pedicle. Selective angiographys is done for transcatheter embolization to reduce bleeding in non-operative management of splenic injury.

Treatment

Emergency Treatment

- Resuscitation and triage regarding associated injuries (ATLS guidelines)
- Blood transfusion and fluid replenishment. Stabilization of the patient
- Monitoring
- FAST.

Further Management

CT scan scoring

Splenic injury < grade I and II—non-operative treatment.
- Continued monitoring
- Continued supportive treatment.

Grade V—need immediate splenectomy and control of hemorrhage.

Grade III and IV injuries—the decision is crucial—on choice on management—to operate or continue with non-operative.

Non-operative treatment is advocated in:
- Hemodynamically stable patients
- Splenic injury gr I, II and III
- No associated injury (polytrauma) to any other organ or system.

Table 28S-2: Classification of splenic trauma.	
Classification of splenic trauma (CT scan based) and management	
Grade I	Hematoma: Subcapsular—non-expanding—<10% surface area. Laceration: < 1 cm deep, capsular tear, no bleed
Grade II	Heamatoma: Subcapsular—non-expanding—10–50% surface area. Hematoma: Intraparenchymal—non-expanding <5 cm in diameter Laceration: Capsular tear 1–3 cm in depth which does not involve trabecular vessel
Grade III	Hematoma: Expanding subcapsular hematoma exceeding 50% of surface area OR ruptured and bleeding OR intraparenchymal haematoma >5 cm Laceration: Parenchymal >5 cm or depth >3 cm, involves trabecular vessels.
Grade IV	Laceration involving segmental or hilar vessels with >25% devascularization
Grade V	Shattered or avulsed spleen; hilar devascularization with entire spleen separation

Advantage of non-operative **treatment**—splenic functions preserved particularly the immunological long-term risk of sepsis with pneumococci and hemophilus are avoided.

But a timely surgery can be life saving.

Q. Indications for emergency splenectomy in trauma.

Emergency Surgery
- Persistent hypotension < 90 Hg systolic BP, tachycardia > 120 despite 2 litres of saline and blood transfusion (2 litres)
- Primary Gr IV or V injury
- Grade III with large subcapsular hematoma when it threatens to leak (delayed rupture)
- Secondary complications—sepsis, peritonitis or hemoperitoneum
- Splenic artery aneurysm—found at Doppler or CT angiography
- Delayed splenic rupture—early surgery is life saving.

Laparotomy and splenectomy or laparoscopic exploration and splenectomy.

Splenic preservation done whenever possible in traumatic rupture—especially in children

Surgery: Choice of Procedures
- Splenectomy.
- Partial splenectomy—upper or lower pole preservation depending (upon the injury to the splenic branch vessel (superior or inferior)
- Splenorrhaphy—capsular repair and suturing of the trabecular vessel (using 4-0 polyglactin) indicated for Gr III or II. Can't be done for Gr IV and V.
- Mesh wrap—spleen is wrapped in hemostatic mesh (oxydised cellulose) to contain hemorrhage and splenectomy avoided.

Complications of Splenectomy/Splenic Surgery
- **Due to injury and surgery**
  - Hemorrhagic shock and death
  - Injury to pancreatic tail and pancreatitis
  - Pancreatic fistula
- **Infective complications**
  - Left subphrenic abscess
  - Empyema thoracis
  - Peritonitis

- **Hematological complications:**
  - Thrombocytosis
  - Erythrocytosis
  - Hypercoagulability—venous thrombosis.

Q. Opportunistic postsplenectomy infection (OPSI).

- **Postsplenectomy immunological consequences:**
- Risk for developing pneumonia, meningitis and major sepsis increased three-fold
- Opportunistic postsplenectomy infection (OPSI)
- Poor opsonisation and phagocytosis
- Susceptibility to pneumococcal and haemophilus influenzae infection
- Risk of overwhelming sepsis is greatest within the first 2-3 years after splenectomy.

Prevention of OPSI
- Prophylactic antibiotics—in immune suppressed
- Vaccination
- Post-splenectomy, a vaccine is given with in 12 hours.of surgery preferably.

Before elective splenectomy—vaccinating against pneumococcus, meningococcus C (both repeated every 5 years) and *H. influenzae* type B (Hib) are considered.

General Indications for Splenectomy
Refer **Table 28S-3**.

Table 28S-3: Indications for splenectomy.

Indications for splenectomy	
Trauma	**Hypersplenism**
• Accidental	• Portal hypertension
• Operative	• Variceal surgery
• Ptosis of spleen	• Splenic neoplasms, large cysts, granuloma(TB)
• Diagnostic or therapeutic procedures	• Abscess
	• Aneurysm of splenic artery
Hematological	• Oncological
• Hereditary spherocytosis	• Part of *en bloc* resection—gastrectomy, colectomy
• Purpura (ITP)	

LIVER

> **SU28.10:** Describe the applied anatomy of liver. Describe the clinical features, investigations and principles of management of liver abscess, hydatid disease, injuries and tumors of the liver.

ANATOMY OF LIVER

Liver develops from the hepatic bud from the endoderm of the foregut, which gives rise to hepatocytes and bile ducts. The endothelium is derived from the vitelline and umbilical veins, the liver sinusoids are formed by the merger of the vitelline and umbilical veins with endodermal bud. The septum transversum, a mesodermal structure, gives rise to the supporting connective tissue, the Kupffer cells and the hemopoietic cells.

Liver is divided into a functional right and left 'unit'. There are two anatomical lobes with separate blood supply, bile duct and venous drainage. Dual blood supply (20% hepatic artery and 80% portal vein); the quadrate lobe is an independent unit.

Arterial supply: Hepatic artery from celiac axis—gives off gastroduodenal and divided into right and left hepatic branches to the respective lobes.

Portal vein divides at the porta hepatis into right and left and accompanies the arterial branch to the respective segments.

Veins: Three hepatic veins—right, middle and the left. Draining segments and inferior hepatic veins which join the vena cava directly—connecting inferior part of the liver (caudate lobe included).

Each hepatic segment has the artery portal vein and the bile duct. Hepatic hilum: Transverse fissure: hepatic artery to the left of bile duct along the free border of hepatoduodenal ligament and the portal vein behind the bile duct.

> **Q. Describe segmental anatomy of liver and enumerate Couinaud's segments.**

Segmental Anatomy of Liver
(Refer Figure 28H-1)

- Important in lever resections and transplantation.
- Two lobes, four sectors and eight segments.
- **The main portal fissure (the Cantlie's line)** divides the liver into two lobes. The line extends from the gallbladder fossa to the left side of IVC.
- **The left portal fissure** divides the left lobe into two sectors, an anterior, with segments 3 and 4 and a posterior sector, with segment 2. The left hepatic vein runs in the fissure.
- The segment 1 - is caudate lobe and is independently supplied by hepatic arteries and portal veins and the venous drainage is directly into the inferior vena cava.
- **The right portal fissure** divides the right lobe into an two sectors—the anteromedial containing segments 5 and 8 and posterolateral sector with segments 6 and 7. The right hepatic vein runs in this fissure.

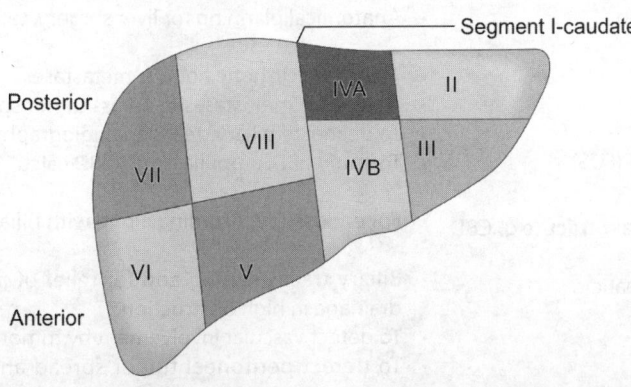

Fig. 28H-1: Couinaud' segments of liver

- Each segment has its own blood supply from hepatic artery, the portal vein, and the draining hepatic vein and the bile duct..
- Surgical importance—the segments can be removed individually without prejudice to the remaining for surgical remedy.

Q. What are the functions of the liver?

Functions of the Liver

Synthesis of albumin and clotting factors.

Metabolism and Excretion

- Glucose—glycolysis, gluconeogenesis.
- Protein catabolism to form urea.
- Hemoglobin—breakdown and formation of bilirubin.
- Metabolism of hormones
- Metabolism and excretion of drugs.

Homeostasis

- Core body temperature
- pH balance and correction of lactic acidosis
- Detoxification: Removal of gut endotoxins and foreign antigens.
- Storage: Glycogen, iron, copper, vitamins A and B12.

Liver Function Tests

- Hepatocyte function;
  - The cellular enzymes levels in blood—increase in acute hepatocyte damage.
  - Aspartate transaminase (AST- SGOT) and alanine transaminase (ALT-SGPT)
  - The gamma-glutamyl transpeptidase (GGT) level,
- Biliary canalicular state obstruction leads to elevated levels of enzymes;
  - ALP (alkaline phosphatase) and 5-nucleotidase.
- Synthetic function: Bilirubin—unconjugated and conjugated
  - Serum albumin, clotting factors vit K dependent, prothrombin time.

Q. Role of radiology and imaging in liver disease.

Radiology and Imaging in Liver Disease (Refer Table 28H-1)

Q. Short notes on alfa-fetoprotein.

ALFA-FETOPROTEIN

- A glycoprotein with a carbohydrate moiety.
- Fetal yolk sac secretes it to protect the fetus from maternal estradiol.
- Its levels reduce in the first year after birth.
- Normal value is up to 10 ng/mL.
- It is a tumor marker for hepatocellular carcinoma (levels reach 100–1000 ng/mL)
- Helps in follow up to suspect recurrence in post-resection state.
- AFP is also seen elevated in:

Table 28H-1: Imaging in liver disease.

Non-invasive imaging	**Application**
• Ultrasound—first imaging	• Cysts, nodules, dilated IHBD, calculi
• Multi slice spiral CT scan	• Anatomical planning for liver surgery, tumors or metastases
• CT angiography	
• MRI	• Tumor v/s cirrhotic nodule, metastases.
• PET scanning	• To look for metastases or assess tumor spread.
• MRCP	• To delineate biliary tree (cholangiography)
• Endoscopic ultrasound (EUS)	• To study CBD, ampulla, small CBD calculi + biopsy
Invasive imaging	
• ERCP Imaging the biliary tract (e.g. CBD stones)	• For endoscopy recording along with biliary intervention
• Percutaneous transhepatic cholangiography PTC	• Biliary tract imaging and for relief of jaundice by biliary drainage in high obstruction.
• Angiography	• To detect vascular involvement by tumor
• Laparoscopy	• To detect peritoneal tumor spread and superficial liver metastases
• Laparoscopic ultrasound	

- Non-seminomatous testicular tumors
- Ovarian tumors in females—yolk sac tumors
- Benign hepatoblastoma.

ACUTE LIVER FAILURE

Causes

- Viral hepatitis (hepatitis A, B, C, D, E)
- Weil's disease (leptospirosis)
- Shock and multiorgan failure
- Acute cholangitis:
  - Drug hypersensitivity or toxicity: Paracetamol, non-steroidal anti-inflammatory drugs, anesthetic agents, isoniazid, antidepressants.
  - Acute Budd-Chiari syndrome.
  - Poisoning, fatty liver in pregnancy, Wilson's disease.

Clinical Features

Early stage may be silent and signs are seen in late stages (severe failure):
- Clinical jaundice, fetor hepaticus.
- Signs of hepatic encephalopathy:
  - A flapping tremor
  - Drowsiness, confusion
  - Leading to hepatic coma.

Treatment of Acute Liver Failure

Supportive Therapy

Monitoring and correction of:
- Acid-base balance and blood glucose
- Fluid and electrolytes imbalance.
- Nutritional requirement—glucose, albumin.
- Cerebral edema—mannitol—infusion for osmotic diuresis with monitoring.
- Renal insufficiency—monitoring and treatment—hemofiltration
- Respiratory dysfunction—ventilatory support.
- Treatment of bacterial and fungal infection.

Transplantation in Acute Liver Failure

Transplantation is indicated when irreversible liver failure is anticipated—severe metabolic acidosis (pH,7.3), encephalopathy grade 4, protrombin time 100 sec, serum bilirubin >300 mg% and creatitinine >300 mmol/L, children below 10 years and adults above 40 years of age, drug idiosyncracy as etiology.

Chronic Liver Disease

Hepatic reserves are abundant and clinical features are seen only when over 75% of the functioning liver is compromised.

Clinical Features
- Asthenia and lethargy
- Fever
- Features of liver failure appear
- Jaundice
- Wasting (Protein catabolism)

Signs of Hepatic Failure
- Coagulopathy (bruising)
- Cutaneous: Spider naevi and palmar erythema
- Cardiac—hyperdynamic circulation.
- Cranial: Neurological—hepatic encephalopathy—drowsiness, stupor, flapping tremor, fetor.

Portal Hypertension
- Ascites, esophageal varices
- Splenomegaly
- Engorged periumbilical veins (caput medusa).

> Q. Describe the Child-Turcotte-Pugh (CTP) classification of liver function as per severity.

The parenchymal destruction leads to cirrhosis, which is classified as per severity (refer **Table 28H-2**):

Patients with liver disease are at greater risk of surgical and anesthetic complications.

For a given procedure, the risk is higher by 10% for a CTP A, 30% for a CTP B and 75-80 % for CTP C class of liver disease.

> Q. Discuss the etiology, classification and management of liver trauma.

LIVER INJURIES

Penetrating

- Stabs
- Bullet and missile injuries
- Fall or hit against sharp objects

Table 28H-2: CTP classification of hepatocellular function in cirrhosis.

Child–Turcotte–Pugh (CTP) classification of hepatocellular function in cirrhosis.

	Points	1 point	2 points	3 points each
1.	Bilirubin (mg/100 mL)	<2	2–3	>3
2.	Albumin (g/100 mL)	>3.5	2.5 to 3.5	<2.5
3.	Ascites	None	Well controlled	Uncontrolled
4.	Encephalopathy	None	Grade I–II	Grade III–IV
5.	INR	<1.7	1.7–2.2	>2.2
	Prothrombin time prolonged by	<4 sec	4–6	>6

Child's (CTP) score—A = 5–6 points, B = 7–9 points, C = 10–15 points

Table 28H-3: Classification of liver trauma in severity

Grade	Hematoma Subcapsular	Hematoma Parenchymal	Laceration
1	<10% of liver surface	—	Capsule tear, < 1 cm deep
2	10–50%	Size:< 10 cm	Capsular laceration 1–3 cm deep
3	>50%	> 10 cm	> 3 cm deep
4	Rupture of expanding hematoma, active bleed		Parenchymal disruption **25–75%, of a lobe** affects >3 segments in one lobe—R or L
5	**Vascular injury** Major hepatic veins or retrohepatic vena caval injuries		Parenchymal disruption **> 75%** of a lobe or more than 3 couinaud segments
6	Hepatic avulsion		

Blunt Injuries

- Fall from height
- Road traffic accidents—steering wheel
- Crush injuries—buildings, industries
- Natural disasters.

Classification of Liver Trauma on Severity

Refer **Table 28H-3**.

Management of Liver Trauma

Guidelines

Consider poly trauma—attend associated injuries.

Emergency resuscitation (as per principles of advanced trauma life support (ATLS): Airway, breathing and circulation.

High-risk categories:

- Crush injury with multiple rib fractures
- Stabbing/gunshot in lower chest or upper abdomen.

Assessment of injury

Focused assessment with sonography in trauma (FAST)—in emergency room and emergency — CT chest and abdomen with contrast.

Decision on Managing Liver Injuries: Non-operative or Operative

- **Non-operative management with active monitoring:** For Injuries Grade I, II and III with active USG /CT monitoring, if they are hemodynamically stable and in good general condition.
- **Emergency surgery for:**
  - Injuries Grade IV, V and VI
  - Deterioration of the patient despite resuscitation in those under non-operative group.
  - Emergency laparotomy if hemodynamically unstable.

Specific surgical steps at laparotomy
- **Pringle maneuver**: For Initial control of on table bleed by holding and compressing the free border of lesser omentum (hepatoduodenal ligament) between thumb in front and two fingers (index and middle) behind in the foramen of Winslow—this will minimize the bleeding by occluding the portal vein and hepatic artery.
- Suturing of the lacerations
- Resection for torn major hepatic vessels.
- **Packing** if diffuse parenchymal injury—perihepatic packing—above, behind and below with radio tagged mops—removed after 2 to 3 days.
- Packing with absorbable hemostatic mops—oxidized cellulose and allowed to get absorbed. Here a reopening is avoided if patient stabilizes.
- **Interventional radiography**: Hepatic arterial embolisation—for effective control of hemorrhage from aneurysm or pseudoaneurysm. Massive hepatic necrosis and failure can complicate.

Damage control surgery (DCS): In an unstable patient—to save life.
- Initial laparotomy, packing and control of bleeding
- Resuscitation to continue concurrently and postoperatively and specific measures to correct hemodynamic instability (transfusions). Coagulopathies (frozen plasma, platelets), systemic dysfunction (renal failure) and electrolyte and acid base defects along with antibiotic cover.

Complications of Liver Trauma
- Parenchymal
  - Intrahepatic hematoma
  - Liver abscess
- Biliary canaliculi and ducts
  - Within liver—bile collection
  - Biliary peritonitis due to leak.
  - Biliary fistula
- Vascular
  - Tear of hepatic or portal vein—hemoperitoneum and shock
  - Hepatic artery aneurysm
  - Arteriovenous fistula
  - Arteriobiliary fistula
- Liver failure—due to acute massive hepatic necrosis.

Results and Prognosis
- Good trauma management has improved the outlook.
- Overall mortality is around 10% in isolated liver trauma and 25 - 30% when associated with other major trauma, 40 to 50% in Gr IV and V injuries
- Nonoperative management succeeds in over 80% of Gr I-III injuries.
- Gr IV and V injuries have 40% success and are employed only by the tertiary centers.
- Damage control surgery in non specialised centers can save lives and shift the patients to specialized centers for specific complications like biliary or vascular disruptions.
- Emergency approach is for polytrauma, unstable patients, and isolated liver injuries grade IV, V and VI.

INFECTIOUS CONDITIONS OF THE LIVER

> Q. Etiopathogenesis, complications, clinical diagnosis and management of amebic liver abscess.

AMEBIC LIVER ABSCESS

Amebiasis continues to be a major health problem in tropical countries, but its incidence is lower than in last century.

Etiology: Protozoa: *Entamoeba histolytica*.

Pathogenesis and pathology of amebic liver abscess

Route of entry: Feco-oral route—through food contaminated by feces with amebic cysts.
- The cysts evolve into trophozoites in the large bowel and inhabit the crypts of colonic mucosa (mostly cecum and sigmoid),
- Where they secrete the histolytic enzyme to digest mucosal cells to form ulcers—flask shaped with overhanging margins, wherein the amebae thrive.

- From here they gain access to the portal vein and reach the liver, where they cause liquefaction necrosis of hepatocytes, and thrombosis of blood vessels, leading to formation of the amebic abscess.
- The pus is chocolate brown colored and odorless—the typical "anchovy sauce".
- The lesions are initially multiple small micro-abscesses (amebic hepatitis—as it is erroneously called) which coalesce to form larger abscess or abscesses.
- Site of preference—right lobe—segments—VII and VIII, although any segment may be involved and both lobes may be affected.

Note: There is very little inflammatory reaction to the amebic lysins and hence the abscess is initially free from pain or inflammatory symptoms and signs, (until it is complicated). Unlike a pyogenic abscess, amebic abscess has no wall made of a pyogenic membrane and a fibrotic wall; the amebic trophozoites are seen in the wall of the abscess with a free access into blood vessels. The absence of a fibrotic wall makes ir easier for the amebicidal drugs to reach the abscess (unlike hydatid). The condition heals without much of fibrosis ; hence with least risk of cirrhosis.

Complications
- Secondary bacterial infection; (bowel microbes travel via portal vein)
- Rupture into pleural cavity—empyema most common (70%)
- Bronchus—broncho pleural fistula
- Peritoneal cavity—peritonitis
- Bile duct—sepsis and jaundice
- Pericardium—cardiac tamponade
- Through skin—amebiasis cutis and ulcer
- Chronic granuloma—"ameboma"of cecum or rectum (mimics carcinoma.
- Brain—amebic encephalitis—multiiple abscesses (blood spread—to brain)
- Ameboma of brain.
- Septicemia—in cirrhotics.

Clinical Features
- Males outnumber females by 10 times; more common in alcoholics
- A history of an amebic dysentery may be ewlicited in some, but not a must.
- Pain in the right upper quadrant is very common.
- Shoulder pain on right side in some.
- Fever, chills and rigors, loss of weight, and a dry cough may be present.

Common Signs
- A tender hepatomegaly is seen in most.
- Right sided intercostal tenderness.
- Right sided pleural effusion.
- Abdominal wall edema in right hypochondrium in acute cases.
- Tenderness and rigidity.

Chronic long-standing silent abscesses—a hard smooth, firm or hard liver may be palpable, mimicking a hepatocellular carcinoma.

Differntial Diagnosis
- Acute pyogenic abscess—alcoholics, diabetics and elderly—more common
- Cholecystitis
- Subphrenic abscess
- Hepatocellular carcinoma (when it is a chronic abscess)
- Pleurisy and pleural effusion.

Investigations
- **Liver function tests:** Mild alteration—elevated bilirubin, ALP and prothrombin time
- Leukocytosis may not be there unless secondarily infected with bacteria
- Chest X-ray
- Elevated right dome of diaphragm, effusion
- Ultrasonography—accurate in assessing the liver abscess, pleural complications biliary tree complications.
- CT to evaluate in multiple abscesses.

Treatment of Amebic Liver Abscess
Medical treatment: Micro-abscesses and small abscesses of 2.5 to 3 cm respond well.
- Nitroimidazoles
  - *Severe cases:* Injection metronidazole dose (40 mg/kg/day = about 500 mg Q8H or Tinidazole 600 8 hourly divided doses for 10-14 days.

- *Milder cases:* Tab. metronidazole 800 mg Q8H or Tinidazole 600 mg Q 12 H -5 days.
- *Others:* Secnidazole and ornidazole.
• Antibiotics for 5-7 days to control associated bacterial infection.
  - *Intravenous:* Amoxycillin, 1 g Q8H, Ceftriaxone 1 g Q12H or
  - Ciprofloxacin 200 mg Q12H
  - Oral cefixime 400-600 mg daily or Amoxycillin 1-2 g/day or cipro 1 g/day.
  - Tetracycline or oxytetracycline 1 g, daily.
• Injection dehydroemetine 1.5 mg/kg/day IM for 5 days, under monitoring for cardiotoxicity.
• Chloroquine 250 mg twice a day; (for 14 to 21 days with monitoring for optic nerve toxicity and cardiotoxicity).

Aspiration of Abscess
Indications
- Abscesses larger than 10 cm
- Abscesses >5 cm persisting, refilling and those enlarging despite medications
- Aspiration of left lobe abscess
- Aspiration of pericardial tamponade
- Aspiration of pleural effusion or empyema.

Open Surgery
- Laparotomy—rupture and peritonitis.
- Thoracotomy—for empyema not amenable for aspiration or
- For repair of a bronchopleural fistula not responding to medical therapy.
- Emergency relief of pericardial tamponade.

> Q. Short note on pyogenic abscess of liver.

PYOGENIC ABSCESS
Increasing incidence—alcoholics, drug abusers, diabetic and immunosuppressed.

Etiology
- Ascending infection through biliary tract
  - Cholangitis
  - Gallbladder empyema
  - Obstruction of CBD by stone, stent
- Through the portal vein; sepsis in the portal vein bed—pericolic abscess, infection in colon, small intestines.
- Through the hepatic artery:
  - Bacteremia
  - Pneumonia
  - Bone sepsis (osteomyelitis)
  - Soft tissue sepsis.

Pathology: More common in right lobe than in the left.
- Solitary or multiple
- Abscess cavity has a pyogenic membrane and with time a thick fibrotic wall develops—heals with scarring (unlike amebic abscess)
- Rupture and septicemia may ensue.

Clinical Features
- General—fever, chills, asthenia
- Local—pain right upper quadrant or tip of right shoulder.
- Tenderness over the liver area or intercostal spaces on right 9th and 10th space.

Differential Diagnosis
- Amoebic liver abscess, hydatid cyst
- Subphrenic abscess.

Investigation
- Leukocytosis
- Ultrasonography
- CT scan.

Treatment
Aggressive antibiotics—against gram negative and anerobic organisms (piperacillin and tazobactum with metronidazole, or a cephalosporin -ceftriaxone +metronidazole).

Supportive Treatment
Early drainage: Ultrasound guided aspiration. And drainage with a thick pig tail catheter for most abscesses in liver and for thoracic collections.

Surgery: Rarely indicated—laparoscopic or laparotomy drainage.
- For rupture and peritonitis.
- Abscess caudate lobe (rare)

Q. Short notes on pylephlebitis.

PORTAL PYEMIA (SYN: ACUTE PYLEPHLEBITIS)

A life threatening septic condition of liver due to septic emboli from infective thrombosis in veins draining into portal vein. Any infective condition in organs drained by portal vein can lead to pylephlebitis.

Etiopathogenesis

Acute peritonitis, appendicitis, diverticulitis, abscesses in colorectal bed, infected hemorrhoids, perianal abscess.

The above cause infective thrombosis in the colonic veins; the thrombus gets dislodged and carried by the portal vein to the liver causing multiple abscesses. Immunocompromised states contribute to etiology.

Microbiology

Mixed infection: *Esch coli*, anaerobic streptococci and bacteroids, clostridia (from bowel).

Diagnosis:
Clinical features
- High fever with rigors, jaundice, signs of liver failure—drowsiness.
- Systemic toxicity.

Blood culture: May grow organisms.
Imaging: Gas and thrombus in portal vein.
Liver function: AST and ALT elevated.

Treatment

Antibiotics: Combination of piperacillin and tazobactum with metronidazole.
Aminoglycosides: Amikacin + ceftazidime + metronidazole.

Supportive Treatment

Treatment of primary cause.
- Prognosis: Very high mortality
- Cause of death: Liver failure or septicemia and, multiorgan failure.

Prognosis is worse than that of an amebic abscess due to the poorer condition of the patient.

Q. Describe parasitology, pathology, clinical diagnosis and management of hydatid cyst of liver. (long answer)

HYDATID CYST OF LIVER

Hydatid cysts occur in any tissue of the body and liver is among the commonest sites.

It is caused by the "dog tapeworm" *Echinococcus granulosus* a parasite, whose life cycle involves th dog and definitive host and the humans as the intermediate host.

Life Cycle

Dog eats the infected offal of the sheep
↓
The adult worm grows in the dog's intestines. It has a head (scolex), neck and proglottids (three segments), having about 500 eggs in the proglottid.
↓
The dog's excreta spills ova into grass and vegetables
↓
These ova are ingested by sheep, cattle or man (intermediate host)
↓
Carried through portal vein into the liver in larva form
↓
Larvae develop into hydatid cyst slowly over a few years

Hydatid Cyst has Three Layers

1. **Outer—pericyst (adventitia):** It is an inseparable fibrous membrane as a reaction of the hepatic stroma to the parasite.
2. **Middle—ecto cyst (laminated membrane):** Secreted by the parasite. It is elastic and pale white and can be easily peeled off the pericyst contains the hydatid fluid.
3. **Inner—endocyst (germinal epithelium):** The only live part of the cyst which it lines from inner aspect The endocyst secretes the brood capsules with scolices (head of future worms) and hydatid fluid.

The brood capsule disintegrates and releases scolices to develop in to daughter cysts.

Consequences
- Calcification of the pericyst, death of the parasite.
- Progression and enlargement of the cyst.
- Acute rupture into peritoneal cavity—anaphylaxis and death.
- Slow rupture and peritoneal hydatidosis
- Rupture into biliary ductal radicles
- Pressure on bile ducts and jaundice
- Liver dysfunction
- Suppuration and infection—septicemia
- Formation of retroperitoneal cyst, lung cysts, mediastinal cysts.

Clinical Features
- Painless hepatomegaly—most common
- Pain and fever in case of infection
- Jaundice in those with obstruction.

Diagnosis
Sonography
- It is diagnostic.
- Double contoured membrane of the cyst (detached membrane) water lily sign.
- Calcification of cyst wall and rosettes of daughter cysts.

Intraoperative ultrasound (IOUS)—helps in searching for multiple cysts and during "PAIR".
- X-ray may show calcification.
- CT scan abdomen—"cart wheel" multi-vesicular rosette like appearance.
- MRI—useful in presence of jaundice
- To find the relation of hydatid to biliary tree
- To detect cystobiliary communication.

Casoni test—now replaced by other tests.

Serological tests ELISA
- Indirect hemagglutination or latex agglutination test
- Immunofluorescence antibody test
- Immunoelectrophoresis.

Treatment
Medical Treatment
Indications
- All cysts unless contraindicted (pregnant patient, cyst in brain, bone and eye)
- Prior to intervention—usually 2 weeks prior to interventions and continues for 4 weeks after multiple cysts.
- Albendazole is the drug of choice.
- Three cycles of Albendazole—each 4-week cycle with 2 weeks interval between the cycles.
- It is ovicidal/larvicidal/ vermicidal.
- Dose—400 mg twice daily (10 mg/kg /day).
- Monitor LFT, white cell counts, (leukopenia), fever.
- It penetrates poorly into bone, brain and eyes.
- Praziquantel—60 mg/kg along with albendazole for 2 weeks.
- Adverse effects—bone marrow suppression and aplastic anemia
- Mebendazole—rarely preferred now.

> **Q. What is PAIR with reference to hydatid cyst.**

Puncture-Aspiration-Injection-Reaspiration (PAIR)

A percutaneous procedure performed under CT or ultrasound guidance
- Under guidance—22 G Fr needle is used.
- 50 % of fluid is aspirated and all daughter cysts are punctured.
- Scolicidal solution-cetrimide or hypertonic saline is injected into the cyst and
- Reaspiration is done after 20 minutes of injection of the scolicide.

Double-puncture aspiration and injection (D-PAI) has also been practiced.

Scolicides
- Povidone iodine
- Silver nirate
- Absolute alcohol.

Complications of PAIR (10-30%)
- Anaphylaxis, mortality—1-2%
- Infection
- Recurence of cyst.

Contraindications to PAIR
- Inaccessible (posterior or caudate lobe) cysts.
- Multiple cysts, thick walled and calcified.
- Multiseptate cysts.

- Cystobiliary communication (MRI or a cholangiogram after the first aspiration shows).

Surgery options: The following are done as per the feasibility
- Laparoscopic or open excision of the intact undamaged cyst without spillage.
- Pericystectomy (with liver margin) or hepatic lobectomy for very big cysts, e.g., left lobe
- Marsupialisation in infected cysts.
- Open aspiration of cyst, injection of scolicide and closed drainage.
- Suturing and closure of the biliary communications after evacuation of the cyst.

Malignant Hydatid: Echinococcus multilocularis (multi alveolaris)
- Common in eastern Europe and Turkey
- Multiple cysts, resistant to treatment,
- Poor prognosis—liver failure being the cause of death.

Actinomycosis of liver
- Spread from ileocecal focus (portal vein)
- Cervico facial focus via arterial route (hepatic artery)
- Progressive destruction. of liver and liver failure sets in
- Aspiration under sonographic guidance and staining of the pus -for the "sun ray" appearance
- **Treatment:** Long-term Penicillin G—for 3 to 6 months.

TUMORS OF THE LIVER

Benign Tumors

Hemangioma
- Most common benign tumor of the liver.
- More common in females (3 times the males).
- Solitary or multiple in any lobe.
- Most are asymptomatic until their detection late in life (5th decade).
- **Complications:** Enlargement and compression of duodenum—obstruction, pain and vomiting
- Rupture and hemorrhage
- Thrombosis, infection.

Diff. diagnosis: HCC, metastases.

Diagnosis
- MRI is the most accurate modality.
- Ultrasonography and CT are also helpful.
- Angiographic confirmation—for tumors larger than 8 cm—before surgery is planned.

Treatment
- Observant policy—for smaller ones
- Surgical resection of the lobe—only for symptomatic tumors and in case of diagnostic uncertainty after the imaging study.

Hepatic adenoma: Risk potential for malignancy (HCC)—10%.
- Women aged between 25 and 50 are commonly affected.
- Associated with use of oral contraceptive pills—80% solitary, 20% are multiple.
- **Complications:** Rupture and bleeding (30%), hepatocellualr carcinoma (10%).
- About 60% are found incidentally at imaging.
- Treatment:
  - Asymptomatic tumors found incidentally and those <5 cm. Stopping the contracaptive pills and observation for regression.
  - Larger than 5 cm and symptomatic; surgical resection (lobectomy or segmentectomy).

Focal Nodular Hyperplasia (FNH)
- A benign condition of unknown etiology with no malignant potential.
- **Pathology:** There is a focal hyperplasia of liver tissue having both hepatocytes and Kupffer cells and fibrous stroma.

Clinical Features

Middle-aged females, asymptomatic.

Differential diagnosis: Metastatic cancer.
- Sonography shows—a solid tumor mass.
- Contrast CT or MRI shows—central scarring and a hypervascular lesion.
- MRI with liver specific contrast agents (gadolinium) is done to detect metastases.
- AFP and CEA—levels are normal.
- No treatment is needed if the diagnosis is confirmed and cancer excluded.

Malignant Tumors of the Liver

Metastatic (>80%)
- From portal vein bed—alimentary tract and retroperitoneal.
- Distant—hepatic arterial spread—breast, **urogenital**, bone, head and neck, melanoma.

Primary (20%)
- Hepatocellular carcinoma.
- Cholangio carcinoma
- Hepatoblastoma—infants and children.

Hepatoblastoma
- Affects children below 2 years mostly, with male preponderance.
- Origin: Fetal or embryonic hepatocytes.
- Serum alfa-fetoprotein is elevated.
- CT scan shows vascular mass with speckled calcification.

Treatment
- Resection where feasible.
- Chemotherapy: It is a chemosensitive tumor treated by combination of doxorubicin, vincristine and 5-FU.
- Liver transplantation is also being practiced.

Hepatocellular Carcinoma (HCC)
- Majority of cases in Africa and Asia.
- Rising incidence all over.

> **Q. Enumerate the etiological factors in hepatocellular carcinoma.**

Etiological Factors
- HBV
- HCV
- Chronic alcoholism—the metabolism products act on hepatocytes
- Oxidative metabolites in diabetes and obesity
- Background of hepatic non-alcoholic fatty liver disease (NAFLD)
- Primary biliary cirrhosis
- Clonorchiasis
- Industrial poisons
- Hepatic adenoma.

Pathology
- Unicentric or multicentric
- Spread—within the liver across the lobes
- Extrahepatic—diaphragm, bowel, kidney, adrenal, vessels, spine.
- Hematogenous—lungs, bone, brain.

Histological Variants
- Better prognosis: Fibrolamellar type(FL HCC) and clear cell variant.
- Poor prognosis: Mixed hepatocellular and cholangiocellular; giant cell variant; sarcomatoid variant (carcinosarcoma).

Clinical Features
- Male: Female 4:1
- Right lobe more often involved than left
- Unicentric or multicentric (cirrhotics)
- Enlarged liver
- Features of secondaries.

Investigations
- Blood—hemogram, liver function tests and prothrombin time, alfa-fetoprotein and carcinoembryonic antigen levels
- Ultrasound
- CECT
- MRI—detects metastases
- CT angiography—to evaluate the tumour for possible respectability

Elastography—for fibrotic index.

Evaluation involves:

Tumor stage—to choose the type of treatment.
Tumor size and extent—to determine feasibility of extent resection.
Patient selection for major hepatectomy is decided based on clinical parameters:
- Determination of volume the possible future liver remnant (FLR)—liver to be left behind after resection for HCC.
- Portal hypertension without gastric/esophageal varices, child pugh (CTP) score, A/B
- Platelet count ≥100,000.

Hepatocellular Carcinoma (HCC Staging): AJCC staging (Optional Reading)
Refer **Table 28H-4**.

Oncological Contraindications to Resection
- Extrahepatic metastasis
- Multiple and bilobar tumors

Table 28H-4: Staging of HCC.

Staging of hepatocellular carcinoma (HCC): AJCC staging (optional reading)

Simplified T- stage

T—size, number of nodules, vascular invasion and invasion of neighboring organs

TX—not assessed, T0—no evidence of tumor
T1—solitary tumor without vascular invasion, T1a—<2 cm, T1b—> 2 m

T2—> 2 cm, < 5 cm with vascular invasion or multiple nodules

T3—> 5 cm one or more nodules

T4—invasion of branch of portal vein or hepatic vein.
Extrahepatic visceral spread (other than gallbladder)

N - Nx, N0, N1

M - Mx, M0, M1

Histological Grade: Gx—not assessed

G1—well differentiated, **G2**—moderately differentiated
G3—poorly differentiated, **G4**—undifferentiated

Fibrosis score

F0—fibrosis score—0–4 (nil or mild fibrosis), F1—score 5–6 (severe or cirrhotic)

Stage			
Stage I	TI	N0	M0
Stage II	T2	N0	M0
Stage III	IIIa T3 and IIIb T4	N0	M0
Stage IV	IVa - any T - N1	N1	M0
	IVb - any T - N		M1

Table 28H-5: Definitions of hepatic resections.

	Name of the hepatic resection	Segments resected
1.	Right hepatic lobectomy (right hemihepatectomy)	Segments V to VIII
2..	Left hepatic lobectomy/hemihepatectomy	Segments II to IV
3.	Left bisegmentectomy (anatomical left lobe)	Segments II + III
4.	Right extended lobectomy (trisegmentectomky)	Segments IV to VIII
5.	Left extended lobecotmy (itrisegmentectomy)	Segments II–IV, V, VIII

- Involvement of the main bile duct
- Presence of tumor thrombus in the main portal vein/vena cava.

The Terminology for Hepatectomy

Refer **Table 28H-5** and **Figure 28H-2**.

Portal Vein Embolization (PVE)

PVE is a preoperative procedure designed to increase the safety of major liver resections. The portal vein on side of tumor is embolized, prior to surgery. This diverts portal flow to the future liver remnant (FLR), which undergoes hypertrophy, reducing the risk of liver failure after resection.

Q. Enlist surgical options in treatment of hepatocellular carcinoma.

Treatment of HCC

Anatomic Surgical Resection

Patients with normal liver or with early cirrhosis without portal hypertension **(Child's A)**

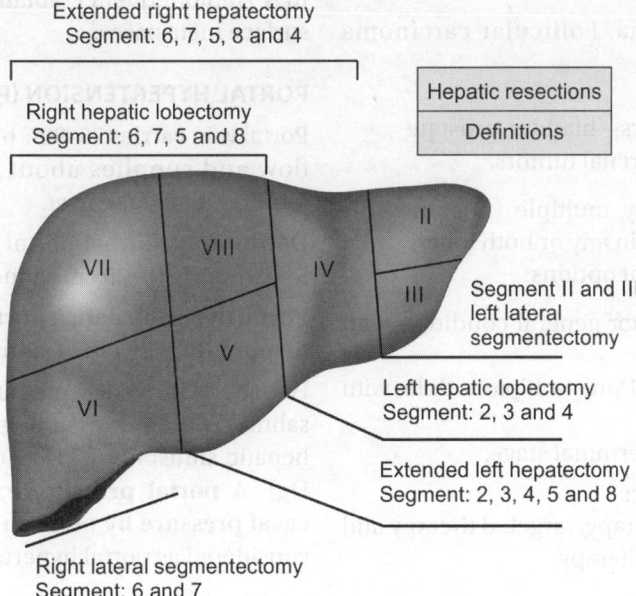

Fig. 28H-2: Types of hepatic resections.

Orthotopic Liver Transplantation (OLT)

Indication: Milan criteria: T 2 tumors.
- Single tumor less than 5 cm or
- Patients with three or less tumors, of size less than 3 cm
- Without vascular invasion or metastases

Bridge therapy before transplantation, with regional therapy—transcatheter arterial chemoembolization [TACE] or yttrium-90 [Y-90]), or

Direct ablation—radiofrequency or Laser.

Non-resectable Tumors or not Suitable for Transplantation

Palliative options of systemic therapy or/along with hepatic-directed therapies.

PALLIATIVE THERAPY FOR HCC

- **Local ablative therapy**
  - RFA ablation—upto 5 cm tumors are ablated.
  - TACE—transcatheter arterial embolization/chemoembolisation
  - Percutaneous ethanol/acetic acid injection
  - Microwave/cryoablation

- **Radiotherapy:** Transarterial radiotherapy—transarterial Yttrium-90 microspheres/I-131 lipiodol.
- **Surgery:** Hepatic artery ligation.
- **Targeted therapy:** Sorafenib: Tyrosine kinase inhibitor—marginal benefit of two to eight months.

Summary of treatment of HCC
- Diagnosis and staging plus evaluation
- Resection—for T1, T2 tumor within one lobe, non-cirrhotic, no portal hypertension.
- Transplantation-orthotopic liver transplantation—T2 tumors or cirrhotic patients /PHT
- TACE—T3 multiple tumors
- TKI-Sorafenib- for T3 T4–N1
- Supportive—all M 1 tumors

Cholangiocarcinoma of Liver

From biliary duct system.

METASTATIC TUMORS

Incidence: Metastatic tumor is almost 20 times more common than the primary lever tumors.

Etiology
GI tumors
- Carcinoma in stomach, colon and rectum, pancreas, small bowel, esophagus and carcinoids

- Melanoma
- Breast carcinoma. Follicular carcinoma thyroid (FCT)
- Lung
- Urogenital cancers—bladder, prostate
- Testicular and adrenal tumors.

Pathology: Generally multiple (uncommonly solitary) and may be in any or both lobes.
Treatment: Treatment options:

Clinical features: Poor general condition with anemia.
Nodular hetomegaly: Hard multiple nodules with umbilication.
Ascites, jaundice in terminal stage.

Treatment: Modalities
Resection, chemotherapy, targeted therapy and intra-arterial chemotherapy.

Resectability means—removal of tumor tissue from the liver with clear surgical margins, leaving adequate normal liver tissue to sustain life.

Indications for Metastasectomy

Site of Primary Tumors

- Colorectal secondaries—best suited for resections and improve survival significantly.
- Neuroendocrine tumors (glucagonoma, carcinoid, gastrinoma)—good results.
- Other malignancies—non-colorectal and non-neuroendocrine tumors—poor prognosis.

Number of Metastases

- Three or less than 4 metastases.
- Should be in a single segment or at worst in a single lobe.
- CEA—below 200 ng/dL.

Work up

- PET/CT scan—for finding metastases—hepatic and extrahepatic
- CEA.

Chemotherapy: 5 FU with irinotecan or oxaliplatin.

Monoclonal antibody (targeted) therapy—bevacizumab (anti-vascular endothelial antibodies)/cetuximab.

RFA (radiofrequency ablation—small (<3 cm) surface metastases.

PORTAL HYPERTENSION (PHT)

Portal vein carries 75–80% of total hepatic blood flow and supplies about 30-35% of oxygen requirement of the liver.

Definition: Normal portal venous pressure is 5–10 mm Hg (8–20 cm saline)

Portal hypertension: A portal venous pressure of more than 20 cm of saline (10 mm of Hg).

Hepatic vein wedge pressure (HVP) is 20 cm saline, with a pressure gradient across the hepatic sinusoid of 11–13 cm saline (5–7 mm Hg). **A portal pressure exceeding the vena caval pressure by more than 5 mm hg is** also considered as portal hypertension.

Compensated PHT

A compensatory increase in porta pressure to overcome hepatic resistance to the portal flow maintains the normal flow (PVP to HVP gradient is restored).

Decompensated PHT: The hepatic resistance to portal flow is more than the portal flow. PVP to HVP gradient is lost. The blood flow is reversed and there is stasis of blood in the portal bed causing the opening of porta systemic collaterals, which divert the blood to the systemic veins, bypassing the liver.

Portasystemic Collaterals

Hepatopetal collaterals (porto-portal)— obstruction is **pre hepatic**, collaterals develop to make the blood flow through the liver (between splenic bed and the hepatic hilar area (portal cavern) in portal vein thrombosis).

Hepatofugal collaterals (porto-systemic) collaterals between portal and systemic veins.

- Esophagogastric junction—left gastric vein to azygos system and to IVC.
- Falciform ligament umbilical vein to abdominal wall veins and to IVC.
- Anal canal—superior hemorrhoidal veins (portal) to inferior hemorrhoidal (systemic) and to the iliac veins.

- Retroperitoneal: Surface of the abdominal viscera to retroperitoneal veins (systemic).

Q. Describe briefly the etiopathogenesis of portal hypertension.

ETIOPATHOGENESIS

Increased resistance/obstruction to the flow of portal venous blood.

Level of Obstruction

Pre sinusoidal—liver function is normal, compensatory collaterals restore hepatic blood flow.
Post sinusoidal—liver function compromised.

Etiology of Portal Hypertension

Refer **Table 28H-6**.

Problems in Portal Hypertension—4 Fold

- Esophageal varices—may cause catastrophic bleed.
- Porta systemic encephalopathy—due to diversion of blood off the liver, the blood returns to the right heart without the being detoxified in the liver. (especially the nitrogenous products including ammonia). These products reach the blood cause encephalopathy.
- Hypersplenism—due to congestive sequestration of blood in the spleen.
- Ascites—hypoproteinemia cases transudation High outflow pressure causes "hepatorrhea'— oozing of fluid from the congested liver.

Clinical Features

- Gastrointestinal bleeding—melena and hatemeis (if severe), anemia (if chronic).

Table 28H-6: Etiology of portal hypertension

Heart	RA ↓	LV ↓ RV ←	Congestive heart failure Chronic constrictive pericarditis IVC Web
IVC 0-4 cm saline	↓		Tumor Invasion /thrombosis
Hepatic veins 2-4 cm	Right mid left ↓		Budd Chiari syndrome Tumor invason
Liver	Post-sinusoidal obstruction		Cirrhosis—biliary, Laennec's, Wilson's Hemochromatosis, post hepatitis poisoning
	Pre sinusoidal obstruction ↓		Sarcoidosis Schistosomiasis Portal space infiltration—Hodgkin's leukemia, congenital hepatic fibrosis
Portal Vein 8-14 cm water	Pre-hepatic		Congenital anomaly: Hepaticoportal A-V fistula Malformation, atresia of portal vein.
	High pressure		Thrombosis of portal vein Umbilical sepsis Splenectomy Pyelephlebitis Idiopathic
	↑ Splenic vein		Increased hepatopetal flow in splenic vein—in pre-sinusoidal PHT (to overcome portal venous obstruction)

- Gastroesophageal bleeding—due to rupture of varices at gastroesophageal junction.
- Portal gastropathy; sub mucous variceal dilatation of capillaries in the stomach
- Gastric antral venous ectasia (GAVE)—venous elements dilate in the mucosa—streaks of superficial vessels " water melon stomach" at gastroscopy
- Splenomegaly—congestive and hypersplenism
- Collateral—dilated veins around umbilical and upper abdominal wall (caput medusa)
- Peripheral edema
- Ascites
- Liver cell failure: Jaundice palmar erythema and clubbing.
  Gynecomastia and testicular atrophy (estrogens are not metabolised by liver).
- Encephalopathy: confusion, altered behavior, drowsiness, flapping tremor.

Q. Discuss principles of management of portal hypertension.

Investigations

- Blood:
  - Hemoglobin and PCV
  - Liver function tests: Platelets
  - Prothrombin time and INR
  - Renal function
  - Blood ammonia (for encephalopathy)
  - Electrolytes.
- Ultrasonography—most important in diagnosis of PHT. Elastography to evaluate fibrosis.
- Contrast CT and MRI- to check nodules, splenomegaly, portal vein thrombosis and collaterals.
- CT angiogram—focusing on SMA and celiac artery.
- MR venography—for extrahepatic portal vein thrombosis. It also delineates hepatic veins and helps diagnose Budd-Chiari syndrome
- Upper gastrointestinal endoscopy—for varices, gastropathy and GAVE.
  Also to rule out peptic ulcer and other causes of bleeding like Dieulafoy lesion.

Treatment of Portal Hypertension

Summary of principles of treatment of portal hypertension

Evaluation of severity—based on child pugh score:

Non specific measures

- Transfusion: Blood—plasma, packed cells, coagulation factors as needed
- Correction of anemia
- Vit K injections vit K1- 10 mg IM or IV for 5 days
- Nutrition and electrolytes—supplementation
- Nutrition supplementation
- Inj. vitamin K-10 mg IM for 5 days.

Specific treatment of portal hypertension

- Treatment of esophageal varices—emergency or elective
- Prevention or treatment of hepatic encephalopathy
- Prevention and treatment of infection
- Treatment of ascites
- Reduction of portal pressure
- Drugs to reduce the portal pressure—emergency or long term beta blockers, nitrates

Surgeries—portosystemic shunt.
- Non-selective
- Selective.

TIPSS followed by:
- Liver transplantation.

Q. Management of esophageal varices. (Long answer)

MANAGEMENT OF ESOPHAGEAL VARICES

- Emergency—acute variceal bleed
- Elective—to control or prevent bleeding and encephalopathy.

Emergency Management of Acute Variceal Bleed

Resuscitation

- Hemorrhagic shock
- Diagnosis
- Inj. vitamin K-10 mg IM for 5 days.
- Blood and blood product transfusions.

Diagnosis: To exclude a non-variceal cause of acute bleed.

Endoscopy at the earliest after resuscitation and stabilization of the patient.

Q. Short note on Sengstaken Blakemore tube.

Hemostasis by Sengstaken-Blackmore tube—balloon tamponade for the varices:

Sengstaken tube: A trilumen tube with two inflatable balloons—gastric and an esophageal and a lumen for irrigaton and aspiration.

It is employed in severe bleeding when endoscopy is not feasible.
- Sengstaken–Blakemore tube is placed for temporary hemostasis
- The gastric balloon is inflated with 300 mL of air and the tube is pulled to fit the gastric fundus; the esophageal balloon is inflated to a pressure of 40 mm Hg
- This provides good tamponade of the varices at the gastric fundus, esophagogastric junction and lower esophagus
- The position of the tube is confirmed by X-ray.
- The balloon is deflated after 12 hours to prevent pressure necrosis of esophagus
- The Senstaken tube can be kept for upto 72 hours for tamponade and control of bleeding after which specific measures are to be taken. The gastric tube is used for saline lavage

Complications: Aspiration, esophageal ulceration and perforation.

Clinical Features of Variceal Bleed
- Hematemesis—from oral end
- Melena—tarry (hematin) foul smelling semi liquid
- Hematochezia—dark (maroon) can be seen in massive upper GI bleed, with the blood passing unaltered through the bowel due or rapid transit (it is typical of lower GI bleed).

EXCLUDE NON-VARICEAL BLEED

Etiology: Upper gastrointestinal bleeding

Refer **Table 28H-7**.

Signs Acute GI Bleed

Hypovolemia: Tachycardia, weak pulse, low BP, pallor, sweat.

Endoscopy
- Upper GI Endoscopy: To assess the bleeding varices and diagnosis.

Table 28H-7: Etiology of upper GI bleed.

Varices	Tumours
Esophagitis	GI cancers
Mallory Weiss tear	Leiomyoma, GIST
DU/GU/Erosions	Lymphoma
Portal gastropathy/GAVE	ANGIOMA
Foreign bodies	Angiodysplasia
Pancreatitis	Telangiectasia
Bleeding disorders	Dieulafoy Lesion

- Portal gastropathy, GAVE, growth, ulcer, angiodysplasia, GI.

Specific Treatment Started along with Evaluation

- Balloon tamponade: Sengstaken-Blakemore tube—for control of bleeding (until endoscopy can be performed safely.
- Endoscopic diagnosis and therapy
- Pharmacotherapy in variceal upper GI bleed
  - Vasopressors—vasopressin/glypressin/terlipressin
  - Continuous infusion—splanchnic vasoconstriction.
  - Somatostatin continuous infusion or
  - Its analogue octreotide—infusion or subcutaneous (reduces splanchnic blood flow and portal pressure and gastric secretary activity)
- Acid inhibitors—PPI/H-2 blockers for stress ulceration and peptic ulcer bleed.
- Antifibrinolytics—tranexamic acid/EACA.

Q. Short note on endotherapy for bleeding varices.

ENDOTHERAPY IN BLEEDING VARICES

Endoscopic variceal band ligation
- Sclerotherapy (largely replaced by band ligation).
- Glue—cyanoacrylate glue injection into varices—particularly—fundal varices.
- Argon plasma coagulation (APC)—for GAVE.
- LASER for varices—not very popular.

Q. Short notes on TIPS.

Transjugular intrahepatic portasystemic shunt (TIPS)—an emergency intrahepatic shunt is created for quick control of bleed.

Complications
- Hepatic vein tear, intrahepatic hemorrhage, liver failure, sepsis.
- Now it is usually used as a bridge for patients waiting for transplantation.

Surgery in Variceal Bleed
Indications
- Continued bleed with requirements exceeding 6 units and 4 units in high risk patients.
- Hemodynamic instability continuing despite therapy.
- Failure of endoscopic localization and/or therapy/rebleed.

Surgery for Variceal Bleed
Emergecy Portosystemic Disconnection
- Laparoscopic or open stapler devascularization (disconnection of gastroesophageal junction and re suture/stapling to cut off the portal back flow).
- Tanner's subesophageal disconnection and resuturing.
- Boerema Crile—transesophageal variceal suturing.
- Sugiura Futagawa—most extensive devascularization—veins along lower esophagus and lesser curvature are divided, gastro-esophageal disconnection (staples or suture) done and coronary vein ligated.
- **Emergency portasystemic shunt:** Commonly porta caval or mesocaval in children.
  - A desparate measure at contain bleeding is infrequently required today.
  - Emergency portacaval shunt.
  - Good control but high morbidity and mortality—due to liver failure and encephalopathy.

Long-term Measures and Control: Portal Hypertension (PHT)
To reduce portal pressure
- **Medical**: Beta blockers—propranolol—20 to 80 mg/day in divided doses
- Nitrates—not as effective.

Q. Name the porta caval shunts to treat portal hypertension.

PORTOSYSTEMIC SHUNTS (REFER FIGURE 28H-3)

Surgery for Portal Hypertension Refer Table 28H-8

TIPS—transjugular intrahepatic portosystemic shunt (already mentioned earlier)

This is done in patients as a bridge therapy while waiting for a hepatic transplantation against recurrent bleeding episodes.

Liver Transplantation: Child-Pugh B or C with PHT

Orthotopic Liver Transplantation
- Recipient hepatectomy
- Donor segmentectomy.
- Placing the liver to position and
- Vascular anastomosis—hepatic artery, hepatic vein and portal vein.
- Bile duct to bile duct.

Management of Ascites

Albumin infusions until liver recovers.

Treatment
- Low salt diet
- Abdominal tapping of ascitic fluid (2-2.5 L at a time) supplementation of albumin
- Diuresis—spironolactone 50 to 100 mg with or without furosemide 40 mg daily
- Propranolol—reduces portal pressure
- TIPS
- Liver transplantation.

Q. Short note on Budd-Chiari syndrome.

Budd-Chiari Syndrome
- This is caused by occlusion of the major hepatic veins or inferior vena cava.
- Mostly by thrombosis or physical block.

Causes
- Thrombosis of hepatic veins
  - Spontaneous thrombosis, e.g., in myeloproliferative diseases—commonest
  - Polycythemia, contraceptive pills.
  - Tumor invasion

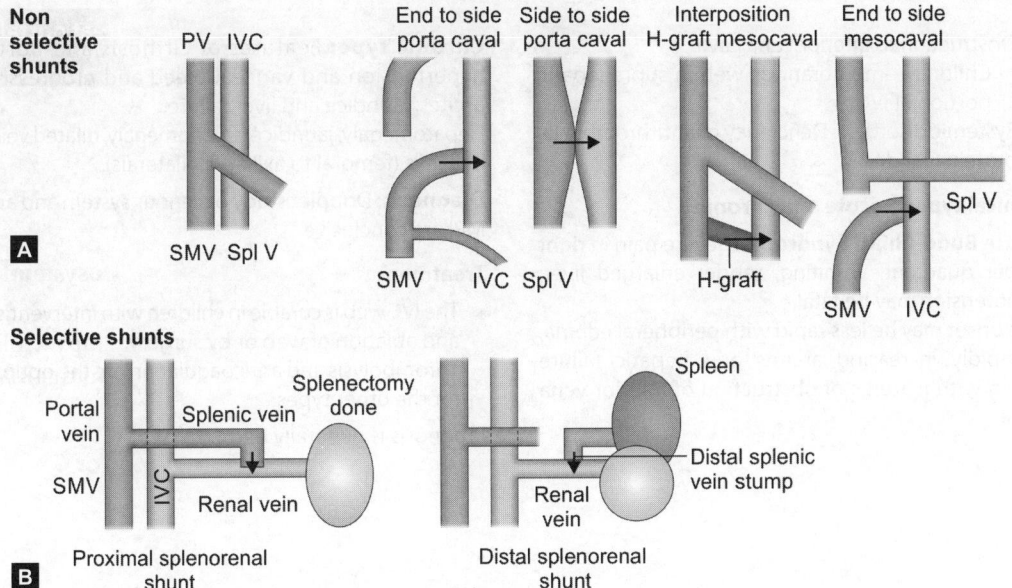

Fig. 28H-3A and B: Types of portosystemic shunts. (A) Non-selective shunt; (B) Selective shunt. (PV: portal vein; IVC: inferior vena cava; SMV: superior mesenteric vein; Spl V: splenic vein;

Table 28H-8: Portosystemic shunts

Elective portosystemic shunt operations

Type of shunt	Anastomosis	Decompression and bleeding control	Risk of shunt closure	Risk of encephalopathy
Portacaval shunt—end to side	Portal vein—end to side inferior vena cava (IVC)	Very effective	Least	Maximum
Side to side Useful in ascites	Portal vein—side to side to IVC	Very effective	Very low	Very high
Mesocaval shunt Done in children	Superior mesenteric vein SMV divided and end anastomosed to IVC—end to side	Very effective	Very low	High
Interposition—H graft mesocaval	H graft is interposed between SMV and IVC	Effective	Very low	High
Splenorenal shunt (proximal)	Splenectomy, proximal end of splenic vein anastomosed to left renal vein	Effective early	High risk	Moderate
Selective shunts Distal splenorenal shunt (DSRS)—Warren	No splenectomy, splenic vein divided. Distal stump anastomosed to left renal vein	Effective early	High risk	Least risk
Inokuchi Shunt	Left gastric (coronary) vein to IVC via a graft	Pre-hepatic PHT	High risk	Least risk

- Obstruction to Inferior vena cava
  - Children—membranous web in suprahepatic portion of IVC
- Systemic disorders: Deficiency of antithrombin III, protein C and S.

Clinical types—acute and chronic

Acute Budd-Chiari Syndrome: Severe pain in right upper quadrant, vomiting, tender enlarged liver, hypotension may be fatal.

The onset may be less rapid with peripheral edema, a rapidly increasing ascites and hepatic failure along with features of obstruction of inferior vena cava.

Chronic type: Features of cirrhosis and portal hypertension and variceal bleed and progressive ascites, jaundice and liver failure.

Hepatomegaly, jaundice, splenomegaly, dilated veins in flanks (femoral to axillary collaterals).

Diagnosis: Doppler study of venous system and and MRI are conclusive.

Treatment

- The IVC web is curable in children with intervention and ablation of web or by surgery.
- Thrombolysis and anticoagulation are the options for the other types.

Prognosis is generally bad.

BILIARY TRACT

> **SU28.12:** Describe the applied anatomy of biliary system. Describe the clinical features, investigations and principles of management of diseases of biliary system.

APPLIED ANATOMY OF BILIARY SYSTEM

Gallbladder along with the bile ducts, develops from the hepatic bud, the endodermal outpouching from the foregut. The adult anatomy is highly variable between individuals.

The gallbladder is a pear shaped hollow organ generally fixed by the fibrous cystic plate to the gallbladder fossa on the inferior surface of the liver - segments 4B and 5. Size—7–12 cm long, 3–4 cm wide at the widest part. Volume—about 25–40 mL.

Parts: Fundus, body, a neck that narrows as the infundibulum and a cystic duct.

Wall of gallbladder—peritoneal covering, thin muscle layer, and mucous membrane lined by glandular epithelium and goblet cells; the mucosa intrudes into muscle layer as crypts of Luschka. The submucosa and muscularis mucosae are absent in the wall.

Cystic Duct

- Variable length (average 1–3 cm) could be sessile gallbladder and width (may vary from an average of 1–4 mm to even 15 mm).
- The mucosa has spiral folds (the Heister's valves), surrounded by the sphincter.
- Hartmann's pouch: The dilated part of infundibulum, proximal to its junction with the cystic, with stasis of bile and impaction of stones.

Bile duct: All the segmental intrahepatic ducts join to form the right and left hepatic ducts.

The hepatic ducts join about 2.5 cm below the porta hepatis to form the common hepatic duct which is joined by the cystic duct 2.5 cm distally, to become the common bile duct (the CBD), the junction of two ducts being highly variable.

The common bile duct (CBD) has 4 parts
- Supraduodenal—2.5 cm
- Retroduodenal (behind first part of duodenum)—2.5 cm
- Infraduodenal—2.5 cm
- Intraduodenal part—0.6–14 mm (variable). It runs through the wall of the second part of duodenum and joins the ampulla of Vater, along with the pancreatic duct, to open through the duodenal papilla.

Arterial supply: Gallbladder; cystic artery from the right hepatic artery—run behind the CBD along cystic duct to enter the gallbladder at neck or distal body (variable) through two branches, the anterior and posterior.

Veins: Drain into 4th and 5th segments of liver (through the cystic plate) and also into portal vein.

Bile ducts: An arterial arborization of twigs from the right hepatic artery supplying the duct. Venous network drains into the portal vein at the porta.

> **Q.** Describe the surgical anatomy of Calot's triangle.

Calot's Triangle (Refer Figure 28B-1)

It is formed by the lower surface of liver, cystic duct and medial border of the gallbladder laterally and common hepatic duct medially.

Contents

- Cystic artery and its branch to the cystic duct.
- Cystic lymph node of Lundh is seen near the junction of infundibulum and cystic duct. It drains the gallbladder and cystic plate. It helps as a guide to locate for the cystic artery.

Lymphatic Drainage

- Gallbladder—submucosal and subserosal lymphatics—to the cystic node of Lundh and to the hepatic nodes in the porta and from there to the hepatic and celiac.
  Subserosal lymphatics drain into the subcapsular lymphatics of liver.

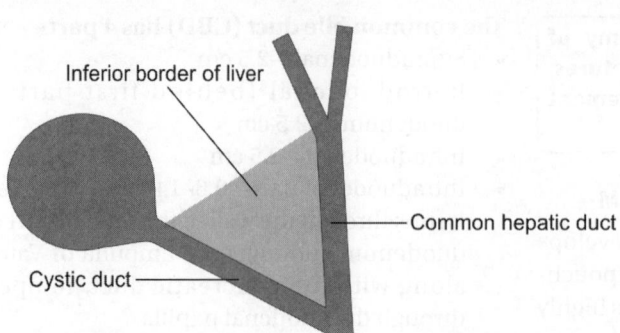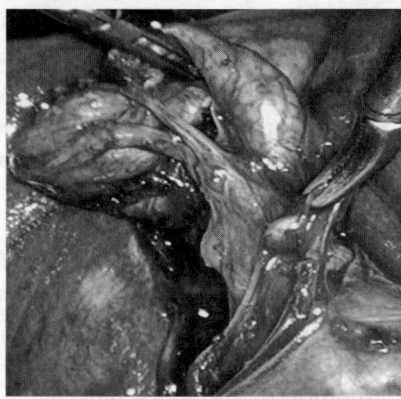

Fig. 28B-1: Calot's triangle.

- CBD—to the nodes in the porta above (then to the hepatic and celiac) and to the pancreatico-duodenal nodes and to the mesenteric from there.

Function of Gallbladder

- A reservoir for the bile—released after food intake due to action of cholecystokinin (duodenal secretion), which contracts the gallbladder and relaxes the sphincter or Oddi.
- Concentration of bile—5-10 times (daily secretion of bile is around 1,000 mL— 98% water) by active absorption of water, sodium chloride and bicarbonate through the mucous membrane, leading to higher concentration of cholesterol, bile salts, bile pigments, and calcium.
- Secretion of mucus—about 20—25 mL/day. A mucocele is the result of obstructed gallbladder due to absence of bile entering the gallbladder and continued secretion of mucus.

Investigation of Gallbladder and Biliary Tract

Blood

Liver function test—indicates the function of liver and obstruction to the biliary tree as elevated alkaline phosphatase.

Liver enzymes are elevated in cholangitis.
Tumor markers: High serum levels of CA 19-9 in pancreatic head cancer, CEA in ductal carcinoma and AFP in hepatocellular carcinoma respectively.

Q. Briefly outline imaging in biliary disease.

Radiology and Imaging in Biliary Disease

Plain X-ray

Radiopacity

- 10% of gallstone are radiopaque, biliary sand (calcium mixed) as limey bile is seen, mixed stones are seen
- Calcification of gallbladder wall (porcelain gallbladder)
- CBD stone.

Radiolucency

- In gallbladder wall—emphysematous cholecystitis
- Free air in gallstone due to air entrapped
- Triradiate (Mercedez sign) or biradiate (Seagull sign)
- Free air in CBD—choledochoduodenal fistula or post ERCP.

Oral Cholecystography and Intravenous Cholangiography are not generally done now.

Ultrasonography: Cornerstone of Biliary Tract Evaluation

Transabdominal Ultrasonography (US)

It is the first imaging modality for biliary system. Advantages: Easy and quick to perform and inexpensive; apart from being absolutely harmless. Disadvantages: Interpreter dependent; poor imaging quality in obese and in presence of bowel gas and gastric food contents.

Findings: Details of gallbladder—measurements of the organ, stone, polyp, wall edema, thickness, pericholecystic inflammation, cystic duct.

CBD and periampullary region along with the details of obstruction (site, extent, details of growth), and to differentiate intrahepatic from extrahepatic biliary obstruction.

Endoscopic Ultrasonography (EUS)

An ultrasound transducer loaded to the tip of an endoscope is used to evaluate the layers of stomach, duodenum and periampullary anatomy or pathology, head of pancreas and the CBD —lower end of CBD, nodes and CBD stones.

Biopsies are taken from pancreas or nodes. Pneumobilia is typical of emphysematous cholecystitis.

CT Scan

- Overcomes the disadvantages of ultrasonography.
- Preferred modality in staging of cancers of the liver, gallbladder, bile ducts and pancreas.
- To assess—extent of the primary tumor and its relation to regional anatomy—the organs and vessels and lymph nodes. Also to assess metastases.
- Disadvantage—25% of gallstones may be missed; poor screening tool for stones.
- Exposure to radiation.

MRI and MRCP

- Magnetic resonance cholangiopancreatography (MRCP) is a noninvasive modality for imaging of the gallbladder and biliary system—obstructive dilatation, strictures and ductal abnormalities.
- Often combined with magnetic resonance imaging of the biliary pancreatic system to evaluate lesions in the head, nodes, ductal lesions like stricture, hilar tumors and metastases in the liver
- Used as an alternative to ERCP and PTC for diagnosis.

Scintigraphy (Radioisotope Imaging of Gallbladder and Bile Ducts)

- The modality is a study of both structure and function of gallbladder.

- Iminodiacetic acid(IDA) is actively taken up and cleared by the hepatocyte through bile which concentrates in the gallbladder.
- A radioisotope (e.g., Tc99) tagged to the IDA salt such as hippuran (HIDA) is injected.
- The same is concentrated in gallbladder and excreted through bile duct. The gamma camera delineates the gallbladder and biliary tree. Useful in diagnosis of dysfunctional gallbladder (acalculous cholecystitis) and ductal abnormalities.

Q. Short note on ERCP.

Endoscopic Retrograde Cholangiopancreatography (ERCP)

An invasive study for diagnosis and therapy of biliary and pancreatic ductal obstructive lesions. Under sedation with propofol or midazolam, a side viewing gastroduodenoscope is passed, duodenal papilla is identified and sphincter of Oddi is cannulated, radiopaque dye is injected. Biliary and pancreatic ductal system is delineated by contrast X ray (C-arm screening).

Therapy

Biliary sphincterotomy (Oddi's sphincter) is performed with a wire and selective cannulation of pancreatic or biliary duct is performed for necessary therapeutic procedure (stone removal by basketing, placement of biliary stents, or pancreatic stents. Laser lithotripsy for ductal stones of pancreas and stones in CBD.

Indications

- Post MRCP uncertainty of diagnosis.
- For sampling of bile and pancreatic juice for cytology and culture.
- Biopsy or brush cytology from tumour site.
- MRCP has reduced the diagnostic indications today as it avoids complications of ERCP.

Therapeutic indications

- Bile duct—extraction of stone
- BIliary stenting—for stricture, tumor or post stone extraction.
- Naso biliary drainage in obstructive jaundice.
- Pancreatic ductal stenting—for strictures
- Lithotripsy of pancreatic ductal calculi

- Endoscopic papillotomy—for papillary stricture
  Acute biliary pancreatitis—to disimpact the ampullary calculus

Preparation: Correction of coagulopathy—vit K-1, 4-5 days prior to procedure.

Contraindications:
- Coagulopathy, bleeding disorder. Renal failure
- Acute pancreatitis not due to biliary calculi

Complications
- Acute pancreatitis; ascending cholangitis, septicemia.
- Duodenal—perforation; late stricture of duodenal papilla.
- Bleeding from pancreaticoduodenal vessels.

Q. Percutaneous Transhepatic cholangiography (PTC)

PERCUTANEOUS TRANSHEPATIC CHOLANGIOGRAPHY

- A flexible and blunt tipped, non-bevelled needle 0.7 mm wide (e.g., Okuda or Chiba needle) is passed by puncturing right 8th intercostal space in midaxillary line, under ultrasound or fluoroscopic guidance into the dilated intrahepatic bile duct.
- After confirming the needle tip in the duct by aspiration, the bile is sampled for cytology and culture.
- A water-soluble iodine dye is injected into the duct to delineate the biliary tree and assess the obstruction (tumor, stricture).
- A therapeutic stent is passed over a guidewire (over the catheter under image guidance).
- The stent is passed across the obstruction—especially the high biliary obstructions, inaccessible for ERCP (e.g., Klatskin tumors, in high strictures of common hepatic ducts in CHD).

Preparation

- Correction of any coagulopathy—vit K or frozen plasma given to correct prothrombin time.

- Transfusion of plasma and red cells if needed.
- Antibiotic prophylaxis (infected biliary tree due to obstruction).

Complications
- Bleeding
- Bile leak into peritoneum and biliary peritonitis.
- Septicaemia.

INTRAOPERATIVE IMAGING TECHNIQUES

Peroperative Cholangiography

- A catheter is inserted into the cystic duct and contrast injected directly into the biliary tree to visualize the same, during a laparoscopic or open operation for biliary pathology. After injection the head end is tilted down 20 degree to allow the dye to fill the intrahepatic biliary tree.
- It is done to evaluate for stones in bile duct and to study ductal anatomy.
- Air bubbles may be mistaken for filling defects of stones and hence should be prevented from being injected.
- After exploration, a T-tube is left in the CBD and incision closed.

Postoperative Cholangiography

Please refer T tube cholangiography (page 440).

Operative Choledochoscopy (Biliary Endoscopy)

A flexible fiber-optic endoscope is passed peroperatively, via cystic duct or directly through an opening made in the CBD (choledochotomy) to identify and remove any residual stones.

Post exploration of the bile duct, a T-tube is left in the CBD to maintain drainage of the biliary tract. A track forms in about 8-10 days allowing passage of the choledochoscope if need be to remove any residual stone particles.

Laparoscopic Ultrasonography

A laparoscopic ultrasound probe is used to image the extrahepatic biliary system.

It is used in staging of biliary and pancreatic tumors by identifying and evaluating relationship of the primary tumor to major vessels such as the portal vein and superior mesenteric vein, hepatic artery and the superior mesenteric artery.

Congenital Abnormalities of the Gallbladder and Bile Ducts

During early fetal life the gallbladder is entirely intrahepatic; it may be absent in a few (agenesis).

The phrygian cap: Mistaken for a pathological deformity of the organ.

Floating gallbladder the gallbladder may hang on a mesentery, prone for torsion.

Double gallbladder, septum of the gallbladder. Diverticulum of the gallbladder.

Variations in Cystic Duct Insertion

Absence of the Cystic Duct

May be congenital or acquired—due to ulceration and erosion of the, CBD by a stone impacted at the lower end of cystic duct.

Low Insertion of the Cystic Duct

A cystic duct joining the CBD very low, often infraduodenal part of duodenum may mimick the CBD.

An accessory cholecystohepatic duct—drains the gallbladder into the liver.

It may be missed at surgery causing bile leaks.

> **Q. Short answer on extrahepatic biliary atresia.**

EXTRAHEPATIC BILIARY ATRESIA

Etiology and Physiology

Incidence: About 1 in 10000 live births affecting both sexes equally.
Associated anomalies are common—seen in about 20% of cases
- Situs inversus absent vena cava and a preduodenal portal vein
- Cardiac lesions, polysplenia.

Pathogenesis

An inflammatory process from the time of birth is believed to cause progressive destruction of the extrahepatic bile ducts leading to biliary obstruction and biliary cirrhosis and portal hypertension. If untreated, the child dies of liver failure before three years.

Classification of Biliary Atresia

Three main types:
1. Type I: Atresia restricted to the common bile ducts.
2. Type II: Atresia of the common hepatic duct.
3. Type III: Atresia of the right and left hepatic ducts.

Clinical Features

- Neonatal jaundice—one third have it at birth and all by one week of birth. It is progressive. Pruritus severe.
- Liver function tests show conjugated hyperbilirubinemia and elevated alkaline phosphatase.
- Stools will be clay colored and urine will be dark.
- Steatorrhea and osteomalacia (biliary rickets).
- Skin xanthomas may be present.

Differential Diagnosis

Obstructive jaundice in a neonate:
- Choledochal cyst
- Neonatal hepatitis—only biopsy and a scintiscan can differentiate
- Inspissated bile syndrome
- Examples are α1-antitrypsin deficiency
- Drug induced and TPN induced, if any.

Treatment

Orthotopic liver transplantation is the best. Others—poor results
- Type I lesions: Roux-en-Y hepaticojejunostomy is done but progressive fibrosis results in poor long-term results.
- Type II and III: Kasai portoenterostomy
- Radical excision of all bile duct tissue up to the porta hepatis and anastomosis of the exposed liver tissue to jejunum (portojejunostomy).

Early operation—at 8 weeks has the best chance of long term survival upto 10 years.
- 50% of long-term survivors develop portal hypertension with variceal bleeding

Q. Short note on choledochal cyst.

CHOLEDOCHAL CYST

- It is congenital dilations of the intra and/or extrahepatic biliary ductal system.
- The pathogenesis: It is no very clear
- It is a premalignant condition with a very high chance of developing a cholangiocarcinoma..

Classification (Depending upon the Level and Parts of the Biliary Pancreatic Junction)

Types of choledochal cysts
- Type 1 fusiform
  - Diffuse
  - Diffuse including the pancreatic duct.
- Type 2 Saccular (diverticulm of CBD)
- Type 3 Choledochocele. Dilated cyst like lower end of CBD
- Type 4 Fusiform + intrahepatic extension
- Type 5 intrahepatic type

Clinical Features

- It may present at any age
- Clinical triad—jaundice, fever, a mass in right upper quadrant, and abdominal pain.
- About 60% of cases are children below 10 years.
- Cholangiocarcinoma should be suspected in adults.

Diagnosis

- Ultrasonography—confirms a cyst and biliary dilatation.
- Magnetic resonance imaging (MRI/MRCP) displays the anatomy of extra and hepatic biliary ducts and also pancreatic duct.

Treatment

- Complete excision of the cyst
- With a Roux-en-Y bilioenteric anastomosis (hepatico-docho-jejunostomy en Y).
- This is to avert risk of recurrent cholangitis, stricture and a cholangiocarcinoma.

Congenital Dilatation of the Intrahepatic Ducts (Caroli's Disease)

- Congenital anomaly with multiple irregular saccular dilatations of the intrahepatic ducts
- Separated by segments of normal or stenotic ducts
- With a normal extrahepatic biliary system.

Caroli syndrome: The biliary dilatation is associated with congenital hepatic fibrosis.

Clinical Features

- Age of presentation—30 years affects both sexes equally.
- Abdominal pain, cholangitis or end-stage liver disease.

Complication: Cholangiocarcinoma.

Management

- Antibiotic therapy for cholangitis
- Relief of jaundice by endoscopic biliary stenting or radiological intervention.
- Hepatic resection for localized disease. Hepatic transplantation for diffuse disease with fibrosis.

GALLSTONES (CHOLELITHIASIS)

General Considerations

Bile Acids

- **Unconjugated:** Cholic acid, deoxycholic acid, chenodeoxycholic acid
- **Conjugated:** Glycocholic acid, taurocholic acid.

Composition of Luminal Bile

About 97% water, 1-2% bile acid and salts, pigment, protein, carbonate, phosphate\, calcium, sodium, potassium, enzymes (glucuronidase, phosphatase).

GALLSTONES

- The most common biliary pathology.
- Affects almost 10 percent of population (75% are asymptomatic).

Types of Gallstones (Fig. 28B-2): Cholesterol Stones, Pigment Stones and Mixed Stones

Cholesterol Stones

They form in aseptic bile and make 10% of all stones.

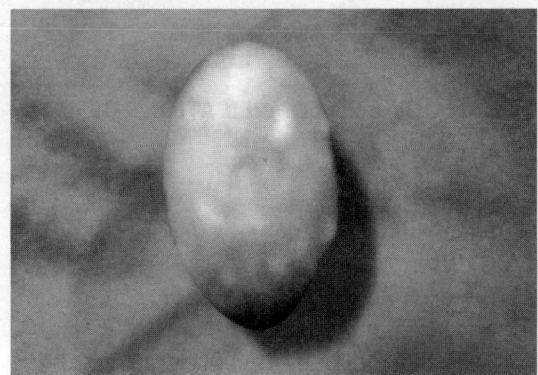

Fig. 28B-2: Pure cholesterol stone.
(For color version see Plate 1)

Solitary, oval, light weight, pale yellow, cut section—radiating lines from centre to periphery with laminar layers. They get embedded in infundibulum forming the Hartmann's pouch.

Pigment Stones

Contain less than 30% cholesterol (make 12-15% more in Asian countries).

Two types: Black and brown

- **Black stones**: Insoluble bilirubin pigment mixed with phosphate and bicarbonate of calcium black, small, irregular shaped, multiple putty masses (sludge)
- **Brown stones**: Calcium bilirubinate, calcium palmitate and calcium stearate, Brown stones are formed in the bile duct and are related to bile stasis and infected bile. Stone formation is related to the deconjugation of bilirubin diglucuronide by bacterial β-glucuronidase.

Mixed

About 75-80%, the are formed in septic bile.
- Multiple faceted stones, cut section—shows laminated central core (debris and bacteria) and alternating layers of cholesterol and bilirubinate (bile acids, bile pigments) and phospholipids and/or carbonate of calcium.

PATHOGENESIS OF GALLSTONE FORMATION

Cholesterol Stone (Refer Figure 28B-2A)

Admirand and small traingle explains the interrelation of the bile acids and phospholipids in keeping the cholesterol in soluble form.

Cholesterol is secreted by the liver from the canalicular membrane in insoluble form. It is kept in soluble form by phospholipid and bile acid forming the "micelles".

The relative concentration of phospholipids, bile acids and the cholesterol decide the solubility of cholesterol. Cholesterol crystals nucleate and stones form when the bile gets supersaturated with cholesterol, with low concentration of bile acids due to the unstable phospholipid vesicles as shown by the triangle.

Pigment stones: Bile pigment solubility depends on catalytic activity of glucuronidase.

It is the emergence of cholesterol and bile pigment in crystalline and paracrystalline form due to disturbances of formation of soluble complexes of them.

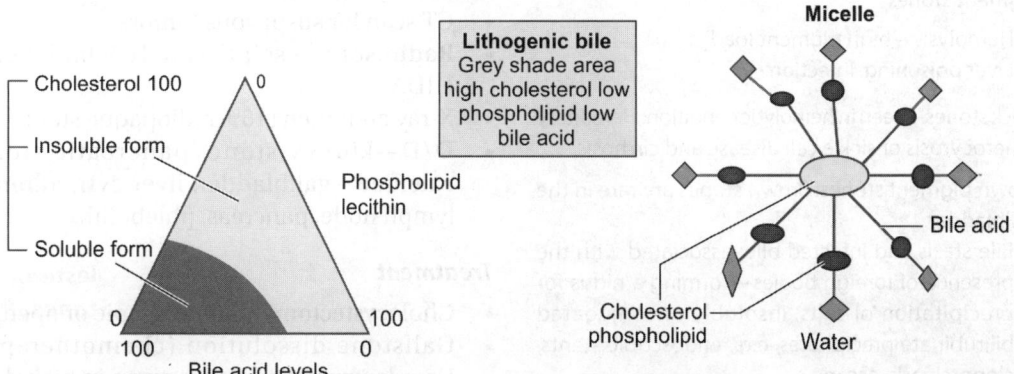

Fig. 28B-2A: Admirand and small triangle

ETIOLOGY OF GALLSTONES

Lithogenic bile:- Supersaturated bile

- Age—advancing age
- Sex—estrogenic effect makes female sex more prone
- Genetics
- Obesity
- Diet medications (e.g. oral contraceptives).
- Starvation
- Pregnancy—stasis and hormones.
- Impaired enterohepatic circulation of bile acids—leads to depletion of bile acids to cause supersaturation and crystallization and nucleation of cholesterol.
  - Resection of the terminal ileum, ileal bypass
  - Gastrectomy, ileal fistula,
  - Crohn's disease—shortened Bowel transit time
  - Cholestyramine binds bile acids and prevents their absorption

Stasis

- Low GI motility, pregnancy, estrogen, vagotomy
- Abnormal emptying of the gallbladder may aid the aggregation of nucleated cholesterol crystals; hence, removing gallstones without removing the gallbladder inevitability leads to gallstone recurrence.

Layering and interfacial tension: Bile enters gallbladder at different times and each time with a different concentration of components. Formati on of layers and the saturation differential may precipitate nucleation of crystals.

Pigment stones: Rovsing theory—all stones start as pigment stones

- Hemolysis—high pigment load
- Liver poisoning, infection

Black stones—seen in hemolytic condition: Hereditary spherocytosis or sickle cell disease and cirrhosis.

Brown pigment stones: Brown stones are rare in the gallbladder.

- Bile stasis and infected bile; associated with the presence of foreign bodies—forming a nidus for precipitation of salts, insoluble unconjugated bilirubinate precipitates, e.g., endoscopic stents, clonorchiasis, ascaris.

Q. Pathology and complications of gallstone.

PATHOLOGY AND COMPLICATIONS OF GALLSTONES

In the Gallbladder

- Silent stones, flatulent dyspepsia
- Gallstone colic
- Acute cholecystitis, perforation, suppuration and gangrene
- Impaction of stone—mucocele and empyema of gallbladder
- Chronic cholecystitis
- Mirizzi syndrome (extrinsic compression of CBD by a stone impacted in the gallbladder)
- Fistulae: Cholecysto-choledochal fistula, cholecystoduodenal fistula.

In the Common Bile Duct

- Obstructive jaundice and liver failure
- Acute ascending cholangitis, white bile and septicemia.

Pancreas: Acute pancreatitis
Intestines: Gallstone ileus due to escape of a large stone through a fistula and impaction at the ileocecal junction.

Saint's Triad: Association of gallstones—colonic diverticulosis—hiatus hernia.

Investigations

- Liver function tests
- Ultrasonography
- MRI and MRCP—for bile duct and periampullary region.
- CT scan for suspicious tumors
- Radioisotope scintiscan-Tc 99m labeled HIDA
- X-ray abdomen (10% radiopaque stones)
- D/D—kidney stone, pancreatic stone, calcified—gallbladder, liver cyst, adrenal, lymph node, pancreas, phlebolith.

Treatment

- Cholecystectomy—laparoscopic or open.
- Gallstone dissolution (chemotherapy): Ursodeoxycholic acids is given in high dose for at least 1-2 years—in pure cholesterol crystals or small calculi.

- But generally formed stones are not suitable nor do they dissolve.

CHRONIC CHOLECYSTITIS

Types
- Calculous cholecystitis
- Acalculous cholecystitis.

Etiology and Pathogenesis

Presence of stone exerts three effects:
1. Pressure on the wall, damage to mucosa and bile irritates the walls.
2. Obstruction of the cystic duct.
3. Increased luminal pressure and ischemia of wall of gallbladder.

Etiological Factors
- Chemical irritation of the mucosa by bile.
- Mucosal damage by the stone.
- Bacterial infection (minor role).

Acalculous cholecystitis—drugs-INH, frusemide, salmonellosis.

Pathology
- The gallbladder may be—fibrosed and small or thick and hypertrophied.
- Chronic inflammatory changes seen on microscopy.
- Bacterial culture of luminal content may be positive only in 20%.

Clinical Features
Right upper quadrant pain—mild to excruciating.

Biliary Colic
Seen in about 25 % of patients with gallstones.

It is a severe right upper quadrant pain with fluctuating severity with associated nausea and vomiting, lasting for minutes or even hours. Pain may radiate to the chest or back.
- Flatulent dyspepsia—accompanies, with intolerance to fatty food and alteration in bowel frequency. It may mimic peptic ulcer or have heart burn.
- Acute presentation—acute on chronic cholecystitis.
- Jaundice—if stone migrates from the gallbladder to obstruct the CBD.
- Gallstone v/s CBD stone—pain is much worse, prolonged episodes, rarely relieved fully, associated with jaundice and fever (cholangitis).

Differential diagnosis—peptic ulcer, hiatus hernia, esophagitis, pancreatic disorder.

Investigations: Refer previous section on gallstones.

Treatment
- Treatment of colic with antispasmodics—dicyclomine or hyoscine/or diclofenac.
- Cholecystectomy: Laparoscopic or open.

> Q. Discuss etiology, pathology, complications and management of acute cholecystitis.

ACUTE CHOLECYSTITIS (REFER FIG. 28.B-3)

Types
Acute calculous cholecystitis—due to obstruction by a calculus.
- It may be acute cholecystitis
- An acute on chronic (existing) cholecystitis (more common)

Acute acalculous cholecystitis:
Infective
- Aerobic: Streptococci, *Salmonella typhi* and para typhi, *Esch coli, Klebsiella*.
- Anerobic: *Clostridium perfringens*, anaerobic streptococci. Bacteroides, propionobacter.

Drugs: Methyldopa, barbiturates, isoniazid, rifampicin.

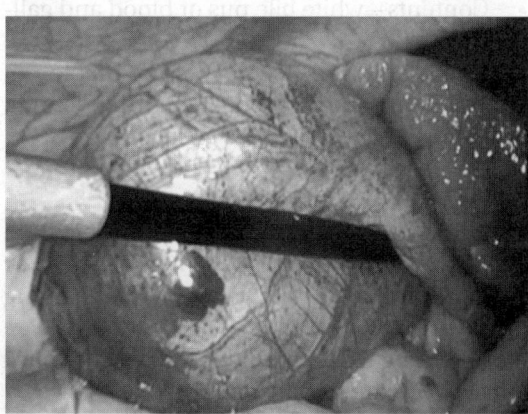

Fig. 28B-3: Acute cholecystitis

Chemical agents: Those in bile and pancreatic juice.

Route of Infection
- Hematogenous—portal vein or arterial route.
- Lymphatic
- Bile: Ascending—along the common bile duct.
  - Descending—through hepatic ducts.
- Local spread through adjacent organs—colon, liver.

Pathology
Obstructive type—more common than the non obstructive (catarrhal) type.
- Obstruction by a calculus at the neck of the gall bladder may lead to resolution (disimpaction of stone) or
- Complications
  - Gangrene (>10%).
  - Empyema of the gallbladder.
  - Perforation of GB—slow (chronic)-- internal fistula - duodenum or colon.
  - Acute - peritonitis—generalized or localized (abscess).
  - Subphrenic abscess.
  - Suppurative pyelephlebitis.

Risk of gangrene and suppuration is high in among diabetics, atherosclerotics and in Immunosupressed.).

Morbid Anatomy
- Gallbladder—thick, edematous, fibrotic (in acute in chronic).
- Mucosa—red, edematous with necrotic areas
- Contents—white bile pus or blood and gallstone.
- Liver—enlarged, edematous and friable.
- Omentum and adjacent organs (duodenum, colon)—adherent to the gallbladder.

Clinical Features
- Age and sex—any age and sex (more females).
- Pain—sudden onset—in right upper quadrant, colicky or vague pain of varying severity.
- Radiating to the shoulder tip or to the back between the shoulder blades.
- Nausea and vomiting and common.
- Fever—usually above 38°C.

Signs
- Febrile and anxious patient.
- Note: Mild jaundice, if present, is due to cholangitis associated with cholecystitis.
- Abdomen: Tenderness and rigidity in ight hypochondrium
- **Murphy's sign (positive):** The patient (in sitting position classically) takes a deep inspiration when the clinician's right hand is held 2–3 fingers below right costal margin. The patient winces and holds the breath due to the inflamed gallbladder hitting the parietal peritoneum under the finger.
- **BOA's sign:** An area of hyperesthesia between 9th and 11th ribs posteriorly.
- A mucocele—felt as a pyriform tender swelling under the right costal margin.

Diagnosis of cholecystitis: Tokyo guidelines TG18/13 criteria:
- Local signs: Pain/murphy sign/guarding.
- Systemic signs: Fever, high CRP, WBC
- Imaging signs GB inflammation.

Differential Diagnosis
- Perforated duodenal ulcer—acute pancreatitis; acute appendicitis.
- Ascending cholangitis—associated with IBD, Crohn's and ulcerative colitis.

Investigations
- Elevation of total WBC and polymorph counts and CRP.
- Ultrasonography: Diagnostic—stone, gallbladder size, wall edema, gas (emphysematous cholecystitis), pericholecystic fluid, free peritoneal gas in perforation, state of the liver, bile duct, pancreas.
- Plain X ray—shows free gas from of perforation of any viscus, a porcelain gallbladder or an radiopaque stones.
- HIDA scan—particularly in acalculous cholecystitis (non-visualization of GB).
- CT scan—helps in assessing the CBD and pericholecystic collections or mass.
- Medical work up—ischemic heart, diabetes, mellitus.
- Rule out associated pancreatitis—amylase and lipase.

Severity Grading of Acute Cholecystitis: Summary as per Tokyo guidelines TG18/13
Grade I: Mild, early episode with no systemic disease.
- Grade II: Moderate—severe inflammation, later than over 72 hours of onset, presence of complications, emphysematous or typhoid cholecystitis.
  Associated moderately severe systemic disease.
- Grade III: Severe inflammation with systemic disease (cardio, neuro, respiratory, renal, hepatic, hematological)—requiring life support.

Treatment
Early cholecystectomy done about 72 hours after initial non-operative therapy. It is done in GR I and selected Gr II before onset of complications.

Nonoperative treatment includes:
- Antibiotic—cephalosporin (Ceftriaxone 1-2 g Q12 H or ciprofloxacin)
- Aspiration—nasogastric tube aspiration to avoid stimulation of gallbladder by CCK.
- Analgesia—Diclofenac or paracetamol.
- Anti acid PPI—omeprazole 20 mg or pantaprazole 40 mg.
- Adequate fluid and electrolyte replacemnent.
- Antiemetic—Ondansetron

EMERGENCY CHOLECYSTECTOMY
- **Emergency surgery (within 24 hours) is indicated for—cholecystitis Gr II, and Gr III:** Performed after a speedy stabilization of patient and work up for comorbidities.
- Presence of complications—gangrene, empyema, mucocele, perforation.
- Patient has long-standing diabetes or atherosclerosis.
- Typhoid cholecystitis.
- Emphysematous cholecystitis.
- Uncertainty of diagnosis.

Surgery: Cholecystectomy
- Laparoscopic route is the gold standard.
- Open cholecystectomy—in patients—unfit for general anesthesia.

Those with low cardiorespiratory reserve to avoid problems of hypercarbia.
Technical reasons—operative or anesthetic challenges on table, laparoscopy converted to open.
Kocher's subcostal incision used (currently smaller incisions than a classical Kocher's classical incision) to access the gallbladder.

Cholecystostomy
- For Gr III—salvage operations: Surgical cholecystostomy under local blocks or image guided cholecystostomy to drain bile.
- **Elective cholecystectomy** after improvement of the condition.

Laparoscopc Cholecystectomy
Classically a four hole—umbilical port for camera and three for the instruments in the subcostal line—one in the high epigastrium, second in midclavicular line and third in right flank.
Calot's triangle is dissected with bipolar diathermy, cystic artery and cystic duct are divided distal to clips. The gallbladder dissected off the fossa and delivered through the epigastric port.
Alternatives: Single incision laparoscopic surgery (SILS)—through umbilicus.
Robotic surgery—laparoscopic surgery with a Robotic arm.

Complications of Cholecystectomy
Intraoperative
- Bleeding—slipped cystic artery, hepatic artery, liver bed from gallbladder fossa, portal vein.
- Bile leak—gallbladder fossa.
- Damage to viscera—CBD or duodenum, colon.
- Diathermy—thermal damage.

Laparoscopic Surgery
- Hypercarbia—due to absorption of carbon dioxide.
- Bile duct damage—transaction, tear, clipping or ligation.

Postoperative

- Reactionary hemorrhage.
- Bile leak—subhepatic collection of bile and hypotension (Waltman Walter syndrome), due to compression of vena cava.
- Bile peritonitis.
- Jaundice—due to bile duct damage and inadvertent ligation.
- Biliary fistula—from accessory ducts, cholecystohepatic duct.
- Fecal peritonitis due to bowel damage.
- Intestinal obstruction.
- Thromboembolism.
- Cardiorespiratory complications.

Late complications—"post cholecystectomy " syndrome, (retained stones, CBD stone or stone in cystic duct stump).

> **Q. Short notes on cholesterolosis (strawberry gallbladder) and gallbladder polyp.**

Cholesteroses (strawberry gallbladder): There are submucous aggregations of cholesterol crystals—seen as yellow specks. It is often associated with cholesterol stones. The wall may be calcified to form porcelain gallbladder.

Cholecystitis Glandularis Proliferans

Pathology
- Gallbladder polyp
- Adenomyomatosis
- Intramural diverticulosis

Gallbladder polyp: A mucosal polyp—fleshy and granulomatous.
- Gallbladder walls may be thickened.
- The polyps may enlarge and some turn malignant (if larger than 6 mm).
- Diff diagnosis—hyperplastic polyp of inflammatory etiology.

Treatment
- Observation and serial scanning is done for polyps upto 5 mm in size.
- Cholecystectomy—for polyp 6 mm and larger; polyps growing as seen at serial sonography.

> **Q. Pathology, clinical features and management of stone in the common bile duct.**

CHOLEDOCHOLITHIASIS (STONE IN THE BILE DUCT)

Types

Primary biliary stones: Form in the bile duct (intra or extrahepatic)—usually pigment.

Causes—stasis in biliary tract.
Impaired physiology—biliary dyskinesia.

Pathology
- Biliary stricture, choledochal cyst, sclerosing cholangitis, Caroli's disease, biliary dilatation.
- Foreign bodies and infestations; ascariasis, clonorchiasis.
- Others: Low-protein diet, malnutrition, obesity, females.

Secondary biliary stones: Form in the gallbladder and migrate into the CBD.

Consequences of Stone in the Bile Duct
- Impaction in the lower CBD (supra or retro duodenal part)—obstructive jaundice
- Biliary cirrhosis and liver failure
- White bile and liver failure
- Ascending cholangitis and sepsis
- Pylephlebitis and liver abscesses and liver failure
- Obstruction at papilla and to pancreatic duct—causing acute pancreatitis
- Chronic fistulation into duodenum or colon (rare).

> **Q. Short note on clinical features of stone in CBD.**

Charcot's triad: Intermittent fever, pain and jaundice.

The impaction of stone in lower CBD causes stasis of bile and causing infection and inflammation.

The stone gets disimpacted and floats causing free flow of bile into the duodenum through the papilla. Thus fever, jaundice and pain subside only to happen again.

Other features: Features of obstructive jaundice but intermittent.

The chronicity of the condition is associated with chronic cholecystitis (thickened or fibrosis of gallbladder, incapable of distension).

The obstruction of CBD calculus is intermittent and hence gallbladder is not palpable clinically.

> **Q. Courvoisier's Law**
>
> **Courvoisier's Law:** If in a case of obstructive jaundice, the gallbladder is palpable, it is not due to a stone in the common bile duct (read above for explanation).
>
> **Exception**; double impaction of stone: a stone in CBD and another in gallbladder neck causing a palpable mucocele.
>
> **Importance:** Helps suspect a cancer of lower CBD or pancreatic head by excluding a stone in patients with obstructive jaundice.

Differential Diagnosis

Carcinoma head of pancreas/peri ampulallay region.
- Bile duct carcinoma
- Bile duct strictures
- Other causes of obstructive jaundice and cholangitis.

Investigations

- Liver function tests—elevation of alkaline phosphatase, conjugated bilirubin.
  - AST and ALT (due to cholangitis)
  - Prothrombin time and international normalized ratio (INR)
- Ultrasosography—detects dilatation of ducts, hepatic texture, abscesses, focal lesions
  - About 75% of CBD stones.
- CT scan—most sensitive for detection of CBD stones.
  - Also detects ductal pathology like stricture, dilatation and growth
  - Hepatic structure, intrahepatic ducts and any abnormality
- MRCP is noninvasive investigation to visualize biliary tree. It is only diagnostic.
- EUS (endoscopic ultrasound)—very useful for lower CBD and head of pancreas lesions.
- ERCP—is invasive and now it is performed mainly for therapy and less for diagnosis.
  - It detects 95% of all obstructive lesions—strictures stones, growth.
  - Used for stenting of bile duct after extraction of stones or Laser coring of stricture.
- Percutaneous transhepatic cholangiography (PTC) is done—for very high obstruction and in cases where ERCP is not possible (previous gastrectomy) or has failed.

Treatment

Preparation of patient for invasive procedure to relieve jaundice.
- Correction of coagulopathy—to correct the prothrombin time
- Injection Vit. K1 10 mg daily for 5 days.
- Frozen plasma transfusion.

IV antibiotics: Ceftriaxone 1-2 g bid or cefoperazone 1 g bid.

Intravenous fluid—to correct dehydration.

Intravenous mannitol (osmotic diuretic)—20% solution—200 mL daily, to prevent renal failure due to hepato renal syndrome.

Relief of Obstruction

ERCP

- **Endoscopic sphincterotomy (papillotomy) and**
- Stone extraction with Dormia basket or balloon catheter; or
  Laser lithotripsy and fragmenting the stone followed by extraction; or
  removal through baby endoscope (choledochoscope)
- CBD stent is placed in situ.

Complications—acute pancreatitis, sepsis and perforation of duodenum.

This is followed by laparoscopic cholecystectomy (or open).

Surgery for CBD Stone

- If ERCP fails in effort.
- Very large impacted stones (depends on the expertise of the gastroenterologist).

Procedures Practiced

- Choledochotomy, extraction of stone and T-tube drainage (T tube choledochostomy).

- Chledochoduodenostomy: CBD is be anastomosed to first part of duodenum for drainage of bile.
  Indication: Very large stones with dilated CBD or stricture of sphincter of Oddi
  Alternatively a choledochojejunal anastomosis can be done.
- Laparoscopic exploration of CBD, operative choledochoscopy and extraction of stone and T tube choledochostomy is done in expert centres

Q. Short note on T-tube cholangiogram.

T-TUBE CHOLANGIOGRAPHY

This is a contrast X-ray study of biliary tree performed 8–10 days after the T-tube is placed in CBD (after exploring the duct), to decide on removal of the T-tube. The dye is injected through the T-tube into CBD and X-ray taken. T-tube is removed if there is free flow of dye into duodenum without any filling defects in the duct which indicate stone or stricture.

BILIARY STRICTURES

Idiopathic:
- Congenital—biliary atresia
- Inflammatory—stones, cholangitis, parasitic, pancreatitis, sclerosing cholangitis.
- Trauma
- Iatrogenic—bile duct injury at surgery cholecystectomy, choledochotomy, gastrectomy, hepatic resection, transplantation
- Malignancy
- Radiotherapy.

Evaluation—is to exclude malignancy and to assess hepatic function apart from evaluating the biliary anatomy.

Treatment
- Short segment strictures are usually stented at ERCP.
- High hilar strictures need PTC and stents.

Surgery
- Excision of the stricture and choledochojejunal anastomosis is performed.
- Long strictures—choledochojejunal or hepaticodochojejunal anastomosis.

Primary sclerosing cholangitis: Autoimmune disorder causing progressive stenosis of CBD. It is also associated with IBD. It has a high risk of leading to cholangiocarcinoma.

Treatment includes ERCP stenting and immunosuppression with steroids, azathioprine.

Tumors of the Bile Ducts

Benign neoplasms causing biliary obstruction may be classified as follows:
- Papilloma and adenoma multiple biliary papillomatosis
- Granular cell myoblastoma
- Neural tumors; leiomyoma; endocrine tumors.

MALIGNANCIES OF BILE DUCTS

Q. Hilar cholangiocarcinoma.

CHOLANGIOCARCINOMA OF BILE DUCTS
- Hilar cholangiocarcinoma (Klatskin tumors), occurring at the bifurcation the CBD, account for 60 to 70%.
- Distal CBD—20-30%
- Intra hepatic—around 5-10%.

Clinical Features

Abdominal pain, early satiety, anorexia and weight loss commonly seen.
Pruritus and jaundice—in a minority of patients.

Signs—jaundice, cachexia and a palpable gallbladder when tumor is in lower CBD.

Treatment
- Choice of treatment depends on the site and extent of the disease.
- 10–15% are resectable, with a chance of long-term survival.

Procedure
- Standard or extended hepatic resection, lymphadenectomy and biliary enteric bypass.
- Pancreaticoduodenectomy (Whipple procedure) for distal common duct tumors.
- Local resection avoided.
- Liver transplantation—for nonmetastatic non-resectable disease.

CARCINOMA OF GALLBLADDER

Etiology
Pre-existing gallstone disease, (porcelain gallbladder), gallbladder polyps.

Pathology
- About 90% of tumors are adenocarcinomas.
- Squamous carcinomas—arise from mucosal squamous metaplasia.
- Gross appearance: It is nodular and infiltrative, with a thickened gallbladder wall.
- Spread: Direct extension into the liver.
- Transperitoneal.
- Lymphatic—perihilar lymphatics and neural plexuses.

Clinical Features
- May look like benign disease (biliary colic or cholecystitis).
- Particularly in older patients.
- Jaundice and anorexia and palpable mass are late features.

Investigations
For biliary obstruction.
- Anemia, leukocytosis, mild elevation in AST, ALT and ALP.
- Elevated inflammatory markers—ESR and C-reactive protein.
- Serum CA19-9 is elevated in approximately 80% of patients.

Imaging—in diagnosis—ultrasonography, and confirmed by a CT scan or MRI/MRCP.

PET scanning for detection of metastatic disease.

Treatment
Cholecystectomy is advised for polyps of gall bladder larger than 6 mm.

For a carcinoma:
Radical en bloc resection—segmentectomy or extended hepatectomy, bile duct resection and regional lymphadenectomy.

Palliation involves relief of jaundice by endoscopic or radiological intervention.

Prognosis: Very poor.

The median survival—6 months–1 year (5 year survival is less than 5%).

> **Q. Etiology and pathology of obstructive jaundice; management of surgical jaundice. (Major question)**

OBSTRUCTIVE JAUNDICE
Obstructive jaundice is due to conjugated hyperbilirubinemia, following obstruction to flow of bile (Refer **Figure 28B-3A**).

Approach to Obstructive Jaundice
- Is this surgical jaundice? Nonobstructive and intrahepatic cholestasis ruled out
- If yes—find out cause, and site/extent of obstruction
- Assess and look for complications
- Build the patient
- Treat complications
- Relief of obstruction—endoscopic/surgical
- Rehabilitation.

Intrahepatic biliary obstruction—from canaliculi upto the porta hepatis—bile ducts.
Extrahepatic biliary obstruction is from the porta hepatis upto the duodenal papilla.

EXTRAHEPATIC BILIARY OBSTRUCTION (SURGICAL JAUNDICE)
Refer **Figure 28B-4**.

Complications of Obstructive Jaundice
- Ascending cholangitis
- Coagulopathy
- Liver failure
- Septicemia
- Hepatorenal syndrome
- Encephalopathy—coma.

History taking in Obstructive jaundice
- Age—congenital/inflammatory cause.
- Sex—carcinoma more in males? Stones—females?
- Occupation - industrial poison.
- Jaundice in community—Weil's, hepatitis.
- Jaundice in family—hereditary - Wilson's disease, congenital spherocytosis, hemolytic anemia.
- Drugs (steroids, estrogen, androgen, nitro drugs).
- Injection/transfusion.

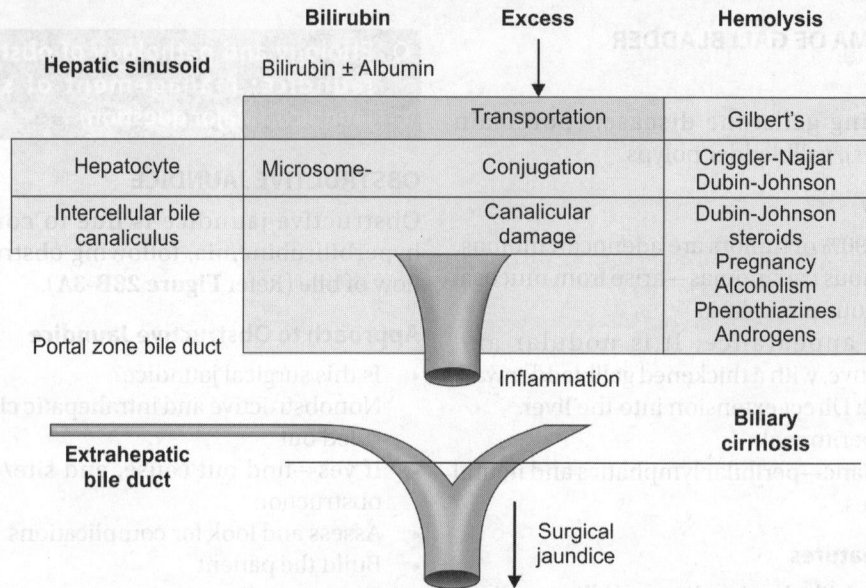

Fig. 28B-3A: Mechanism of jaundice

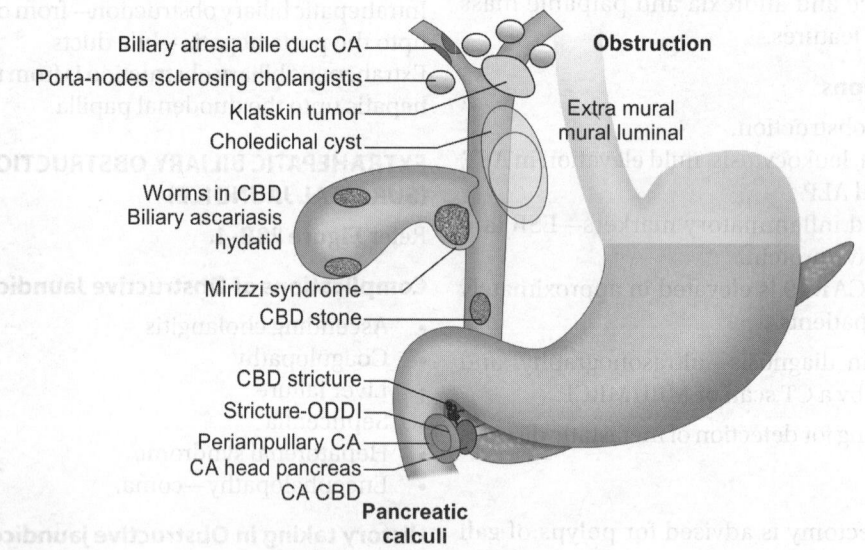

Fig. 28B-4: Etiology of surgical jaundice

Symptoms of Obstructive Jaundice

- **Pain**—stones; painless—carcinoma
- **Fever**—hepatitis/stones
- **Chills and rigors**—cholangitis
- **Pruritus**—obstructive jaundice
- **Dark urine**—conjugated bilirubin
- **Pale stools**—obstructive jaundice
- Vomiting—nausea—obstructive
- Previous—abdominal surgery, colicky pain, dyspepsia.

General Signs in Obstructive Jaundice

- Emaciation—indicates malignancy
- Anemia—and mild jaundice—hemolytic
- Severe jaundice?—carcinoma

- Signs of cirrhosis—gynecomastia, Dupuytren's, Parotomegaly
- Signs of hepatic insufficiency—spider nevi, palmar erythema
- Loss of hair, white nails, bruisability
- CNS—sensorium, flapping tremor, fetor hepaticus
- Search for a primary tumor—breast, thyroid,, stomach, lung, rectum,
- Thrombosed superficial vein/s—**Trousseau's sign** in cancer of pancreas.

Abdominal Signs in Obstructive Jaundice

- Dilated veins—collaterals in portal hypertension
- Ascites—cirrhosis/obstructive hepatorrhea/metastases.
- Liver—nodular—mets
  - Smooth—tender in hepatitis/CCF/alcoholism
  - Nontender in cancer.

COURVOISIER'S LAW

In a patient with obstructive jaundice, if gallbladder is palpable, the obstruction is not due to stone in the common bile duct.
- Exception—double impaction—a stone each in CBD and cystic duct.

Clinical States in Obstructive Jaundice

- Charcot's triad
- Intermittent fever
- Intermittent pain
- Intermittent jaundice.

Pentad of Reynold

- Persistent pain
- Persistent jaundice
- Fever
- Encephalopathy
- Shock.

Investigations in Obstructive Jaundice

Exclude medical jaundice
- Urine—**urobilinogen absent** in total obstruction of over 7 days.
- Stools—**acholic** (no stercobilin); occult blood present in carcinoma
- Liver function tests—high total and direct bilirubin > 45%
- ALP > 3 times; 5-Nucleotidase (5-NT) high only in jaundice due to a pathology in the liver
- Hematology and serology—high WBC count in sepsis
  - Hepatitis markers, A, B and C
- Tumor marker—alfa-fetoprotein - HCC, CA 19-9—pancreas, cholangiocarcinoma, CEA - in cholangiocarcinoma and colonic carcinoma with mets.
- Prothrombin time—raised (depletion of Vit - K clotting factors).

Abdominal Ultrasonography

- Dilated IHBR (**intrahepatic biliary dilatation**)- seen in extra hepatic obstruction
- Dilated bile duct indicates—low obstruction
- Dilated GB means—obstruction distal to cystic duct junction with CBD
- Stones—GB/CBD/pancreas
- **Liver**—size, metastases
- Nodes in porta hepatis
- Ascites
- Other masses—pancreatic head
  - Intraperitoneal/pelvic.

Upper GI endoscopy—to rule out varices, portal gastropathy, gastric/duodenal obstruction.

Endoscopic Ultrasound (Endosonography)

- To evaluate lower CBD and pathology
- To evaluate head masses in pancreas
- To evaluate periampullary cystic lesions
- To evaluate peri pancreatic and retroduodenal nodes
- To take biopsies and aspirate cysts.

Contrast Enhanced CT Scan

- Liver masses/pancreatic masses
- Vascular invasion—mesenteric/porta
- Nodes—celiac/other.

MRI – MRCP – plain/contrast

The best modality to study biliary obstruction—stricture/hilar tumor to study ducts, periductal structures.

Isotope Scanning

Technetium 99-IDA - (HIDA/PIPIDA)—shows biliary excretion.

Invasive Investigations in Obstructive Jaundice—ERCP and PTC

ERCP—localizing lower CBD obstruction

- Filling defect/obstructed CBD/stricture/periampullary carcinoma
- Chain of lake—pancreatic duct
- Bile culture, tumor cytology, stenting for relief of obstruction
- Complications—perforation/pancreatitis/cholangitis.

Percutaneous transhepatic cholangiography (PTC) for localising upper biliary obstruction

Above cystic duct confluence and therapeutic drainage.

Complications—hemorrhage, sepsis/leak/liver failure.

Role of Biopsy in Obstructive Jaundice

- CT/USG—**guided biopsy**
- **Liver**/hilar cholangiocarcinoma/hilar node/pancreatic mass
- EUS guided biopsy—lower CBD/pancreatic head, peri pancreatic and periportal
  - Nodes
- Endoscopic biopsy/periampullary growth—ca stomach/duodenum.

Laparoscopic Biopsy

- Primary lesion
- Secondaries—peritoneum/omentum; nodes.

> **Q. Short note on how do you prepare a patient for surgery for relief of obstructive jaundice?**

Pre-treatment of Surgical Jaundice

- Correct coagulopathy
  - Vit. K-1 10 mg IV daily—3–5 days - monitor INR
  - Platelet concentrate/FFP—before or at intervention
- Build liver glycogen reserve
  - IV 10% glucose
- Nutrition and hydration: Dextrose in water, albumin

- Control sepsis—antibiotics
  - Ceftriaxone + aminoglycoside + metronidazole
  - Piperacillin + metronidazole.
- Intravenous mannitol (to flush kidneys) against hepatorenal syndrome (currently this is not practiced in favor of ensuring adequate hydration and renal perfusion).

> **Q. Briefly enumerate the nonsurgical interventions for relief of extrahepatic obstructive jaundice.**

Nonsurgical intervention—ERCP and PTBD

ERCP

Stent the CBD for stricture
- **Basket** extraction of stones
- **Sphincterotomy** of stenosis of ODDI
- **Life saving**—emergency treatment in cholangitis
- CBD—stenting/sphincterotomy—later surgery

PTBD: Percutaneous Transhepatic Biliary Drainage
  - For high obstructions not amenable to surgery
  - Prograde guidewire stenting of hilar /high biliary obstruction

SURGERY IN OBSTRUCTIVE JAUNDICE

Principle: Bypass or resection of obstructing lesion or liver transplantation.

SURGICAL BYPASS FOR OBSTRUCTIVE JAUNDICE: (Refer Fig. 28B-5 and 28B-6)

- CBD stone—choledocholithotomy
- Benign stricture lower CBD—choledochoduodenostomy
- Malignant lower CBD obstruction—(inoperable) cholecystojejunostomy
- High obstruction—hepaticodochojejunostomy
- Hilar obstruction—portojejunostomy
- Portal obstruction—hepaticojejunostomy
- Cholecystectomy—for Mirizzi's syndrome.

Resectional Surgery in Obstructive Jaundice

- Cholecystectomy—for Mirizzi/cholangitis
- Excision of choledochal cyst
- Excision of bile duct stricture with choledochojejunostomy

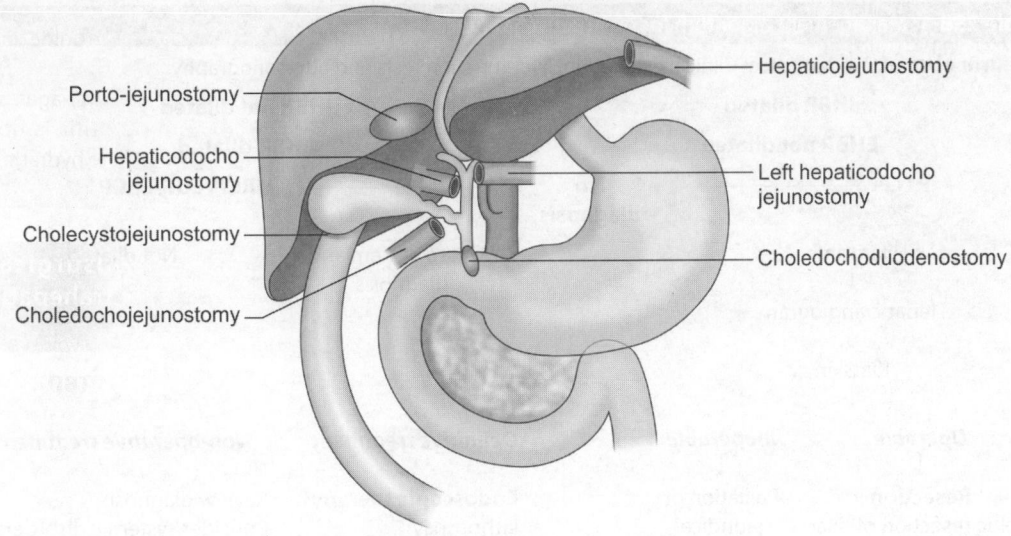

Fig. 28B-5: Surgical bypass for obstructive jaundice.

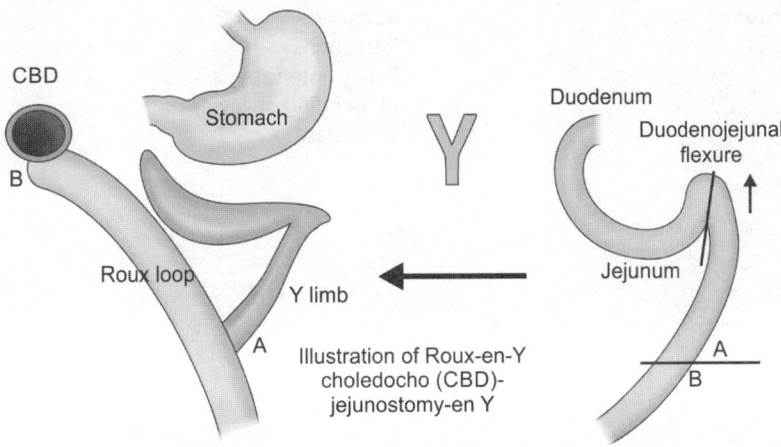

Fig. 28B-6: Roux-en-Y—biliary enteric anastomosis.

- Whipples' pancreaticoduodenectomy—pancreatic/periampullar carcinoma
- Resection of Klatskin tumor with hepaticojejunostomy.

Liver transplantation—biliary atresia.

Q. Describe key steps in managing obstructive jaundice.

MANAGEMENT ALGORITHM FOR SURGICAL JAUNDICE

Refer **Table 28B-1**.

Table 28B-1: Management algorithm for obstructive jaundice.

Confirm obstructive jaundice: Clinical evaluation, liver function tests and ultrasonography.

IHBR dilated			IHBR not dilated	
EHBR not dilated			EHBR dilated	
PTC →		No diagnosis →	MRCP/EUS/ERCP	
Hilar tumor ↓ Hepatic angiogram ↓ Klatskin ↓			Dilated system and diagnosis ↓	Not dilated ↓
Operable ↓ **Resection** Enbloc resection of hilar tumor extended hepatic lobectomy with hilar lymphadenectomy hepaticojejunostomy	*Inoperable* ↓ Palliation of jaundice **PTBD**		*Definitive treatment* ↓ **Endoscopic therapy** Lithotripsy Laser coring Stenting strictures **Surgery** Resections Biliary enteric bypass (depending on level) Transplant	*Non-operative treatment* ↓ Review diagnosis Consider systemic disorders like sclerosing cholangitis. Medical treatment

28.4: THE INTESTINES

SU28.13: Describe the applied anatomy of small and large intestine.

SU28.14: Describe the clinical features, investigations and principles of management of disorders of small and large intestine including neonatal obstruction and short gut syndrome.

SU28.15: Describe the clinical features, investigations and principles of management of diseases of appendix including appendicitis and its complications.

SU28.16: Describe applied anatomy including congenital anomalies of the rectum and anal canal.

SU28.17: Describe the clinical features, investigations and principles of management of common anorectal diseases.

SU28.18: Describe and demonstrate clinical examination of abdomen. Order relevant investigations. Describe and discuss appropriate treatment plan.

SU28.13: Describe the applied anatomy of small and large intestine.

ANATOMY OF SMALL INTESTINE

Embryology: Please Refer Section Congenital Disorders of Intestines

- The small intestine is divided into the duodenum, the jejunum and the ileum (Refer **Table 28S-1**).
- The duodenum has specific functions and subject to diseases peculiar to it, it is usually considered as an entity separate from the jejunum and ileum.
- Excluding the 25–30 cm long duodenum, the jejunum (proximal 40%) and ileum (distal 60%) are together considered as the small intestine from the duodenojejunal flexure, fixed to posterior abdominal wall by the ligament of Treitz, to the ileocecal junction. The length of the small intestine varies from 350 to 800 cm (average of 500 to 600 cm approx).
- The intestinal wall is made of a mucosa, submucosa and the muscle in two layers—the inner circular and outer longitudinal, covered by the serosa.
- Nerves: The Meissner's plexus of nerves are in the submucosa and the Auerbach's myenteric plexus of nerves in intermuscular plane. They receive autonomic innervation from the splanchnic nerves through the sympathetic network around the superior mesenteric artery and its branches.
- The small intestinal pain is referred to T 10 level at the umbilicus.
- Sympathetic supply is from T9-T11 and the vagus supplies the parasympathetic fibers.
- The nerves pass through the superior mesenteric and the celiac plexuses.
- While the vagus stimulates the peristalsis and constricts the sphincters, the sympathetic fibers inhibit peristalsis and relaxes the sphincters.

Table 28S-1: Anatomy of jejunum and ileum compared.

Jejunum	Ileum
- Proximal 40%	- Distal 60%
- Wider lumen	- Comparatively smaller lumen (about 3 cm)
- Thicker wall	- Thinner wall
- Mucosal folds (valvulae conniventes)	- No mucosa folds characterless
- Mesentery; thinner	- Thicker, more fatty
- Single arterial arcades—longer vasa recta	- Shorter vasa recta—complex arterial arcade
- Scanty lymphoid aggregation	- Larger lymphoid aggregates (Peyer's patches)

- The mesentery attaches the intestine to the posterior abdominal wall. The mesenteric root extends from left of the L2 vertebra obliquely downward to the right sacroiliac joint level.
- The blood vessels, nerves and lymphatics run between the mesenteric layers.

Blood Supply
- Arterial supply—from the superior mesenteric artery.
- Venous drainage is through superior mesenteric vein into the portal vein.
- Thus nutrient rich blood from the small intestine is drained into the liver, which carries out the metabolic processing of the nutrients and detoxification.
- The lymphatic drainage of the small intestine follows the arterial supply.

Function of the Small Intestine
- The digestion of food and the absorption of nutrients, water and electrolytes.
- Carbohydrates and proteins are broken down in the intestinal lumen by pancreatic enzymes.
- The jejunal function: Digestion and absorption of fluid, electrolytes, fat, protein and carbohydrate, iron and folic acid.
- Terminal ileum: Absorption of bile salts and vitamin B12 through the specific transporters.

Applied Physiology

Jejunal resection will hamper absorption of the nutrients and iron and folate.

Resection of or diseases of **terminal ileum**:
1. B12 deficiency: Reduction of bile pool and deficiency of fat soluble vitamins—A, D, E and K.

Metabolism of plasma lipoproteins: The small bowel, synthesizes the HDL, LDL, and VLDL, which help the transportation of fats into circulation through the lymphatics.

Hormonal synthesis (Brain gut hormones)
GLP-1 and 2 (glucagon-like peptides), Motilin and peptide YY: These hormones interact with nervous system and modulate the intestinal function and differentiation.

Intestinal secretions: Saliva—1000 mL, gastric 1500 mL, bile 1000, pancreas 1500-2000, intestinal 4000 mL, total 8-9 liters/day.

ANATOMY OF THE LARGE INTESTINE
The large intestine, about 1.5 meter in length (4 ½ to 5 feet) extends from the ileocecal valve upto the anus.

Parts: It is divided into the cecum, ascending colon, right colic (hepatic) flexure, transverse colon with the greater omentum, left colic (splenic flexure), descending colon, sigmoid and rectum.

Wall of the colon: Mucosa, submucosa, muscle inner circular. The outer longitudinal is confined only to sigmoid colon and rectum, the proximal part having the taenia coli.

Taenia coli—are the three longitudinal bands of condensation of longitudinal muscle, running from the base of appendix to the rectosigmoid junction, but spread around the wall of sigmoid.

The longitudinal muscle is shorter in length than the colon invested by the circular muscle and this gives haustral folds like the frill of a curtain, making it conducive to the water absorptive function of the colon.

The cecum and ascending colon is related posteriorly to the right ureter, right gonadal vessels and the 3rd part of the duodenum. The descending colon and sigmoid are related to the tail of the pancreas, left ureter and the left gonadal vessels. The surgical importance lies in avoiding injuries to the said structures during colonic surgery.

Development: The midgut derived parts include the cecum, ascending colon and two thirds of transverse colon; the hindgut derived parts are the distal transverse colon, descending colon, sigmoid and the rectum. This helps to understand the vascular supply and the lymphatics.

The blood supply of the large intestine (Refer Figure 28C-6, Page no. 524)
The superior mesenteric artery through its branches—iliocolic, right colic and the middle colic arteries supplies the cecum, ascending colon and transverse colon upto its distal part.

The inferior mesenteric artery and its branches, viz., the left colic, the sigmoidal and the superior rectal branches supply the distal large bowel.

Communication between superior and inferior mesenteric artery
Marginal artery of Drummond: The anastomoses between adjacent branches of the right colic, middle colic and left colic arteries form a marginal arterial arcade running along the mesocolon. It is the major arterial supply to large bowel from cecum to sigmoid colon.

Applied anatomy: It is important in ensuring arterial supply to colonic anastomoses and segments of colonic conduits in transpositions.

It is narrow near splenic flexure where middle colic and the left colic artery anastomose. (Sudeck's point or watershed area). Splenic flexure is the most vulnerable area in ischemia of large bowel.

Venous drainage: The colonic venous blood drains into the portal vein.

Veins accompany the respective arteries
The venous drainage from the ascending and transverse colon is into the ileocolic, right colic and middle colic veins, which drain into the superior mesenteric vein that forms the portal vein with splenic vein. The blood from left sided part of the colon is into inferior mesenteric vein which joins the splenic vein behind the body of the pancreas. The splenic vein joins the SMV to form the portal vein.

The nerve supply is derived from the splanchnic nerves via a sympathetic plexus around the superior and inferior mesenteric arteries.

Visceral pain from the part of the colon from midgut (supplied by the superior mesenteric) is felt around the umbilicus and pain from colon distal to the transverse (hind gut derivatives) is felt in suprapubic part.

> **Q. Lymphatic drainage of colon. What are lymphovascular units?**

LYMPHATIC DRAINAGE OF THE COLON

The mucosa has no lymphatics and lymphatics deep to lamina propria and through the muscular layer from all parts drain into lymph nodes along their respective arterial branches and the nodes are named after the respective artery (e.g., ileocolic nodes, inferior mesenteric nodes).

The nodes are:
- Epicolic (adjacent to colonic wall)
- Pericolic—near the mesocolic border of wall along the arterial branch
- Intermediate—along the mesocolic branches.
- Central—the main arterial pedicle (ilio colic, right colic, middle colic, left colic and the nodes along inferior mesenteric vein).

Applied Anatomy
The Lymphovascular Units
- The colonic segment, the artery supplying respective segment and the lymphatic field including the nodes, together make a lymphovascular unit.
- Oncological clearance involves resection of a lymphovascular unit.
- Surgical removal of a colonic growth with lymph nodes requires ligation of the main vessels (high ligation) supplying the segment of the colon. Thus the length of colonic segment removed is related to the vascularity of the colonic part.

Function of the Large Intestine
- Absorption of water—about 1500 mL of ileal contents enter the colon every day, condensed into less than 200 mL of feces.
- Active absorption of sodium by a transport system.
- Passive absorption of chloride.
- Dietary fiber in the colon is fermented by normal flora forming short chain fatty acids, necessary for metabolism of colonic mucosa.
- Absorption of some nutrients—glucose, amino acids and fatty acids in a small way.

Motiliy of the colon is variable
- Conon has two types of contractions—segmentation and peristalsis.
- Segmentation—this is to mix the stools in the saccules between the haustrations to facilitate water absorption. And peristalsis is to propel stool towards the anus.

- Generally, after a meal, fecal load reaches cecum in 4 to 5 hours and the anus after about 24 hours.

INTESTINAL DIVERTICULAE

Diverticulae are outpouchings from the bowel wall (all parts of GI tract except rectum may be affected). They may be congenital or acquired.

Congenital diverticulae—all three layers of the bowel are present in the wall (e.g., Meckel's diverticulum) and generally on antimesenteric side.

Acquired diverticulae—muscularis is absent from the wall.

Sites: Mostly in the jejunum **arise from the mesenteric side of the bowel, at the point of entry of the blood vessels** due to mucosal herniation; jejunal diverticulae are more often multiple and variable in size.

Complications

- Bacterial stasis and malabsorption
- Diverticulitis and peridiverticulitis causing peritoneal adhesions
- Perforation and peritonitis/abscess
- Bleeding (rarely)
- Clinical features
- Asymptomatic—found incidentally at imaging or at surgery
- Or symptoms due to complications
- Malabsorption
- Recurrent abdominal pain, bloating, flatulence, or
- Present as an acute abdominal emergency.

Treatment

- Single diverticulum or limited length of jejunum can be resected for treatment of chronic malabsorptive symptoms. But length of bowel resection is kept in mind.
- Perforation of diverticulitis: Intestinal resection is performed and anastomosis carried out (or a temporary stoma in case of severe peritonitis or an unstable patient; but will cause a high output jejunal fistula).

Extensive Diverticulosis

- Prolonged antibiotic therapy for bacterial overgrowth and digestive supplementation.
- Drugs used are usually on rotation—rifaximin, metronidazole, ciprofloxacin, and cefixime.
- **Compromise**: Limited resection of large and complicating diverticula and leaving remaining segments of affected jejunum, and subsequent intermittent antibiotic therapy is a compromise approach between a short gut and a malabsorption.

Q. Meckel's diverticulum.

MECKEL'S DIVERTICULUM

Remember: 2%, 2 feet from ileo cecal junction, 2 inch long. It is the persistent remnant of the vitellointestinal duct.

Pathology

- Congenital diverticulum, it contains all three layers of the bowel wall with its own blood supply, found on antimesenteric side of terminal ileum,
- 2 feet (60 cm) from the ileocecal junction, generally 2 inches long (5 cm)
- Present in about 2% of the population,
- Heterotopic epithelium: found in about in 20% of the cases, usually at its base, having gastric or pancreatic epithelium.

Complications

- Inflammation—diverticulitis
- Perforation, peritonitis.
- Obstruction—due to band of the vitellointestinal duct causing volvulus
- As intussusception or adhesion causing a kink
- Hemorrhage—due to peptic ulceration of the gastric mucosa
- Acute hemorrhage as melena or chronic occult loss.

Clinical Features

- Silent and incidentally found at operation for other cause
- Meckel's diverticulitis (mimics appendicitis)
- Perforation and peritonitis
- Melena or massive rectal bleeding
- Intussusception
- Volvulus or adhesive obstruction

- Chronic peptic ulcer like features—occult blood in stool, and pain
- Littre's hernia—incarceration in an inguinal hernia.

Investigation
- Difficult to diagnose in silent state.
- CT scan may show the Meckel's diverticulum.
- Bleeding from Meckel's diverticulum; detected at radioisotope scanning (99m-technitium).

Treatment
- Incidental finding of a Meckel's diverticulum.
- It is left alone, if it is not thickened and with wide mouth.
- Symptomatic ones are resected.

Meckel's Diverticulectomy
- Resection of the ileal segment and ileoileal anastomosis—procedure of choice.
- Excision of the diverticulum—suture or stapling the base.
- Amputation is avoided for of stricture and missing heterotopic epithelium.

CROHN'S DISEASE (CD)

A chronic full-thickness inflammatory process affecting any part of the alimentary tract.

Etiological Factors
It is complex and involves genetic and environmental factors.
- Genetic factors NOD2/CARD15 gene on chromosome 16q12/is shown to be related. The gene CARD 15 is expressed in Paneth cells of the ileum. Crohn's is genetically transmitted among first degree relatives and monozygotic twins.
- Age—peak incidence between 25 and 40 years although all ages are affected.
- Race—high incidence among Caucasian: The White race and Jewish.

Environmental Factors
- Infection—mycobacterium para tuberculosis is blamed but not proven.
- Food—diet high in refined foodstuffs
- Stress and psychological factors
- Smoking
- Immunological factors.

Clinical Features
(Refer Table 28S-2 and Table 28S-3)

Variable presentation depending on the pattern of the pathology.

Acute CD
- Ileal inflammation and features similar to those of acute appendicitis.

Q. Pathology of Crohn's disease.

Pathology previous name for Crohn's disease was "regional ileitis".
All parts of GI tract are prone to get involved.
- Terminal ileum—70% ("regional ileitis") and proximal ileum.
- Colon—35% (colitis).
- Perianal lesions—fistulae or abscess—25% with ileum.
- The stomach and duodenum are affected in about 5%.

Gross pathology
- Fibrotic thickening of intestinal wall with narrow lumen and fat wrapping of mesentery.
- Stricture with dilated bowel proximally.
- Mucosal—ulceration—linear or serpiginous with intervening mucosal edema giving rise to a cobble stone appearance.
- The transmural inflammation of segments of bowel makes them adherent to each other and to surrounding structures. Also the serosa is thickened and lymph nodes are enlarged.
- The disease is typically intermittent causing "skip lesions".

Microscopy
- Focal areas of chronic inflammation of all the layers—mucosa to serosa.
- Lymphoid aggregates and non-caseating granulomas.
- Arterial occlusions are found in the thickened muscularis propria, and hyperplasia of nerve cells.
- All lesions are separate with normal intestines in between (unlike ulcerative colitis—UC).

Table 28S-2: Crohn's disease and ulcerative colitis compared.

Crohn's disease (CD)	Ulcerative colitis (UC)
Site	
CD can affect any part of the GIT—small and large bowel. Bowel affects full thickness of the bowel wall. Characterized by skip lesions. Causes stricturing and fistulation. Granulomas seen on histology. Associated frequently with perianal disease, recurrence is common after resection. • Anti-saccharomyces cerevisiae antibody (ASCA)—positive • Perineural antineutrophil cytoplasmic antibody (pANCA)—negative	UC affects the colon. Mucosal disease produces confluent disease in the colon and rectum. Stricture and fistula less common. Granulomas not seen. Perianal disease, unusual resection of the colon and rectum is curative. • ASCA—negative • pANCA—positive

Table 28S-3: The Montreal classification of Crohn's disease.

The Montreal classification of CD: Age, location, behavior		
Age of onset • A1 <16 • A2 17–40 • A3 >40	Location • L1—Ileal • L2—colonic • L3—ileo-colonic • L4—Isolated upper GIT	Behavior of disease (inflammation with or without stricture or/and penetration) • B1—non stricturing and non penetrating • B2—stricturing • B3—penetrating-leads to phlegmon/abscess/fistulae • B4—peri anal disease

- As perforation of small bowel and local or diffuse peritonitis.
- As abscesses.
- Fulminant colitis. CD may present with fulminant colitis but this is considerably less common than in UC.

Q. Differentiate ulcerative colitis from Crohn's disease.

Refer Table 28 S-2.

Abdominal Features

- Intermittent fever, anemia and weight loss, colicky pain often postprandial, mild chronic diarrhea.
- A tender mass in right iliac fossa, secondary
- Progressed disease—intra-abdominal abscesses and fistulae
- Stenosis and adhesion causing obstructive features
- Fistulation—enteroenteric or interloop fistulae—ileosigmoid, ileovesical or into female genital tract. Colonic CD presents as colitis or proctitis.

Perianal Lesions

- Superficial ulcers with undermined edges.
- Deep ulcers in the upper anal canal—cause perianal abscesses and fistula.
- Fistulae—recto vesical or rectovaginal fistula.
- The perineum becomes fibrotic, rigid and with multiple discharging sinuses.

The Extraintestinal Manifestations of CD

- Gallstones (due to reduced absorption of bile salts from the diseased ileum)
- Primary sclerosing cholangitis, less common than in UC
- Amyloidosis is common
- Renal calculi
- Chronic active hepatitis
- Metastatic CD can occur in the vagina and/or skin
- **Skin nodules** with ulcers, they are non-caseating granulomas on microscopy
- CD may look like hidradenitis suppurativa.
- Erythema nodosum, pyoderma gangrenosum
- Sacroiliitis, arthropathy
- Aphthous ulceration
- Uveitis.

Investigations
Blood Counts
- Anemia, B12 and folate deficiency, iron deficiency.
- Serum albumin, magnesium, zinc and selenium.
- Acute phase protein measurements (C-reactive protein) and ESR.

Stool—calprotectin levels (it is a marker of inflammation).

Colonoscopic Examination
- Areas of normal mucosa in between irregular areas of inflammation and ulceration.
- Surface exudates with aphthous ulcers.
- Crohn's stricture (common in terminal ileum) with polypoid mucosa—looks like malignancy.

IMAGING IN CROHN'S DISEASE
Ultrasonography
It can detect thickened intestinal loops bowel loops and fluid collections/abscesses.

The small bowel enema (or barium follow through previously)
- Strictures and proximal dilatation.
- Terminal ileum: The 'string sign' of Kantor—narrowing of lumen.

CT with oral contrast: Shows thickened intestinal loops, dilatation, intra-abdominal abscesses and fistulae.

MRI (magnetic resonance imaging) is used to delineate small bowel as well as perianal complications like fistula. MRI is useful in assessing complex perianal disease.
- MR enterography (oral contrast)/MR enteroclysis—to detect a stricture in small bowel enterocutaneous fistulae. The contrast is given through a nasoduodenal tube.

CT or MR Fistulography—to depict and plan treatment of an enterocutaneous fistula.

Endoscopy
- Colonic and ileocecal disease is assessed best. Biopsies taken from lesions.
- Capsule endoscopy—for evaluation of jejunal and ileal disease.

Serology
- Anti-saccharomyces cerevisiae antibody (ASCA)—positive.
- Perinuclear anti-neutrophil cytoplasmic antibody (p-ANCA)—negative.

Complications
- Strictures and bowel obstruction
- Abscess—intraperitoneal, pericolic
- Perforation and peritonitis
- Fistulae- internal and external
- Perianal sepsis and fistulae
- Carcinoma—small and large.

Treatment of CD
- Involves a multidisciplinary team of physician, surgeon, gastroenterologist and immunologist
- Mainly medical treatment
- Role of for surgery—largely in managing complications; but not for a cure or control.

Q. Indications for surgery in Crohn's disease

Indications for surgery in CD
- Free perforation of the bowel
- Persistent or massive acute bleeding
- Malignancy—happens more often in colonic and less frequently in small bowel disease
- Perianal disease (abscess, fistula, stenosis)
- Recurrent intestinal obstruction
- Intestinal fistula—with high output and sepsis.

Relative indications
- Failure of medical therapy
- Steroid dependent disease

Medical Treatment

- Steroids—for getting a remission not for maintenance
- Aminosalicylates 5-ASA—for colonic disease—no use for small bowel
- Immunomodulators—azathioprine, cyclosporine
- Monoclonal antibodies—murine infliximab IV every 8 weeks
  - Human adalimumab
  - 3rd gen—integrin inhibitors—vedolizumab and etrolizumab
- Nutritional support: Oral, enteral, TPN

Steroids

Induces remission in 70–80% of cases with moderate to severe disease.
- But Ineffective in obstructive disease
- Should not be used for maintenance therapy of CD Immunomodulatory drugs are used.

Aminosalicylates

- Colonic symptoms can be treated by 5-ASA but not useful in small bowel CD.

Antibiotics: Metronidazole and ciprofloxacin.

Immunomodulatory Agents

- Azathioprine—a purine analogue, metabolized to 6-mercaptopurine (6-MP). It works by inhibiting cell-mediated immune responses.
- Cyclosporin helps in achieve short-term therapy remission.

Monoclonal Antibodies

- Target tumor necrosis factor alpha and other key pro-inflammatory mediators.
- Infliximab, a murine chimeric monoclonal antibody—intravenous administration every 8 weeks.
- Adalimumab, an entirely human monoclonal antibody is administered subcutaneously every 1–2 weeks,
- Third-generation monoclonal antibody therapies-integrin antiibodies (vedolizumab and etrolizumab).

Nutritional support—supplementation Enteral or parenteral in complications or as preoperative preparation.

Endoscopic Dilatation in Crohn's Disease

- Endoscopic dilatation and stenting of strictures accessible to endo—guidewire.
- Balloon dilatation of strictures done.

Surgery for Crohn's Disease
(Refer Table 28S-4)

- Aim is to preserve healthy gut to have adequate function, by minimising removal of gut and preserving the length of intestine.
- Surgery does not cure CD.
- The course of CD after surgery is unpredictable, but recrudescence is common.

The surgical procedures depend upon the pattern and severity of disease as summarised in Table 28S-4.

Q. Short note on ileostomy.

Ileostomy

Surgically made stoma by opening the ileum to exterior through the anterior abdominal wall.

Types
- Temporary or permanent
- End ileostomy: Cut end is brought to the exterior. Or
- Loop ileostomy: A loop is brought out and an opening is made on the side (antimesenteric border)

Indications
Temporary

Loop ileostomy—performed in patients in critically ill condition due to acute intestinal conditions:
- Multiple ileal perforations
- Typhoid perforations
- Ileal gangrene, sepsis
- Fistulae.

End ileostomy: Temporary or permanent
- After total proctocolectomy for ulcerative colitis, Crohn's disease
- Total colonic Hirschsprung's diseases
- Total colectomy for carcinomas.

Site: In right ileac fossa-the loop is brought through the right rectus muscle.

End Ileostomy

Continent ileostomy, the ileal loops are anastomosed to make a "continent intra-abdominal pouch" before draining the effluent to exterior into a bag, preventing the soiling,.

Ileostomy Care
- Fluid and electrolyte management, avoiding sepsis, nutritional support
- Ileostomy bag, skin and ileostomy stoma care.

Complications
- Diarrhea, sepsis, hemorrhage
- Necrosis (gangrene), retraction, prolapse.

Table 28S-4: Surgery for Crohn's disease.

Surgical procedures for Crohn's	Indication: Pattern of the disease and extent
Ileocecal resection or right hemicolectomy, colectomy with ileoanal anasotmosis	For terminal ileal disease and strictures of small and large bowel
Subtotal colectomy and ileostomy	Acute Crohn's colitis
Temporary loop ileostomy	In acute colonic or anorectal Crohn's disease to allow remission
Proctectomy (abdominoperineal resection) with permanent colostomy	Severe anal disease failing to respond to medical treatment
Proctocolectomy with permanent ileostomy	For severe colonic and anal disease
Strictureplasty: Multiple strictureplasties can be performed along with resection and hence length of resection kept to minimum.	Strictures without inflammation Multiple strictures and long length of ileal disease.
Anal disease is treated by simple drainage of abscesses and insertion of setons through fistula. Infliximab or adalimumab therapy combined with seton insertion. The seton can be removed after the fistula has dried up (after the mAb therapy). Laying open of fistulae (fistulotomy) should be avoided.	Severe anal disease with abscess/fistula

TUBERCULOSIS OF THE INTESTINES

> Q. Etiopathology of ileocecal tuberculosis, its clinical features and management.

- Caused by *Mycobacterium tuberculosis*
- Tuberculosis can affect all parts of body and any part of alimentary tract.

The ileum, proximal colon are preferred sites although less common sites include distal colon, rectum, duodenum, jejunum, stomach and esophagus also the omentum and peritoneum.

Intestinal Tuberculosis

Ileocecal region: (a) Ulcerative–60%, (b) Hyperplastic, (c) Ulcero-hyperplastic.

Route of Infection

Usually secondary to swallowed tuberculous bacilli—from swallowed sputum in pulmonary tuberculosis (human strain) or from infected milk (bovine strain).

Pathology

- Ulcerative tuberculosis: 50–60%
- Hyperplastic tuberculosis: 10–15 %
- Combined ulcerohyperplastic: 25–30%.

Ulcerative Tuberculosis

- Affects patients who mount a low inflammatory response
- Terminal ileum is seen with multiple transverse ulcers and later multiple transverse (napkin ring) strictures in the ileum
- Serosal nodules and thickening with bowel adhesions
- Enlarged nodes with caseation and abscess.

Clinical Presentation

- Fever, diarrhea, weight loss and partial obstruction.
- Sinuses and fistula due to perforation.
- Features of pulmonary TB may be seen.

Hyperplastic Tuberculosis

- Seen in patients mounting a stronger inflammatory response; affects ileocecal region and nodes presenting as a mass.
- The infection occurs in the lymphoid follicles leading to thickened intestinal wall and narrowed lumen.
- Multiple granulomas may form along the intestine.
- Obstructive features are common; fistula and perforation are uncommon.

Clinical Presentation

- Fever (60–70%), anemia and loss of weight
- Abdominal pain—80–90%
- Mass in the right iliac fossa in about 35%
- Obstructive features: Incomplete ileal obstruction, steatorrhea.

Differential Diagnosis

- An appendix mass
- Carcinoma of the cecum
- Crohn's disease
- Actinomycosis
- Lymphoma.

Investigation

CECT or barium follow through:
- A long narrow filling defect in the terminal ileum
- Pulled up cecum, obtuse ileocecal angle (due to fibrosis),
- Multiple strictures and dilatation of ileum
- Ulcerative tuberculosis: Absence of filling of distal ileum (narrowed) and ileocecal region is seen in (due to intestinal hurry).

CT—shows proximal distension and enlarged lymph nodes calcification, collections.
Blood—ESR
NAAT (nucleic acid amplification test)
Peritoneal biopsy.

Treatment

Medical therapy: Patient without obstruction:
- Antituberculous therapy started.
- Nutritional and supportive treatment accompanies the ATT.

Indications for Surgery

- Obstructive symptoms
- Residual lesion after antituberculous therapy.
- Diagnostic dilemma (lymphoma or a carcinoma)-preferably by diagnositic laparoscopy.

Surgery

- Ileocecal resection or right hemicolectomy
  - For obstructive lesion
  - Mass RIF
- Resection of segment and anastomosis
  - Ileal strictures
  - Perforative peritonitis
- Iliotransverse colostomy is indicated in:
  1. Ileocecal mass with fixity.
  2. Patient not fit for resection.
  3. Perforated ileal lesion—as a supplement to ileal resection and anastomosis
- Stricturoplasty (incise longitudinally and suture transversely to widen lumen)
  - For ilial stricture/s—with healthy ileal wall and no active disease.
- Ileostomy after resecting an unhealthy ileum and delayed reanastomosis after treating the disease.

> **Q. Surgical complications of typhoid; management of acute enteric perforation.**

SURGICAL COMPLICATIONS OF TYPHOID

Etiology

- *Salmonella typhi* and paratyphi (paratyphoid). Gram-negative flagellated bacilli.
- Mode of transmission is faeco oral route.
- Transmission: Faeco-oral route is commonest mode of spread.

Pathology

Intestinal Peyer's patches, mesenteric lymph nodes, spleen, gallbladder, liver and bone are involved.

Clinical presentation: Fever, abdominal pain.

Abdominal complications

- Paralytic ileus—most common
- Intestinal hemorrhage—from ulcerated Peyer's patches.
- Perforation
- Cholecystitis (leads to chronic career state)
- Typhoid lesions - abscess like collections in liver and spleen.

Extra-abdominal complications

- Myocarditis
- Meningitis and encephalopathy
- Airway obstruction—due to perichondritis and laryngitis
- Osteomyelitis and arthritis

- Myositis
- Venous thrombosis
- cystitis, and epididymo-orchitis.

Typhoid (Enteric) Perforation

- Perforation usually occurs in 3rd week of the infection in ileal Peyer's patches.
- Typhoid ulcers are multiple, on the anti-mesenteric side, in the longitudinal axis.
- Multiple ulcers may perforate serially, one after other, rather than simultaneously—due to the progressing degeneration of muscle of bowel wall.

Clinical Presentation

- Severe toxicity
- Severe diarrhea
- Soft abdomen (no rigidity myopathy)
- Relative bradycardia (heart rate is lower due to myocardial depressant effect)
- Soft abdomen
- Obliterated liver dullness

Investigations

- Plain X-ray—shows free gas
- Ultrasound abdomen may not be rewarding
- Blood culture may be positive culture (90% +ve) and stool cultures are required. Marrow culture is useful
- Widal test may be positive
- WBC may be low (neutropenia).

Treatment

Aggressive antibiotics are started (high dose ceftriaxone with quinolone (ciprofloxacin or ofloxacin).

Surgery

Emergency: Procedures
- Laparotomy. Closure of perforation and peritoneal toilet and drainage.
- Resection of ileum for multiple perforations.
- Seromuscular sutures for impending perforations of Peyer's patches
- Exteriorisation of ileum—done in a critically ill patient: Loop ileostomy—for draining toxins out of ileum.

Second stage: Surgery—for restoration of continuity of the bowel after recovery of the patient: Reanastomosis of ileal loops and closure of stoma.

Supportive care
- Intensive monitoring
- ICU care, blood transfusion, fluid and electrolyte managemen
- Parenteral nutrition given and later enteral feeding started.

SURGICAL COMPLICATIONS OF ROUNDWORM (ASCARIS LUMBRICOIDES)

Clinical Presentation of Ascariasis
- Worm colic
- Toxicity—fever, tachycardia
- Recurrent incomplete intestinal obstruction
- Acute intestinal obstruction (mass of round worms may be felt in some)
- Perforation-common in the ileum, intraperitoneal abscess
- Dyspepsia, malabsorption, iron deficiency anemia
- Migration of worm into the CBD/pancreatic duct
- Ascending cholangitis (Charcot's triad; fever, jaundice and upper abdominal pain) or features of pancreatitis).

Investigations
- Ultrasonography—shows the bolus of worm/s; worm the bile duct or pancreatic duct.
- Blood—eosinophilia, anemia, hypoalbuminemia.
- LFT for features of obstruction or cholangitis.

CT/MRI will detect worm/s or dilated CBD or pancreatic duct.

Treatment
- In cases with obstruction: Piperazine citrate 60 mL is given thorugh naso gastric tube in case of obstruction. (30 mL orally at night in non obstructing case). Usually worms are passed in 48 hours and obstruction gets relieved.
- Intravenous fluids are given for support.
- Albendazole, mebendazole or pyrantel pamoate are other drugs used for non obstructive cases.

Surgery: When obstruction persists or worsens or in case of perforation.
- Laparotomy and milking worms into the cecum is done
- Enterotomy is done for removal of a large bolus of worms and is closed with non absorbable sutures.
- Perforation (mostly in ileum): Removal of any free worms in peritoneal cavity, closure of perforation and peritoneal lavage for peritonitis.
- CBD obstruction: ERCP, worm extraction and stenting.

Q. Pneumatosis Cystoides Intestinalis (PCI).

PNEUMATOSIS CYSTOIDES INTESTINALIS (PCI)

A condition with presence of gaseous cysts containing nitrogen, hydrogen and carbon dioxide in the submucosal and subserosal plane of the intestinal wall.

Etiology
- It is associated with pathological conditions or iatrogenic.
- Associated conditions—duodenal ulcer, chronic pulmonary disease, bowel obstruction.
- Scleroderma, necrotizing enteritis—in children.
- Iatrogenic causes—colonoscopy, air contrast enema, laparoscopic surgery.
- Positive pressure ventilation.

Pathogenesis: Many theories have been proposed—mechanical, bacterial and pulmonary.

Mechanical theory: High intraluminal pressure forces gas through a mucosal breach into lymphatics which spread the gas. But fails to explain the hydrogen content on the cysts.

Bacterial theory: Submucosal localization of fermenting *Clostridia* and *Escherichia Coli* causing production of gas and its retention in the submucosa.

Proved by its therapeutic response to administration of metronidazole.

The pulmonary theory: Asthmatics and COPD—rupture of the alveoli and release of air through the mediastinum into the retroperitoneal space; its subsequent movement through the perivascular spaces in the intestinal wall.

Carbon dioxide during laparoscopy can also escape through mediastinum to reach intestinal wall through subadventitial plane of the mesenteric vessels.

Pathology
- Gaseous bubbles spread through the layers by peristalsis.
- Sites: Any part of the gastro intestinal tract may be involved—jejunum most commonly, later ileocecal and colonic walls layers of mesentery.

Clinical Presentation
Any of the following:
- Abdominal pain, intestinal obstruction and rectal bleed and perforation.
- X-ray or CT scan are diagnostic.

Treatment
- Oxygen administration per nasally—70% saturation for 5–7 days.
- Hyperbaric oxygen: At 2.5 times the atmospheric pressure for 2 hours every day for 3 days.
- Intravenous metronidazole and ceftriaxone.

Treatment of the causative factors:

Surgery indicated uncommonly in—
- Perforation or peritonitis
- PCI refractory to treatment.

Resection of the involved segment is performed.

Q. Etiology and management of ileal strictures.

ILEAL STRICTURES

Causes
- Tuberculosis of ileum/jejunum
- Crohn's disease
- Radiation enteritis
- Ischemic strictures after bowel ischemia, necrotising enterocolitis
- **Garrey's stricture:** Ischemic stricture at the constricting band of a long-standing

incarcerated hernia. The hernia is reduced at surgery but ischemic damage persists.
- Drug induced: Potassium chloride tablets.
- Nonspecific causes

Investigation
- Contrast Enhanced CT scan is the modality for accurate localization.
- Systemnc investigations fro diagnosis—like tuberculosis and Crohns.

Treatment
- Treatment of the primary disease.
- Resection of bowel segment and anastomosis.
- Strictureplasty.

Q. Blind loop syndrome and principles of its management.

BLIND LOOP SYNDROME
The small intestinal peristalsis clears the contents and prevents stasis. If there is stasis resulting in delayed bacterial clearance, the bacterial colonization happens in the stagnant contents and it can cause deficiency states together referred to as a "blind loop syndrome".

The stasis promotes bacteria overgrowth preventing breaking down of fats.

Etiology
- Chronic intestinal obstruction (stricture or tuberculous adhesions), jejunal diverticulosis
- Distal gastrectomy blind loop in duodenum an jejunum
- Ileo transverse anastomosis; ileocolic and ascending colon
- Ileosigmoid fistula—entire large intestine from cecum to sigmoid is the blind loop.

Impact on Nutrition
- Stasis in upper jejunum—fat absorption, distal ileum—vit. B12 deficiency.
- Steatorrhea, glossitis, osteomalacia, paresthesia and peripheral neuropathy.

Treatment
Intermittent oral antibiotics therapy rifaximin, metronidazole, ciprofloxacin, tetracycline and cifixime are used on rotation. And improvement is seen for some time.

Surgery: Only when the anatomical abnormality can be corrected, e.g., resection of the segment with diverticulosis.
- Resection of the blind loop of the intestine.
- Resection of colonic fistula with colon.

Q. Short answer on enterocutaneous fistula.

ENTERO CUTANEOUS FISTULA

Etiology
- Post-traumatic
- Radiotherapy
- Crohn's disease
- Tuberculosis
- Postoperative—leak from anastomosis
- Damage to intestinal loop during surgery
- Repeat laparotomies.

Pathology
- Loss of water
- Electrolytes
- Protein and nutrients
- Infection—systemic
- Skin—infection and excoriation/digestion by digestive juices.

High output fistula: >500 mL of effluent per day—challenging and highly morbid.
Low output fistula: < 500 mL of output per day.

Factors Preventing Healing of an Intestinal Fistula
High output fistula:
- Specific disease like Crohn's disease, tuberculosis
- Distal obstruction
- Epithelial continuity from gut to skin.
- Presence of intervening abscess.

Management of Fistula

Evaluation and investigations:
- For causative disease, evaluation of general systemic and nutritional status.
- CECT abdomen and CT fistulography studying the anatomy of the fistula to define bowel length and plan a surgical strategy.

Low Output Fistulas

Heal on their own after correction of nutrition if there is no distal obstruction or specific disease.

SNAP: Principles

- **S:** Sepsis—is treated and eliminated; skin—protection—collection of leak fluid in bags and care of skin (e.g., with zinc paste).
- **N:** Nutrition—total parenteral nutrition or supportive.
- **A:** Anatomical assessment—CT/fistulography
- **P:** Definitive planned surgery—resection, a re do anastomosis or a bypass.

SMALL INTESTINAL TUMORS

Benign tumors (majority of small bowel tumors)

Lipomas, neurogenic tumors adenomas and hemangiomas.

Clinical Presentation

- Asymptomatic
- Intussusception
- Small bowel obstruction
- Bleeding—sudden or chronic and occult (causing anemia)
- That may cause anemia or may even be overt.

Investigation

- Difficult to diagnose by CT
- Capsule endoscopy
- Small bowel endoscopy are helpful.

Treatment

Resection and anastomosis for all symptomatic tumors.

PEUTZ–JEGHERS SYNDROME

- An autosomal dominant disease
- Multiple hamartomatous polyps in the small bowel and colon and melanosis of the mouth and lips, digits and perianal skin.
- The gene STK11 on chromosome 19 is detected in some of the affected persons.

Complications

Bowel obstruction and malignancies of bowel.

Management

- Colonic surveillance
- Female patients are advised to get screening of breast and cervix.
- Polyps are observed for malignant change.
- Polypectomy - endoscopic or surgical is done for intussusception or bleeding from polyps.
- Bowel resection—for multiple polyps.

MALIGNANT TUMORS OF SMALL BOWEL

Less common and present late or diagnosed after resection of small bowel for obstruction.

Types

- Epithelial—adenocarcinoma
- Neuroendocrinal: carcinoid tumors
- Lymphomas
- Mesenchymal tumors (gastrointestinal stromal tumors [GIST]).

Adenocarcinoma: Affects the jejunum more frequently than the ileum.

Predisposing Conditions

Crohn's disease, familial adenomatous polyposis (FAP), HNPCC syndrome (familial non polyposis colon cancer, Peutz–Jeghers syndrome and coeliac disease.

Clinical Presentation

- Anaemia or acute gastrointestinal bleeding
- Intussusceptions
- Obstruction.

Treatment

Surgical resection of lesion with 5 cm of tumor free bowel on either side with the mesentery. Right hemicolectomy: Distal ileal tumors.

Prognosis: Poor

Carcinoid Tumors (Also Refer Carcinoid of Appendix)

> **Q. Clinical features and management of carcinoid syndrome.**

- These are neuroendocrinal tumors arising from Kulchitsky cells (ECL cells) at the base of crypts of Leiberkuhn.

- Ileum is the second most common part after appendix. Other sites—rectum, pancreas, stomach.
- Extraintestinal—bronchus, mediastinum.

Pathology
- Small tumors, may be multiple with distortion and scarring of the bowel and mesentery.
- Lymphatic metastases early and metastasize through portal vein into liver.
- They produce vasoactive peptides, 5-hydroxytryptamine (serotonin—most common)
- Histamine, prostaglandins and kallikrein, which are inactivated in the liver.

Carcinoid Syndrome: Liver metastases release unmetabolised peptides into circulation and produce the systemic effects including pulmonary and tricuspid stenosis.

Often the symptoms are induced by intake of alcoholic drinks.

Clinical features of carcinoid syndrome
- Flushing -sudden attacks—involves face and chest area
- Diarrhea.and borborygmi
- Asthmatic attacks—due to bronchospasm
- Reddish—blue cyanosis
- Palpitations
- Features of pulmonary and tricuspid stenosis

Investigations
- Serum study for chromogranin - A
- Octreotide scanning—to detect otherwise asymptomatic multiple tumors and secondaries.

Treatment
- Surgery is mainstay and octreotide is for control of carcinoid syndrome.
- It is a chemoresistant and radio resistant tumor.

Surgery for primary tumor—resection.
But multiple and secondaries cause recurrence.

Treatment of Carcinoid Syndrome
- Preoperative octreotide coverage and surgery: Resection of primary tumor.

- Liver metastases: Hepatic lobectomy (metastasectomy) if limited to one lobe.
- Non resectable disease: Long-term octreotide coverage.
- Long-term prognosis: Slow growth of secondaries and survive for many years.

Q. Short note on gastrointestinal stromal tumors (GIST)

Gastrointestinal Stromal Tumors
- These are mesenchymal tumors—benign and malignant types
- Criteria for malignancy—**c-kit (CD 117)** staining and size of tumor
- Associated conditions—neurofibromatosis

Sites
- Stomach—most common site
- Other parts of the gut are also involved

Clinical Features

Age group: 50- to 70-year age group most commonly
Asymptomatic and incidentally found at abdominal imaging
Symptomatic
- Mass per abdomen and pain with nausea
- GI bleeding—hematemesis or melena
- Asthenia and lethargy

Treatment: Modalities: Surgery and/or TKI (tyrosine kinase inhibitor)
Radioresistant and chemoresistant
- **Surgery**: Resection of the part of bowel is the treatment of choice
- **Tyrosine kinase inhibitor:**
  Imatinib—is effective in advanced cases:
  – As adjuvant therapy after surgery
  – Preoperative to obtain resection in an non resectable tumor
  – Reducing incidence of recurrence.
  – As primary therapy for advanced tumors
Sunitinib—for recurrences or imatinib resistant

Lymphoma
- Small bowel lymphoma may be primary or part of a systemic NHL. They may be of B-cell type (mostly) or T-type.
- Predisposing conditions: Crohn's disease, immunodeficient states, post transplant state and HIV infection.

Clinical Features

- Anemia, anorexia and weight loss, bleeding or perforation.
- Diarrhea and pyrexia of unknown origin and local obstructive symptoms.
- Burkitt's lymphoma arises from in ileocecal region, particularly in children.

Treatment

Mainly chemotherapy.
- **Surgery**—for complications:
- Bleeding, obstruction or perforation—involves bowel resection followed by chemotherapy.

> **Q. Short note on short gut syndrome.**

SHORT GUT SYNDROME (SGS)

Refer **Table 28S-5**
After resection of long lengths of intestine, (as in midgut volvulus, necrotising enteritis, mesenteric infarction Crohn's disease or in case of radiation enteritis) digestive and absorptive function becomes defective.

Pathophysiology

The loss of length of the bowel, loss of absorptive area of the bowel and loss of valves leads to severe nutritional deficiencies, often not sustainable. To some extent ileum can compensate for jejunal loss but not the converse. Loss of terminal ileum and colon are crucial in causing SGS.

Consequences of Short Gut

- Formation of gallstones
- Excessive secretion of gastric acid
- Fatty infiltration of liver leading to fulminant hepatic failure
- Urinary stones
- Dehydraton, depletion of sodium (salt) and potassium
- Osteomalacia, tetany (hypocalcemia)
- Hypomagnesemia
- Bleeding diathesis
- Peripheral neuropathy

The consequences of bowel resection depend upon the anatomical part (jejunum or terminal ileum) and the length of the resected bowel.

The infants and young children tolerate resection better owing to intestinal compensatory hyperplasia.

Adaptation

- Enteroglucagon is secreted causing compensatory hyperplasia of mucosal ville (and length of intestine in infants), thus increasing transit time and absorptive function.
- Also colonic absorption of water and sodium improves.
- Adaptation is better in patients whose ileum and caecum are preserved.

Treatment

Difficult and prolonged.

Early Phase

- Total parenteral nutrition (TPN).
- Water and electrolyte replenishment.
- Low fat and high protein diet.
- Oral cholestyramine to bind bile salts.
- Loperamide to control diarrhea.

Table 28-S-5: Short gut syndrome.

Massive bowel resection leads to short gut syndrome (residual bowel < 200 cm)	
• Low transit time • Low absorptive surface • Malabsorption of fat • Malabsorption of calcium and magnesium • Formation of soaps and unabsorbed fatty acids • Alteration of pH	• Ileal resection causes the following: • Poor enterohepatic circulation • Poor absorption of bile salts • Bile salts enter colon • Colonic bacteria—act on bile salts • Secondary bile salts are formed • Poor Absorption of water and electrolytes • Diarrhea

- Parenteral vitamin B12 injection regularly.
- Proton pump inhibitors to reduce acid secretions.
- Octreotide—to reduce—secretions in stomach, liver and pancreas and bowel motility.

Adaptive (Late) Phase

- Enteral nutrition (this will stimulate intestinal adaptation).
- TPN supplement—as often as needed.
- Hormones and glutamine supplement.

Surgery

- Bowel lengthening—to increase the intestinal length and absorptive surface.
- Various procedures have been tried, each with limited success.
- Bowel transplantation—under experimental trial stage.

INTESTINAL OBSTRUCTION

> SU 28.14: Intestines—small and large (continued)

INTESTINAL OBSTRUCTION (REFER TABLE 280-1)

Q. Definition, and classification and pathophysiology of intestinal obstruction.

Definition: Interference with forward propulsion of intestinal contents.

Classification—dynamic, adynamic (also included vascular).

Depending on clinical presentation, the obstruction may be:
Acute—usually small intestinal
Chronic—usually large intestinal

Acute on chronic—the acute presentation of small bowel obstruction in a colonic obstruction.

Intestinal obstruction may be:
High small bowel (jejunal) obstruction
Low smal bowel (ileal) obstruction
Large bowel obstruction.

Intestinal obstruction may be:
Simple—blood supply to the segment intact.
Strangulated—vascularity to the segment is compromised causing ischemia of the bowel.

PATHOPHYSIOLOGY OF INTESTINAL OBSTRUCTION (DYNAMIC)

Refer **Table 280-2**.

Table 280-1: Etiology and classification of intestinal obstruction.

Dynamic	*Adynamic*
Mechanical obstruction—increased peristalsis against obstruction	Failure of peristalsis

• Lumen of gut
  – Bolus, foreign body
  – Worms, Gallstone
• Wall
  – Polyp, growth, stricture
  – Volvulus
  – Intussusception
• Outside the gut
  – Adhesions, band, kink
  – Tumor
  – Hernia
	• Vascular occlusion
	  – Mesenteric artery thrombosis; embolism
	  – Mesenteric vein thrombosis
	• Paralytic ileus
	  – Post operative
	  – Reflex
	      Trauma—abdominal
	      Fracture spine, plaster jacket
	      Retroperitoneal bleed
	  – Infective and toxic—bacterial
	  – Mechanical (later stage)—adhesions form
	  – Metabolic
	      Uremia, hypokalemia
	  – Drug induced:
	      Anticholinergics, an antidepressants
	      Antiperistaltic agents (tramadol)

Table 280-2: Pathophysiology of intestinal obstruction.

Summary: Pathophysiology of intestinal obstruction (dynamic)

Simple obstruction	Strangulated obstruction
• Hyperperistalsis • Distension • Fluid electrolyte loss • Absorption of toxins	• Toxemia and septicemia • Peritonitis • Gangrene of bowel and extension • Blood loss due to gangrene

Details

Simple Obstruction

- **Changes in peristalsis** - Colicky pain
  - Bowel proximal to obstruction: Initial hyperperistalsis and later failure of peristalsis (aperistalsis)
  - Obstructed segment - blocked
  - Distal segment: Normal peristalsis and emptying follwed by collapse of distal bowel after luminal emptying.
- **Distension: Adaptive to luminal contents—** abdominal distension.
  - Gas: 70% is swallowed air (mainly N_2)
    - 20% Nitrogen diffusion from blood
    - 10% bacterial degradation of food (H_2S) -hydrogen sulfide.
  - Fluid:
    - Normal secretions stagnate proximal to obstruction in the bowel lumen
    - Saliva: 1500 mL/day/4L
    - Gastric secretion: 2500 mL/day/4L
    - Bile and pancreatic: 1000 mL/4L
    - Intestinal secretion: 3000 mL/4L
  - **Total**: Upto 8 L of fluid and electrolyte loss into the lumen daily.
    - Excess of intestinal secretion ("exsorption") into the lumen and
    - Decreased absorption ("insorption")
- **Fluid and electrolyte loss**
  Net result: Hypovolemia due to
  - Defective absorption,
  - Vomiting and
  - Third space loss—sequestration of fluid in bowel lumen.
  - Early and worst in high (jejunal) obstruction
  - Late and bad in low (ileal) obstruction.
  - Slow and minimal in large bowel obstruction.
- **Absorption of intestinal luminal toxins**:
  - Bacterial toxins accumulate and get absorbed from the stagnant fluid.
  - More profound absorption of toxins occurs after release of obstruction, due to their release into distal bowel.
  - Contains endotoxin.

STRANGULATED OBSTRUCTION

- **Obstruction with interference with vascularity**.
  - **Compression of veins:** This causes **Bowel congestion**—edema of bowel—increased compression on wall and
    - Increased luminal secretion (increased exsorption)
    - Bowel distension and
    - Increased intra luminal pressure
  - **Arterial obstruction**—causes arteriolar and then arterial occlusion and
  - **Gangrene of the segment**—gangrene
- **Loss of blood into the lumen**—blood loss
- **Distension**
  - First in the gangrenous bowel.
  - Then—the bowel segments distend—both proximal and distal to the gangrenous part due to infective thrombosis spreading into the proximal part of the vessels, thus devascularizing the healthy bowel.
- **Translocation of bacteria and bacterial toxins**—across the gangrenous bowel—and absorption into blood stream from the peritoneal membrane.

PARALYTIC ILEUS (DISCUSSED AT THE END)

Etiology: Refer Table 28O-1 for Etiology

Clinical features: Painless silent abdomen, massive distension no pain, no feces, no flatus, no peristalsis (tinkling sounds heard due to movement of fluid in distended loops).

As the time passes, adhesions develop between the bowel loops and the obstruction now turns mechanical.

> **Q. Short note on closed loop obstruction.**
>
> **Closed loop obstruction: (Refer Figure 28O-1)**
> - A situation when bowel loop is closed at both ends, resulting in rapid changes in the lumen and wall and early strangulation and gangrene, if not released in time.
> - For example: An obstructive growth at hepatic flexure distally and the competent ileo cecal valve proximally resulting in a closed loop of cecum and ascending colon.
> - A volvulus (twisting) of a loop of intestine (small bowel or sigmoid).

Closed loop obstruction examples

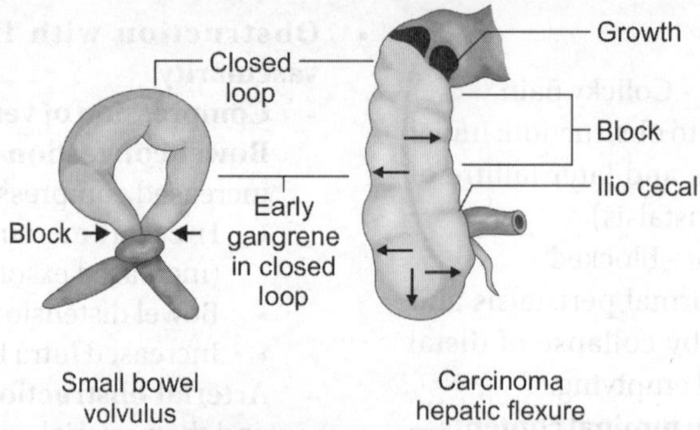

Fig. 280-1: Closed loop obstruction

Q. Describe clinical features of intestinal obstruction.

CLINICAL FEATURES OF ACUTE INTESTINAL OBSTRUCTION

Cardinal Features

Refer **Table 280-3**.

Table 280-3: Cardinal features of acute intestinal obstruction.

Symptoms: Pain vomiting distension constipation

Signs: Tenderness, rigidity, distension
- Rebound tenderness (in strangulated obstruction)
- Visible "step ladder" peristalsis
  - Features of dehydration and electrolyte imbalance
  - Toxemia/septicemia
  - Blood loss due to gangrene in strangulation

SIMPLE V/S STRANGULATED OBSTRUCTION

Refer **Table 280-4**.

CHRONOLOGY OF SYMPTOMS RELATED TO LEVEL OF OBSTRUCTION

Refer **Table 280-5**.

Order of presentation of cardinal symptoms—numbered as 1 to 4.

Q. Explain X-ray findings in acute intestinal obstruction.

Radiology in Intestinal Obstruction (Refer Figure 280-2)

Plain X-ray abdomen: AP (antero posterior) view - erect or lateral decubitus view.
- **Distended bowel loops**—helps in localising the level of obstruction.
  Note: Size of bowel loop is not the feature to localize the part, but the mucosal pattern is.
    - Jejunum: Valvulae conniventes—parallel lines run from one wall to the other
    - Ileum: Featureless (characterless)—no features.

Table 280-4: Clinical features: Simple obstruction and strangulated obstruction.

Feature	Simple obstruction	Strangulated obstruction
Pain Pain free intervals	Short spells of colicky pain Intervals common and long	Severe, long, continuous spells Short intervals or absent
Vomiting Vomitus	Follows pain (except high obstruction) Food, bilious	Accompanies pain and severe, Blood stain/dark
Toxemia	Absent or mild and late	Early and profound
Shock	Absent or /mild	Profound
Rigidity—rebound tenderness	Absent Absent	Present Present

Chapter 28: Abdominal Cavity, Hernia and Digestive Tract

Table 280-5: Chronology of symptoms as per level of bowel obstruction.

Type of obstruction		Pain	Vomiting projectile	Distension	Constipation
Acute Small bowel	High (jejunal)	1st	1st (with pain)	Absent	+ or nil
	Low (ileal)	1st	3rd	2nd	4th
Acute on chronic		4th	3rd	2nd	1st
Chronic (large bowel)		2nd/3rd	+/-	Usually 1st or 2nd	1st
Paralytic ileus		Absent	2nd or 3rd regurgitant	1st	2nd

X Ray finding for level of intestinal obstruction

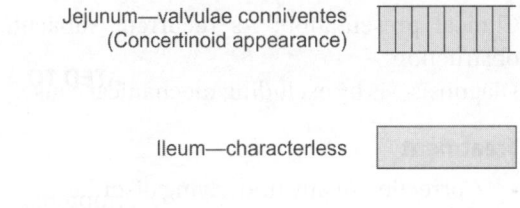

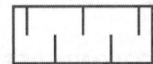

Fig. 280-2: X-ray findings to identify level of bowel obstruction

- Colon: Haustration—mucosal fold—runs across the lumen but stops short of opposite wall.
- Multiple air-fluid levels
  - Normal air fluid levels: one at duodenal cap, second at ileo cecal junction.
  - More than three levels indicates intestinal obstruction.

  The number of levels will be more in more distal obstruction.
- Ground glass opacity—shows free fluid (fluid/purulent liquid/blood/ascites).
- Free gas in peritoneal cavity—perforation
- Any radiopaque finding—gall stone or a swallowed foreign body.

CECT (contrast enhanced CT scan)—very accurate—in localizing, identifying strangulation and identifying any etiological factor.
- Blood: Hemoglobin
- Electrolyte levels (sodium, potassium, bicarbonate, chloride)
- Blood gas analysis—to identify acidosis.
- Urea and creatinine.

Q. Describe principles of treatment of intestinal obstruction.

Treatment of Acute Intestinal Obstruction

- Gastro intestinal aspiration—to decompress the bowel of gas and toxic luminal fluid.
- Replacement of fluid and electrolytes and blood.
- Anti bacterials—cephalosporins and metronidazole; carbopenems (meropenem or piperacillin) are preferred if strangulated obstruction.
- Surgery:
  - To relieve obstruction
  - To prevent strangulation
  - To remove strangulated bowel loop
  - Peritoneal toilet and drainage.

The non-operative measures are started together with diagnostic evaluation and active monitoring. Hourly measurement of abdominal girth is important.

Early Surgery if

- Strangulation is suspected or anticipated
- High (jejunal) obstruction, (heavy electrolyte loss can be fatal)
- No response to 4 to 6 hours of conservative measures
- Acute on chronic obstruction
- Obstruction due to a hernia incarceration.

Principles of Surgery

- Relieve the obstruction.
- Decompress the bowel proximal to obstruction and prevent absorption of toxic fluid.
- Deal with cause of obstruction.

Goal of Surgery in Intestinal Obstruction

- Relieve obstruction
- Restore bowel continuity
- Suck out toxic stagnant fluid
- Peritoneal drainage.

Q. Discuss paralytic ileus.

PARALYTIC ILEUS

Neuro muscular conduction fails in myenteric and submucous plexuses of nerves.

Etiology

- Post operative—reflex.
- Post-traumatic—reflex—spinal fracture, plaster jacket, retro peritoneal bleed.
- Infective—reflex and toxic factors.
- Metabolic—uremia and hypokalemia.
- Drugs—anti cholenergics.

Clinical Features

- Distension
- Silent (aperistaltic)
- No pain—but may be felt due to distension
- Regurgitant vomiting
- Absolute constipation (obstipation) no feces, no flatus, no peristalsis.

Mechanical obstruction follows prolonged paralytic ileus due to formation of adhesions.

Investigation

- CT abdomen: To check for possible contributing intra abdominal cause.
- Treatment: "Don't flog a tired horse"
- Nasogastric aspiration
- Intravenous fluid and electrolyte replacement
- Correct metaboiic and/infectious causes.

Surgery

- Only in late cases when mechnical obstruction has set in
- Prolonged paralytic ileus (indicating sepsis)
- To relieve: To decompress the bowel respiratory distress due to distension.

Q. What is intestinal pseudo-obstruction?

PSEUDO-OBSTRUCTION

Associated with a variety of syndromes with neuropathy and/or myopathy.

Small Intestinal Pseudo-obstruction

- **Primary (idiopathic)** or associated with familial visceral myopathy or
- **Secondary** to metabolic and iatrogenic factors (medications).

Clinical presentation: As recurrent subacute obstruction.

Diagnosis—is by excluding mechanical cause.

Treatment

- Correction of any underlying disorder.
- Metoclopramide and erythromycin are used.

COLONIC PSEUDO-OBSTRUCTION

This may occur in an **acute or a chronic form**.

The functional obstruction is seen in elderly—as acute large bowel obstruction with massive distension of cecum **(Ogilvie syndrome).**

Complication: Cecal perforation.

Diagnosis: Urgent confirmation by colonoscopy or a CT to exclude mechanical cause.

Treatment

- Treatment of any known co morbid cause.
- Intravenous neostigmine—1 mg, repeated after a few minutes.
- Colonoscopic decompression.
- Cecal perforation is more likely when cecal diameter is over 14 cm.
- **Surgery**—carries a high morbidity.
  - **A colostomy** is performed to relieve distension.
  - Cecostomy: It was in practice previously for preventing a cecal perforation.

VOLVULUS OF INTESTINES
(REFER TABLE 280-6)

Acute twisting of a segment of bowel around its axis (mesentery) is called volvulus. The lumen of the bowel gets occluded if the torsion exceeds

Table 280-6: Classification of volvulus of intestines.

Etiological classification

Primary volvulus	Secondary volvulus
• Congenital malrotation of the gut volvulus neonatorum • Congenital bands or abnormal mesenteric attachments, e.g., cecal volvulus and sigmoid volvulus	• More common • Due to rotation of a bowel loop around an acquired band or adhesion or stoma

180 degree and vascularity gets compromised when the rotation is full (360°).

This causes closed loop obstruction, with its rapid changes to strangulation. The bacterial gases and venous congestion add to the luminal distention and worsening of distention. Thrombosis of vessels follows causing bowel ischemia and gangrene.

Volvulus Neonatorum

A life threatening neonatal emergency secondary to intestinal malrotation.

Q. Write a note on volvulus of sigmoid colon.

Sigmoid Volvulus

More common in Africans and Asia.

Predisposing Causes

- Idiopathic megacolon in African individuals.
- Associated with dilated sigmoid due to chronic constipation in old age or due to high fiber diet.
- Drug induced constipation due to long-standing use of psychotropic drugs.
- Anatomical factors as in the figure given below:

Anatomical factors (Refer **Figure 280-3**)
- Narrow attachment sigmoid mesocolon
- A fibrous band or adhesion
- Overloaded (fecal) colon
- Long axis of sigmoid mesocolon
- Younger patients present earlier and the prognosis worsens with delay in diagnosis.
- Rotation occurs in the anticlockwise direction.

Classification

- Simple volvulus
- Gangrenous volvulus.

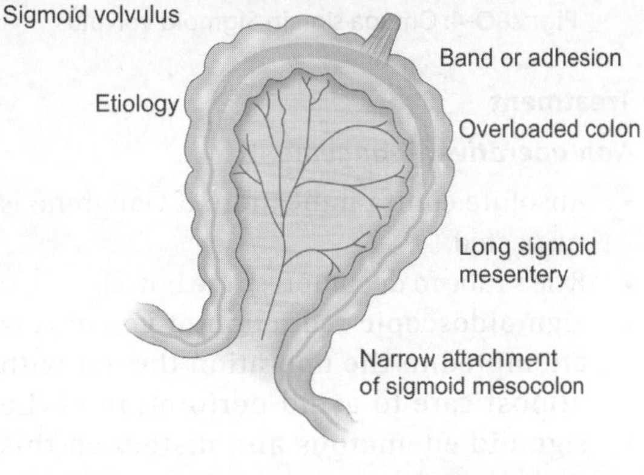

Fig. 280-3: Predisposing factors of Sigmoid volvulus.

Also classified clinically as:
- **Fulminant (acute):** Sudden onset, severe pain, early vomiting, rapid regression to gangrene and clinical deterioration.
- **Indolent (progressive):** Insidious onset, slow progressive course, less pain, late vomiting.

Acute Presentation

- Generally elderly patient or those with chronic constipation.
- Sudden and severe abdominal pain with progressive distension of abdomen.
- Hiccough and retching.
- Vomiting due to reflex and projectile type, with gastric contents.
- Absolute constipation.

Diff. Diagnosis

- Colonic pseudo-obstruction
- Acute gastric dilatation.

X-ray: Shows "bent tube appearance" the "omega sign" due to the massively dilated sigmoid colon. Refer **Figure 280-4**.

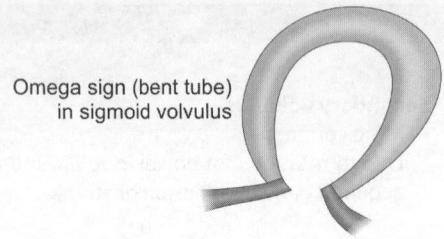

Fig. 280-4: Omega sign in Sigmoid volvulus

Treatment

Non-operative Management

- Absolute contra indication: if Gangrene is suspected.
- Ryle's tube to decompress the bowel.
- Sigmoidoscopic reduction of volvulus is attempted in the operation theater with utmost care to avoid perforation of the sigmoid edematous and distended this walled.

Surgery

- Aim: Derotate the volvulus and prevent recurrence.
- Emergency laparotomy: Lower midline incision.

Surgical Procedure

- **Volvulus without strangulation**:
  - **Sigmoid colectomy: Derotate and resect the sigmoid—removes the cause** like the narrow attachment of mesocolon and long mesocolon.
  - Sigmoidopexy is not recommended (it has a very high recurrence—it fixes an abnormal sigmoid).
- **Gangrenous sigmoid: Resect the volvulus without derotation** (toxic contents not allowed to get absorbed into circulation).

Options for restoration of continuity of sigmoid after resection:

- Primary anastomosis—of colonic ends during the operation (one stage)
- Two-stage approach—indication—in gangrene and those with comorbidities
  - 1st st—double barrel colostomy. Proximal and distal loops are brought out as a in the left iliac fossa; 2nd stage: Anastomosis 8 weeks after the first
  - (Hartmann's operation: Proximal loop—as a left iliac end colostomy and distal lop closed) in patient with poor general condition—The bowel continuity can be restored after 8 weeks when the patient is fit (2nd stage).

ILEOSIGMOID KNOTTING (COMPOUND VOLVULUS)

During a sigmoid volvulus, an ileal loop encircles the sigmoid and volvulus of sigmoid tightens the ileal loop further around the base of the volvulus strangulating both the sigmoid and the encircling the loop of ileum. The condition rapidly progresses to cause gangrene of sigmoid or /and ileum endangering the life.

Clinical Presentation

- Acute intestinal obstruction (small bowel obstruction type) with milder distension of abdomen (due to vomiting).
- Early toxicity causing the patient sick.
- Plain X-ray—shows distended ileal loops amidst distended sigmoid colon.
- CT scan helps to confirm.
- The condition has high morbidity and an early surgery to relieve the strangulation is rewarding.

Surgery

Early laparotomy can save a resection of the ileal loop by undoing the knot and resection of sigmoid colon. But in most cases it is not possible to undo the knot and hence a combined resection of the ileo sigmoid knot is performed. This involves decompression of bowel with resection of ileal loop and sigmoid followed by colocolic and ileo-ileal anastomosis.

CECAL VOLVULUS

- About 25–30% of all cases of adult volvulus.
- A congenital mobile cecum (failure of fixation) is more prone for volvulus.
- Often associated with malrotation of gut.
- Common in late pregnancy due to pushing up of a mobile cecum.

Clinical Presentations: Acute pain a distended cecum, a potentially closed loop obstruction and prone for gangrene. Examination may show a palpable resonant swelling in the midline or left upper quadrant of the abdomen.

CT and X-ray are helpful to Diagnosis

A massive dilatation of cecum(more than 14 cm) is an urgent indication for surgical remedy.

Aims of Surgery: Derotate and prevent recurrence:

- Right hemicolectomy - is the choice.
- Cecopexy after derotation and appendicectomy is less popular (recurrence rate of about 20%). Here cecum and ascending colon are fixed to the paracolic peritoneum.
- Cecostomy - in patients with poor general condition, a decompression will serve. Any recurrence is dealt with later with a resection.

Any gangrenous changes requires a right hemicolectomy.

Obstruction by Adhesions and Bands

Adhesions or band may be:

- Congenital bands—obliterated persistent vitello intestinal duct.
- Omental band—due to omental adhesion to an inflamed organ.
- Post-operative adhesions and/or band (almost always involve the small bowel, spare colon).
- Post peritonitis—septic
- Freeing bodies like talk, polypropylene mesh.
- Chronic inflammatory diseases—tuberculosis, Crohn's.
- Post radiation.
- The post-operative and post infective adhesions are most common cause of adhesion related obstructions.
- The severity presentation decides the treatment approach.

Prevention

- Laparoscopy—has a lower propensity to form adhesions formed than laparotomy.
- Minimal handling of bowel, avoiding tissue ischemia and ensuring serosal cover are advised.

> **Q. Define and classify intussusception. Describe the etiology, pathology, clinical features and management of acute intussusception.**

INTUSSUSCEPTION

A condition when one part of the intestine invaginates into immediately adjacent part.

Classification: Based on—chronology, direction and vascularity

- Chronology: Acute or chronic
- Direction
  - Antegrade; proximal to distal loop.
  - Retrograde: Distal to proximal (jejunogastric type after a gastro jeunostomy).
- Vascularity
  - Simple or strangulated.

ACUTE INTUSSUSCEPTION

Anatomical types: Refer **Figure 28O-5.**

- Jejuno ileal, ileo ileal, ileo colic, colo- colic, ilio ilio colic or 'retrograde'
- Common in children (mostly in infants between 5 months and 1 year).

Etiology

- Idiopathic—80–90% of all - infants with intussusception.
- Generally considered as due to hyperplasia of Peyer's patches in the terminal ileum, as the triggereing event most cases are preceded by gastroenteritis or upper respiratory tract infection.
- Weaning, loss of passively acquired maternal immunity may contribute to susceptibility to viral infections.
- Older children (>2 years).
- Meckel's diverticulum, intestinal duplication.
- Polyp, invagination of appendix.
- Henoch–Schönlein purpura.

Adult cases: Have clear lead point:

- Sub-mucous lipoma. A polyp, any tumor—like a carcinoma or gastrointestinal stromal tumor (GIST).
- Colo-colic type is more common—in adults and elderly—usually a polyp or growth.

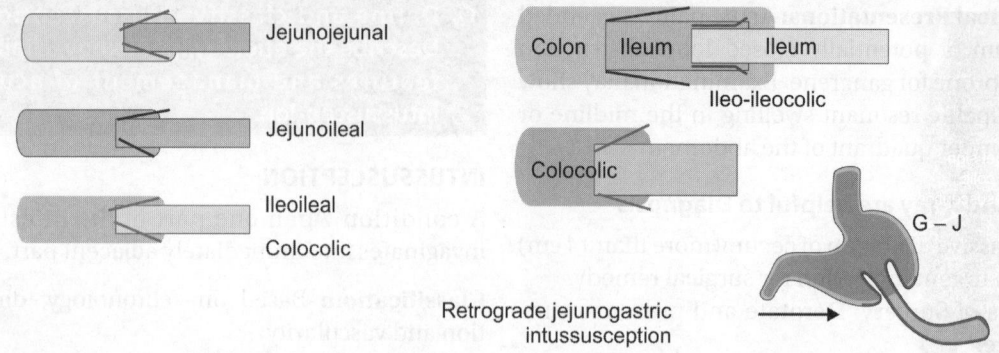

Fig. 280-5: Types of intussusception

Parts of Intussusception (Refer Figure 280-6)

The mass is the intussusception.
An intussusception has three parts:
1. The intussuscipiens—the sheath or outer tube.
2. The intussusceptum—the entering or inner tube and the returning or middle tube.
3. The Apex: The part that advances is the apex.
   - The neck is the junction of the entering layer with the mass.

The degree of ischemia is proportionate to the tightness of the invagination (e.g., maximum at the ileocecal valve) with the risk of gangrene in the intussusceptum.

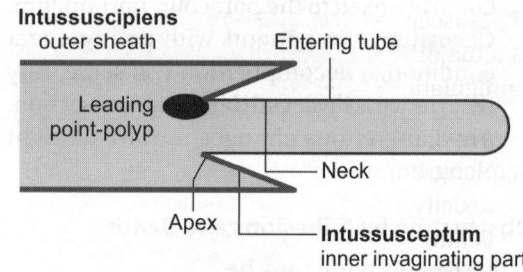

Fig. 280-6: Parts of intussusception

Clinical Features
Infants
- Spells of crying (colicky pain) and blanching with pain free sleep in between.
- Children cry incessantly and have pain free intervals.
- The child passes " currant jelly stools" due to strangling effect.
- Examination reveals a sausage shaped around the umbilicus that changes position as time progresses. Finally an intussusception may protrude per anally.
- Differential diagnosis is a prolapsed of the rectum in children—a finger probe can be passed around the protruding intussusception.

Gangrenous intussusceptions: Suspected if there is toxicity, blood in stool and tenderness.

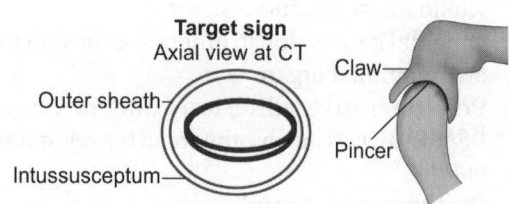

Fig. 280-7: Radiological signs of intussusception

Diagnosis (Refer Figure 280-7)
- Ultrasonography
- CT (with water soluble luminal contrast)
- The "target sign" in axial and a "claw" in coronal section **(refer Fig. 280-8)**.
- Barium enema (previously)—shows a "claw sign". With a "pincer" shadow of the intussusception.

Treatment of Intussusceptions
Conservative
- Treatment of respiratory infection in children.
- Hydrostatic reduction: Only for non strangulated

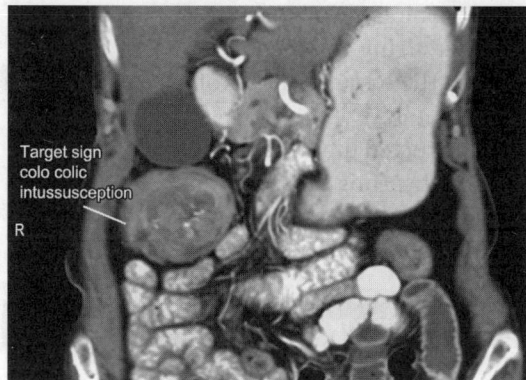

Fig. 280-8: Target sign of intussusception

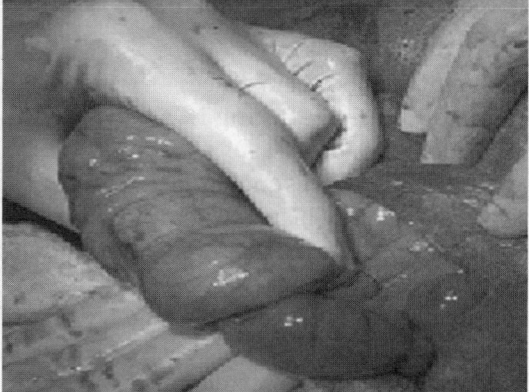

Fig. 280-9: Acute ileo-ileo colic intussusception.
(For color version see Plate 4)

Image guided—hydrostatic reduction of intussusception with the help of enema succeeds in a majority of cases intussusception without strangulation.

Surgery: Indicated in:
- Gangrenous intussusceptions suspected—toxicity, blood in stool.
- Failure of hydro static reductions.
- CT shows specific pathology like diverticulum, polyp or a tumor **(Figs. 280-8 and 28 O -10)**.

Laparotomy
- **Reduction** of intussusception (usually ileo-colic), appendectomy.
- **Resection** of the mass and anastomosis done if
  - There is any specific pathology found
  - Irreducibility
  - Gangrenous intussusception.

Adults
- Always a definite pathology is found. Meckel's diverticulum in young adults, and polyp, lipoma or neoplastic pathology as the patients' age advances.
- A majority are colo-colic type but others are also seen depending on the type and site of the pathology.

Colo-colic—intussusception: Generally it presents with recurrent attacks with is intermittent and milder pain.

Obstruction is rarely complete and hence vomiting is rarely seen.

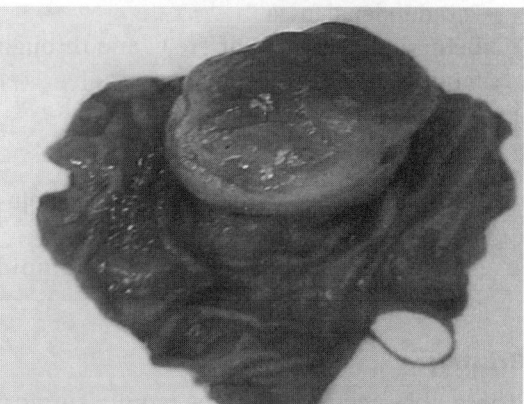

Fig. 280-10: Submucous lipoma in intussusception.
(For color version see Plate 4)

Rectal bleed is due to a carcinoma or a polyp (not to intussusception).

A mass in right lumber region with an emptiness in right iliac fossa, mass contracts under the palpating fingers and also one which changes position with time, are pathognomonic signs.

Diagnosis: Ultrasonography and CT scan are diagnostis.

Treatment: Surgery
- Laparoscopy or laparotomy, reduction of ileal segment (if possible) and resection anastomosis
- Colo-colic type—usually a growth is responsible and a formal colonic resection is done, e.g., right or left hemicolecomy or sigmoid colectomy.

INTESTINAL OBSTRUCTION DUE TO INTERNAL HERNIAS

Entrapment of bowel in spaces or orifices within the abdomen resulting in occlusion and strangulation of bowel.
- Congenital spaces and normal passages
- Diaphragmatic hiatus—sliding hernia
- Paraesophageal hernia herniation through diaphragmatic hernia
- Foramen of Bochdalek, Morgagni, dome of the diaphragm
- Mesenteric and mesocolic defects
- Defect in broad ligament.

Around the duodenum:
- Paraduodenal fossa
- Behind the ligament of Treitz and through foramen of Winslow (into lesser sac).

Iatrogenic
- Postoperative adhesions causing gaps
- Through mesocolic rent after a gastrojejunostomy
- Thorough paracolic space of a sigmoid colostomy or transverse colostomy.

Treatment

These obstructive conditions require surgical release after a CT diagnosis to avoid or to deal with a gangrene. The definitive diagnosis is made mostly on operative table.

As there are vessels running along borders of anatomical spaces hepato duodenal ligament in case of Winslow's foramen or mesocolic rent, blind division of the strangulating structure should not be done. Bowel is decompressed and resected if necessary.

NEONATAL INTESTINAL OBSTRUCTION

Q. Enumerate causes of neonatal intestinal obstruction

Common Causes
- Congenital atresia and stenosis
  - Duodenal atresia, jejunal and ileal atresia
- Malrotation of midgut
  - Midgut volvulus
- Meconium ileus
- Necrotizing enterocolitis
- Obstructed congenital groin hernia (inguinal or femoral)
- Obstructed umbilical hernia
- Hirschsprung's disease
- Anorectal atresia and imperforate anus
- Intestinal atresia and stenosis.

Q. Write short notes on duodenal atresia.

DUODENAL ATRESIA

Commonest Jejunum and ileum are next.

Duodenal atresia is due to failure of fusion of foregut with midgut and failure of developmental recanalization of the gut.

Associated with—anorectal malformations, congenital heart diseases, trisomy syndromes.

Three Types of Duodenal Atresia (Refer Figure 280-11)

Complete separation, fibrous cord, stenosis and/or a wind sock (membranous web).

Windsock type—membranous partition which is pliable and opens proximally but not distally like a windsock.

Clinical Features
- Neonatal—vomiting— vomitus is bilious when stenosis is distal to duodenal papilla (80%) and non bilious when it is proximal to the papilla (20%).
- Dehydration and electrolyte loss.
- Plain X-ray of abdomen shows a double-bubble sign.

It is a surgical emergency.
- Preoperative preparation—evaluation for associated anomalies.
- Correction of fluid and electrolytes.
- Gastric decompression.

Surgery: Duodenoduodenostomy is performed and associated anomaly like malrotation is corrected.

Jejunal and ileal atresias—vary from simple stenosis through fibrous bands to multiple

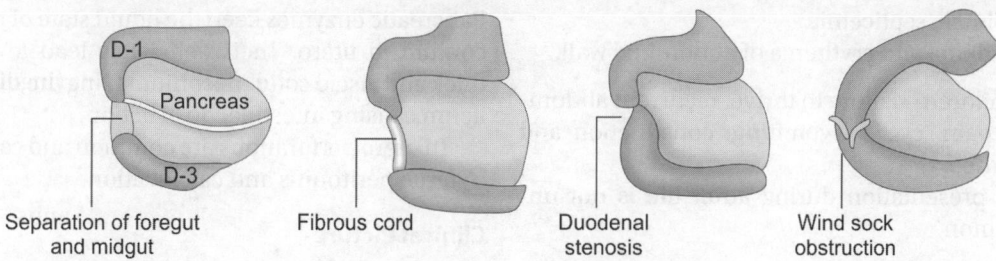

Fig. 280-11: Types of duodenal atresia

segmental atresias with mesenteric separation. Treatment involves restoration of continuity.

> **Q. Describe pathogenesis of midgut malrotation and treatment.**

MIDGUT MALROTATION

Embryological Basis

The midgut gives rise to the GI tract distal to second part of duodenum, upto the distal third of transverse colon. The endodermal tube lengthens and undergoes 270 degree clockwise rotation along with foregut, thus bringing duodenum to right side.

Any abnormality in the rotation and fixation of the midgut in the fetus leads to malrotation.

Rotation: During Intrauterine Life

- **Stage 1:** In 4th-8th week: Protrusion of midgut: Midgut with its main artery superior mesenteric artery (SMA), grows rapidly and protrudes through the umbilicus into the cord.(physiological hernia).
- **Stage 2:** In 10th-12th week, return of midgut into the coelomic cavity happens:
  - The small bowel returns to the left side of the abdomen followed by:
  - Ceco-colic loop (also to the left side)
  - Rotation of midgut—270° clockwise.
  - The ceco-colic segment rotates to occupy right iliac fossa.
  - Duodenojejunal segment—rotates 270 degree and moves behind and to the left of the superior mesenteric artery.
- **Stage 3:** Fixation of bowel and fusion of parts of mesentery.

Anomalies of Rotation of Midgut (According to the Stage of Rotation)

First Stage Anomalies

- Exomphalos major/minor or
- Gastroschisis.

Second Stage Anomalies

Errors of rotation in this stage
- Nonrotation: Entire small bowel is on right side and the colon on the left side with the cecum in mid line as suspension.
- Incomplete rotation—the most common type of malrotation.

  Caecum is located in subhepatic
  - A wide peritoneal band (Ladd's band) bridges the ceco-colic loop to posterior abdominal wall compressing the 2nd part of the duodenum. The entire midgut is seen hanging without fixation with a narrow based mesentery along with superior mesenteric artery. This causes midgut volvulus(neonatorum).

  Reverse rotation: Final 180° rotation occurs clockwise and colon lies posterior to duodenum.
- Third stage anomalies of fixation
  - Subhepatic cecum
  - Mobile cecum and ascending colon leading into cecal volvulus.

ASSOCIATED ANOMALIES 20-25%

- Congenital diaphragmatic hernia of Bochdalek
- Duodenal atresia; esophageal atresia.

Midgut Volvulus (30%) (Clockwise Rotation)

- Features of strangulation, perforation, peritonitis.

- Shock, septicemia
- Edema and erythema of abdominal wall.

In children—failure to thrive, recurrent abdominal pain, cyclical vomiting, constipation and diarrhea.

Late presentation during adult life is not uncommon.

Investigations

- Plain X-ray abdomen shows multiple air fluid levels, often showing the colonic shadows mainly on left side. Barium meal (dilute/microbarium) and follow through X-ray is preferred.
- CT abdomen—only if needed (to avoid radiation)
- Blood parameters including hemoglobin and electrolytes.

Treatment

- Resuscitation—nasogastric aspiration
- Fluid and electrolyte replacement, blood transfu;sion as needed
- Antibiotic cover
- Surgery: Ladd's operation
    - A transverse laparotomy above umbilicus (transpyloric plane)
    - Derotation of the volvulus
    - Division of the Ladd's band
    - Widening of duodenocolic isthmus (widen the root of the mesentery)
    - Pushing the small bowel to right and entire colon to the left (convert into a non rotation)
    - Appendicectomy (to avoid confusion in case of appendix lying on left side).

If the bowel is gangrenous—massive bowel resection is needed; (has a poor prognosis). Resection and enterostomies are done with both ends of bowel be reanastomosed later.

Q. Meconium ileus.

MECONIUM ILEUS

Also Refer Meconium peritonitis (under chapter Peritonits).

Etiology: Cystic fibrosis, autosomal recessive genetic disorder.

Pancreatic enzymes keep the liquid state of meconium in utero. Their deficiency lead to the thick and viscid solid meconium filing the distal ileum causing intestinal obstruction.

In utero perforations are common and cause a sterile peritonitis and calcification.

Clinical Picture

- A non thriving baby with high salty content of sweat and abdominal distension is typical.
- Progressive obstructive features precipitate acute obstruction.
- Dilated bowel loops are visible and palpable in the newborn.

Investigations

- X- ray of abdomen—shows:
    - A dilated small bowel loops.
    - Fluid levels are not seen. Peritoneal calcification may be seen.
- Contrast enema—with gastrografin—shows a micro colon (collapsed and narrow)
- Sweat test—high sodium and chloride levels (>70 mmol/L).
- Gene mutation analysis.

Treatment

Non-surgical Treatment

For uncomplicated meconium ileus:
- Hyperosmolar gastrografin enema; (draws fluid into intestinal lumen and liquefies the viscid meconeum by its saponifying property.
- Extra intravenous fluids to compensate for the diffusion into bowel lumen.

Surgical Treatment

For Complications of meconeum ileus:
- Intestinal perforation, volvulus or atresia
- Failure of therapy with hyperosmolar enemas.

Surgical Procedures

- Intestinal resection and temporary stoma formation
- Resection and primary anastomosis
- Bishop Koop operation (less often done now)—resection of blocked ileal segment, anastomosis of proximal ileal end to side of distal ileum with a stoma of distal loop like a "chimney".

CHRONIC LARGE BOWEL OBSTRUCTION

Refer chapter on large intestinal diseases.

Causes

Organic

- Intraluminal—fecal impaction
- Intramural—growth, diverticulosis, strictures—ischemia and Crohn's post radiation.
- Anastomotic stenosis and stenosis of colostomy stomal stenosis
- Extra mural—metastatic deposits from stomach or ovary, endometriosis, hernia.

Functional: Idiopathic megacolon, Hirschsprung's disease, pseudo-obstruction.

MESENTERIC VASCULAR INSUFFICIENCY (WITH/WITHOUT OCCLUSION)

Q. Causes of mesenteric vascular ischemia.

Classification

Acute intestinal ischaemia
- **Arterial**—with or without occlusion
- **Venous**
- **Chronic arterial**—central or peripheral
- Common sites:
  - The superior mesenteric vessels
  - Embolization—most common cause and lodge at origin of middle colic artery
  - Thrombosis—at root of superior mesenteric artery (SMA)
  - Inferior mesenteric artery—collaterals mask clinical picture
- **Embolism (50%)**
  - Thromboembolism:
    Thrombus from left atrial appendage in atrial fibrillation.
    Post-myocardial infarction: Thrombus from a mural infarct.
    Thrombus from an atheroma of aorta or aortic aneurysm.
    Vegetations from heart valves in endocarditis.
  - Thrombosis:
    Atherosclerosis
    Hypercoagulative state
    Vasculitides—thromboangiitis obliterans (TAO), polyarteritis nodosa

Superior mesenteric vein obstruction
- Primary thrombosis—portal hypertension, portal pyemia, sickle cell disease and oral contraceptive pill (women).

Non-occlusive mesenteric ischemia (NOMI)
- Due to variation in splanchnic circulation; Associated with critical illness.
- Hypotension, hypoperfusion or/and vasospasm due to *shock*.

Pathogenesis of Acute Mesenteric Ischemia

Any mesenteric occlusion, arterial or venous, leads to rapid hemorrhagic infarction of bowel.
- Mucosal ischemic injury
- Edema of the bowel wall and mesentery (more with venous occlusion)
- Hemorrhagic exudation into bowel lumen and peritoneal cavity.

Changes vary from mucosal necrosis and sloughing, to full infarction, occur in a few hours.

Area of infarction depends upon the site of occlusion—main trunk—bowel necrosis from duodenojejunal (DJ) flexure to left colic flexure.

Clinical Features

- Sudden onset of severe abdominal pain—in a patient with atrial fibrillation or atherosclerosis.
- The central abdominal pain, disproportionate to the physical signs.
- Early: Persistent vomiting and defecation.
- Later: Passage of frank altered blood.
- Abdominal rigidity is a late feature.
- Shock—combined—hypovolemic and septic.
- Digital examination of rectum—blood in stool or frank blood.

Investigation

WBC—polymorphonuclear leukocytosis.

CT Abdomen

Intestinal wall thickened and gas absent from lumen of the bowel.

Gas (some cases)—in wall of intestine or mesenteric and portal veins.

Treatment

Depends on the state of the individual patient.
- Resuscitation
- Laparotomy with embolectomy via the ileocolic artery or revascularization of the SMA by vascular bypass.
- Anticoagulation—early in the postoperative period.
- Ischemic bowel should be resected
- Mortality is very high.

Q. Short notes on mesenteric angina.

CHRONIC MESENTERIC ISCHEMIA (MESENTERIC ANGINA)

- Atherosclerosis and affects the proximal superior mesenteric and coeliac vessels.
- Mesenteric angina.
- Post prandial central abdominal pain (within 30-60 minutes of eating).

Clinical Features

- Weight loss and diarrhea
- Differential diagnosis—mistaken for those of peptic ulcer disease or irritable bowel syndrome.

Diagnosis: Doppler study of abdominal vessels and CT angiography.

Treatment

- Selective visceral angiography and stenting/angioplasty.
- Surgery: Bypass graft—aorto-celiac or mesenteric bypass.
- Prohibition of smoking.
- Anticoagulation.

28.5: THE VERMIFORM APPENDIX

> **SU28.15:** Describe the clinical features, investigations and principles of management of diseases of appendix including appendicitis and its complications.

DISEASES OF THE VERMIFORM APPENDIX

It is a tubular blind organ, 4–10 cm long and 3 to 6 mm thick (lumen 2–3 mm) projecting from the cecum at the junction of the three taenia coli, about 2 cm below th ileo-cecal valve. It is shot and wide based at birth and it grows longer during first and second year. The differential growth of the cecum rotates it to the retrocecal position (70-75%) within the peritoneum question.

Anatomical Positions of the Appendix (Refer Figure 28A-1)

It may lie in different positions due to anomalous cecal rotation: Retro cecal 70-75%, pelvic 20%, subcecal 2%, paracecal 2%, preileal 1-2 % and post ileal 3-5%.

In an undescended cecum the appendix lies in the right iliac fossa while it may be on left upper quadrant in malrotation of midgut. Also appendix lies in left iliac fossa in situs inversus.

The appendix is made of mucosa, thick submucosa with a very rich lymphoid tissue and two layers of muscle, the inner circular and outer longitudinal, (the tenia coli fuse and continue as longitudinal muscle).

Mesoappendix

- It is the mesentery of the appendix arising off the lower mesentery—contains blood, fat and lymphatic channels that join the ileocecal lymph nodes.
- The appendicular artery is a branch of the lower division of the ileocolic artery.
- From the base of the appendix along the free border of the mesoappendix.
- An accessory appendicular artery may arise from posterior cecal branch.

Microscopy

- Mucosa—columnar epithelium of colonic type but the crypts are ileal type.
- The base of the crypts have argentaffin cells (Kulchitsky cells)
- The submucosa contains numerous lymphatic aggregations or follicles.

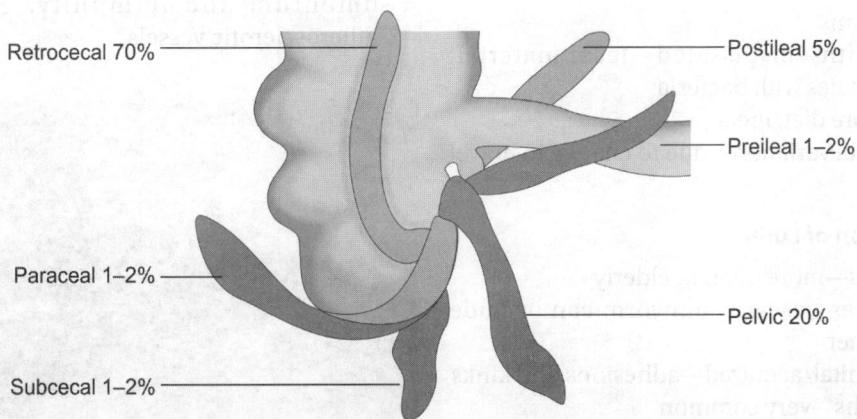

Fig. 28A-1: Anatomical positions of the appendix

Summary of applied anatomy of appendix
- Develops from midgut, blind muscular tube
- Variable position
  - Retrocecal 70–75%
  - Pelvic 21%
  - Paracecal 2%
  - Pre-ileal 1%
  - Post-ileal 5%
  - Subcecal
- Base of appendix is constant
- Artery—branch of ileocolic
- Vein—into ileocolic—superior mesenteric
- Lymph nodes—ileo colic, superior mesenteric
- Microscopy—rich in sub mucous lymphatic tissue (abdominal tonsil), muscular layer, serosa
- Mesentery of appendix is the mesoappendix
- Distal 1/3 of appendix is usually bare
- Appendicular artery runs in its free edge and terminates on the bare area of appendix
- Thrombosis can result in gangrene.

> **Q. Discuss etiology, pathology, clinical diagnosis, and management of acute appendicitis.**

ACUTE APPENDICITIS
- Rare in infants, common in children
- Most common in 2nd/3rd decade, no age exempt, less common in elderly.

Etiology
- The exact cause is unknown
- Infective—both anaerobic and aerobic organisms
- Faecolith—inspissated—fecal material, phosphates with bacteria
- Low fibre diet, meat
- Seasonal variation—due to change in bowel flora.

Obstruction of Lumen
- Tumors—more often in elderly
- Parasites—ascaris, pinworm can occlude the lumen
- Congenital/acquired—adhesions and kinks
- Fecoliths—very common
- Foreign bodies in ingested food.

Bacteriology: *Esch. coli*, Enterococci *Cl. welchii*, bacteroides, anaerobic streptococci.

Pathology
Course
- Localization of infection—by omentum or
- Spread of infection across the peritoneum—by perforation or
- Bacterial translocation across the inflamed wall of appendix.

Two Types of Appendicitis
Non-obstructive (or catarrhal) 65% and obstructive 35%.

Commences in the mucosa and the submucous lymphatic follicles.

Inflammation may lead to:
- Resolution
- Ulceration—fibrosis
- Suppuration.

Reattack: Gangrene
Refer Fig. 28A-2: Gangrenous tip of appendix.

Obstructive Appendicitis
- In the lumen—foreign body, worm, fecolith
- Wall—inflammatory stricture, carcinoma, carcinoid, tuberculosis
- Outside the wall—adhesions, hernia strangulation (Littre's hernia).

Pathogenesis (Refer Table 28A-1)

Risk Factors for Perforation of the Appendix
- Extremes of age; infants—ill developed omentum and immunity, elderly—atherosclerotic vessels

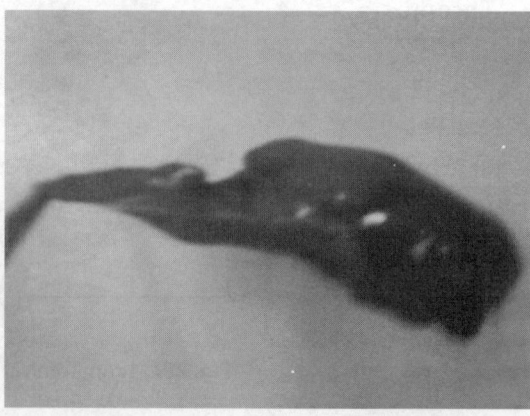

Fig. 28A-2: Gangrenous appendix

Table 28A-1: Pathogenesis of acute appendicitis.

Non obstructive appendicitis
Inflammation may resolve or cause submucosal fibrosis; OR →
It may lead to → infection → thrombosis of artery → gangrene of tip →

Obstructive appendicitis:

Occlusion of lumen ↓	Complete gangrene ↓	
Mucocele →	Perforation	
	Pseudomyxoma peritonei	Peritonitis

- Immunosuppression
- Diabetes mellitus
- Fecolith obstruction
- Pelvic appendix
- Previous surgery.

Complications of appendicitis
- Suppuration and gangrene
- Perforation
- Peritonitis—generalized or localized pus collection
- Appendix abscess
- **Appendix mass:** A complex mass of appendix, cecum omentum, ileal loop (all adherent to iliac fossa)
- Mucocele of appendix
- Pseudomyxoma peritonei
- **Intra-abdominal abscess**
  - **Subphrenic**
  - **Pelvic**
- Liver abscess
- Portal pyaemia
- Septicemia
- Thrombosis of neighboring mesentery of ileum and ileal gangrene (in post ileal appendicis).

Clinical Features
- Rare before 2 years of age
- Commonest—20-30 years
- No age is however an exception.

Murphy's triad of symptoms—pain, fever and vomiting.

Pain
- Peri-umbilical colic, pain shifts to the right iliac fossa, non radiating due to peritoneal irritation.

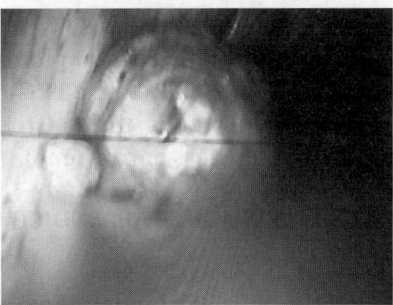

Fig. 28A-3: Fecolith in peritoneum from perforated appendix.
(For color version see Plate 2)

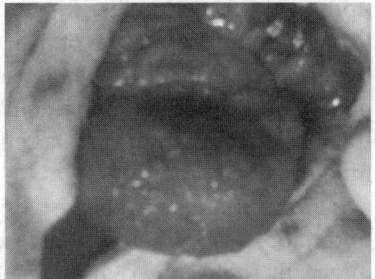

Fig 28A-4: TB ileum and appendicitis.
(For color version see Plate 2)

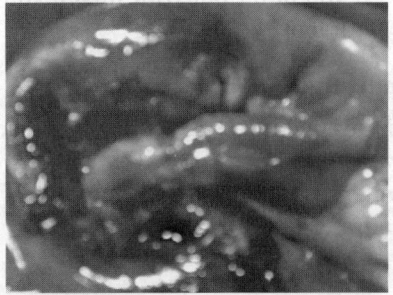

Fig. 28A-5: Ileal gangrene due to thormbosis of mesentery in post-ileal appendicitis.
(For color version see Plate 2)

- Anorexia, nausea/vomiting
- Symptoms commence any time, usually early hours of the morning.

Obstructive appendicitis: Pain is colicky and accompanied by vomiting.

Vomiting
- More of nausea, vomiting due to reflex pylorospasm.
- Usually follows pain in mild attack but accompanies pain in obstructive type.

Fever
- Appears after the other two symptoms
- Low grade fever (usually below 39°C)
- No chills and rigors unless there is complication (abscess or gangrene).

CLINICAL SIGNS IN ACUTE APPENDICITIS

Pyrexia
- Localised tenderness in the right iliac fossa
- Muscle guarding
- Rebound tenderness
  - Rovsing's sign—pain felt in right fossa upon pressure on left iliac fossa.
  - Cope's Psoas sign: Spasm of psoas upon hyper extension of the right thigh with the patient lying on left side and extending the thigh caused by irritation of a retrocecal inflamed appendix.
  - Cope's obturator sign: Severe pain due to obturator spasm when patient flexes and internally rotates the right thigh.
  - Digital rectal examination(P/R)—tender high on right wall
  - "If you don't put your finger, you'll put your foot".

Appendicitis in Special Situations

Retrocecal appendix: Less tender right iliac fossa (RIF).
- Tenderness mainly in loin, guarding over the quadratus lumborum.

Pelvic appendix
- Diarrhea may be the symptom
- Tenderness on P/R

Post ileal: Diarrhea and retching and vomiting.

Q. Short note on Alvarado score in appendicitis.

Alvarado (Mantrels) score for diagnosis of acute appendicitis.

Symptoms score
- Migratory RIF pain   1
- Anorexia   1
- Nausea and vomiting   1

Signs
- Tenderness (RIF)   2
- Rebound tenderness   1
- Elevated temperature   1

Laboratory
- Leukocytosis   2
- Shift to left (leukocytic segmented count)   1

Total score - 4 or below rules out 5–6 - suspicious 7 and above confirms diagnosis of acute appendicits. Currently inflammatory response score is followed.

Q. Differential diagnosis of acute appendicitis.

DIFFERENTIAL DIAGNOSIS OF ACUTE APPENDICITIS

A lot of clinical conditions mimick acute appendicitis. Refer **Table 28A-2** and **Fig. 28A-4**.

Investigation

Urine analysis to rule out urinary infection
Pregnancy test to exclude a ruptured ectopic.
Leucocytosis: Total count and polymorph counts are elevated.
C-reactive protein-level is elevated.
Urea, creatinine, blood sugar and liver function tests.

Ultrasound examination—appendix thicker than 6 mm, non-compressible.
   Very useful in children and thin adults and in excluding a gynaecological condition.
   Also to evaluate for abscess and collections.
CECT (Contrast enhanced CT) scan—very sensitive and specific (> 95%).

Treatment of Acute Appendicitis

Surgery for Uncomplicated Appendicitis
The treatment is laparoscopic appendicectomy or open appendicectomy.

Chapter 28: Abdominal Cavity, Hernia and Digestive Tract

Table 28A-2: Differential diagnosis of acute appendicitis.

Lower Abdomen:	Upper abdomen:
• Acute enterocolitis • Acute amebic typhlitis (cecal inflammation) • Acute diverticulitis (cecal diverticulitis) • Acute Meckel's diverticulitis. • Acute Crohn's enteritis • Acute mesenteric lymphadenitis • Acute torsion of appendices epiploicae	• Acute cholecystitis • Acute perforated duodenal ulcer. • Acute pancreatitis • Acute poisoning
Pelvis	**Extra abdominal conditions**
• Acute salpingitis • Acute torsion of ovarian cyst • Ruptured ectopic gestation • hemorrhage into cyst in endometriosis • Mittelschmerz (ovulation pain)	• Acute tonsillitis • Acute pleurisy • Acute basal pneumonia
	Medical conditions
	• Acute viral hepatitis • Acute porphyria • Diabetic keto acidosis • Henoch's purpura • Herpes zoster—T10–12
Retroperitoneum	
• Acute right sided pyelonephritis • Acute ureteric colic	
Spine	
• Tuberculosis of spine	

Anesthesia: General anesthesia for laparoscopic and preferably for open too.

Incision for open operation:
- McBurney's grid iron incision—perpendicular to the spinoumbilical line. Muscle splitting— each abdominal wall muscle is split between the fibers.
- A low transverse incision along the skin crease 2 cm below the McBurney's point extending laterally for 3-4 cm.
- Muscle cutting incision (Rutherford Morrison).

Antibiotics are started before surgery—ceftriaxone and metronidazole.

Intravenous fluid and electrolyte supplementation.

NSAID—preferably only after confirmation of diagnosis or else the diagnosis may be masked.

Non-operative treatment - for -
- Subsiding attack of appendicitis
- Appendix mass
- A mild non-obstructive appendicitis in an elderly patient with significant medical comorbidities.

Treatment
- Rest to bowel—intravenous fluids and nutrition.
- Intravenous antibiotics—metronidazole and ceftriaxone.
- Ertapenem and meropenem for peritonitis due to gangrene and perforation.

Disadvantage: 25–30% get a relapse within a year—require appendicectomy.

Q. Complications of appendicectomy.

Complications after Appendicectomy

General
- Deep vein thrombosis and thromboembolism
- Respiratory infection
- Hypercarbia in laparoscopic procedure.

Abdominal
- Hemorrhage—from slipped ligature or displaced clot from the appendicular artery
- Paralytic ileus
- Wound sepsis

- Intestinal obstruction due to formation of adhesions.
- Intra abdominal abscess—pelvic, paracolic inter bowel, subdiaphragmatic)
- Faecal fistula
- Pylephlebitis (portal pyaemia)
- Late—incisional hernia
- Right inguinal hernia—injury to ilioinguinal nerve.

Laparoscopic Appendicectomy
- Port hernia
- Atypical mycobacterial infection at port sites.

Q. Discuss appendix mass (appendicular phlegmon).

APPENDIX MASS (APPENDICULAR PHLEGMON)

A mass in right iliac fossa forming usually after 48 hours of onset of an attack of acute appendicitis as the natural response to contain and keep the infection localized, by forming adhesions between the appendix, greater omentum, small bowel loops and cecum and the posterior peritoneum/abdominal wall.

Clinical Features
- A mildly tender lump in RIF, with vague borders.
- It may undergo resolution over 3–5 days.
- It may form an abscess.

Differential Diagnosis
- Acute pericolic abscess—secondary to— diverticulitis, perforation
- Carcinoma cecum—nontender, anemia, blood in stools
- Tuberculosis (ileocecal)—irregular, nontender lump; history of chronic symptoms.
- Crohn's disease
- Iliac adenitis—abscess—over inguinal ligament, causes psoas spasm.
- Ameboma—less common than before, h/o amebic dysentery.
- Actinomycosis
- Tubo ovarian mass (females)
- Ovarian cyst (females)
- Unascended kidney
- Undescended testis (males).

Diagnosis
Clinical and CT scan imaging, white cell count for monitoring.

Q. Discuss the Ochsner Sherren Regimen.

Treatment of Appendix mass
Non operative treatment with active observation and elective appendectomy after 8 weeks.

Why?: Surgery at this stage is hazardous:
- Due to the risk of spreading infection and damaging the colon and general peritonitis
- Therefore join hands with the nature in localizing the infection and allow resolution.
- Interval appendicectomy after 6–8 weeks.

Contraindications
- Presence of complications—gangrene, perforation or signs of peritonitis/abscess
- Doubtful diagnosis
- Infants, children, elderly.

Measures under Ochsner-Sherren Regimen:
Patient is kept nil per oral until improvement (NPO)
- Intravenous fluids
- Antibiotics: Ceftriaxone or piperacillin +tazobactam with metronidazole.
- **Measure and mark size of mass daily**— review with ultrasound if needed.
- Nasogastric aspirations - if needed.
- Charts: Abdominal girth monitoring
- Intake output, pulse, BP, temperature 6 hourly.

Further action depends on the course of the mass (Refer **Table 28A-3**).

Q. Write a short note on appendix abscess.

APPENDIX ABSCESS
- It is due to perforation, suppuration or gangrene of appendix following acute appendicitis.
- Also, abscess may form following failed Ochsner-Sherren regime (conservative treatment)
- The abscess may lead to generalized peritonitis or systemic sepsis.

Table 28A-3: Clinical course of appendix mass, and plan of treatment.

Appendix mass—course	Resolution	Forms abscess/peritonitis
• Pain	• Gradual reduction	• Increase
• Size of mass	• ---Do --	• Increase
• Temperature	• Returns to normal	• Rising
• Heart rate	• No tachycardia	• Tachycardia
• Diarrhea	• Normal bowel movement	• Present
• Bowel sounds	• Normal peristalsis	• Ileus may set in
• WBC count	• Normal counts	• Counts increase
• Ultrasound	• No collection/free fluid	• Abscess or peritoneal fluid
Ochsner-Sherren Regimen	Continue until full resolution of mass	**Stop - the regimen, and perform emergency surgery**—appendectomy (when possible) and drain OR drain abscess and peritoneal cavity
Interval appendectomy (interval before the next attack)	Appendectomy after 6–8 weeks	

Clinical Features

- Swinging temperature, tender mass in right iliac fossa (RIF) or increase in size of an appendix mass.
- Tachycardia, abdominal distension or paralytic ileus may be present.
- Diagnosis is confirmed with ultrasound exam/CECT and polymorphonuclear leukocytosis.

Treatment

- Antibiotics—combination of piperacillin and tazobactam or meropenem with metronidazole
- Emergency surgery to drain the abscess.

Drainage of abscess - under general anesthesia

- **Extraperitoneal drainage:** Most abscesses are abutting the iliac fossa (retrocecal appendix) and secluded from general peritoneal cavity and hence drainage can be accomplished from a flank incision and draining the retrocecal collection without entering the peritoneal cavity.
- **Transperitoneal drainage:** (Laparotomy or laparoscopic) required when abscess is in relation to pelvis or ileocecal junction/retro-ileal or between bowel loops.

Appendicectomy: Done when there is a gangrenous or suppurated appendix.

Any adherent appendix can be left behind for an interval appendectomy.

Edematous bowel and omentum are least disturbed to avoid damage to bowel a fistula.

> **Q. Write a short note on mucocele of appendix.**

MUCOCELE OF APPENDIX

Cystic dilatation of the appendix by luminal accumulation of epithelial mucinous secretion. The lumen is blocked at the base of appendix.

- Age: Mostly—50 and 60 years.
- Sex: More common in females.
- Etiology neoplastic (AMN): Appendiceal mucinous neoplasms, OR non neoplasitc.
- AMN may be low grade (LAMN) or high grade (HAMN) or mucinous adenocarinoma.
- Non-neoplastic (appendicitis or fecolith blocking the lumen).
- Course: Resolution (only in some non neoplastic) or perforation - pathological during surgery. The cells are spilled into peritoneal cavity, causing diffuse peritoneal mucoid deposits (pseudo myxoma peritonei). Malignancy should be excluded by histopathology in all mucoeles.
- Clinical presentation—may be like acute appendicitis or a silent mass in right lower quadrant. Ultrasound or CT are useful in diagnosis.
- Treatment: Appendectomy—excision of intact mucocele without rupture.
- Right hemicolectomy—if base of appendix is involved or lymph nodes are enlarged

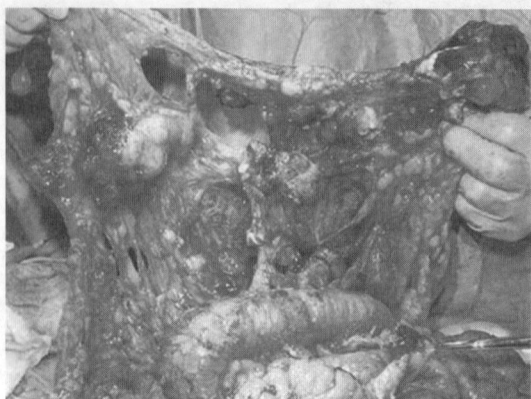

Fig. 28A-6: Pseudomyxoma peritonei.

- If there is spillage, treat the case as a pseudo myxoma peritonei.

Tumors of Appendix
- Carcinoids
- Epithelial tumors—mucinous—adenomas/adenocarcinomas.

> **Q. Write a short note on pseudomyxoma peritonei (PMP).**

PSEUDOMYXOMA PERITONEI (PMP)

Please refer **Figure 28A6**.
The peritoneal cavity is filled by tumor deposits, mucinous ascites, and omental masses. The etiology includes - perforation of a mucocele and mucinous tumor of appendix or ovary.

Pathology of PMP (Carr's classification)
- Acellular mucin
- Low-grade mucinous carcinoma peritonei
- High-grade mucinous carcinoma peritonei
- High-grade mucinous carcinoma peritonei with signet ring cells

Clinical feature: Progressive and massive abdominal distension, symptoms of bowel dysfunction and anorexia and at times features of partial obstruction. The condition progresses rapidly to death, if untreated.

Treatment epithelial tumors of appendix:
- Colonoscopic surveillance for 5 years and surgery for doubtful situation: For low grade tumors without PMP and with a low-risk of developing PMP.
- Aggressive surgery indicated for tumors with high-risk of PMP (high-grade tumors, invasive adenocarcinoma, goblet cell tumor and those with nodal spread).

Preventive surgery for epithelial tumors—right hemicolectomy omentectomy with prophylactic right parietal peritonectomy, (bilateral salpingoophorectomy in female) and intraperitoneal chemotherapy.

Principles of treatment of PMP: Cytoreductive Surgery (CRS) + Chemotherapy with HIPEC.
Cytoreductive surgery—laparotomy, appendectomy, salpingo oophorectomy Clearing the mucoid jelly, release of obstruction plus omentectomy peritonectomy and multivisceral resectioms.

HIPEC: Hyperthermic intraperitoneal chemotherapy (mitomycin/5 FU) (or gemcitabine) chemotherapy—regimen: Cisplatin, mitomycin C, 5-fluorouracil, and paclitaxel.

Prognosis:
Poorer outcomes: In males, patients with high-grade or invasive tumors and elevated tumor markers.
Survival after CRS + HIPEC: 5 year—85% and 10 year 70%.

> **Q. Write a short note on carcinoid of the appendix.**

CARCINOID OF THE APPENDIX—SYN: ARGENTAFFINOMA

- **Cell of origin:** Kulchitsky cells in crypts of Leiberkuhn - The enterochromaffin-like (ECL) like cells (amine precursor uptake and decarboxylation [APUD] origin).
- **Sites:** Arise any where in the gastrointestinal (GI) tract. Most common sites - appendix followed by ileum.
  Others: Bronchus, pancreas or ovary
- Age: 10-70 years, more common in females.
- Occurs in any part of the appendix, but most are in distal part or tip (75%).
- Size 1 cm or more, hard yellow tumor.
- 5% metastasize. To liver.

- Produces 5-HT, kinins, histamine and prostaglandins.
- These are detoxified in liver.
- Metastases in liver function and release the products into circulation which reach the right heart causing tricuspid stenosis.
- **Carcinoid syndrome**—only if it metastasizes.
- Cyanosis, hot flush, diarrhea and asthma like spells.

Investigations:
- Urine: Urinary HIAA levels >1000 ng/mL (normal 2–9 ng/mL
- Serum chromogranin B levels or immunohistochemical staining of tumor for chromogranin.
- In carcinoid syndrome—octreotide scintiscan tagged helps in locating the tumor.

Treatment
- Most tumors are found incidentally in appendectomy specimen:
- Follow up with serum Chromogranin B, for Tumors smaller than 2 cm and at least 2 cm away from base
- Right hemicolectomy is done - for tumors larger than 2 cm and less than 2 cm from base of appendix.
- Oligometastases: 3 or less and in a single lobe: Hepatic lobectomy.
- Polymetastatic disease—control of carcinoid symptoms—long term octreotide and previously cyproheptadine.
- Prognosis—generally good, even in metastatic disease with octreotide.

GIST (gastrointestinal stromal tumor).
- Uncommon in appendix.
- Seen as a mural thickening like an ileal tumor.
- Immunohistochemistry (IHC) staining of appendectomy will confirm.

Treatment
- Hemicolectomy—for tumor at base or invading cecum/mesentery.
- Imatinib.
- Sunitinib.

Q. Differential diagnosis of mass in the right iliac fossa.

MASS IN THE RIGHT ILIAC FOSSA

Appendicular Mass
- Preceding history of pain, vomiting and fever 2 or 3 days
- Tender mass in RIF
- Leukocytosis.

Carcinoma of Cecum
- Anemia, h/o hematochezia
- Irregular mass—mobile or fixed.

Ileocecal Tuberculosis
Barium enema or colonoscopy
- Pulled up caecum, filling defect
- Obtuse ileocecal angle
- Small bowel strictures
- Peritoneal nodules, ascites.

Amoebic Typhlitis
- History of amebic dysentery
- Mass is soft, tender, gurgling, tenderness at amebic point (Manson-Bahr)
- Stool examination.

Intussusception
- Colicky pain
- Red currant jelly stool
- Empty right iliac fossa (RIF), mass contracting under palpating hand
- Barium enema
- Coiled spring appearance.

Tubo-ovarian Mass
- Mass arising out of pelvis
- Gynecological symptoms
- Pelvic examination
- Ultrasound examination.

Others
- Iliac lymphadenitis
- Crohn's disease
- Enlarges unascended right kidney
- Tumour of undescended right testis
- Psoas abscess
- Tumors from iliacus muscle, bone.

THE LARGE INTESTINE

> SU 28.16: Large intestinal disorders congenital, non-malignant obstruction.

CHRONIC LARGE BOWEL OBSTRUCTION
Causes
Organic
- Intraluminal—fecal impaction
- Intramural—growth, diverticulosis, strictures—ischemia and Crohn's post-radiation
- Anastomotic stenosis and stenosis of colostomy stomal stenosis
- Extra-mural—metastatic deposits from stomach or ovary, endometriosis, hernia

Functional

Idiopathic megacolon, Hirschsprung's disease, pseudo-obstruction.

HIRSCHSPRUNG'S DISEASE (CONGENITAL MEGACOLON)

> Q. Discuss the pathology, diagnosis and principles of management of Hirschsprung's disease.

Hirschsprung's Disease (HD)

It is due to the congenital absence of ganglion cells from—Auerbach's and Meissner's plexus in anorectum and colon. The aganglionosis may extend proximally to involve the entire colon. Affects newborn infants. And may present later child hood or in adult life.

Incidence: 1 in 5000 births, generally male child, 10% are familial. Gene mutation described in chromosome 10.

Pathology
Three zones—aganglionic, transitional and dilated (proximal)
1. **Aganglionic zone**—spastic segment.
   - The internal anal sphincter and rectum are involved (partly or entirely).
   - This segment is narrow, non-relaxing and spastic.
2. **Transitional zone**—cone of the HD.
   - Proximal to it—contains sparsely distributed few ganglion cells with formation of cone.
3. **Proximal dilated zone**—colon is grossly dilated.
   - Mucosa—hyperemic with multiple ulcers
   - Hypertrophied circular muscle fibers.

Classification of Hirschsprung's Disease (HD)
- Ultrashort-segment HD—aganglionic part—in only anal canal and terminal rectum.
- Short-segment HD—aganglionic anal canal and full rectum (80%).
- Long-segment HD—aganglionic part—anal canal, rectum and part of the colon are (10%).
- Total colonic aganglionosis—HD—total absence of ganglions from anal canal, rectum and full length of the colon.

Clinical Presentations and Complications
- Neonatal intestinal obstruction (most common presentation).
- Severe, often fatal, enterocolitis.
- Perforation, peritonitis and septicemia.
- Late growth retardation.

Chronic course of the disease with constipation, abdominal distension and malnutrition.

At times may present in late childhood or adult life with the above history.

Neonatal presentation—within 3 days of birth (90% present in neonatal period).
- Failure to pass meconium.
- Passes toothpaste stools—narrow and sticky stool when a finger is introduced into the anal canal.
- Distension of the abdomen.

Digital examination of rectum: It is a super-continent baby.

Digital examination—anal tone high, gripping the finger and a ballooned rectum above, with the baby passing gas and meconium with loud flatus.

Differential diagnosis
- Other causes of neonatal intestinal obstruction like anorectal malformation.
- Acquired megacolon—rectum is loaded with stool, anal tone is low.
- Meconium plug syndrome—failure or pass meconium, but anal tone is normal.

Older children: The mother reveals history of passing pellet like stools, straining at stool, malnutrition and abdominal distension.

Adults: Rare—h/o chronic constipation and rarely still as a pseudo-obstruction of colon.

Diagnosis
Investigation:
- Gastrografin enema (or thin barium).
- Contrast enhanced CT scan. Shows the megacolon with a conical segment joining the distal spastic part above the levator ani (unlike in acquired megacoon where the dilated segment is upto the anal canal below the levator ani).

Full thickness rectal biopsy—for histopathological confirmation of agangliolosis.

Treatment
Surgical correction—done generally in stages and less often in a single stage.
- **Stage I:** Surgery—transverse colostomy, rectal full thickness biopsy to prove diagnosis. Post op: Supportive care—for nutrition and general health.
- **Stage II:** Definitive surgical procedure after child weighs 10 kg of weight.

Principles
- Resection of aganglionitic colon.
- Coloanal anastomosis for restoration of colonic continuity.
- Closure of colostomy later.

The Surgical Procedures for HD
Modified Duhamel Operation
- Resection of aganglionic colon and upper rectum (lower third retained)
- Anastomosing the proximal colon to posterior wall of the rectal stump.
- Here the anastomosis is between the rectum without ganglions, which is insensitive to defecatory sensation anteriorly and a proximal ganglionated and sensate rectum posteriorly; this ensures the continence through an intact levator ani and internal sphincter.

Soave's Procedure
- Resection of the aganglionic segment
- Mucosectomy of the ano rectal stump
- Endorectal pull through of the proximal colon.

Total proctocolectomy and ileo-anal anastomosis: For total aganglionosis of colon.

Swenson's operation: Resection of HD segment and coloanal anastomosis.

Anorectal myectomy: Indicated in ultra short segment and short-segment Hirschsprung's disease

> **Q. Short note on pathology and complications of diverticulosis coli.**

DIVERTICULOSIS COLI
Colonic diverticula are acquired:

Contributing Factors
A low fiber diet, ageing with altered collagen structure of bowel wall causing motility abnormality and increased intraluminal pressure.

This results in herniation of mucosa through the circular muscle at the points of penetration of blood vessels into the bowel wall. It is seen maximally seen in sigmoid colon (90%).

Saint's Triad: Association of diverticulitis, gallstones and (esophageal) hiatus hernia.

Pathology
These diverticula are thin without full three layers and allow stagnation of fecal mater with resulting bacterial overgrowth and complications.

Complications
- Infection and diverticulitis, peridiverticulitis
- Perforation: Causes—
  - Pericolic abscess
  - Generalized peritonitis.

- Intestinal obstruction:
  - **Fibrosis and stricture** of large bowel and obstruction.
  - **Adhesions**—between small bowel loops and inflamed large bowel.
- Haemorrhage: Profuse and recurrent hemorrhage due to erosion of vessels adjacent to a diverticulum.
- Fistula formation (colocutaneous, enterocolic, colovesical or colovaginal).

Clinical Features

- Progressive constipation or with diarrhea, pain—colicky or later continuous, commonly in the left iliac fossa, flatulence, heaviness and distension of lower abdomen.
- The symptoms worsen with progression.
- Examination may reveal a tender sigmoid colon.

Complications

Present with their respective features
- Diverticulitis: Severe pain, tenderness and guarding.
- Peridiverticular abscess—same as above but may be with fever.
- Perforation: Generalised peritonitis—systemic features—generalized tenderness and guarding.
- Hemorrhage—painless and heavy bleeding is common.
  - Torrential bleed may be due to angiodysplasia.
- **Fistula**—resulting from diverticular disease—depending on the site of disease.
- Colovesical fistula (the most common)—causing recurring urinary tract infections
- Pneumaturia (flatus in the urine) or even faeces in the urine.
- Colovaginal fistulae—common after hysterectomy.
- Fecal fistula—colocutaneous fistulation.

Hinchey Classification of Complicated Diverticulitis

- Grade I - Mesenteric or pericolic abscess
- Grade II - Pelvic abscess
- Grade III - Generalised (purulent) peritonitis
- Grade IV - Fecal peritonitis.

Investigation

- X-ray abdomen—shows a pneumoperitoneum in perforation.
- Spiral CT—detects bowel wall thickening, abscess formation and extraluminal disease.
  - Helps CT guided percutaneous drainage of localized abscesses, avoiding a laparotomy or laparoscopy.
- Contrast study of colon and endoscopy are performed—to assess the extent of diverticulosis, to exclude a carcinoma, other causes of constipation.
- Contrast CT—for delineating a fistula.
- Colonoscopy—to identify diverticula, to exclude carcinoma, angiodysplasia.
- Therapeutic—to control bleeding—injection or photocoagulation/laser.

Treatment

Uncomplicated Diverticulosis

- To promote free purgation and avoid constipation—high fiber diet, ispagula psyllium husk.
- Antispasmodic—for control of acute pain (dicyclomine or hyoscine, drotaverine).
- Acute diverticulitis: Intravenous antibiotics (metronidazole and ceftriaxone).
  - A CT scan is done for confirming diagnosis and to evaluate for complications (abscess or peritonitis).
  - Evaluation of bowel after the acute attack.
  - Colonoscopy and CT virtual colonoscopy.
- **Pericolic abscess:** Percutaneous drainage for pericolic abscesses larger than 5 cm in size after antibiotics.

> **Q. Short notes on surgical treatment for diverticulosis Coli.**

Surgery for Diverticulosis

Emergency surgery is to control peritoneal infection.

Indications
- Generalised peritonitis
- Failure of medical management to contain the infection and acute bowel obstruction.

High morbidiy and mortality and hence the need for due care in decisions regarding the procedures to be performed.

Procedures done at Laparotomy
- Hartmann's operation: Resection of the inflamed colonic segment (sigmoid) and closure of distal rectal stump; and subsequent second operation after 2-3 months for colonic reanastomosis.
- Colonic resection, anastomosis and a proximal defunctioning ileostomy (closed after 6 weeks).
- Simple proximal defunctioning ileostomy (not generally preferred).

Elective Surgery
- Pericolic abscess—drained
  - Fistulae and colonobstructing strictures —need resection of the affected bowel.
  - Colovesical fistula—resection of the sigmoid colon with a sleeve of the bladder wall containing the fistulous opening.
- Haemorrhage - treated by resection after—
  - Endoscopy to distinguish from angiodysplasia
  - CT angiography or selective angiography.
- Recurrent attacks of diverticulitis.

ULCERATIVE COLITIS (UC)
- Crohn's disease and ulcerative colitis are considered under inflammatory bowel disease.
- UC affects colon and rectum and has extraintestinal manifestations.
- The incidence is much higher in India than in the west.
- Affects both sexes equally in early life, usually diagnosed between 20 and 40.

Etiology
- Complex and partly understood.
- Genetic and familial background.
- 10-20% of patients have a first-degree relative with inflammatory bowel disease.
- Stress and emotions play a role and so do the food habits.
- Smoking is claimed to be protective.
- Autoimmune mechanisms—**cytotoxic** T lymphocytes against colonic epithelial cells and UC is associated with HLA - B27 genotype.

Q. Short note on pathology of ulcerative colitis.

Pathology
- The pathological process starts in the rectum to progress proximally **in continuity** (unlike skip of CD). The inflammation in the colon affects mucosa and superficial submucosa—seen as superficial and diffuse.
- 'Pseudopolyposis' is seen in 25-30% of cases.
- Strictures are unusual and indicate a carcinomatous change.
- Dysplasia associated lesions or mass [DALMs]: Irregular mucosal masses indicating a carcinoma coexisting.

Histological examination
- Lamina propria and crypts: Increased inflammatory cells.
- "Crypt abscesses" are typical.
- Goblet cells are depleted of mucin.
- Dysplasia follows with time. High grade dysplasia usually turn carcinomatous in 10-20 years.
- Generally risk of cancer increases with duration of the disease and the risk is higher with earlier onset of disease. Generally it is related to the duration of disease after onset—taken as 1%—at 10 years, 10-15% at 20% at 30 years.
- Synchronous cancers and/or DALMS (Dyplasia Associated Lesion/Mass) arise frequently.

Clinical Features of UC: Related to Extent of Disease (Refer Table 28C-1)

Q. Classify ulcerative colitis based on severity of clinical features.

Proctitis/Colitis/Proctocolitis and Complications

Severity classification—based on stool frequency and presence of systemic illness.

Q. Enumerate extracolonic manifestations of ulcerative colitis.

- **Extraintestinal manifestations of UC**
- Arthritis—15% of patients—affecting knees, ankles, elbows and wrists.
- Sacroiliitis and ankylosing spondylitis are 20 times more.
- Sclerosing cholangitis and progress to cirrhosis and hepatocellular failure.

Table 28C-1: Classification of severity of ulcerative colitis.

	Intestinal/Abdominal	Systemic	Extraintestinal
Isolated proctitis (10-15%) Rectal disease	Rectal bleeding, tenesmus mucous discharge	Usually absent	Absent
Colitis	Bloody diarrhea, urgency, tenesmus, pain less common	Anemia Hypoproteinemia Malaise, anorexia, and fever	Present

	Stool frequency	Bleeding/abdominal signs	Systemic signs
Mild disease	< 4 stools/day	With or without bleeding	No systemic signs of toxicity
Moderate disease	> 4 stools/day	Abdominal pain may be present	Mild systemic\features
Severe disease	> six bloody stools/day	Abdominal pain ++ bleeding +	Inflammatory markers, high C-reactive protein High ESR
Fulminant disease	> 10 stools/day	Continuous bleeding distension, abdominal tenderness needs blood transfusion progressive colonic dilation progresses -to **toxic megacolon'** suggestive of **disintegrative colitis,** perforation	Tachycardia Hypoalbuminemia High fever, ESR, CRP fever, tachycardia, anemia, hypoalbuminemia

- Greater risk of development of large bowel cancer.
- Cholangiocarcinoma—risk not influenced by colectomy.
- The skin lesions-erythema nodosum
  - Pyoderma gangrenosum resolve with good colitis control.
  - Uveitis and episcleritis.

Q. Write a note on acute toxic megacolon.

Acute Fulminant Colitis (Toxic Megacolon)

Incidence is 5%.
Etiology (**Common causes**):
- Ulcerative colitis
- Ischemic colitis
- Acute fulminant amebic colitis
- Clostridium difficile enterocolitis
- Diabetic abdomen.

Clinical features
- Over ten bloody stools per day and later stool frequency reduces along with severe abdominal pain and progressive distension.
- X-ray shows a colonic width more than 6 cm

Treatment
- Steroids
- Fluids and blood transfusion
- Intensive medical therapy—two thirds of patients respond and go to remission
- A third of them need emergency surgery to avoid colonic perforation.

Surgical treatment: Emergency resection (subtotal colectomy with ileostomy) or a cecostomy to decompress the colon.

Indication for emergency surgery
- Progressive increase in colon diameter despite medical therapy
- Colonic perforation (very high mortality) 40 to 50%
- Severe hemorrhage (rare).

Q. Describe the investigations and principles of treatment of ulcerative colitis.

Investigations in Ulcerative Colitis

Endoscopy: Colonoscopy with biopsy, chemoendoscopy and narrow band imaging for early findings. Contraindicated in acute colitis (perforation may happen).

Indications
- To make a diagnosis
- To determine the extent of involvement
- To look for dysplasia-associated lesion or mass (DALM) and malignant change
- To differentiate from Crohn's
- To monitor the response to treatment.

Radiology

X-ray in toxic megacolon
CECT
- Featureless colon (no haustrations)
- Significant thickening of the colonic wall and stranding in the colonic mesentery in pancolitis.

Medical Therapy
- The 5-aminosalicylic acid (5-ASA) and derivatives are given orally or topically. They act by inhibition of the cyclo-oxygenase enzyme system.
- Corticosteroids—for acute exacerbations—topically or systemically.
- Immunosuppressive drugs azathioprine and cyclosporin for maintaining remissions.
- Monoclonal antibodies—infliximab and adalimumab—act against anti TNF alpha.
- **"Colonic rescue therapy"** vedolizumab, is used in fulminant colitis to avoid emergency surgery.

Indications for Surgery
- Severe or fulminating disease not responding to medical therapy
- Chronic disease with anemia, frequent stools, urgency, and tenesmus
- Inability of the patient to tolerate medical therapy azathioprine-induced pancreatitis, steroid psychosis
- Steroid-dependent disease—failure to maintain remission even with steroids
- Severe dysplasia or malignancy
- Extraintestinal manifestations
- Severe hemorrhage
- Stenosis causing obstruction.

Surgery

Emergency Surgery

Subtotal colectomy with ileostomy and distal rectal mucous fistula.

Elective surgery (see above for indications)
- Subtotal colectomy and ileostomy
- Proctocolectomy and permanent end ileostomy.

Restoration of bowel continuity :
- Proctocolectomy with ileoanal pouch reconstruction—to restore bowel continuity
- Subtotal colectomy and ileorectal anastomosis.

Colonic Crohn's disease:
- Medical therapy is almost along the lines of ulcerative colitis
- Rectum is also affected and hence needs to be resected. Therefore, total proctocolectomy with permanent ileostomy required.

> Q. Discuss surgical manifestations of intestinal amebiasis.

SURGICAL MANIFESTATIONS OF INTESTINAL AMEBIASIS

Etiology

Entamoeba histolytica: The amebic trophozoites emerge from the swallowed cysts.

The trophozoites digest the mucosa and submucosa of large bowel (most commonly the sigmoid and rectum and ileocaecal region of the colon in others. This forms typical ulcers with shape of flask in the sigmoid, rectal, cecal and ileal mucosa.

Clinical consequences and complications:
- Acute amebic dysentery
- Acute hematochezia—bloody diarrhea
- Secondary bacterial infection
- Fulminant colitis
- Colonic perforation and peritonitis, pericolic abscess, perianal abscesses
- Toxic megacolon (rare)
- Amebic granuloma—mimicking a carcinoma.

Chronic amebiasis causes chronic abdominal pain, loss of appetite, intestinal colic.

Extraintestinal amebiasis (discussed under chapter liver)
- Amebic liver abscess (most common)
- Pericarditis
- Amebic empyema
- Cutaneous amebiasis
- Amebic encephalopathy and brain abscess and very rarely.

Clinical Features
Amebic dysentery:
- Abdominal colicky pain with diarrhea
- Tenderness in left iliac fossa (Amebic point of Sir Philip Manson Bahr).

Acute fulminant amebic colitis—often life threatening
- Severe bloody diarrhea, worsening to torrential bleeding
- Toxicity and sloughing of colonic mucosa.

Amebic typhlitis (inflammation of cecum)
- Pain and tenderness in right iliac fossa—similar to that in acute appendicitis.
- Mass in right iliac fossa.

Differential diagnosis:
- Appendix mass
- Carcinoma colon
- Crohn's mass
- Ileocecal tuberculosis.

Investigations
- Stool examination: Saline wet mount of fresh stool—to demonstrate trophozoites and cysts in chronic presentation.
- Serology—indirect hemagglutination test
- Polymerase chain reaction (PCR).

Treatment
In acute cases
- Metronidazole IV or metronidazole retention enema may also given in addition.
- Intravenous fluid supplementation.
- Antibiotic like tetracycline or ciprofloxacin to treat superadded bacterial infection.
- Antispasmodics to treat spasmodic pain.

Chronic cases:
- Tab metronidazole (400–800 mg) 3 times daily is given for 10 days

- Tablet Tinidazole 2 g daily for 3 days.
- Secnidazole—as a single dose of 2 g.
- Diloxanide furoate—against cysts in chronic amebiasis (500 mg thrice daily for 10 days).
- Tab. dehydroemetine is reserved for resistant cases (in view of cardiotoxicity).

Toxic megacolon (refer under ulcerative colitis)
An emergency state colon with acute severe and progressive distension of colon with severe pain and systemic toxicity, which may lead to necrosis and perforation of colon.

Q. Short note on angiodysplasia of colon.

Angiodysplasia of colon
- It is a vascular malformation made of dilated tortuous submucosal veins.
- Presents with bleeding from the colon in patients over the age of 60.
- It may be mild bleeding with anemia or sudden and massive bleeding.
- More common in right colon.

Diff. Diagnosis: Diverticular bleeds.

Investigations
- Colonoscopy
- Selective angiography (superior or/and inferior mesenteric artery) seen as a " blush"
- Technetium-99m (99mTc)-labelled red cell scan
- It may still be elusive.

Treatment
When found at colonoscopy
- Endoscopic—argon plasma coagulation (APC)
- Coagulation with cautery or argon laser
- Angiographic embolization to stop bleeding followed by surgery (bowel undergoes necrosis).

Surgery: Resection of colonic segment.
- Bleeding can't be controlled by endoscopy
- After angio- embolization
- "Blind resection" to control incessant bleeding despite nonsurgical measures.

Q. Write a note on ischemic colitis.

ISCHEMIC COLITIS
- Colonic ischemia may be acute or chronic.
- Common in atherosclerotic persons and those with heart diseases.

- Other causes include Thrombosis, embolism, vasculitis and hypercoagulable states like polycythemia.
- Diabetes, renal disease, immunological disorders contribute to the pathogenesis.
- Area near splenic flexure is most prone for ischemia. It is the "watershed" point of Griffith, marking the junction of superior and inferior mesenteric branches.

Clinical Presentation

Mainly three clinical settings:
- Intermittent mucosal ischemia and nerosis/ulceration—recurrent bleeding.
- Chronic muscular ischemia—ischemic stricture—obstruction.
- Full thickness infarction—acute -gangrenous colon—peritonitis.

Symptoms
- Pain—left iliac or hypochondrial—intermittent or colicky.
- Hematochezia.

Acute presentation: Usually embolic episode—severe pain disproportionate to the signs of peritonism, vomiting, bloody stools hemodynamic instability and peritonitis.

Differential diagnosis: Other causes of lower GI bleeding.

Carcinoma colon: Ulcerative colitis; Crohn's disease.

Investigation

Acute ischemia/acute abdomen
- Plain X-ray reveals: Free gas under diaphragm—due to perforation 'thumb printing sign' caused by submucous hemorrhage and mucosal edema.
- CT scan shows colonic wall thickening.
- CT angiography may show a vessel block.

Chronic Ischemia

Colonoscopy and contrast enhanced CT scan are done.

Treatment

Acute ischemic event:
- Resuscitation
- Emergency laparotomy—resection of gangrenous bowel and diversion colostomy. Anastomosis is done after recovery of the patient from the acute event.
- Mortality is extremely high.

Chronic Progressive Ischemia
- Conservative treatment leads to improvement in three fourths of patients
- Measures include—intravenous fluids and nutrition and avoidance of oral feeds
- Antibiotics and antiplatelet drug like aspirin.

Indications for Surgery (Resection and Anastomosis)
- Gangrene, peritonitis
- Stricture
- Segmental ischemia.

CHRONIC CONSTIPATION

- **Organic: Obstructing surgical diseases**
- **Medical disorders**
  - Neurological conditions: Parkinson's disease, multiple sclerosis
  - Diabetic neuropathy
  - Spinal cord lesion
  - Endocrine conditions—hypothyroidism, hypercalcemia.
- **Drugs that can cause constipation**
  - Benzodiazepines, carbamazepine
  - Tricyclic antidepressants, phenothiazines (chlorpromazine)
  - Opiates, particularly codeine and morphine
  - Statins
  - Cholestyramine
  - Iron
- **Functional Disorders**
  - Syndrome of impaired rectal emptying associated with pelvic floor dysfunction.

Investigations
- Colonoscopy
- CT virtual colonoscopy or barium enema
- Whole-gut transit time
- Defecating proctography may show impaired pelvic floor relaxation, rectal intussusception and/or rectocele
- Anorectal manometry—confirm an abnormal pattern of straining.

TREATMENT OF CHRONIC CONSTIPATION AND COLOPARESIS

- Dietary fiber.
- Laxatives—bulk, osmotic and stimulant.
- Prucalopride—selective agonist of serotonin (5HT-4) receptors.
- Rectal irrigation.
- Biofeedback: This involves training in pelvic floor function.
- Sacral neuromodulation—sacral nerve stimulation.
- Surgery: The results of surgery are relatively poor.
  - STARR—stapled transanal rectal resection—full thickness resection of a rim of rectum with the device.
  - Total colectomy and ileorectal anastomosis—unpredictable results and high complication rate.
  - Colostomy—in moribund patients unfit for any resections.

> **Q. What is colostomy? Describe types, indications and complications and write a note on stoma care.**

COLOSTOMY

Colostomy is the surgery for fecal diversion through a stoma on anterior abdominal wall.

Types

Refer **Figure 28C-1**.
- Colonic part diverted
  - Transverse colostomy
  - Sigmoid colostomy
  - A cecostomy (rarely done now)

- Design of the colostomy
  - Loop colostomy
  - End colostomy
  - Double barrel,
  - Spectacle colostomy (Divine's)

Purpose of diversion: Temporary - defunctioning colostomy (sigmoid or transverse) and permanent.

Temporary—defunctioning colostomy

- To allow distal healing—after colorectal resections, perineal trauma, anorectal fistula.
- Relief of acute distal obstruction—obstructing cancer
- Pelvic tumors
- To facilitate pelvic irradiation.

Permanent colostomy:

If anal sphincters destroyed:
- Local/neurological disease/trauma/surgery
- After surgical removal of distal anorectum.

Types of colostomy (Refer **Figure 28C-1**)
Loop colostomy (generally temporary):
- Transverse or sigmoid colostomy.

Double barrel colostomy

Here both open ends of divided colon brought out together.
- Paul Mikulicz sigmoid colostomy - the walls of colonic segments adjoining the ends are sutured.
- Devine's method - a skin bridge intervenes between the openings.

End Colostomy

- After abdominoperineal resection or Hartmann procedure.

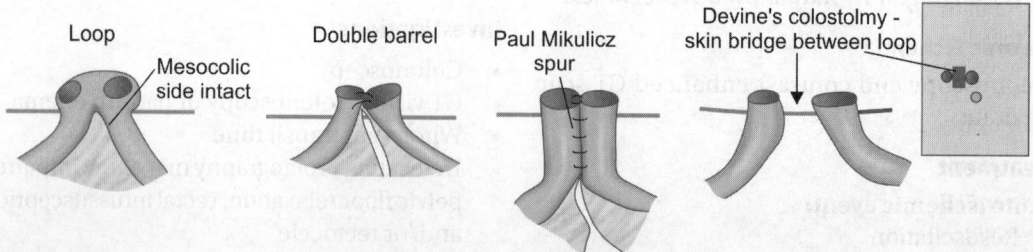

Fig. 28C-1: Types of colostomy

- Palliation of distal rectal cancer.
- Incontinence after spinal injury or neurological disease.

Complications of Colostomy
(Refer Table 28C-2)

Closure of Colostomy
After maturation of colostomy at least 3 months—for better healing.

Intraperitoneal Closure
- Mobilization
- Closure in layers
- Resection and anastomosis
- Advantage: Complete mobilization and no kinking/obstruction.

Extraperitoneal Closure
- Colon is mobilised and ends anastomosed without opening peritoneum.
- Advantage—no peritoneal contamination in case of leak.
- Disadvantage—kink and obstruction to colonic propulsion.

LOWER GASTROINTESTINAL BLEEDING

Q. Classify gastrointestinal bleeding.

Gastrointestinal bleeding—definitions
Site of bleed
- Upper GI bleed: Proximal to ligament of Treitz
- Lower GI bleed: Distal to ligament of Treitz.

Presentation
- Acute or chronic
- Occult or overt.

Nomenclature of the bleed
- Hematemesis: From oral end
- Melena: Tarry (hematin) foul smelling semi-liquid
- Hematochezia: Dark (maroon) unaltered blood, usually colonic tumors, diverticula, ulcers; also massive proximal or intestinal bleed
- Fresh blood: P/R—piles, fissure, polyp, severe proximal bleed.

Symptoms of GI bleed

Upper GI Bleed
- Acute—hematemesis/melena
- Chronic—melena/occult blood in stool—anemia/palpitation, asthenia

Table 28C-2: Complications of colostomy.

Complications of colostomy	
• Infection	• Retraction
• Bleeding	• Loss of colostomy
• Strangulation—necrosis or gangrene	• Prolapse of colostomy
	• Paracolostomy hernia
	• Internal herniation—through paracolostomy space of Goligher
• Obstruction	
• Diarrhea	

Lower GI Bleed
- Fresh blood—continuous/intermittent—rectum/anus
- Dark blood—colon/distal ileum
- Melena—Generally from upper GI tract but can be from proximal colon/ileum
- Severe upper gastrointestinal bleeding (UGIB) can also present as dark blood/clots
- Infectious—HIV, *Salmonella*, *Shigella*, tuberculosis

Q. Discuss etiology and management of acute lower gastrointestinal Hemorrhage.

Refer **Table 28C-3** and **Table 28C-4**).

Etiology of Lower GI Bleed
90% is colorectal, 10% is jejuno ileal (Refer Table 28C-4).

Signs of GI Bleed

Acute GI bleed
- Hypovolemia—tachycardia, weak pulse, low BP, pallor, sweat.

Chronic GI bleed
- **General**—anemia, exertional dyspnea, tachycardia.
- Iron deficiency anemia, koilonychia.

Signs of specific diseases
- Hepatic—caput medusae, splenomegaly
- Dermatocutaneous angioma, telangiectasia bullae, ulcers in mouth
- Rheumatoid arthritis (history of in NSAID intake bleed)
- Bleeding diathesis, e.g., petechiae.
- Vascular.

Table 28C-3: Etiology of lower gastrointestinal bleeding.

Etiology—age-wise

Specific disease distinctive for different age groups

Adolescents/young adults	Older adults
• Inflammatory bowel disease • Polyps • Meckel diverticulum • Bleeding diatheses • Upper gastrointestinal bleeding (e.g. peptic ulcer)	• Colonic diverticula • Angiodysplasia • Colorectal carcinoma/polyps • Rectal trauma/fissure/hemorrhoids • Upper gastrointestinal bleeding (e.g. peptic ulcer) • Anticoagulation therapy

Table 289C-4: Etiology of lower gastro intestinal bleeding—pathology-based.

Colorectal bleed	Small bowel bleed (10%)
• Diverticulosis coli • Hemorrhoids • Fissure in ano • Acute infective colitis • Inflammatory bowel disease (IBD)—ulcerative colitis/Crohn's • Ischemic colitis • Radiation colitis • HIV associated colitis • Solitary rectal ulcer syndrome (SRUS) • Polyps/colonic/rectal cancer • Angiodysplasia • Portal hypertension—rectal varices	• Meckel's diverticulum • Crohn's • Tuberculosis • Intussusception • Ischemic enteritis/gangrene of bowel • Lymphoma/GIST • Angiodysplasia • Heterotopic gastric mucosa • Worms • Jejunal ulcers/typhoid ulcers • NSAID

Clnical features suspicious of HIV in lower GI bleed.

Lower GI (LGI) Bleed

History: Important

Remember - **Cancer and HIV**

IBD: Stool + blood

CMV Infection

Lower gastrointestinal bleeding (LGIB) with pain. Isch. colitis/IBD/Infective

Severe pain is suspicious of: Toxic megacolon/perforation

Cancer—usually occult blood or chronic intermittent bleed.

LGI bleed: Examination

- A higher lesion should not be missed by finding a distal lesion
- Rectal exam—digital/proctoscopy is important.

Investigations

- Blood—for anemia, bleeding diathesis
- Fecal occult blood positive.
- Sigmoidoscopy/colonoscopy and biopsy.
- MDCT/scan or CT angiography.
- Scintigraphy (radioisotope) in acute bleeds.
- Barium enema—largely replaced by CT.
- Diagnostic endoscopy—in LGI bleed.
- Upper GI endoscopy—to look for upper gastrointestinal bleeding (UGIB) (10-15%).

Colonoscopy—in acute/chronic lower GI bleeds (except massive bleeds and hemodynamically unstable)

- Will show angiodysplasia radiation proctopathy
- Peroperative endoscopy.

Capsule endoscopy—jejunal tumors or ulcers.

Double lumen enteroscopy/push enteroscopy.

Radiology in GI Bleed

- **Diagnosis**
  - MDCT/CT angiography: Locate arterial/venous bleed
  - Radioisotope scintigraphy: To locate bleeder/lesion—99m Tc.
- **Therapy**
  - Selective angiography and embolisation
  - Cannulating celiac/inferior mesenteric artery.

CT angiography

- Useful in diverticular bleed
- Small bowel telangiectasia.

Gastrointestinal bleeding scintigraphy (GIBS)—technetium-99m-labeled RBC

It is non-invasive and helps in diagnosis of GI bleeding; to see if it is active, to assess its severity and to localise site of bleeding.

LGI bleed—right colic artery

- Superior mesenteric arteriography
- Selective catheter angiography on right colic
- Selective embolisation with Polyvinyl alcohol particles to embolize the bleeding artery.

Therapeutic endotherapy in lower GI bleed

Injection

- Into bleeding lesion
- Sclerotherapy, adrenaline injection, cyanoacrylate glue or thrombin.

Thermal

- LASER: Argon, Nd: YAG
- Heater probe, electrocoagulation
- Argon plasma coagulation
- Photodynamic therapy

Endoscopic polypectomy

- **EMR (endoscopic mucosal resection) others**: Mechanical devices; topical spray, microwave coagulation

Management of Acute Gastrointestinal Bleeding in High Risk Patients

Refer **Table 28 C-5**.

SURGERY IN ACUTE GI BLEED: GENERAL PRINCIPLES

Indications for Surgery in Lower Gastrointestinal Bleeding

- Active persistent bleeding with hemodynamic instability, not responding to aggressive resuscitation
- Persistent, recurrent bleeding
- Transfusion of more than 4 units of packed red blood cells (PRBCs) in a 24-hour period, with active or recurrent bleeding
- Transfusion of more than 6 units of PRBCs during the same hospitalization

Table 28C-5: Management of acute GI bleeding—high risk patients.

Acute GI bleed—management—high risk patients:
- Hospitalisation—resuscitation and stabilization of the patient in intensive care unit
- Restore the normovolemic state by correction of hypovolemia—infusion and/or transfusion
- Monitoring of—CVP arterial line, intravenous line, monitor vitals, urine output

Stabilized patient		Unstable patient Despite resuscitation
Stable? Emergency endoscopy		Unstable? Emergency surgery
No diagnosis?	Diagnosis—treatment	With on table endoscopy
Angiography— CT angio/ selective angiography	Diagnosis—embolization	
No diagnosis? scintigraphy	Diagnosis—surgery and resection	
No diagnosis?	**Blind surgery**	

- Failure of endoscopic localization and/or therapy/rebleed
- Failure of angiographic control/localization
- Resection of necrosed part after embolization
- "Blind" exploration—for search and act on bleeder (laparotomy and search for bleeder—resect the bleeding part or colonic segment/entire colon) refer below under "blind resection".

Resection for Localized Lesions
- Diverticulum
- Polyp/tumor—carcinoma/GIST
- Meckel's diverticulum
- Vascular lesions
- After control of bleeding with angioembolization (the segment of bowel undergoes infarction) or endoscopic therapy.

Undiagnosed LGI Bleed? - "Blind Resections"

First, a right hemicolectomy—helps in controlling 60-75% of the bleeds (from right side of colon).

Subtotal colectomy is done if bleeding continues, (20-30% bleed from left side).

Mortality of operation is very high but it is **less than** in not operating.
- Overall—10-15% in acute LGI bleeds
- Factors contributing to high mortality—bleed, hypovolemia, transfusions, multiorgan failure and the delay in operating.

ANORECTAL SURGERY

> **SU28.16:** Describe applied anatomy including congenital anomalies of the rectum and anal canal.
>
> **SU28.17:** Describe the clinical features, investigations and principles of management of common anorectal diseases.

SURGICAL ANATOMY OF RECTUM

- The length of the adult rectum is about 15 cm. It is divided into three parts:
  - The upper third, covered by peritoneum anteriorly and laterally and it is not fixed.
  - The middle third with the peritoneal cover over the anterior side and partly the lateral.
  - The lower third, which lies below the peritoneal reflection in the pelvis.
- The rectum lies over the sacral hollow end ends at anorectal junction, with three lateral curves, with the convexities of the upper and lower curves to the right and that of the middle to the left.
- The opposite side on the curve is marked on the mucosa by semicircular folds (Houston's valves).
- The puborectalis muscle makes the anorectal angle of 120 degree, by encircling the rectum on its lateral and posterior aspects.
- Denonvilliers' fascia separates the lower third of the rectum from the prostate or vagina.
- Waldeyer's fascia separates the rectum from the coccyx and lower two sacral vertebrae.
- These tough fascial layers are barriers against infiltration of malignancies.
- They form the fascial envelope for total mesorectum excision (TME) (oncological clearance)—preventing intra operative spillage of cancer cells in surgery for rectal cancer.

Rectum and Anal Canal: Muscles

- Internal sphincter—continuous with circular muscle of rectum, ends 6-8 mm above anal orifice
- External sphincter—continuation of longitudinal muscle
- Anorectal ring—puborectalis, external and internal sphincter.

Rectum and Anal Canal: Mucosa

- Terminal portion of large intestine
- Upper mucosal and lower cutaneous part
- Junction is marked by anal valves of Morgagni—dentate line or pectinate line, marking the junction of hindgut with proctodeum.

Anal Canal

Anal Crypts and Valves

- Anal crypt—above each anal valve. Space for foreign body to lodge.
- Columns of Morgagni
  - 8 to 14 connected by valves—anal valves
  - Anal glands are in intersphincteric space—open into crypt by penetrating the sphincter.

> **Q. Short note on anal cushions.**

Anal cushions

- Mucosal humps overlying the superior hemorrhoidal plexus
- Fibroelastic strands pass through venous plexus anchoring the mucosa to internal anal sphincter
- They assist internal sphincter in anal continence for flatus (have receptors)

EMRYOLOGY OF RECTUM AND ANAL CANAL

Refer **Figure 28AR-1 to AR-5**.

> **Q. Surgical importance of dentate (pectinate) line?**

Refer **Table 28AR-1**.

Anatomy of Rectum and Anal Canal

Refer **Figure 28AR-4**.

Anal Canal and Rectum: Coronal Section View

Refer **Figure 28AR-5**.

Anal Sphincters

Refer **Figure 28AR-6**.

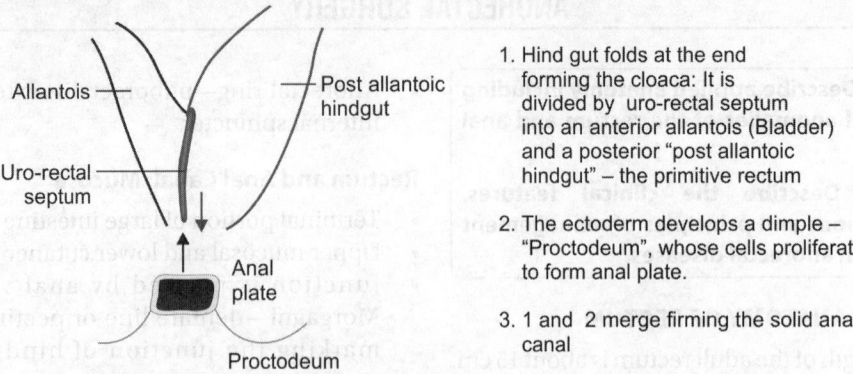

1. Hind gut folds at the end forming the cloaca: It is divided by uro-rectal septum into an anterior allantois (Bladder) and a posterior "post allantoic hindgut" – the primitive rectum

2. The ectoderm develops a dimple – "Proctodeum", whose cells proliferate to form anal plate.

3. 1 and 2 merge firming the solid anal canal

Fig. 28-AR-1: Embryology of rectum and anal canal

Development of rectum and anal canal

Cloaca is split by the uro-rectal septum into anterior allantois (later forms the bladder) and a posterior post allantoic gut, latter forming the rectum

The post allantoic gut meets the proliferating plate of ectodermal cells at the anal dimple, the proctodeum to form the anal membrane

The recanalisation of proctodeum form the anal canal and the anal membrane ruptures to form the dentate line

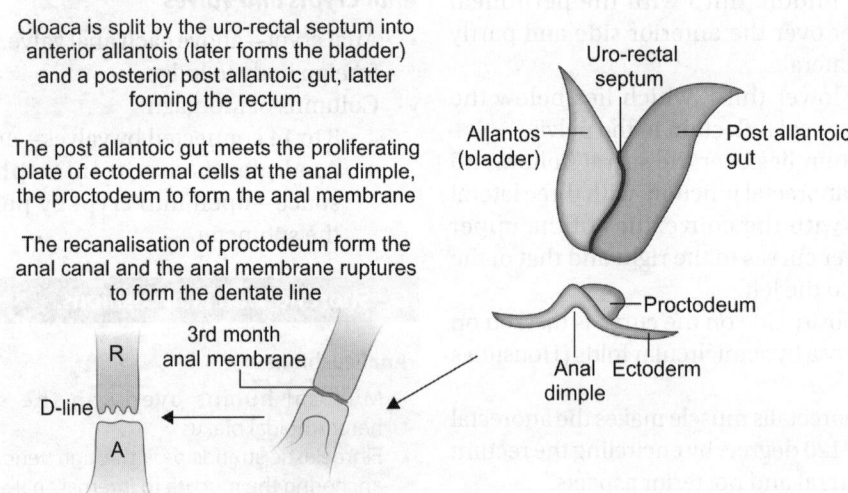

Fig. 28AR-2: Development of rectum and anal canal

Proctodeum meets post allantoic hindgut at **Anal membrane**—at 3 months. The same ruptures to leave behind **Dentate line**—after 7th month.

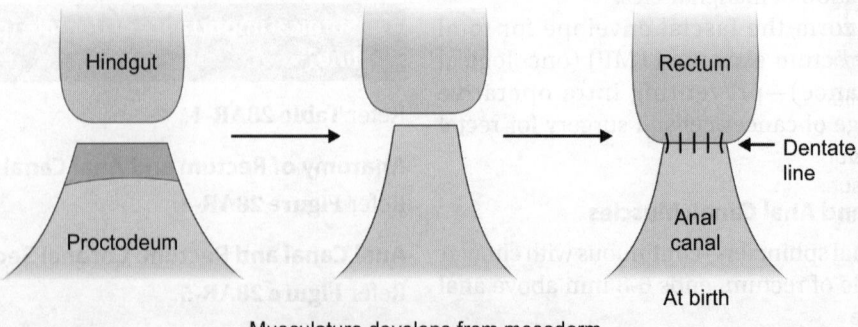

Musculature develops from mesoderm

Fig. 28AR-3: Development of anal canal

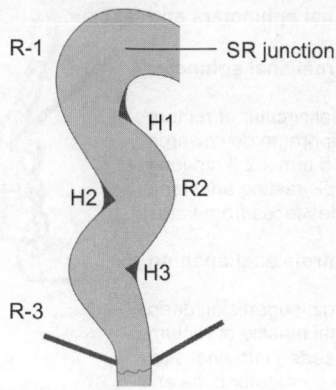

Fig. 28AR-4: Anatomy of rectum and anal canal

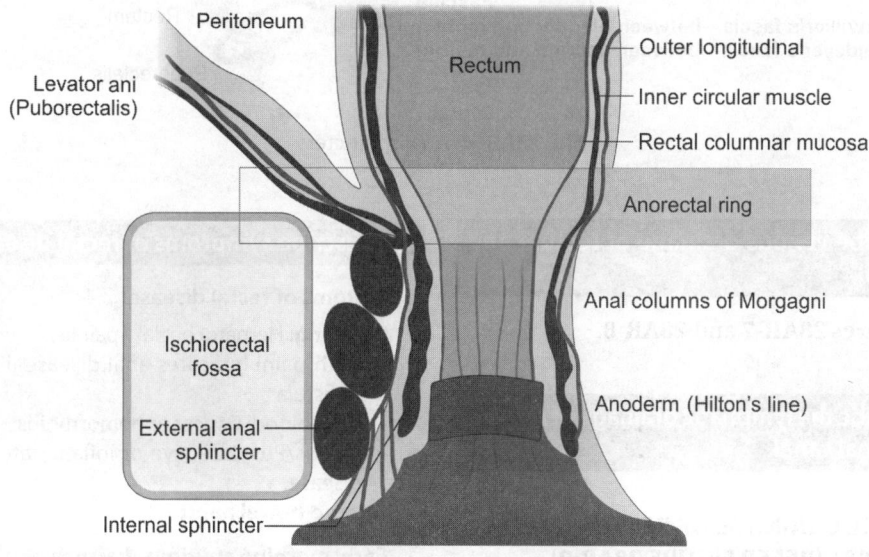

Fig. 28AR-5: Coronal view of anal canal and rectum

Table 28AR-1: Surgical importance of dentate line.		
Pectinate line (dentate)	*Above*	*Below*
• Epithelium • Color • Venous drainage • Nerve supply • Lymphatic	• Columnar/cuboidal • Pink • Portal vein • Sympathetic and parasympathetic • No somatic pain • Inferior mesenteric nodes	• Squamous • Skin • Inferior vena cave • Somatic • Pain sensitive • Inguinal nodes

Anal sphincters and fascia

Internal anal sphincter

Continuation of internal circular of rectum from pelvic diaphragm downwards
2.5 mm x 2.5 cm long
Keeps anus closed—resting anal tone differentiates feces from flatus

External sphincter controls anal opening

Three parts—subcutaneous, superficial, deep continuation of longitudinal muscle of rectum below puborectalis—inserted into anal skin through corrugator cutis ani
Puborectalis (levator ani)—most important for fecal continence

Fasciae
Denonvillier's fascia—between bladder and rectum
Waldeyer's fascia—between sacrum and rectum

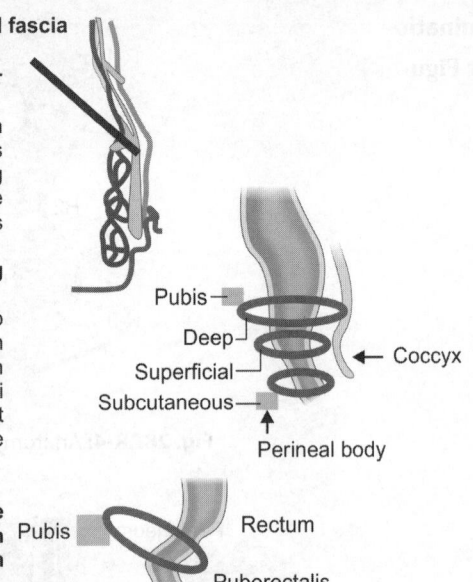

Fig. 28AR-6: Anal sphincters

Q. Describe venous drainage of rectum and anal canal.

Refer **Figures 28AR-7** and **28AR-8**.

Q. Describe the lymphatic drainage of rectum and anal canal.

LYMPHATIC DRAINAGE OF RECTUM AND ANAL CANAL (REFER FIGURE 28AR-9)

- Rectum surrounded by peri and pararectal nodes enclosed in the mesorectal sheath (primary nodes). Secondary nodes are along vessels.
- Lymphatics from upper third drain into nodes along into superior rectal nodes.
- Middle third—mainly into superior rectal nodes and partly through middle rectal nodes —into internal iliac nodes.
- Lower third—along inferior rectal vessels to inguinal nodes.

Q. Describe symptoms of rectal disease.

Symptoms of rectal disease

- **Bleeding:** Hematochezia—painless
  - With pain: Indicates anal disease like fissure or fistula
  - With blood: Cancer or hemorrhoids
  - Mucus/Pus: Infective or inflammatory bowel disease.
- Altered bowel habit

- **Early morning spurious diarrhea**
  - The patient wakes up from sleep with an urge for passing stools but—passes blood (not stools)
  - Due to the bleeding that collects in rectal ampulla overnight
  - **Sense of incomplete defecation**—the growth causes sense of distension.
- **Tenesmus:** Typically in a cancer
- **Discharge:** Mucus or purulent or blood stained
- **Prolapse: Hemorrhoids or a prolapsed**
- **Pruritus:** Anal discharge anorectal pathology, enterobiasis, tinea cruris, eczema.

Examination of Anal Canal and Rectum

Refer **Figures 28AR-10 and 28AR-11**.

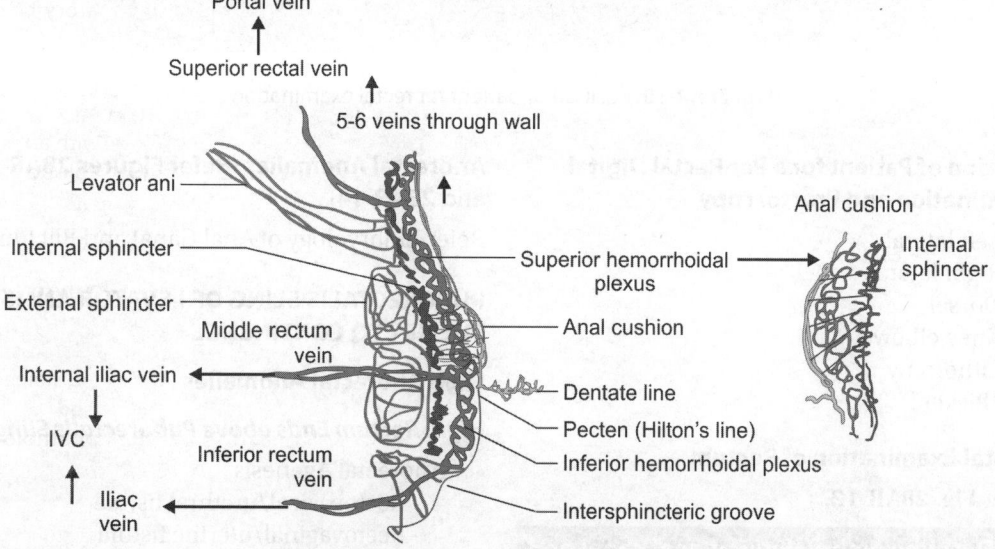

Fig. 28AR-7: Venous drainage of rectum and anal canal

Fig. 28AR-8: Anorectal venous drainage

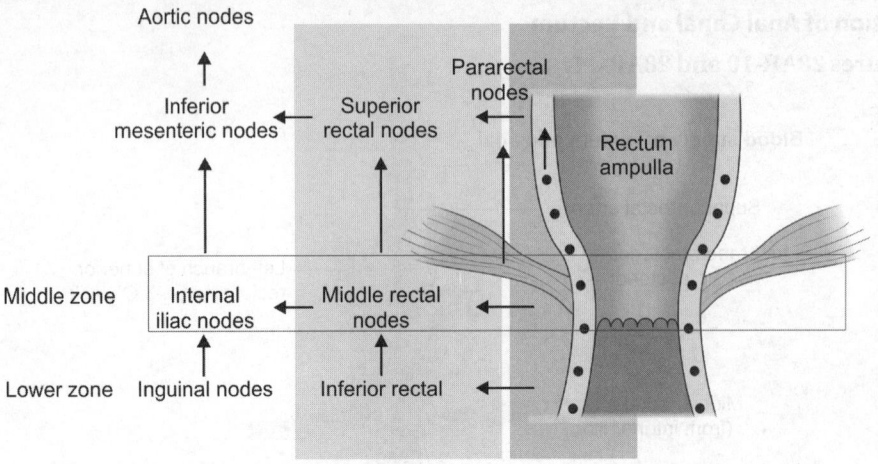

Fig. 28AR-9: Lymphatic drainage of anal canal and rectum

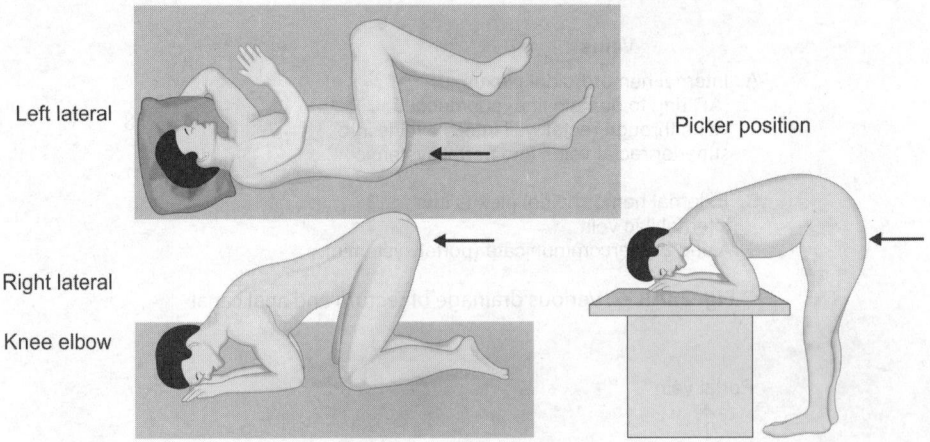

Fig. 28AR-10: Position of patient for rectal examination

Position of Patient for a Per Rectal Digital Examination and Proctoscopy

- Left lateral
- Right lateral
- Dorsal
- Knee elbow
- Lithotomy
- "Picker".

Digital Examination of Rectum

Refer **Fig. 28AR-12**.

> **Q.** Describe embryology of anal canal and classify ano rectal anomalies.

Anorectal Anomalies (Refer Figures 28AR-13 and 28AR-14)

Refer Embryology of Anal Canal and Rectum

PUBORECTALIS SLING OF LEVATOR ANI IS THE KEY TO CONTINENCE

High Anorectal Anomalies

High: Rectum Ends above Puborectalis Sling

- Anorectal Agenesis
  - Rectovesical/urethral fistula
  - Rectovaginal/uterine fistula
- Rectal agenesis
- Cloaca

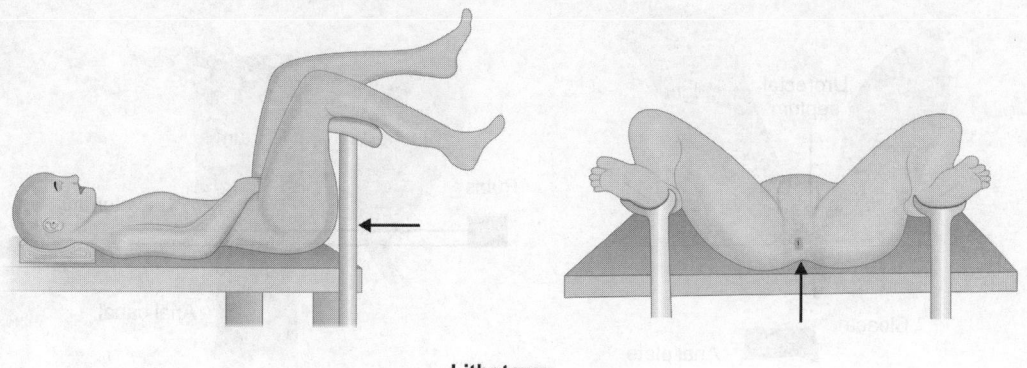

Lithotomy

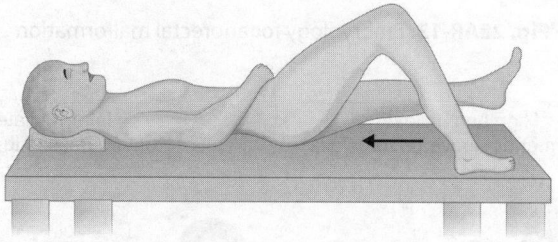

Dorsal

Fig. 28AR-11: Positions for digital examination of rectum

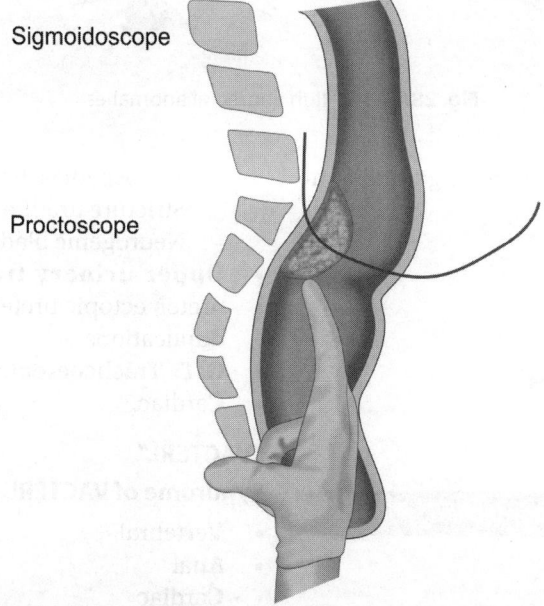

Sigmoidoscope

Proctoscope

Fig. 28AR-12: Digital examination of rectum

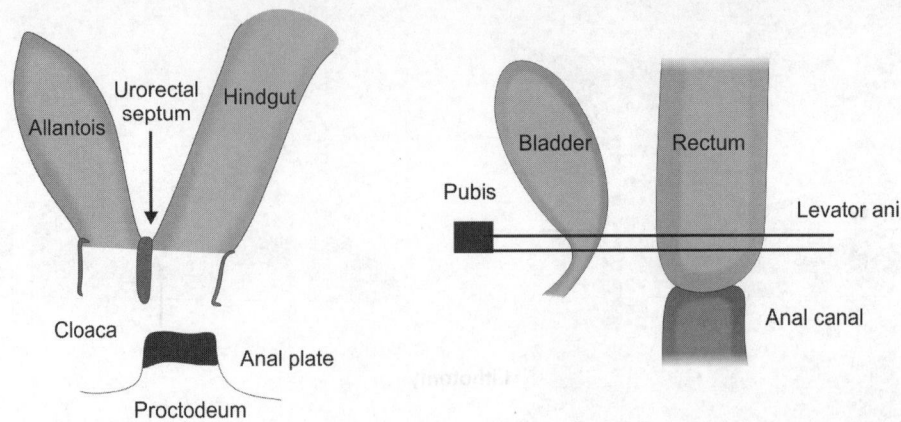

Fig. 28AR-13: Embryology for anorectal malformation

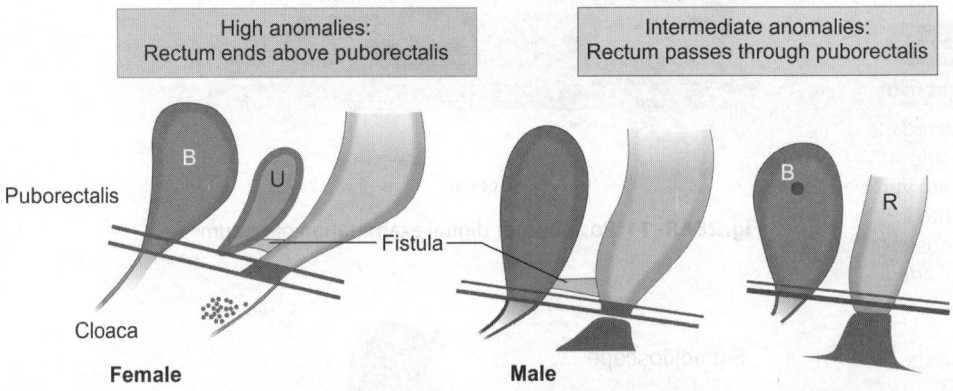

Fig. 28AR-14: High anorectal anomalies.

- Vesicointestinal fissure: Split genitalia, no pubic symphysis.

Low Anomalies

Refer **Figure 28AR-15**.

Low Anorectal Anomalies

Refer **Table 28AR-2**.

Q. What are VACTERL anomalies?

Associated Anomalies

- Sacral agenesis: Partial or complete with or without neurological deficit
- Urological defects
- **Lower urinary tract**
  - Hypospadias; bifid vagina
  - Stricture urethra
  - Neurogenic bladder
- **Upper urinary tract**: Hydronephrosis, ureter, ectopic ureter, cystic kidney, aplasia, duplications
- **GIT**: Tracheoesophageal fistula (TOF)
- Cardiac.

"VACTERL"

Syndrome of VACTERL Anomalies

- Vertebral
- Anal
- Cardiac
- Tracheal
- Esophageal
- Renal
- Limb

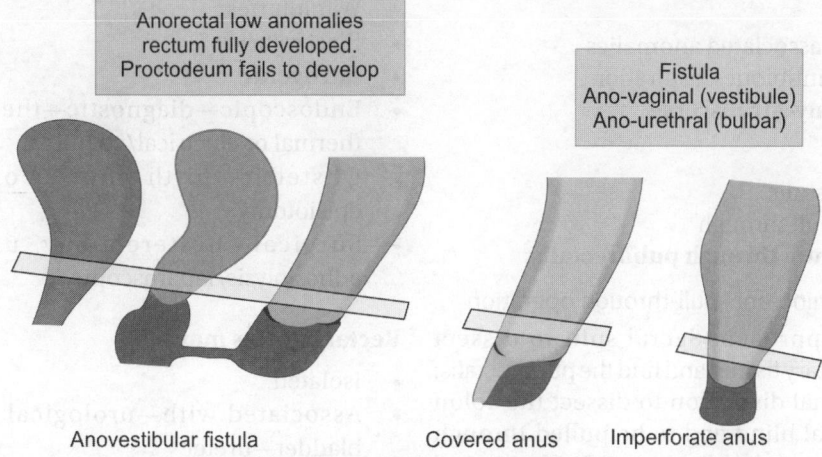

Fig. 28AR-15: Low anal rectal anomalies

Table 28AR-2: Anorectal anomalies.	
Without fistula	**With fistula (commonly intermediate type)**

• Covered anus: Normal anus but a skin cover
• Ectopic anus
   – Into vulva
   – Into vestibule
• Stenosed anus: Partial recanalisation
• Anal agenesis: Failed proctodeum
	• Anorectal stenosis
	• Agenesis with
	   – Rectobulbar fistula
	   – Rectovesical fistula
	   – Rectovaginal fistula/anovaginal fistula

Diagnosis

Failure to pass meconium.

Q. Short note on invertogram.

INVERTOGRAM

Invertogram is used to differentiate high from low anomaly.

- A lateral view X-ray is taken of the baby held inverted, with buttocks pointing uppermost and hips flexed. Air appears in the bowel 6–12 hours after birth and ascends to the upper most part of the patent bowel.
- The pubococcygeal (PC) line is an imaginary line from tip of coccyx to the pubic symphysis drawn (denotes level of puborectalis).
- If air seen seen above the PC line, it denotes a low anomaly.
- An air shadow stopping below the PC line is usually due to a high anomaly.

Further clarification is obtained by injecting a radiopaque dye through anal membrane to delineate any fistula.

Counting of Sacral Vertebrae

- 5 vertebrae are normally seen at birth
- < 4 segments at birth—abnormal
- < 3—risk of neurogenic bladder.

CT scan helps in assessment
MRI to study puborectalis.

Treatment

Low Anorectal Anomalies

- Stenosis: Dilate/anoplasty
- Ectopic anus: "Cut-back" operation
- Membrane: Divide/rupture
- Fistula: Correction of fistula—anal approach usually.

High Anorectal Anomalies

Aim: Ensure a continent passage.

Stage I
- Look for associated anomalies
- Airway, antibiotics, aspiration
- **Colostomy—transverse**.

Stage II
- Divide fistula
- Rectal "pull through"
  Pull rectum through puborectalis.

Sacro-abdomino-anal pull-through operation
- Sacral approach: Sacral split to dissect rudimentary tissues and find the puborectalis;
- Abdominal dissection to dissect the colon and rectal blind end to be pulled through the puborectalis, divide any fistula (vesical or uterine).
- **Anal phase—dissect through the perineum and create the anal canal**
  - Pull the Rectal stump through the pubo rectalis sling into the "new anus".

Stage III
- **Close colostomy**
- Tackle associated anomalies.

> **Q. Short note on sacrococcygeal teratoma.**

- From primitive knot (of notochord), as a tumor between rectum and the sacrum.
- Seen in infants ages below 3 months, affecting more males than females.
- High potential to turn malignant
- Ulceration/infarction/obstruction-rectum/urinary tract
- D/D: Post-anal dermoid
- Sacral chordoma
- Treatment: Removal without delay.

RECTAL INJURIES
Mechanism of Rectal Injuries
- Fall on perineum
- Penetrating
- War injuries
- Blast injuries
- **Iatrogenic**
- Endoscopic—diagnostic—therapeutic—thermal or electrical/chemical
- Obstetric—birth injuries or forceps, episiotomy
- Surgical—hysterectomy, urological, adhesiolysis, laparoscopic.

Rectal injuries may be
- Isolated
- Associated with—urological injuries—bladder—ureter
- Associated gynaecological injuries
- With hemorrhagic shock
- Other injuries.

Rectal Injuries: General Approach
- General—follow advanced trauma life support (ATLS) guidelines—airway, breathing, circulation (ABC) of trauma
- Look for shock and treat—resuscitation
- Look for associated injuries—attend
- Rectal injury: Laparotomy, suture defunctioning colostomy
- Perineal Injury: Debride, pack drain
- Delayed re-look and definitive repair
- Colostomy closure.

Iatrogenic Injuries
Prepared bowel—simple injuries
- Suture close
- Ensure liquid stools with laxatives.

Complex lacerations unprepared bowel?
- Suture laceration
- Defunctioning colostomy and peritoneal drainage
- Closure of colostomy after 3 months.

28.6: Tumors of Colon, Rectum and Anal Canal

TUMORS OF LARGE INTESTINE

> SU 28.16 to SU 28.18: Colorectal cancers: Colon and rectum and anal canal.

TUMORS OF LARGE INTESTINE
Refer **Table 28C-6**.

Benign Tumors

Polyps are mucosal protrusions:
- Solitary, multiple—synchronous or or asynchronous, sessile or pedunculated.
- They may be part of a syndrome.

> **Q. Name the types of colonic polyps and their complications.**

Colorectal Polyps (Refer Table 28C-7)
- A polyp is a mass from surface of intestinal epithelium projecting into lumen
- **Neoplastic polyps**
- Familial adenomatous polyposis (FAP)

Malignant—adenocarcinoma and carcinoid tumor

Hamartomatous—low potential for neoplasia juvenile polyposis syndrome (JPS)

Peutz-Jeghers (PJS)—oral pigmentation, bowel polyps

Cronkhite-Canada—polyps, alopecia, cutaneous pigmentation, nail atrophy

Cowden—hamartomas of 3 germ layers-facial trichelemmal swellings, breast cancer, thyroid disease, GI polyps.

Inflammatory
Associated with—inflammatory bowel disease (IBD) amebic, ischemic schistosomal colitis.

Hyperplastic polyps
Usually < 5 mm, non-malignant; but large ones >2 cm may harbour adenomatous tissue and hence turn malignant.

Colorectal adenomatous polyps:
- Sessile type, pedunculated type
- Flat type and serrated type.

Complications
- Bleeding
- Obstruction
- Intussusception
- Malignant transformation.

Table 28C-6: Benign tumors of large intestines.

Non-neoplastic polyps	Neoplastic epithelial polyps	Mesenchymal lesions
• Hyperplastic polyps • Hamartomatous polyps • Juvenile polyps (juvenile polyposis syndrome) • Peutz Jeghers' polyp • Inflammatory polyps • Lymphoid polyps	• Tubular adenoma • Tubulovillous adenoma • Villous adenoma	• Lipoma • Leiomyoma • Neuroma • Angioma • Hemangioma • Lymphangioma

Table 28C-7: Microscopy of colonic polyps.

Microscopic features of polyps	Risk of cancer	
	Type	Size
• Tubular 75%— "berry on a stalk" • Villous 10%—flat spreading, can cause mucus discharge, diarrhea, hypokalemia and hypoalbuminemia • Tubulovillous 15%	• 5% • 40% • 20%	• 5% if < 1 cm • 35% if < 1–2% • 50% if >2 cm

Invasiveness of polyps – Haggitt's levels
0- Ca in situ- above muscularis mucosae
1- Penetrates muscularis mucosae
2- neck of polyp (junction of head to stalk)
3- invades stalk
4 - invades submucosa below stalk

All sessile polyps are level 4.
Level 4 has > 10% risk of lymphatic spread.

Colorectal Polyps: Treatment
- Colonoscopic snare excision for colonic pedunculated polyps.
- Transanal operative excision for rectal polyps.
- Endoscopic mucosal excision for rectal and sigmoid polyps—sessile or flat.

Surgery: Colectomy—sigmoido rectal resection
- Indications—cases with large, flat polyps or failure at attempt of endoscopic snare polypectomy.
- Histologically invasive cancer.

Q. Short note on familial adenomatous polyposis (FAP).

HEREDITARY POLYPOSIS SYNDROMES
Familial Adenomatous Polyposis (FAP)
- **Auto dominant**—polyps in hundreds to thousands >100 are diagnostic of FAP.
- **Attenuated FAP (recessive)**—mainly right side; fewer polyps
- **MYH** mutation—MAP-recessive trait.

Familial adenomatous polyposis (FAP)
- **Autosomal dominant**—polyps in hundreds to thousands
- Lifetime risk of colorectal cancer—100% over 50 years

Mutation in APC gene—on chromosome—5q.

Associated lesions of FAP
- Endodermal: Colorectal carcinoma (CRC), duodenal polyp, small bowel polyps, periampullary carcinoma.
- Ectodermal:
  - Congenital hypertrophy of the retinal pigment epithelium (CHRPE).
  - CNS tumors (Turcot), skin—cysts, tumors
- Mesodermal: Desmoids, mandibular osteoma (gardner).

Age of presentation—usually present by 15 and all by 30 years.
Treatment of FAP is prophylactic surgery.

The aim: To prevent the development of colorectal cancer.

The following are the options:
- **S**ubtotal colectomy with ileorectal anastomosis (IRA);
- **R**estorative proctocolectomy (RPC) with an ileoanal anastomosis (with an ileal pouch (with an ileal pouch)
- **T**otal proctocolectomy and end ileostomy

Follow up—for other tumors and lesions—with surveillance for life.

Q. Write short note on HNPCC syndrome.

Lynch Syndrome
HNPCC: Hereditary non-polyposis colorectal cancer syndrome.
- The most common (2–5%) inherited CRC with Autosomal dominant trait due to germline mutation in DNA mismatch repair (MMR) gene.
- Occurs in early age (40–45 years), often multiple (20%), in common in proximal colon and has a better prognosis.
- Associated with other malignancies: Endometrial/ovarian/pancreas/stomach/biliary/small bowel/urological malignancies.

Amsterdam II: Criteria for HNPCC
- CRC in three I degree relatives with a HNPCC related cancer (colorectal, renal, ureter, endometrial) (modified to include other cancers—see above)
- Involvement of at least 2 generations
- At least one of them is < 50 years at diagnosis
- FAP excluded
- Tumors confirmed by pathological examination.

Treatment—regular endoscopic surveillance. Family members are screened by genetic study of index case and members for the mutated gene.

COLORECTAL CANCERS
Colonic and rectal cancers are considered together.

Q. Briefly outline pathogenesis of colorectal carcinoma.

Advice to reader: Read the summary, "additional reading" is optional to boost knowledge.

Pathogenesis of Colorectal Carcinoma

Summary of genomics in pathogenesis
- Mutations play a major role in causing colorectal carcinoma.
- Major mutations in Tumor suppressor genes, genes repairing replication errors, cause genomic instability and this along with failure of apoptosis lead to genomic uncontrolled proliferation of cancerous cells.

Additional optional reading: Pathogenesis of colorectal carcinoma

1. Genomic Instability
- Micro satellite instability (MSI)
- Chromosomal instability (CIN)—in 85%
- Chromosomal translocation
- Epigenomic instability—aberrant methylation of tumor suppressor genes.

2. Genetic pathways
- Mutations in tumor suppressor genes—APC, DCC, P-53 and t-suppressor, and in K-ras proto-oncogene.
- **LOH** (loss of heterozygosity) pathway
- **APC** tumor suppressor gene mutational defects (FAP).
  - 80% of sporadic cancers—show
  - Polyp formation after mutation of both alleles
- **K-Ras**—proto-oncogene produces G-protein for cellular signal transduction. Binds GTP; hydrolysis of GTP to GDP, inactivates G-protein.
  - Mutation of K-ras results in failure of hydrolysis– G-protein remains in active form in GTP–leads to uncontrolled cell division
- **DCC**—tumor suppressor gene? Cell differentiation—fails after mutation in the T- suppressor gene
- **P-53**
  - **t- suppressor**—initiates apoptosis in cells with genetic damage
  - But mutation leads to **to failed apoptosis**.

3. RER (Replication Error) pathway
- Genes repairing replication errors – hMSH2, hMLH1, hPMS2 hMSH6 mutations in Mismatch repair genes result in accumulation of errors, genomic instability, carcinogenesis.
- Microsatellite instability (MSI) of RER pathway have better prognosis than tumors of LOH—that are MSS (stable).

Q. Short note: Describe the adenoma-carcinoma sequence.

Refer **Table 28C-8** and **Table 28C-9**.

ETIOLOGICAL FACTORS FOR COLORECTAL CARCINOMA

Age—steady increase in risk after 50 years.
Hereditary—20 % of all CRC.
Environment and dietary factors.

Favorable:
- Oleic acid in oils (coconut, olive, fish oil)
- Selenium, Vit A, C, E, carotenoids are protective.

Unfavorable:
- PUFA and SFA are considered as unfavourable.
- Obesity and sedentary style are said to be unfavourable.
  - IBD: Ulcerative colitis and Crohn's disease.
  - Cigarette smoking.

Table 28-C-8: Adenoma-carcinoma sequence.

Adenoma-carcinoma sequence 7–10 years

Normal epithelium

- Hyperplastic epithelium (dysplasia)
- Early adenoma
- Intermediate adenoma
- Late adenoma
- Carcinoma metastases

- 5q loss APC (initiation)
- Altered DNA methylation
- 12p activation K-Ras (promotion)
- 18 q loss DCC
- Malignant conversion (17 p loss p53)

Table 28C-9: Multistep adenoma carcinoma sequence.

Multi-step adenoma to carcinoma sequence

Loss of heterozygosity: LOH and APC mutation	→	Normal ↓ Dysplasia
K-Ras mutation	→	↓ Small adenoma
LOH and DCC mutation	→	↓ Large adenoma
LOH and p53 mutation	→	↓ Carcinoma

Table 28C-10: TNM staging of colorectal carcinoma.

TNM classification of CRC (must read)

Tumor (depth of invasion)	Nodal spread	Metastasis

• T0: Tumor not evident
• TIS: In situ
• T1: Into submucosa
• T2: Muscularis, propria
• T3: Invades through muscularis propria
• T4-A: Penetrating— visceral peritoneum
• T4B: Invades adjacent organs
	• N0: No nodes
	• N1: 1-3 nodes
	  – N1a: 1
	  – N1b: 2–3 nodes
	  – N1c: No node, but surface deposits—wall or mesentery
	• N2–4 or more positive
	  – N2a: 4 to 6 nodes
	  – N2b: 7 or more nodes
		• M0 - No Metastases
		• M1: Metastases present
		• M1a: One site/organ
		• M1b: 2 or more site/organs
		• M1c: Peritoneal/serosal spread with or without other organs

Stage AJCC	Mod. Astler Coller	Depth of invasion T0 –tumor not evident TIS - In situ	Nodal status	Metastases
I	A	T-1, T-2	N0	M0
II	B	T-3, T-4	N0	M0
III	C	Any T	N1–2 a, b	M0
IV		Any T	Any N	M 1 a, b, c

Note: The above is abridged version of AJCC staging: Substaging of each of the stages II, III and IV into a, b and c is not described here.

- Urinary diversion into sigmoid (uretero sigmoidostomy).
- Acromegaly (high GH levels).
- Pelvic irradiation.

Q. Staging of colorectal cancers.

TNM staging is followed, but Duke's and Astler Coller staging also compared here for exam purpose.

SPREAD OF COLORECTAL CARCINOMA

Refer **Table 28C-10, Figure 28C-2.**
- **Direct spread in the bowel wall or to adjacent organs.**
  - In bowel wall
    - Circumferential *"around"*
    - Longitudinal (submucous): *"Along"*
    - Through (deep): "Across" The Wall
    - Through lumen: Seedling

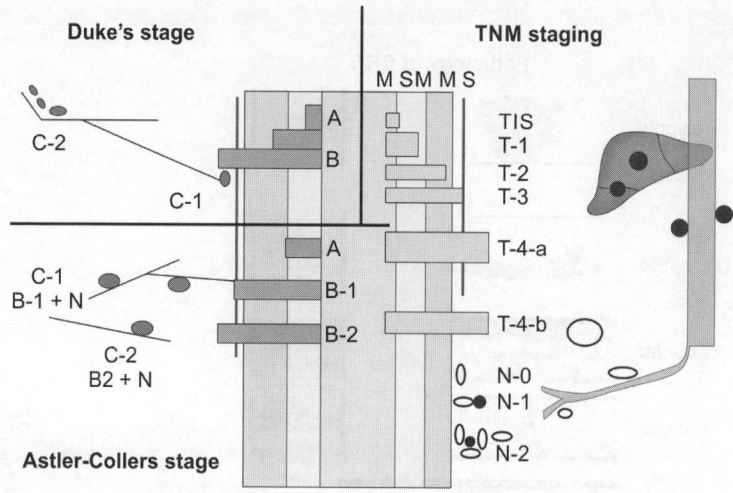

Fig. 28C-2: Staging of colorectal carcinoma: Dukes/Astler-Coller and TNM staging.

Table 28C-11: Comparison of Dukes, Astler Colle and TNM classification of CRC.			
	Duke's	Compared to TNM	Astler-Coller's
Tumor in bowel wall	A	Tumor (T1-2) In muscularis tumor Upto serosa (T3)	A B1
Tumor beyond bowel wall	B	Tumor beyond serosa/(T4a) Adjacent structure /organ(T 4b)	B2
Pericolic nodes	C-1	B-I + Lymph nodes involved	C1
Nodes along vessels	C-2	B-2 + Lymph nodes	C2

- **Lymphatic**—epicolic, paracolic intermediate and central nodes.
- **Transperitoneal**—mesentery, omentum, peritoneal membrane—diaphragm to pelvis.
- **Blood spread**—portal vein—liver.

Duke's v/s Astler-Coller's Staging of Colorectal Cancers

Refer **Table 28C-11**.

Pathology of Colorectal Carcinoma

Refer **Figure 28C-3**.

Incidence and Distribution of CRC

Refer **Figure 28C-4**.

Q. Describe the pathology of colorectal malignancies.

Depicted in page 90 Figure 28C-5A to F.

Macroscopic types of colorectal carcinoma

- Polypoid growth—common in rectum and cecum.
- Ulcerative—mostly in cecum, also seen in rectum, ascending colon.
- Tubular—common in descending colon, rectum rectosigmoid area.
- Annular (napkin ring)—most common in sigmoid and descending colon
- Diffuse infiltrative (linitis like)—cecum, rectum.
- Synchronous multiple growths—mostly associated with HNPCC syndrome.

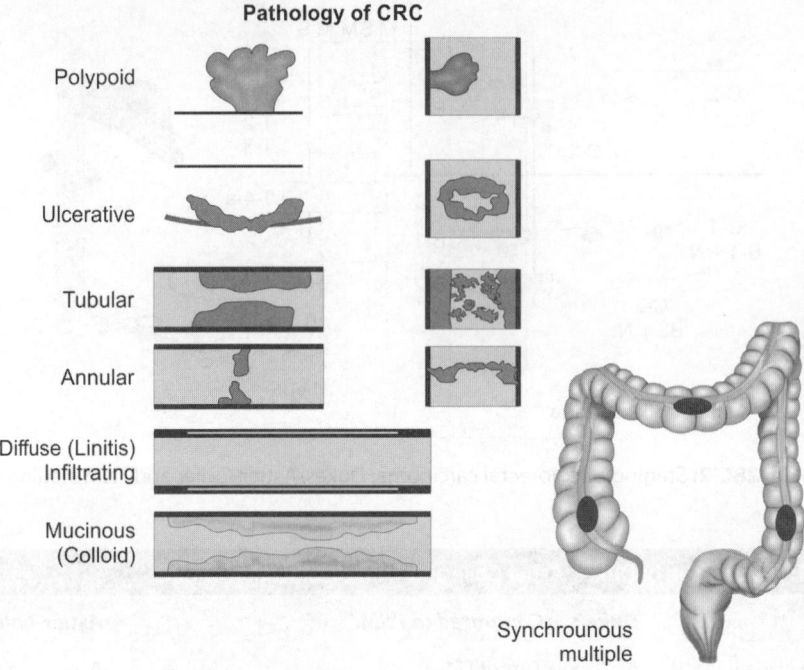

Fig. 28C-3: Macroscopic types of colorectal carcinoma

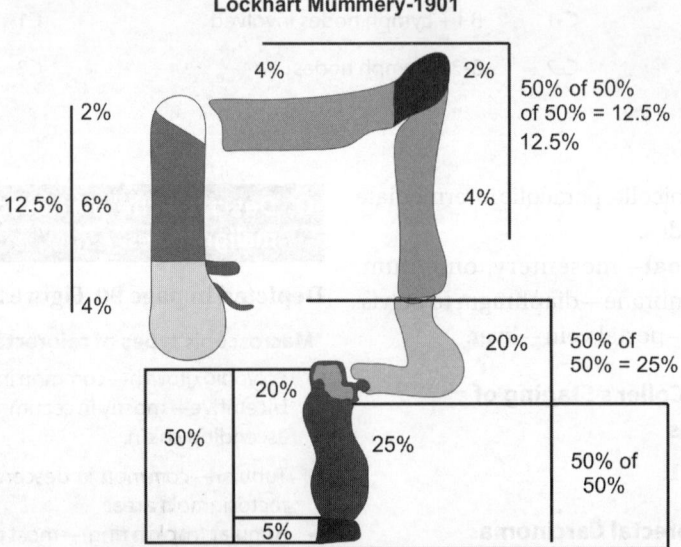

Fig. 28C-4: Distributon of colorectal cancers

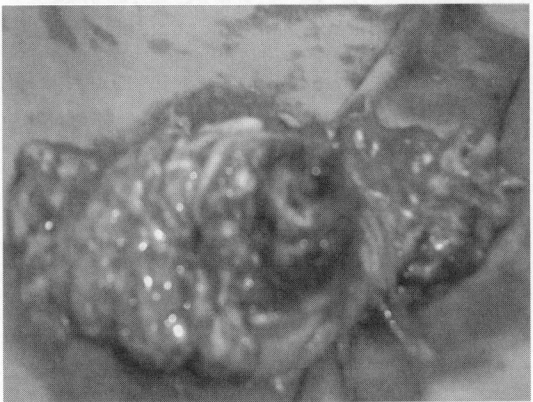

Fig. 28C-5A: Polypoid colonic carcinoma.
(For color version see Plate 3)

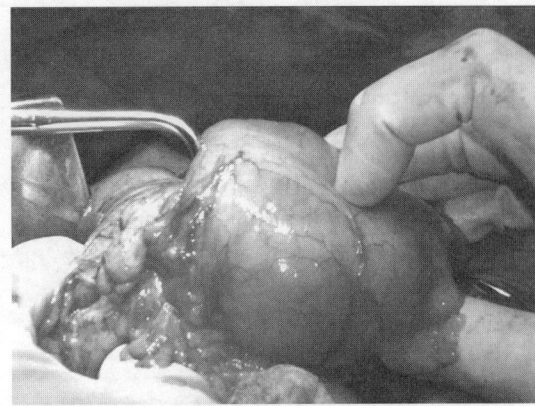

Fig. 28C-5B: Intussusception.
(For color version see Plate 3)

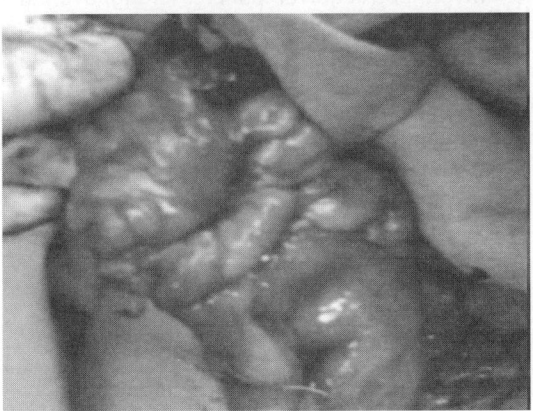

Fig. 28C-5C: Annular sigmoid carcinoma.
(For color version see Plate 3)

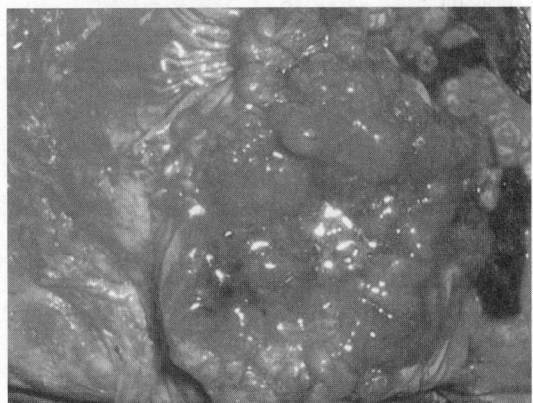

Fig. 28C-5D: Ulcerative carcinoma cecum.
(For color version see Plate 3)

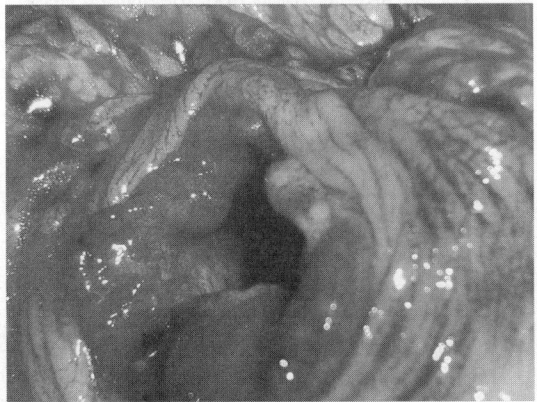

Fig. 28C-5E: Annular carcinoma descending colon.
(For color version see Plate 3)

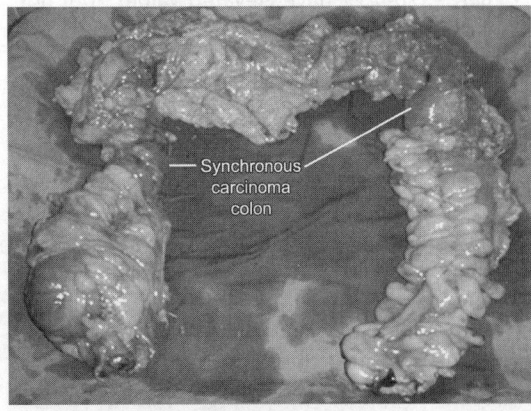

Fig. 28C-5F: Synchronous carcinoma ascending and descending colon.
(For color version see Plate 3)

Histopathology: CRC

Epithelial:
- **Adenocarcinoma:** Broder's types
  - Well differentiated
  - Moderately differentiated
  - Poorly differentiated.
- Mucinous (colloid)—signet ring cells pseudo mucin.
- Squamous cell carcinoma—anal canal

From muscle/stroma
- Gastrointestinal stromal tumors (GISTs)
- Leiomyosarcoma

Melanoma
- Lymphoma (extremely rare)

Secondary carcinomas—spreading from urogenital.

Note: Colonic carcinoma and rectal carcinoma are discussed separately from here.

Q. Describe complications, clinical diagnosis and treatment of colonic carcinoma.

Complications, Clinical Diagnosis and Treatment of Colonic Carcinoma

Refer **Table 28C-12**.

CRC—investigations
Proctoscopy/ sigmoidoscopy/colonoscopy—biopsy
• Blood examination
• For anemia
• CEA – (70–75% have elevated value) - but not diagnostic
• Normal upto 3.5–4 units/mL
• Raised levels indicative but may also be raised in carcinoma pancreas, stomach and cholangio-carcinoma
– Mainly prognostic, for follow up to detect recurrence/metastases
• Ultrasonography—abdomen
• Transrectal ultrasonography (TRUS)—in rectal cancer
• Endoscopic ultrasound (EUS)—staging T and N
• CECT—abdomen/chest ;and PET CT for metastatic work up and follow up
• MRI—to assess pelvic floor muscles and recurrences/response to irradiation
• CT—colonography/MR-colonography (virtual c-scopy)
• Chest—X-ray
• PET—(FDG enhanced)—to detect invisible tumor recurrence and metastases.
• Barium enema – double contrast.

Q. Short notes on carcinoma embryonic antigen (CEA)

- Carcinoembryonic antigen (CEA) is a glycoprotein found normally in of embryonic endodermal epithelium. Serum levels in normal adults are 0–3 ng/mL (upto 5 in smokers). It is increased in cancers and non-malignant conditions too.
- Increased levels are seen in patients with 75% of colorectal cancers; (also in carcinomas of stomach, intestinal tract, liver, pancreas, lung, ovarian, breast, prostate and medullary thyroid carcinoma).
- It is not diagnostic and not specific of a colorectal carcinoma.
- It is used for monitoring of those with elevated pre-treatment levels, after therapy
- To monitor response to therapy and to detect early recurrence.

Q. Principles of surgery in carcinoma colon.

SURGERY FOR COLONIC CARCINOMA

Surgical principles in colonic carcinoma
- Radical segmental colectomies (lympho vascular units)
  - The length of resected colonic segment bearing the cancer is determined by the extent of colonic arterial supply from the divided vessel of "lymphovascular field"
  - The carcinoma with colonic segment, nodes along the artery, omentum are resected.
- Total colectomy with ileorectal/anal anastomosis
  - For hereditary/familial cancers
  - Multiple polyps with cancer
  - Synchronous cancers
  - Metachronous cancers in patients on follow up
- Palliative surgery: Segmental resection
  - Omentectomy
  - Ileo-transverse/sigmoid bypass
  - Proximal colostomy/ileostomy
- **Metastasectomy**
  - Hepatic lobectomy
  - Lung resections

Table 28C-12: Complications, clinical diagnosis and treatment of colonic carcinoma.

Complications of colonic carcinoma
- Bleeding
- Obstruction
- Intussusception
- Volvulus (rare)
- Perforation—peritonitis
- Peri colic abscess
- Internal fistula: Gastrocolic, colovesical

Clinical Features of Colonic carcinoma

Symptoms depend on site and type of growth.

Generally:
- Left-sided growths are annular (napkin ring)
- Right-sided growth are ulcerative/ proliferative
- Rectal growths are proliferative or tubular

• Bleeding
  – Hematochezia
  – Occult—secondary anemia
• Obstructive
  – Progressive constipation—may be alternating with diarrhea
  – Acute obstruction
  – Acute intussusception
  – Volvulus
	• Abdominal mass: Features due to local spread
	  – Ureteric obstruction
	  – Fistula – anorectic/anal, internal (colovesical/rectovaginal)
	• Metastatic features
	  – Para aortic nodes, omental mass, liver nodules, ascites
	  – Skin nodules: Lung, brain, bone deposits

Differential diagnosis of carcinoma colon

• Mass abdomen • Appendix mass • Pericolic abscess • Lymphoma/TB • Hematochezia • Ischemic colitis • Crohn's/ ulcerative colitis • Differential diagnosis of anemia	• Intestinal obstruction • Pseudo obstruction • Volvulus/Intussusception. • Ascites • Other causes of ascites. • Hepatomegaly

Colonic Resections (Refer Figure 28C-6)

Specific Resections

Right colonic growth—radical right hemicolectomy
- Terminal ileum—20–30 cm, cecum, ascending colon and the proximal 2/3s of transverse colon (supplied by middle colic artery)
- Arteries ligated: Ileo-colic, right colic and right branch of middle colic artery
- The root of middle colic artery is ligated in growth of hepatic flexure.

Carcinoma of transverse colon

Radical—extended right hemicolectomy

Right hemicolectomy + transverse colectomy

Carcinoma of descending colon or left colic flexure
- Radical left hemicolectomy is performed
- Arteries ligated: Left branch of middle colic
- Ascending branch of left colic
- Upper one or two sigmoid branches of left colic

Carcinoma of sigmoid colon: Sigmoid colectomy
- All sigmoidal branches are ligated at their origin from left colic and inferior mesenteric artery.

Surgical palliation of colonic cancer
- Palliative resection—of primary
- Debulking of primary/omentectomy
- Metastasectomy (hepatic lobectomy)
- Release of obstruction
- Ilio-transverse or sigmoid by pass/proximal
  – Colostomy/ileostomy
- Resection after angiographic embolisation

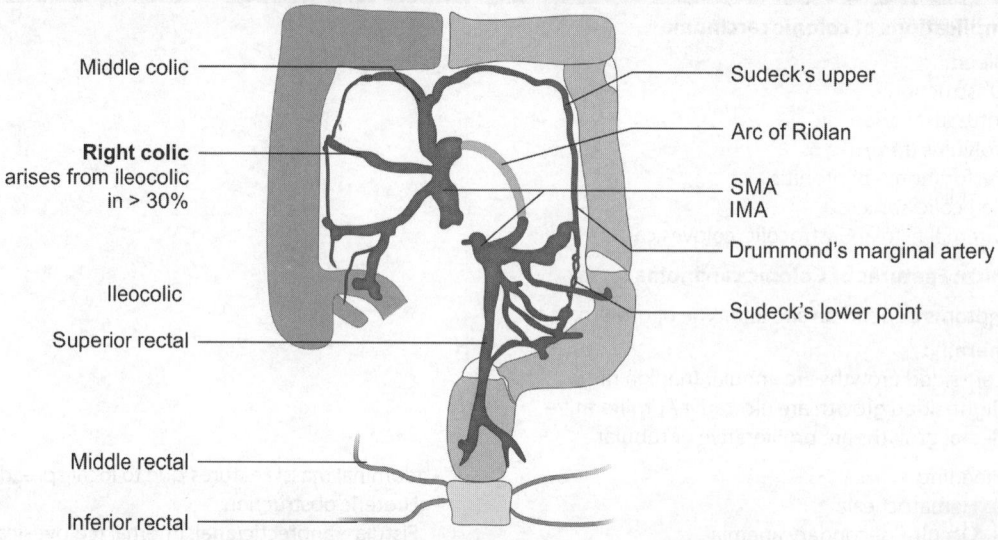

Fig. 28C-6: Applied arterial anatomy in colorectal resections
(SMA: superior mesenteric artery; IMA: inferior mesenteric artery)

Non surgical palliation of colonic cancer

Q. Non-surgical palliation of colonic cancer.

Endoscopic palliation

- For obstruction
  - Stenting: Self-expanding metallic stents—successful in transverse, descending, sigmoid and rectosigmoid junction.
  - **Laser** coring of primary tumor and recanalization.
- For bleeding
  - Endoscopic coagulation: Photodynamic or laser
  - Angiographic embolization
- For metastases
  Liver mets: Radio frequency ablation RFA
  - Of liver metastases if < 3 cm, accessible
  - Cyber knife for liver/lung metastases
  - Transarterial chemoembolization (TACE) (chemotherapy)
  - Transarterial radioembolization (TARE)
  Pleural Effusion: Pleurodesis
  Cerebral metastases: Radiotherapy
  Pathological fractures: Chemo/radiotherapy + fixation
- **Targeted biotherapy**
  - Monoclonal antibodies: Bevacizumab, cetuximab.

CARCINOMA RECTUM

Refer **Table 28C-13**
Refer previous section for etiopathogenesis and pathology of colorectal cancers.

Q. Stage carcinoma rectum (refer previous section) and complications.

Q. Describe lymphatic drainage of rectum with reference to carcinoma rectum.

RECTAL LYMPHATICS (REFER FIGURE 28C-7)

Q. Principles of treatment of rectal carcinoma.

Treatment of Rectal Carcinoma: Must know

- Surgery is the mainstay
- Chemotherapy and radiotherapy are adjuncts—as adjuvant or neoadjuvant
- Targeted biotherapy—for metastatic disease (anti VEGF, EGFR monoclonal antibodies.

Surgery for carcinoma rectum

Intent

- **Curative:** It may be
  - **Conservative** (for local early cancer)
  - **Radical** (for locoregional cancer)
- **Cytoreductive**
- **Palliative.**

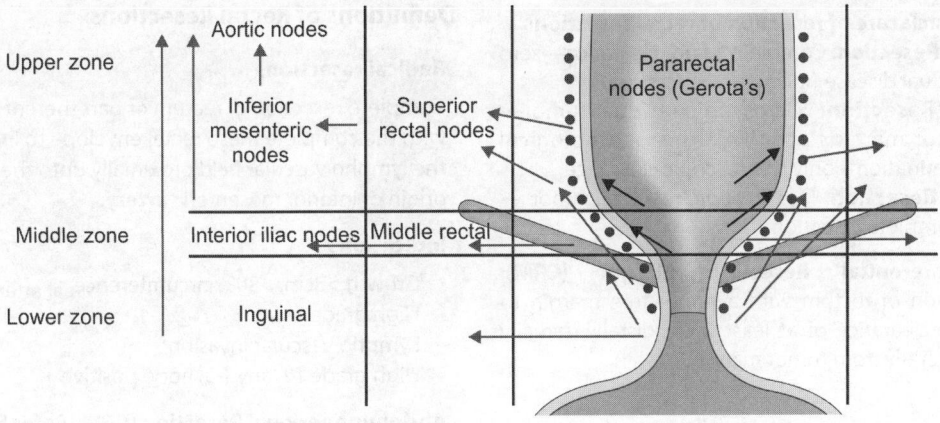

Fig. 28C-7: Rectal lymphatics with reference to rectal carcinoma

Table 28C-13: Complications, clinical features and differential diagnosis of rectal carcinoma.

Complications of rectal carcinoma
- Perforation
- Hemorrhage
- Secondary hemorrhoids
- Fistulation: Rectovaginal/urethral/vesical peri anal/ perineal
- Obstruction: Rectal/ureteric infiltration into sacral plexus

Clinical features:–CA-rectum
- **Bleed** – fresh /dark - rectum/anal
- Obstructive symptoms
  - Altered bowel habit
  - Recent or progressive constipation
  - Intestinal obstruction—obstipation
- Irritative symptoms
  - Incomplete defecation
  - Tenesmus (similar to strangury)
  - Early morning spurious diarrhea)
- Symptoms of spread
  - **Pain** – sacral plexus/anal canal
  - **Dysuria** – anterior spread to urethra/ bladder
- Digital rectal examination: Approx 90% are palpable with in 10 cms of anal
  - Verge; finger stained with mucus and blood

Differential diagnosis of carcinoma rectum
- Hemorrhoids
- Fissure
- Ulcerative colitis/Crohn's
- Tuberculosis
- Benign tumours
- Amebic granulomas
- Carcinoma colon

Investigations (Refer Colonic Carcinoma)
Proctoscopy, sigmoidoscopy
- CECT - for staging; MRI of pelvis to study pelvic floor invasion.
- Ultrasonography - for preliminary evaluation of abdomen (nodes and liver in particularly)
- TRUS - for evaluation of T1 T2 lesions and peri rectal nodes
- FDG - PET - for metastases
- Serum CEA

Nomenclature of resection of rectal resections

- **R-0 Resection:** Complete tumor clearance—zero residual disease (macro and microscopic)
- **R-1 Resection:** Microscopic residual tumor—tumor margins positive at histopathological examination – only macroscopic clearance
- **R-2 Resection:** Macroscopic residual tumor — incomplete resection.

Circumferential Resection Margin (CRM): Resection of rectum with a tumor free margin to ensure clearance of at least 2 cm distally, radially and laterally from tumor margin.

Summary of treatment of carcinoma rectum: Stagewise (AJCC)—Must Read

Stage I

T1-low Gr, <3 cm, < 1/3 of circ. - ESMR: Endoscopic submucosal resection.

T2-N0-low Gr: Local wide resection of rectal wall with 1 cm margin.

TAMIS: Trans anal minimally invasive surgical resection of rectal wall and mesorectum.

Stage I High Gr or T2, T3 low gr -N0/ N1: Radical rectal resection is must.

Rectum full or part with meserectal envelope (contains nodes and fat)

The selection of surgical procedure is decided by site and grade of growth. Please refer **Table 28C-14** given.

T4, T3 high grade, N2

Neo adjuvant chemoradiation (NACT/RT) followed by **Radical surgery—LAR or APR**

T4b-NACT/RT—followed by cytoreductive resection followed by adjuvant therapy.

Definitions of Rectal Resections

Radical resections

Complete resection of rectum or part thereof along with the complete meso rectal envelope to include the lympho vascular field proximally upto the origin of inferior mesenteric **artery.**

Indications

- Growth >3cm, >30% circumference
- High grade
- Lympho vascular invasion
- High grade T2, any T-3, node positive +

Abdominoperineal Resection (APR) (Refer Figure 28C-8)

- Anal sphincters sacrificed
- Abdominal and perineal mobilisation with resection
- Permanent colostomy

Transabdominal restorative resections (anterior resection)

Here rectum is resected and bowel continuity restored by suturing the proximal colon to rectal stump. The patient is continent for feces.

Types

- High and low/ultra low. High anterior resection (HAR)—rectum divided above peritoneal reflexion (upper half)
- Low anterior resection (LAR)—rectum divided below peritoneal reflexion (lower third)

Anterior resection (**LLAR**—low low - anterior resection)—total mesorectal excision (**TME**) with colo-anal anastomosis (**CAA**).

Rectum is divided below below the levator ani, leaving the external anal sphincters intact. Hence the patient is partly continent.

Table 28C-14: Surgical procedure in rectal carcinoma— T1 high gr, T2, T3 /No-N1.

	Low grade (margin 2 cm)	*High grade (margin 5 + cm)*
Upper 1/3	LAR	LAR
Middle 1/3	LAR St III- NACTRT + LAR	St I, II-LAR ST IIIA- NACTRT + LAR St IIIB, NACTRT -APR
Lower 1/3—upper half Lower of lower 1/3	TME/CAA APR	APR

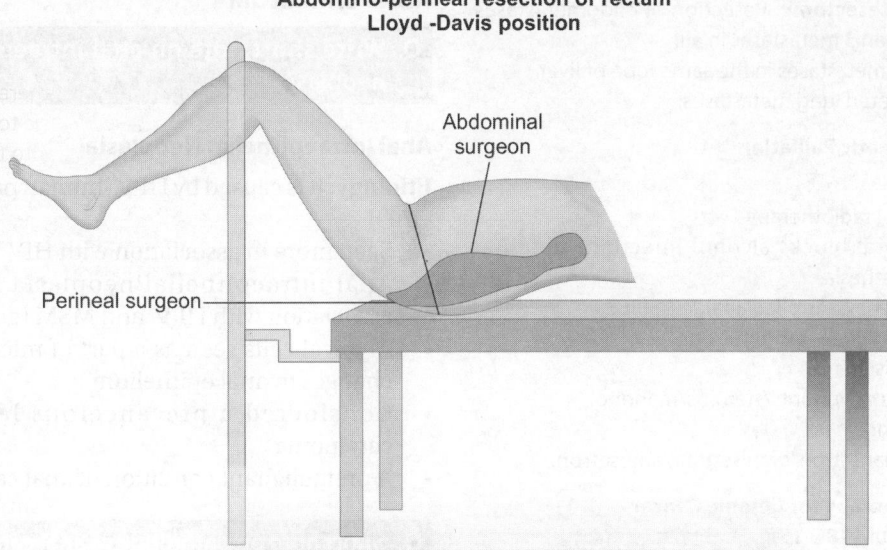

Fig. 28C-8: Abdomino-perineal resection of rectum.

TAMIS (trans anal minimally invasive surgery): Through a single port

Transanal resection of rectal wall and mesorectum for nodal clearance) for T1/T2 lesions <3 cm and less than a third of rectal circumference

Super Radical Options
- Resections with regional "add on"
- APR—with pan hysterectomy
- APR with metastasectomy for oligo metastases
  - Hepatic lobectomy—right or left
- APR—with cystectomy/ureteric reimplantation

Pelvic excenteration—Brunschwig's operation.

Recommended for additional reading.

Operative Approach to Restorative Rectal Resections

- Trans abdominal
- Abdomino-sacral
- Transphincteric
- Abdomino-anal pull-through.

Curative—local/conservative rectal resections

Indications for conservative resections (curative)

- Growth < 3cm size
- Within 8 cm of anus
- Involves less than 30% circumference
- Stage: T-1, T-2
- Histologically low grade.

Procedure

The lesion is resected with + 1 cm margins along with full thickness of rectal wall.

Approach for local resections:

- Trans anal (Park's)
- Trans sphincteric (York-Mason)—post anal approach through the sphincters.
- Trans sacral (Kraske') - splits the sacrum and coccyx.
- Endo—anal pull-through and resection (CV Mann).
- ESMR—endoscopic submucosal resection—for rectal and recto sigmoid lesions—T1.
- TAMIS—treansanal minimally invasive surgical resection with mesorectal excision.

Transanal Endoscopic Microsurgery (TEM)

- For T-1 growth above 13 cm from anus, (high rectal; Recto Sigmoid junction, distal sigmoid)

Q. Principles of palliative surgical and non-surgical treatment carcinoma rectum.

Palliative surgery—rectal cancer

- Resection (R-2) with proximal colostomy
- Hartmann's operation
  - Division of the sigmoid: Closure of the distal rectal stump, left in the pelvis
  - Proximal colostomy.
- Colostomy only
- Omentectomy

- **Metastesectomy:** Resection of oligometastases (less than 3 metastases in all)
  - < 3 metastases in the same lobe of liver.
  - Isolated lung metastases.

Symptomatic Palliation

- Pain
  - Local radiotherapy
  - Neural blocks alcohol injections epidural anesthesia.
  - Patient-controlled analgesia (PCA)
  - Morphine—tab/infusions
- Convulsions
  - Anticonvulsants/steroids/mannitol
- Vomiting
  - Ondansetron/granisetron/ramosetron.

Chemotherapy for Colonic Cancer (Refer Table 28C-15)

Chemo radiation for rectal cancer

Table 28C-15: Chemo-radiation for rectal cancer.

Adjuvant	Neoadjuvant (preoperative)
• For T3, T4 (St II/ Astler-Coller- B-2) • For node positive (St. III/ Astler Coller - C) • For high grade • For M-I—metastatic disease	• T4 - all tumors • T3 high grade (?) • Locally non resectable • Prior to cytoreduction

Chemotherapy regimens: Reduce/prevent local recurrences/metastases

- 5-FU+ LV+ Oxaliplatin (FOLFOX) - FOLFOX 6 regimen
- 5-FU+ LV + Irinotican (FOLFIRI
- 5- Fluorouracil (5-FU):
- (1) Oral Capecitabine; (2) 5- FU + Levamisole; (3) 5-FU+ Leukovorin

Targeted therapy: Gives survival advantage in metastatic disease with/without chemotherapy:
- VEGF inhibitors: Bevacizumab, Ramucirumab
- EGFR inhibitors: Cetuximab, (if mutantion negative for BRAF and KRAS)
- Kinase inhibitors: BRAF inhibitors: Encorafenib.

ANAL CARCINOMA

> Q. Write short note on anal intraepithelial neoplasia.

Anal Intraepithelial Neoplasia

Etiology: It is caused by HPV (human papilloma virus)
- Seen more in association with HIV
- Anal intraepithelial neoplasia (AIN)—association with HPV and MSM (gay)
- Atypical cells seen as a part of microscopic changes in anal epithelium
- Considered a precancerous lesion of carcinoma
- A premalignant condition of anal cancer.

> Q. Short note on pathology of anal cancer and treatment of anal carcinoma.

Pathology of Anal Cancers

- Squamous cell carcinoma (SCC)
- Transitional
- Glandular (adenocarcinoma)
- Melanoma.

Anal Carcinoma

- Origin from anal epithelium—squamous cell carcinoma
- Lymphatic spread: To inguinal and iliac nodes
- Painful lesions.

Treatment

It is mainly chemo radiation (CT-RT).

Surgery: The following are the procedures performed after chemo radiation.
- Post CTRT—wide excision + bilateral ilioinguinal lymph node dissection.
- Colostomy for obstruction
- APR (abdominoperineal resection of anorectum with permanent pelvic colostomy) after chemoradiotherapy.

ANAL CANAL

> SU 28.17–18: Anorectal suppurations: Abscesses and fistulae.

ETIOLOGY AND PATHOGENESIS OF ANORECTAL ABSCESSES

Anorectal Abscess (Refer Table R-1)

> Q. Etiology and pathogenesis of anorectal abscesses; write a note on cryptoglandular sepsis.

ETIOLOGY OF ANORECTAL ABSCESSES

Table R-1: Etiology of anorectal abscess.

Cryptoglandular abscess (non-specific)	Predisposing causes
• Cause not seen—80% • Cause seen—20% • Sepsis through anal fissure • Anal lining tear during defecation • Sepsis from thrombosed prolapsed piles • After sclerosant injection • Post hemorrhoidectomy	• Septicemia/bacteremia • Diabetes mellitus • Leukemia • Immunosuppression • HIV
Specific abscess • Crohn's • Ulcerative colitis • Tuberculosis	

PATHOGENESIS: ANORECTAL ABSCESS
Theory of Cryptoglandular Sepsis

- Infection from anal crypt spreads to anal gland causing suppuration and spread of sepsis along intersphincteric space.
- Then to other perianal spaces.

Specific abscesses result from disease process and secondary sepsis.

- Pelvic/intraperitoneal sepsis causes supralevator sepsis.

> Q. Classify anorectal abscesses; discuss pathology and clinical features of anorectal abscesses.

Anatomical Classification of Anorectal Abscesses

Refer **Figure 28R-1**.

Types of Anorectal abscesses

- Perianal—60%
- Ischiorectal—30%
- Intersphincteric—5% high and low (above dentate line or below dentate line)
- Sub mucous
- Sub cutaneous
- Pelvirectal (suprelevator).

Pelvirectal: Secondary to Pelvic Sepsis

- Salpingitis
- Peridiverticular abscess
- Rectal injuries.

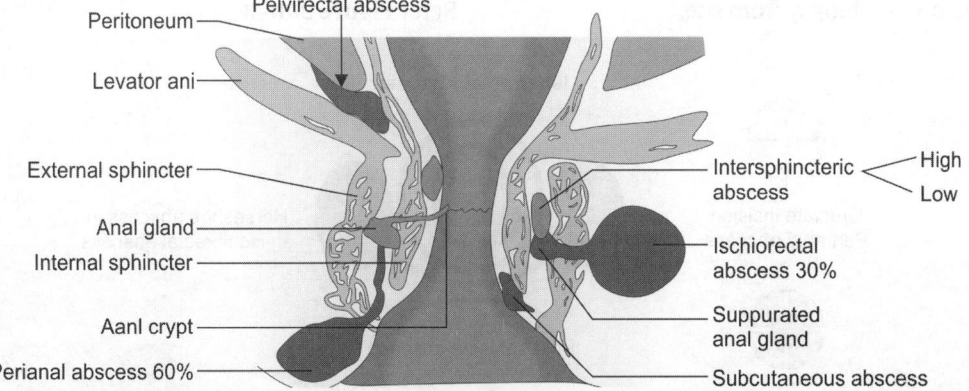

Fig. 28R-1: Anorectal abscesses:

Complications

- Rupture
  - Into anus
  - Outside
- Fistula in ano
- **Ischio rectal**—spread to opposite side— through post sphincteric space (**horse shoe abscess**)
- Pelvi rectal - peritonitis
- Septicemia
- Portal pyemia.

Clinical Features and Differential Diagnosis

- Throbbing pain
- Fever with chills
- Features of sepsis
- Thrombosed external piles
- Carcinoma anus
- Condyloma lata.

> Q. Investigations and treatment of perianal and ischiorectal abscesses.

Investigations

- General health indices
  - For example: Hb%, WBC counts, renal function
  - HIV
  - Diabetes
  - Immunosuppression.
- Ultrasound
- Transrectal ultrasound (TRUS)
- CT scan
- MRI
- Specific - diseases?- tuberculosis or Crohn's—biopsy from site.

Treatment of Anorectal Abscess (Refer Figure 28R-2)

Antibiotic/analgesic
Drain the abscess early
Wound care

Perianal abscess: Cruciate incision over the abscess, drain all pus and trim the skin edges.

Ischiorectal—treated in 2 stages:

- Acute stage: Cruciate incision, drain the pus and break the septa.
  - Excise skin over the ischiorectal fossa
- Later - after 3–5 days - It is re explored and a search is specifically carried out for a fistula in ano, which can be tackled.

ANORECTAL FISTULA

> Q. Describe etiology and classifications of anorectal fistulae.

A track lined by granulation, which opens:
- Externally: In the peri anal and/or perineal skin
- Internally: In anal canal/rectum.

Etiology of Anorectal Fistulae
Refer **Table 28R-2**.

Milligan Morgan Classification of Anorectal Fistulae

Based on the relationship of level of tract to the ano- rectal ring and dentate line.
(Refer **Table 28R-3**).

Classification of Anorectal Fistulae
Refer **Figure 28R- 3**.

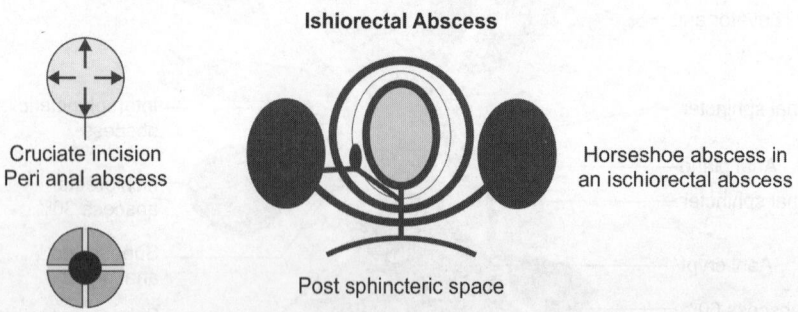

Fig. 28R-2: Drainage of perianal and ischiorectal abscess

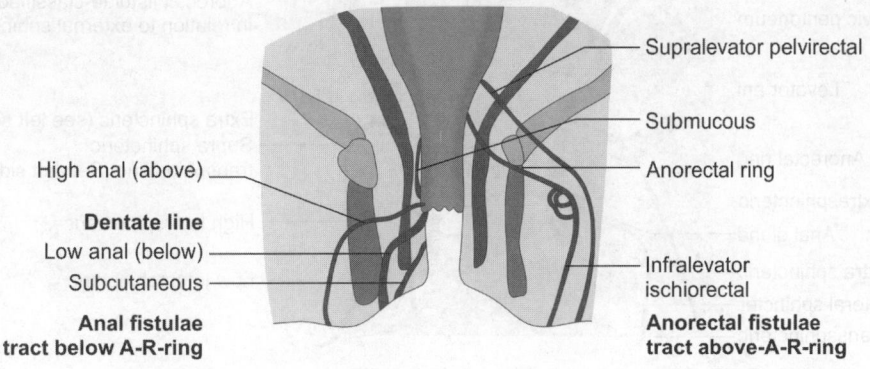

Fig. 28 R-3: Milligan Morgan classification of anorectal fistulae

Park's Classification

- Based on relationship of the fistulous tract to the external anal sphincter
- Based on the theory of crypto glandular origin of all anorectal sepsis:

Table 28R-2: Etiology of ano rectal fistulae.

Cryptoglandular	Secondary/specific
• Following – abscess • Spontaneously ruptured • Inadequate drainage	• Previous surgery • TB/ulcerative colitis/Crohn's • Acute abdominal sepsis **Pelvirectal abscess** • Carcinoma rectum/anus • Actinomycosis • Human immunodeficiency virus (HIV) • Lymphogranuloma venereum (LGV)

Table 28R-3: Milligan Morgan classification of anorectal fistulae.

The tract is above AR ring: Anorectal fistula	Pelvirectal(supralevator) Ischiorectal (infra-levator) Submucous
Replace by a line (to differentiate rectal from anal)	
Fistula tract below AR ring Anal fistula	Tract above dentate line— • High anal
	Tract below dentate line
	Low anal Subcutaneous

- Anorectal sepsis—starts in the intersphincteric space
- Spread of fistulous tract in relation to external sphincter and
- Relation to rectal and anal wall

Park's Classification – Tract Relation to External Sphincter (Refer Figure 28R-4)

Types

- Intersphincteric: High and low
- Transsphincteric
- Suprasphincteric
- Extrasphincteric.

Milligan Morgan classification—refers to level of relation of tract to anus and rectum.

Park's classification—refers to relation to the external sphincter based on crypto glandular abscess concept.

> **Q. Short note on Goodsall's rule.**

GOODSALL'S RULE (REFER FIGURE 28R-5)

- Fistulae with an external opening in front of transverse anal line have a direct tract opening into anal canal.
- Fistulae with an external opening posterior
- to the transverse anal line or beyond 3.5 cm of anus, have a curved tract and internal opening in the posterior midline.

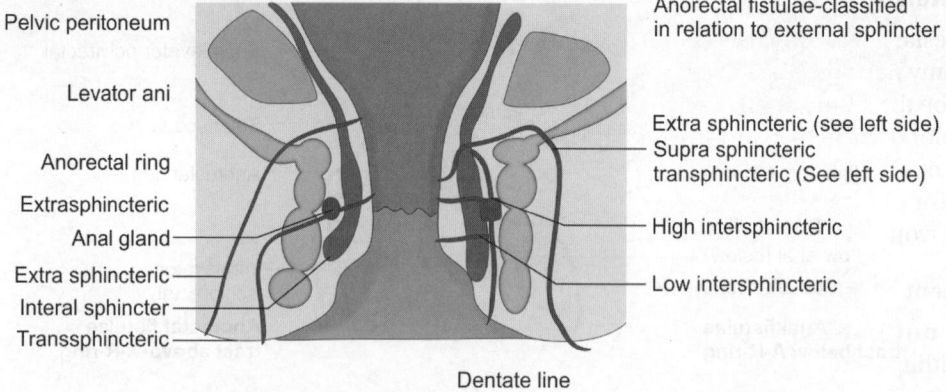

Fig. 28R-4: Park's classification of anorectal fistulae

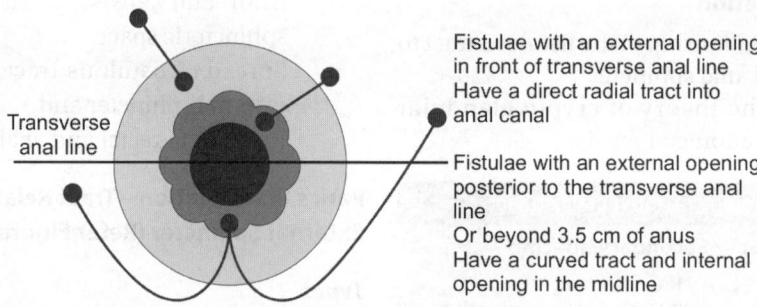

Fig. 28R-5: Goodsall's rule

Q. Enumerate clinical features and complications of anal fistulae.

Clinical Features

- Persistent sero-purulent discharge
- Acute exacerbations of sepsis
- Openings—one/more
- Goodsall's rule—to identify high/low
- Per rectal examination reveals—one internal opening
- Probing dangerous.

Goodsall's rule does not apply ato Fistulae of specific pathology like TB.

Complications of Fistula

- Recurrent abscesses
- Multiple fistulous openings
- Septicemia
- Bleed
- Spread to portal system
- Malignancy.

Q. Evaluation and treatment of fistula in ano.

Investigations: Anal Fistula

- Pus culture and sampling for actinomycosis
- **HIV**
- Proctoscopy/colonoscopy—for evaluation for inflammatory bowel disease
- Chest X-ray—for tuberculosis
- Perianal USG
- **Transrectal ultrasound (TRUS)** to get a clear axial, coronal and sagittal views in understanding the anatomy of the complex fistulae
- **MRI** with contrast
- Fistulography, CT fistulography
- **Biopsy** from fistula.

Treatment: Surgery

Antibiotics are only to control sepsis.

Low Fistula

Anesthesia: Local, spinal, epidural or general
Lithotomy position
- Probe the fistula under anesthesia. Or inject a color dye (methylene blue) into the tract.
- Lay open tract
- Excise—biopsy

Post op would toilet to open wound.

Treatment of Anorectal Fistula

- **Do not cut anorectal ring open**—for avoiding incontinence.

Lay open the track partially and insert a seton.

Seton: Insert a **seton**
- A thread/silk ligature to induce fibrosis in the anorectal ring in sides of fistula tract—can be cut later
- Herbal (caustic) seton.

PELVIRECTAL (SUPRALEVATOR) FISTULA (EXTRASPHINCTERIC)

- Usually secondary to: Tuberculosis/carcinoma ulcerative colitis or Crohn's.
  - FB damage to rectum GE
- Treat specific cause, e.g. infliximab infusion in Crohn's, antitubercular therapy [ATT] in tuberculosis.

Surgery – in Stages

- 1st: Colostomy—wait for healing
- 2nd stage; seton insertion and wait for healing.

If the fistula fails to heal, a staged operation with colostomy cover is planned.

Other Procedures

Alternatives to Fistulotomy (Sphincterotomy)

- Ligation of intersphincteric fistula tract (LIFT)—tract curetted, ligated in intersphincteric space at its entry across the internal sphincter into anal canal.
- Video-assisted anal fistula treatment (VAAFT)—endoscopic curettage and fulguration.
- Video-assisted LIFT (VA-LIFT)
- Fibrin sealant
- Endorectal advancement flap
- Dermal island flap anoplasty
- Laser: "FiLaC": Fistula Laser Closure
- Proximal superficial cauterization, emptying regularly fistula tracts and curettage of tracts (PERFACT procedure).

> **Always to be remembered**
> - Preserve continence
> - Not every fistula needs fistulotomy
> - Recurrence preferable to incontinence
> - Do no harm

> Q. Write a note on pilonidal sinus.

PILONIDAL SINUS

Syn: Jeep bottom (Pilos – hair; nidus - nest).

Classification

- Congenital
  - Sinus in a post-anal dermoid
  - Persistent neural canal sinus
  - Notochordal anomaly?
- Acquired
  - Barber's finger web (interdigital)
  - Natal cleft—common in—hairy men
  - Toilet paper users.

SACRO-COCCYGEAL PILONIDAL SINUS

> Q. Pathogenesis and pathology.

Etiological Factors

- Male preponderance—74 % are males, hormone effect, hairy body, more sweat and maceration
- Most common in age 20-30 years.
- Dark haired—stiff hairs, rare in negroes
- Obese and overweight—deep natal cleft
- Prolonged sitting—jeep driver's disease.

Pathogenesis

Hair shed—from over the neck and back → travels in intergluteal cleft → Skin softens → abscess forms and the cavity which is formed sucks in loose hair from the furrow → causes abscess → bursts → and forms → sinus-tract → re-abscess → Bursts open to form another new sinus

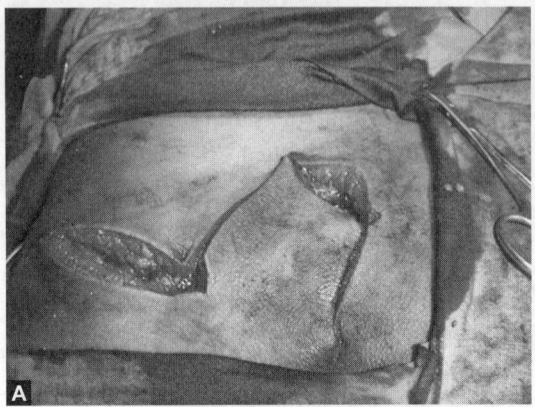 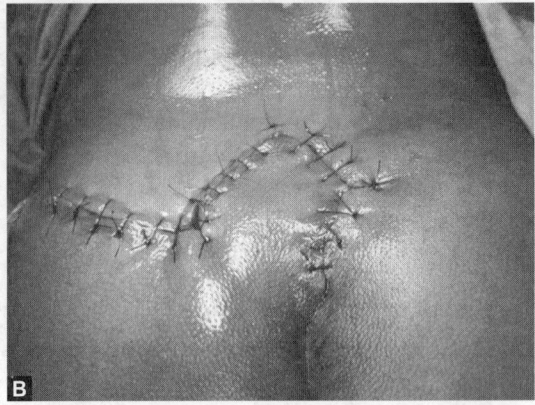

Figs. 28R-6A and B: Steps of rhomboid flap reconstruction for pilonidal sinus

Pathology

- Subcutaneous tract with side tracts
- Stratified squamous cell tissue
- Hair shafts lie loose or stuck in granulation tissue of wall of sinus
- Stops short of sacral fascia and periosteum.

Clinical Features

- Discharging sinus or sinuses
- Remissions and acute exacerbations
- High rate of recurrence after surgeries.

Differential Diagnosis

- Osteomyelitis of sacrum
- Tuberculous sinus
- Infected post anal dermoid.

> **Q. Principles of treatment of pilonidal sinus of sacro coccygeal area.**

Treatment

Acute Exacerbations

Localbath/dressing/drain abscess/antibiotic.

Definitive Surgery (During Remissions)

General Principle

- Radical excision of infective tract and all diseased tissue

- Drainage of subcutaneous plane
- Closure of wound away from midline—to obliterate and flatten the midline intergluteal cleft.

Surgery for Pilonidal Sinus

- Radical excision
- Primary closure
- Split skin graft
- Secondary healing by granulation and epithelialization
- Karydakis' procedure—asymmetric closure
- Bascom procedure: Radical excision of sinus tract through paramedian incision and midline closure of sinus openings (Refer **Fig. 28R-7**).

Plastic Reconstruction with Flaps

Refer Figures 28R-6A and B.

Local gluteal flap advancement/rotation

- Rhomboid flap/Limberg's flap
- V-Y plasty/advancement
- Z-plasty—single
- Multiple Z-plasty.

Non-surgical therapy:

- Sclerotherapy
- Irradiation.

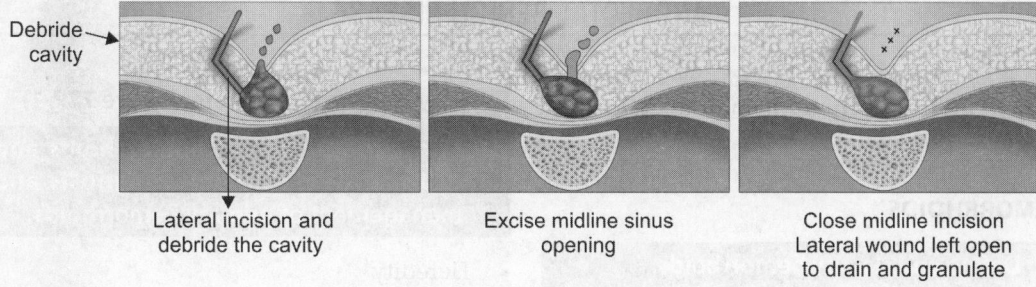

Fig. 28 R-7: Bascom procedure for pilonidal sinus

ANORECTAL BENIGN DISEASE

SU 28.17-28.18: Rectum—hemorrhoids, fissure, prolapse, pilonidal sinus.

HEMORRHOIDS

Q. Define and classify hemorrhoids.

Hemorrhoids—the dilated venous plexus of the anal canal.

Classification

Anatomical—in relation to the dentate line
- Internal (superior and middle hemorrhoidal plexus)—above dentate line
- External (inferior hemorrhoidal plexus)—below dentate line.

Pathology—based on structure—vascular of mucosal
- Vascular (arterial component of superior rectal artery)
- Prolapsing (mostly in elderly) mucosal.

Etiological—based on cause
- **Primary**—without a demonstrable illness
- **Secondary**
  - Rectal carcinoma
  - Pregnancy
  - Portal hypertension
  - Vascular malformations

Primary Hemorrhoids (Refer Figure 28P-1)

Q. Etiopathogenesis of hemorrhoids and discuss the pathology, diagnosis and management of primary hemorrhoids.

- Heredity
- The vertically placed venous columns are vertical and subject to effect of gravity
- Constipation—low residue diet
- Venous radicles in superior hemorrhoidal plexus lie in loose areolar tissue
  - They pierce through rectal muscular wall and get compressed during defecation. As a result, the veins get engorged and dilated.

Pathogenesis of Hemorrhoids

Internal anal Sphincter (IAS) Dysfunction

- Increased IAS activity
  - Obstruction to venous outflow
  - Congestion and engorgement
  - Symptomatic piles
- Straining
- Stretching
- Fragmentation of muscularis submucosae ani muscles

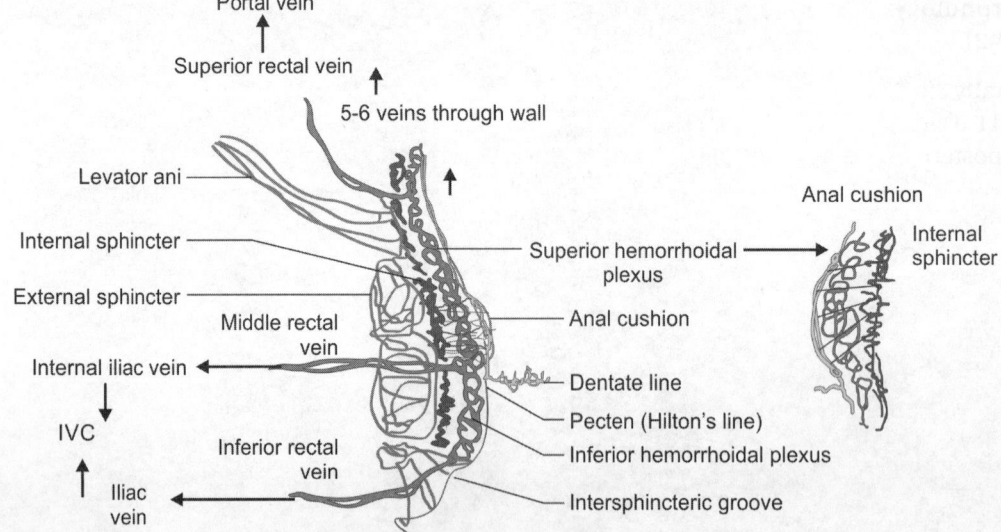

Fig. 28P-1: Venous anatomy of rectum and anal cushions

- Sliding down of anal cushions
- Engorgement
- Symptomatic piles—prolapse of mucosal cushions.

> Q. Describe the "anal cushions" and their importance in hemorrhoids.

ANAL CUSHIONS " CORPUS CAVERNOSUM RECTI" OF STELZNER

- These are submucous venous plexus containing arterial twigs, venules, smooth muscles, elastic tissue and connective tissue.
- Symptomatic anal cushions are called " piles" or hemorrhoids.
- Anal cushions get pushed during defecation by fecal ball against muscular tone.
- Breaking of elastic bands—separation of veins off the muscular base.
- Prolapse beyond dentate line.

Pathogenesis of Prolapsing Piles

- Attenuation of submucosal muscle fibers
- Detachment from internal anal sphincter
- Mucosa/submucosa/vascular plexus become more mobile. They fall anteriorly (at defecation) and prolapse.
- Engorgement, prolapse and strangulation.

> Q. Morphology of primary hemorrhoids.

Morphology of hemorrhoids (Refer **Figure 28P-2**).

Usually 3 masses
- 11 o'clock (right anterior), 7 o'clock (right posterior) and 3 o'clock (left lateral)

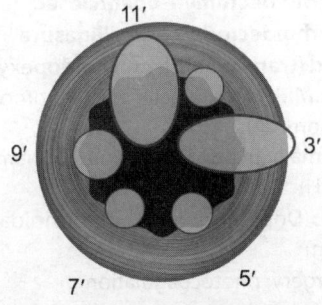

Fig. 28P-2: Primary hemorrhoids.

- Corresponding to superior rectal arterial branches.

Three accessory piles (in 30%)—at 1", 5" and 9"

Each hemorrhoidal mass is made of:
- Pedicle—above ano-rectal ring—pink color (made of veins + arterial branch)
- Internal pile mass—anorectal ring—dentate line
- External pile—below dentate line (seen on anal margin).

Clinical Features of Hemorrhoids (Refer Table 28P-1) and Complications

Complications
- Hemorrhoge and shock
- Acute thombosed hemorrhoids
- Acute prolapse
- Thromobosis
- Suppuration
- Gangrene (refer **Figure 28 P-3**)
- Portal pyemia
- Septicemia

> Q. Clinical features and differential diagnosis of hemorrhoids.

> Q. Management of hemorrhoids.

Investigations
To exclude secondary causes for hemorrhoids and to rule out differential diagnosis.
To stage hemorrhoids.
- Proctoscopy and Sigmoidoscopy
- Ultrasonography —to detect intra-abdominal mass/fluid
- Portal hypertension and cirrhosis
- Liver function

Conservative Treatment: Hemorrhoids
- High fiber diet
- Avoid irritant food
- Ispaghula husk
- Treat associated infections and infestations (deworming and amebicides).

Table 28P-1: Clinical features and differential diagnosis of hemorrhoids.

Clinical features of hemorrhoids	
<ul><li>Bleeding—painless</li><li>Prolapse of the pile mas—at stools or persistent later/</li><li>Discharge—mucous or watery.</li><li>Pruritus</li><li>Secondary anemia</li><li>Per rectally—impalpable and painless unless complicated</li></ul>	
Differential diagnosis of hemorrhoids **Mass**<ul><li>Peri anal or subctaneoous hematoma or abscess</li><li>Sentinel pile in fissure</li><li>Anal warts</li><li>Thrombosed external piles</li><li>Prolapsing polyp</li><li>Rectal mucosal prolapse</li><li>Total rectal prolapse</li></ul>	***Bleeding***<ul><li>Fissure</li><li>Rectal polyp</li><li>Malignancy—carcinoma.</li><li>Pruritis</li><li>Unnoticed trauma</li><li>Inflammatory bowel disease (IBD)</li><li>Bleeding disorders</li><li>Medications</li><li>HIV</li></ul>

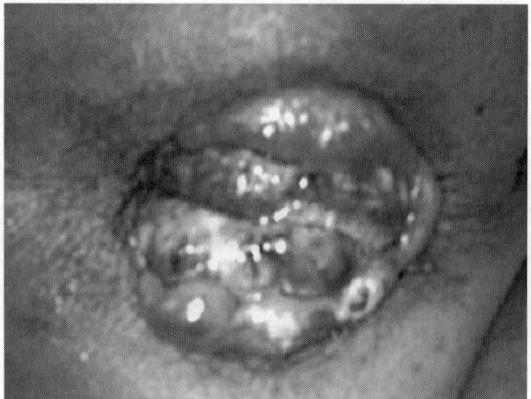

Fig. 28P-3: Acute prolapsed hemorrhoids with gangrene

Medical measures
- Flavonoids
- Calcium dobesilate
- Diosmin
- Steroid ointment—doubtful value.

Laxatives—to relieve strain on sphincter
- Stool softeners: Liquid paraffin
- Irritant purgatives: Milk of magnesia, senna, castor oil
- Bisacodyl; sodium phosphate/sodium picosulfate; lactulose, lactitol.
- Polyethylene glycol.

Ointments: Symptomatic
- Steroids: Hydrocortisone acetate; beclomethasone dipropionate
- Local anesthetics: Lignocaine hydrochloride, cinchocaine hydrochloride
- Local hemostatics: Feracrylum
- Anti coagulant: Heparin sodium and heparinoid ointments—for thrombosed piles.
- Astringents—zinc oxide.

Options for treatment of hemorrhoids
- Symptomatic - diet, laxative, flavonoids, local application (see above
- **Sclerotherapy**
- **Banding (Barron)**
- Infrared radiation
- **Hemorrhoidectomy—open/closed**
- **Hemorrhoidectomy—laser/ligasure**
- **Stapled (transanal)hemorrhoidopexy**
  - **Syn: MIPH**—minimally invasive procedure for hemorrhoids
  - Minimally nvasive procedure for hemorrhoids (MIPH)
- DGHAL (Doppler guided hemorrhoidal arterial Ligation)
- Cryosurgery; photocoagulation
- Lords anal dilatation

General Principles in Treatment of Hemorrhoids (Refer Table 28P-2)

Principle of Open Hemorrhoidectomy

High ligation of hemorrhoidal pedicle and excision along with skin covering the external pile and leaving the wound open to heal.

Generally three pile masses are excised—at 3, 7 and 11 o'clock position.

Closed Hemorrhoidectomy

The piles are dissected in submucous plane and excised amnd the would edges closed.

PRINCIPLES OF STAPLED HEMORRHOIDOPEXY (SYN: MIPH)

Syn: Minimally invasive procedure for hemorrhoids (MIPH).

The MIPH Device is a Branded Instrument

- Repositioning: The prolapsed mucosa is brought up into its original position by lifting the hemorrhoidal tissue into place.
- Retracting: The stapling device to retract excess mucosal tissue.
- Restoring; after retracting excess tissue, the device removes the excess tissue, reconnects by stapling the edges and restores the anal canal wall.

Doppler Guided Hemorrhoiodal Artery Ligation (DGHAL)

This aims at blocking hemorrhoidal artery and causing shrinking of the pile mass. It is done under control of a doppler probe fitted on a proctoscope.

Q. Thrombosed external pile.

THROMBOSED EXTERNAL PILES (SHORT NOTES)

"5- day painful lesion"
- Peri-anal hematoma
- Ruptured external hemorrhoids
- Precipitated by strain
- Sudden painful swelling
- Tense and tender

Table 28P-2: Summary of treatment for hemorrhoids.

Grade I **Injection sclerotherapy:** For grade I • Phenol in almond oil • Ethanolamine oleate • Sodium tetradecyl sulphate (STD) *Complications* • Ulceration/hemorrhage • Portal pyemia • Perirectal extravasation	*Gabriel Syringe is used* • 1–3% phenol in almond oil • 1–3 cc injected into each of • 1–3 pile masses in • 1–3 sittings • 1–3 weeks apart
Grade II • Baron's rubber banding • Laser hemorrhoidectomy • Cryosurgery • Infrared coagulation • Radiofrequency ablation are less popular	

Grade III and IV
 • Hemorrhoidectomy
   – Open (Milligan-Morgan procedure: Ligation excision
   – Closed (Park's)
 • Laser hemorrhoidectomy
 • Thermal sealants–e.g. ligasure.
 • Doppler guided hemorrhoidal artery ligation (DGHAL)
 • **Stapled hemorrhoidopexy (minimally invasive procedure for hemorrhoids)**	

- May be associated with interno-external hemorrhoids.

Differential Diagnosis
- Carcinoma anus
- Condyloma.

Natural History and Complications
- Resolution
- Suppuration—abscess/fistula
- Fibrosis—skin tag
- Rupture and bleed.

Treatment: Thrombosed Piles
Small hematomas may resolve over 5 days and are observed.

Emergency
- Incision and evacuation of hematoma
- Excise skin over the external pile mass

If it is associated with interno external piles.
- Treat with local paraffin and NSAID
- Antibiotics
- Manual dilatation to relax the strangulating sphincter.
- Definitive surgery for hemorrhoids after 6 weeks.

> **Q. Define, describe the pathology, clinical diagnosis and treatment of fissure in ano.**

FISSURE IN ANO (REFER TABLE 28P-3)
Definition: Longitudinal ulceration/tear in anal canal.

Etiology of Anal Fissure (Refer Table 28P-4)
Multiple fissures and non-midline fissures seen in:
- IBD – Crohn's; TB; syphilis
- Sexual injury
- HIV
- Blood dyscrasias.

Pathology of Anal Fissures
Refer **Figure 28P-4**.

Clinical Features of Fissure in Ano
Refer **Table 28P-5**.

Treatment of Anal Fissure
Aim: To break the vicious cycle of pain – spasm – strain – tear – pain.
- Relieve pain—jelly/ointment—lignocaine 2%
- Relieve edema - sucralfate or steroid cream
- Relieve constipation—paraffin, isphagula granules

Table 28P-3: Distribution of anal fissures.

Midline	Posterior	Anterior	Ant + post
Male	90%	10%	10- 15%
Female	60%	40%	Overall

Table 28P- 4: Etiology of anal fissures.

Primary	Secondary
• Sphincteric spasm—high resting anal tone • ? Trauma • Strain at stool • Tear on anal mucosa • Pain • Spasm of internal sphincter	• Post op (constipation) • Post-partum • Crohn's • Tuberculosis • Anal sexual injury • Anal cancer—may present as fissure • Secondary syphilis

Chapter 28: Abdominal Cavity, Hernia and Digestive Tract

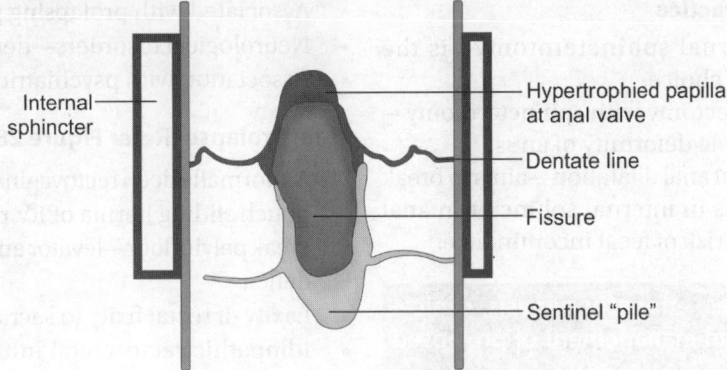

Fig. 28P-4: Pathology of fissure in ano

Table 28P-5: Clinical features of fissure in ano.	
Symptoms	**Signs**
• Painful defecation • Bleeding – only in acute - bright red. • Streaked stool - streak of blood on the stool • Discharge • Pruritus ani • Dysuria and frequency	• Anal spasm • Puckered anus • Sentinel pile (skin tag) • Ulceration at anal verge (on spreading buttocks apart
Differential diagnosis	
• Carcinoma anus • Multiple fissures of Crohn's • Tuberculous ulcer • Anal chancre	• Multiple fissures with pruritus ani • Multiple fissures with patulous anus – Gay • Proctalgia fugax

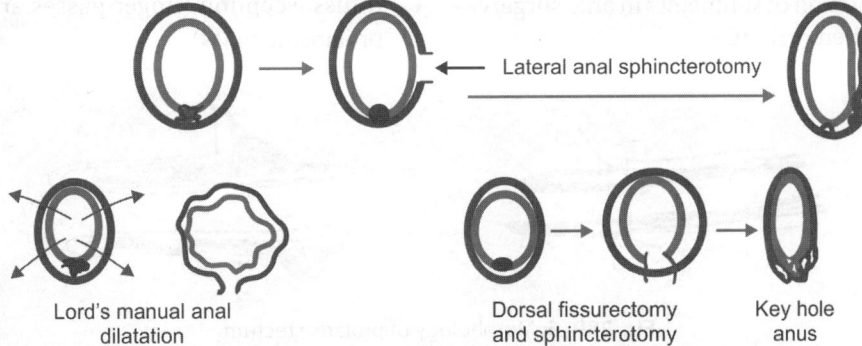

Fig 28P-5: Surgical procedures for anal fissure

- Relieve sphincteric spasm
  - Nitroglycerin 5% jelly, isosorbide, nifedipine
  - Diltiazem 2% ointment.
- Pharmacological sphincterotomy
  - Botulinum toxin injection into sphincter.

Surgery for Anal Fissure (Refer Figure 28 P-5)

For all chronic fissures—not responding to conservative measures or botulinum injection and recurrent fissures after non-surgical measures.

Procedure in practice

- Lateral internal sphincterotomy—is the procedure of choice.
- Dorsal fissurectomy with sphincterotomy—causes key hole deformity of anus.
- Lord's manual anal dilatation—aims to break fibrous bands in internal sphincter in anal pectin. High-risk of fecal incontinence.

> **Q. Discuss types, etiopathogenesis, clinical diagnosis and management of prolapsed rectum.**

PROLAPSE OF THE RECTUM

Refer **Figure 28P-6** and **Table 28P-6**.

> **Q. Etiology of prolapsed rectum.**

Etiology

Partial Prolapse

Children

- Absent sacral curve.(straight sacrum)
- Diminution in supporting ischiorectal fat (acute diarrhea, malnutrition)
- Increased intra-abdominal pressure (e.g. cough).

Adult

- After division of sphincters in anal surgery—fistula/hemorrhoids
- Associated with prolapsing piles
- Neurological disorders—demyelination
- Association with psychiatric disorders.

Total Prolapse (Refer Figure 28P-7)

- Abnormally deep rectovaginal/vesical (RV)—pouch sliding hernia of RV pouch
- Weak pelvic floor—levator ani or neurological deficit
- Laxity of rectal fixity to sacral hollow
- Idiopathic recto-rectal intussusceptions—anterior/posterior/circumferential.

> **Q. Clinical features and differential diagnosis of prolapsed rectum.**

- Clinical features—prolapse
- Mass per anus
- Discharge
- Constipation
- Ulcer, bleeding
- Gangrene (rare)
- Low sphincteric tone

Differential Diagnosis

- Prolapsed piles
- Mucosal piles
- Polypoid tumor
- Intussusception (finger passes around the prolapsing mass).

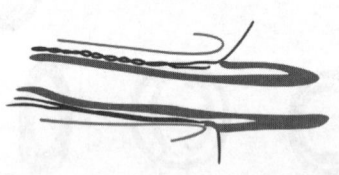 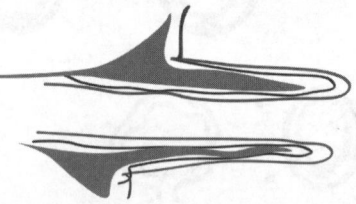

Fig. 28P-6: Morphology of prolapse rectum

Table 28P-6: Prolapse of the rectum.

Partial	Complete
• Usually children (affects adults too)	• Commonly adults (children also affected)
• Only mucosa	• Full thickness
• < 4cm	• > 4 cm
• No peritoneal hernia	• Peritoneal herniation present

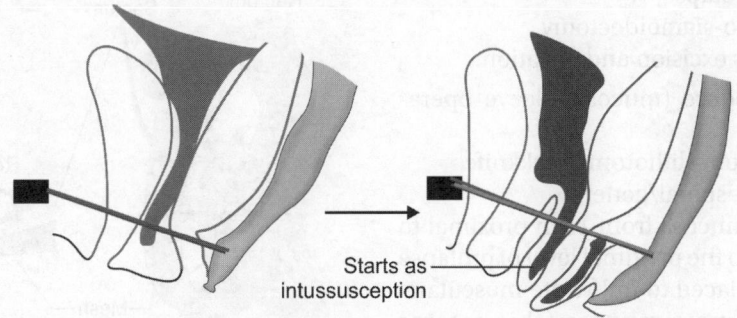

Fig. 28P-7: Pathogenesis of prolapse rectum

Q. Investigations and principles of treatment of prolapsed rectum.

Investigation
- Sigmoido-colonoscopy to exclude growth
- EMG to assess pelvic floor strength
- General indices of nutrition and systemic health
- Gynecological and urological evaluation
- MRI of pelvic floor
- Anal manometry
- General measures
- Correct anemia malnutrition
- Avoid constipation.

Strengthen Pelvic Floor
- Levator exercise
- Electrical stimulation.

Surgical Treatment: Any of the Following
- Narrow the anal orifice - in children - Thiersh's operation
- Obliterate Douglas pouch
- Levator repair to restore the strength of pelvic floor
- Resect the prolapsing segment
- Suspend the prolapsing rectum.

Q. Describe the principles of treatment of prolapse rectum in children and adults.

Children
Non-operative Methods
- Correction of constipation, diarrhea, respiratory tract infection
- Institution of proper habits of defecation

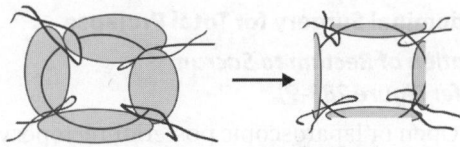

Fig. 28P-8: Goodsall's suturing

- Improve nutrition
- Supporting the anus manually or by strapping
- Levator exercises

Treatment: Partial Prolapse
- Sclerotherapy: Peri-anal injection of sodium tetradecyl sulfate (STD)
- Thiersch's wiring: Perianal circumferential purse string.

Adult
- Sclero-therapy
- Thiersch's operation
- Mucosal excision
- Goodsall's suturing (Refer **Figure: 28P-8**)
- Stapled transanal rectal resection (STARR).

Treatment of Total Prolapse

Objectives
- Obliterate the deep rectovesical pouch
- Fix rectum to sacrum
- Repair the pelvic floor
- Resect redundant sigmoid, (if needed).

Surgery for Total Prolapse

Perineal Procedures
- Pelvic floor muscle strengthening—perineorrhaphy/levotor repair.

- Excision of prolapse
  - Miles' recto-sigmoidectomy
  - Delorme's excision and plication.

Delorme's procedure (mucosal sleeve operation)
- Patient position—lithotomy/jackknife
- Anaesthesia—spinal/general
- Excision of mucosa from 1 cm proximal to dentate line to the proximal level of prolapse
- Sutures are placed to imbricate muscularis and approximate mucosa (this creates plication of redundant rectal muscular wall).

Abdominal Surgery for Total Prolapse

Fixation of Rectum to Sacrum (Refer Figure 28P-9)

- Open or laparoscopic posterior rectopexy—most preferred
  - Polypropylene mesh wrap and fixation—most preferred
  - Polyvinyl sponge wrap (induces fibrosis).
- Roscoe Graham rectopexy
  - Extensive dissection/levator repair and posterior suture fixation to sacrum
  - High incidence of impotence due to damage to nerves.

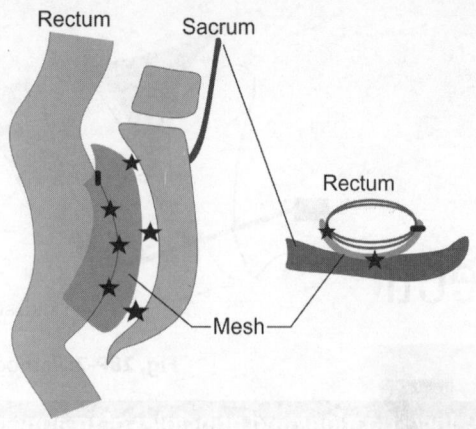

Fig. 28P-9: Posterior mesh rectopexy

- Lahout's extraperitonisation of sigmoid
- Ripstein's sling fixation of rectum to sacrum
- Anterior sigmoidopexy

Sigmoidectomy with Rectopexy

Bulky sigmoid is resected and colorectal anastomosis done, rectum is fixed to sacrum with a polypropylene mesh.

Section 7

Urogenital Surgery

29. Kidney, Ureters and the Bladder
30. Scrotum, Testis and the Penis

Kidney, Ureters and the Bladder

Chapter 29

SU29.1–29.4: Hematuria, Congenital Disorders, Infections and Obstructive Pathology	
SU29.1	Describe the causes, investigations and principles of management of hematuria.
SU29.2	Describe the clinical features, investigations and principles of management of congenital anomalies of genitourinary system.
SU29.3	Describe the clinical features, investigations and principles of management of urinary tract infections.
SU29.4	Describe the clinical features, investigations and principles of management of hydronephrosis.
SU29.5–29.6: Renal Calculi and Renal Tumors	
SU29.5	Describe the clinical features, investigations and principles of management of renal calculi.
SU29.6	Describe the clinical features, investigations and principles of management of renal tumors.
SU29.7–29.11: Bladder, Prostate and Urethra	
SU29.7	Describe the principles of management of acute and chronic retention of urine.
SU29.8	Describe the clinical features, investigations and principles of management of bladder cancer.
SU29.9	Describe the clinical features, investigations and principles of management of disorders of prostate.
SU29.10	Demonstrate a digital rectal examination of the prostate in a mannequin or equivalent.
SU29.11	Describe clinical features, investigations and management of urethral strictures.

SU29.1-29.4: Hematuria, Congenital Disorders, Infections and Obstructive Pathology

SU29.1: Describe the causes, investigations and principles of management of hematuria.

Q. Classify hematuria and enumerate the causes. Describe management of hematuria.

HEMATURIA

Refer **Table 29U-1** and **Figure 29U-1**.

Definition

Hematuria is presence of blood in urine.
- **Visible hematuria (VH)**—overt
- **Non-visible hematuria (NVH)**—occult (microscopic).

Hematuria may be:
- Intermittent or continuous.
- Hematuria with pain (painful hematuria) or without pain (painless hematuria).

Strangury

It is an intense desire to pass urine associated with severe and unbearable pain referred to urinary meatus with inability to pass urine even as the person passes a drop or two of blood at the end of the momentary act. It signifies an intense irritative focus in the trigone or the prostatic urethra.

Causes of Hematuria

Refer **Table 29U-1**.

Table 29U-1: Causes of hematuria.

Kidney	Ureter
• Renal injury	• Ureteric stone
• Renal stones	**Bladder**
• Wilms' tumour	• **Carcinoma**
• Polycystic disease	• Schistosomiasis
• Tuberculosis	• Cystitis
• Renal cell carcinoma	• Tuberculosis
• Glomerulonephritis	• Bladder stone
• Renal Infarct	
General	**Prostate**
• Blood dyscrasias	• BPH
• Coagulopathy anticoagulant drugs	• Carcinoma prostate
	Urethra
	• Injury, urethritis
	• Tumors

History

Intermittent or continuous.

Pain: Hematuria is painless in pathologies of upper urinary tract and painful in those of lower tract.

Timing of hematuria with in relation to voiding:
- Initial—urethral pathology.
- Through the stream—pathology in bladder or upper tract.

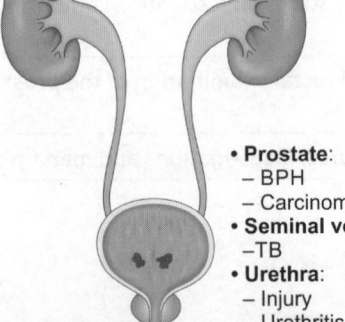

Fig. 29U-1: Causes of hematuria

- Terminal—pathology in bladder neck; prostate or proximal urethra.

Remember Mnemonic - TIN
- Trauma
- Infection
- Neoplasm—all levels of the urinary tract
  - Anticoagulant therapy.

Clinical triad of a renal tumor—haematuria, loin pain and a palpable loin mass.

Investigations
Urine Test
- For blood—benzidine in glacial acetic acid.
- Microscopy.
- Urine culture and sensitivity.
- Urinary cytology for diagnosing urothelial malignancy.
- Coagulation profile.
  Bleeding time; clotting time; prothrombin time; platelet count.
- Renal function tests—blood urea, serum creatinine.

Ultrasound
Stones, tumors, prostate.

Doppler—to look for any bleeding lesions (e.g. renal aneurysm) or renal infarct.

Cystourethroscopy to look for bladder or urethral pathology.

Contrast enhanced computed tomography (CECT) abdomen—has replaced intravenous urography (IVU).

CT- angiography—if any specific pathology is suspected at Doppler study and to plan for angio embolisation.

Treatment
- Treatment of systemic causes and hemorrhagic shock, stabilization of hemodynamics, blood transfusion and correction of hypovolemia.
- Antibiotics if there is any clue of infection
- Establishing the cause, e.g.,nephritis
- Correction of coagulation disorders and of bleeding diathesis.
- **Treatment of the cause:** Depending on the pathology, e.g., radical nephrectomy for renal cell carcinoma: Removal of calculus for a renal or bladder calculus or a fulguration of a bleeding bladder tumor.

> **Q. Short note: Describe LUTS (lower urinary tract symptoms).**

Lower urinary tract symptoms (LUTS)

Are classified as storage, voiding or post-micturitional
- **Storage LUTS** are frequency, nocturia, urgency and urge incontinence
  - Storage LUTS are typical of an overactive bladder
  - Failure of the bladder to act as a functioning reservoir
  - Overactive bladder or a bladder neuropathy.
- **Voiding LUTS** are hesitancy, a reduced stream and straining
  - Voiding LUTS are typical of bladder outlet obstruction
  - Some patients may have storage and voiding LUTS in combination.
- **Post-micturitional**—incomplete emptying and post micturitional dribbling.
  - Voiding and post-micturitional LUTS are commonly seen in males with bladder outlet obstruction (BOO) and may have storage LUTS due to the overactive hypertrophied bladder. Investigation—urodynamic studies.

Urinary symptoms as defined by the International Continence Society (ICS):
- **Frequency**—frequent voiding during day.
- **Nocturia**—patient wakes at least once at night to void.
- **Strangury** is a sensation of constantly needing to void; most commonly due to a lower urinary tract infection (UTI).
- **Urgency**—urgent desire to pass urine and inability to hold for long time.
- **Urge incontinence (UI)** is involuntary voiding or leakage after an urgent sensation. Urgency and urge incontinence are seen with an overactive bladder or a neuropathy.
- **Stress incontinence** is involuntary urinary leakage with rise in intra-abdominal pressure (e.g., during coughing, sneezing or laughing) commonly in females after vaginal deliveries.

- **Nocturnal enuresis**—is involuntary leak of urine during sleep—an overflow incontinence.
- **Hesitancy**—difficulty in initiating micturition—a delay in the onset of voiding (seconds to several minutes)—a symptom of bladder outlet obstruction (BOO).
- **Reduced urinary stream**—compared with previous urinary stream (BOO).
- **Intermittency**—urine flow which stops and starts, once or more during micturition.
- **Straining**—it is the muscular effort used in order to initiate, maintain or improve the urinary stream.
- **Incomplete emptying**—the sensation after voiding that bladder fullness persists.
- **Post micturition dribble (PMD)**—the bulbar urethra fails to empty during micturition and this leads to involuntary dribble immediately after one has completed micturition. PMD is not usually remedied by TURP.

> SU29.2: Describe the clinical features, investigations and principles of management of congenital anomalies of genitourinary system.

EMBRYOLOGY OF UROGENITAL SYSTEM

Genital Tract

- **The mesonephric (Wolffian) ducts**—from mesoderm, give rise to male organs on each side—epididymis, vas deferens, ejaculatory duct and seminal vesicles (the duct regresses in females); the testicles develop from the intermediate cell mass and descend distally.
- **The paramesonephric (Mullerian) duct** develops into the female genital organs forming the fallopian tubes at their cranial ends and fusing to form the uterus and upper part of the vagina at their caudal ends (The Wolffian ducts regress in the female due to lack of testosterone).

Urinary Tract

- Each kidney develops from the metanephric blastema (mesoderm). The ureteric bud arises from the distal Wolffian duct to form the ureter and pelvicalyceal collecting system.
- The growth of the abdominal cavity allows the kidneys to **ascend cephalad** into the renal pouches from the pelvic position.
- The fetal hindgut gets divided by the urorectal septum into posterior rectum and anterior bladder with the urachus draining through umbilicus. Cloaca receives both the rectal and urinary component. The male urethra develops into the phallic tissue to form the bulbous and penile urethra.

Summary
- Kidneys develop from the metanephros (mesoderm)
- Ureter sprouts from the mesonephric duct (mesoderm)
- Mesonephric duct regresses in females
- Paramesonephric duct regresses in males

CONGENITAL ABNORMALITIES

Bilateral Renal Agenesis: Incompatible with Life

Unilateral renal agenesis—associated with pulmonary hypoplasia.
- An autosomal dominant trait with incomplete penetrance.
- Due to failure of the ureteric bud to connect with the metanephric blastema.
- Incidence: 1 in 500–1000 births.
- Generally, the ureter and the hemi-trigone are also not developed on the same side.
- The contralateral kidney is usually hypertrophic (may be dysplastic in some).
- The ipsilateral testis and vas deferens (ovary or Fallopian tube in the females) and the adrenal may be absent too.

Renal aplasia is a small dysplastic kidney and not absence of one.

Multicystic Disease

- The kidney is made of multiple cysts (different size) in a loose stroma.
- Due to severe dysplasia.
- Not compatible with life if bilateral.
- It is diagnosed during a prenatal ultrasound scan and presents as a mass in the newborn.
- Often associated with atresia of ureter and obstruction of contralateral PUJ.

Treatment

Some cysts may regress and hence makes a case for observation and relief of obstruction of pelvi ureteric level.

> **Q. Write a note on ectopic kidney and horseshoe kidney.**

ECTOPIC KIDNEY/CROSSED RENAL ECTOPIA

Ectopic kidney: Partial or complete failure of the ascent of the fetal kidney from the pelvis to its normal position.

Renal ectopia is associated with rotational abnormality of pelvis, which should rotate with ascent of kidney (anterior to medial).

Horseshoe kidney: The kidneys are fused at the lower pole.

Crossed renal ectopia: In crossed renal ectopia—both kidneys are on the same side and fused vertically with the ureter on one of the sides crossing the midline to join the bladder on the correct side of the bladder.

The uncrossed kidney is usually above the crossed kidney with its pelvis of facing medially while that of the crossed unit faces anteriorly or laterally.

HORSESHOE KIDNEY

- Incidence: 1 in 1000 autopsies and is more common in males (2:1).
- The two lower poles of the developing kidneys fuse to form an isthmus with two functioning renal units. The inferior mesenteric artery prevents the fused unit from further ascent.
- Arterial supply—variable and unpredictable—may be from neighbouring major vessels.
- or a common artery to supply both renal units. Renal angiography is always—done before any resectional surgery to exclude anomalous arterial supply.

Complications

They are more prone for:
- Stones
- Obstructive uropathy (pelvi ureteric junction obstruction)
- Infection including tuberculosis
- Reflux nephropathy.

Treatment

The obstructive pathology or infection is treated as the case may be.

CYSTIC DISEASES OF THE KIDNEY

> **Q. Enumerate the types of cystic kidney and discuss autosomal dominant polycystic kidney disease (ADPKD).**

Types

Genetic

- Autosomal dominant: Adult polycystic kidney disease
- Autosomal recessive: Infantile polycystic kidney disease is fatal.

Sporadic and dysplastic: Simple cyst, multicystic kidney, medullary sponge kidney.

Acquired renal cystic disease: May develop in patient on long-term dialysis.

AUTOSOMAL DOMINANT POLYCYSTIC KIDNEY DISEASE (ADPKD)

Syn: Adult polycystic kidney disease (PCKD)
- Consists of: Bilateral multiple renal cysts, pancreas liver and arachnoid membranes and berry aneurysm in circle of Willis.
- Caused by genetic mutation in either of the genes—PKD1 and PKD 2 (two different genes)
- Expressed as autosomal dominant pattern.
- It is more common in females. Presents in age group 30–40. May present on one side first.
- Cyst formation occurs at the junction of the distal tubule and the collecting duct.
- Grossly it contains multiple cysts with a clear or brownish fluid (due to hemorrhage).

The differential diagnosis of ADPKD
- Autosomal recessive PKD.
- RCAD syndrome: Tuberous sclerosis complex, von Hippel–Lindau disease, renal cysts and diabetes syndrome.
- Orofaciodigital syndrome type 1, medullary sponge kidney and simple renal cysts.

- The ADPKD proteins, polycystin-1 and polycystin-2, playing a critical role in function of a cilium of tubular epithelium is deficient here in ADPKD.
- Screening: Renal USS used for asymptomatic high risk individuals.
- Diagnosis is made when there are three cysts found—2 on one side and one on the other.
- At least 3 (unilateral or bilateral) renal cysts.

Clinical Manifestations of ADPKD: Renal and Extrarenal

Renal Manifestations

- **Enlarged kidney 10%**
  - A flank or abdominal mass.
  - Cysts contain clear fluid, thick brown material or coagulated blood.
- **Pain**
  - Dull loin ache.
  - Hemorrhage into a cyst causes a more acute severe pain
- **Hypertension 75%:** The most common manifestation of ADPKD; Onset after the age of 20 years, major contributor to progression of the disease and cardiovascular events
- **Hematuria and cyst hemorrhage:** Visible hematuria—40%.
  - Hemorrhage occurs into cyst, which communicates with collecting system causing hematuria.
- **Urinary tract infection and cyst infection:** As sterile pyuria is common in these patients.
- **Nephrolithiasis—20%** of uric acid or calcium oxalate or both.
  - Calcification of cyst wall and parenchyma add to difficulty of diagnosis of stones by imaging in ADPKD.
- **End-stage renal disease:** The 4th to 6th decade of life.

Extrarenal Manifestations

- **Polycystic liver disease:** Cysts are usually asymptomatic;
  Symptoms: Due to a mass effect or due to cyst complications.
- **Intracranial aneurysms:** Occur in approximately 10% of patients
- **Valvular heart disease:** Mitral valve prolapse in up to 25%.
- **Berry aneurysm of circle of Willis**

Investigations

- Urine shows low specific gravity <1.010.
- Blood urea and serum creatinine to assess renal function.
- Ultrasound confirms the cysts.
- CECT or IVU: Spider leg pattern with an elongated compressed renal pelvis, narrowed and stretched calyces.

Treatment

Observation and treatment of hypertension.

Symptomatic Cysts

Image (ultrasonographic) guided aspiration.
Surgery: For pain, hemorrhage, infection.
- **Rovsing operation: Deroofing of the cysts.**
  - Exposure of kidney, puncturing of the cyst and marsupialization of the cysts.
  - Approach—open surgery, retroperitoneoscopic or laparoscopic.
- **Renal transplantation**: For end stage renal disease.
  - Bilateral nephrectomy with renal transplantation after preparation with hemodialysis.

Ureterocoele

A ureterocoele is a cystic enlargement of the intramural ureter, due to atresia of the ureteric orifice.
- Females more often affected than males (4:1)
- 10% are bilateral.
- Often associated with dysplastic or nonfunctional renal tissue.

Complications

- Bladder neck obstruction
- Obstruction of contralateral ureteric orifice.
- Stones in the lower ureter.
- Intravenous urography: 'cobra head'.

Treatment

- Simple ureteroceles—surgical excision with re-implantation of the ureter.
- Endoscopic incision for a calculus stuck in the ureterocele. But it may cause vesicoureteric reflux.

- Unilateral hydronephrosis or pyonephrosis may need nephrectomy.

Duplex Ureters
- Not uncommon.
- More often. Unilateral and in girls.
- May be complete or incomplete duplication.
- Associated with vesico-ureteric reflux in children.

Ectopic Ureters
- Usually associated with duplex ureters; seven times more common in females.
- May cause incontinence in females—because they join the urethra below sphincter.
- Males are continent as the ureter opens above the external urethral sphincter.

Treatment
- Ureteric reimplantation
  - For incontinence
  - For VU reflux.
- Resection of ureter and kidney for ureter draining an infected or dysplastic or atrophic kidney.

> **SU29.3: Describe the clinical features, investigations and principles of management of urinary tract infections.**

URINARY TRACT INFECTIONS
- More common in lower UT
- Females more often affected than men

UTIs are classified as:
- Uncomplicated
- Complicated—an infection with an high risk of serious complications or treatment failure.

> **Q. Discuss the etiopathology, diagnosis and management of acute pyelonephritis.**

ACUTE PYELONEPHRITIS
Acute suppurative inflammation of renal parenchyma and pelvicalyceal system.

Hematogenous infection
- From cutaneous infection—boil or carbuncle, tonsil, infected dental root.
- From lymph nodes in the neck, chest or abdomen.

Ascending infection—the most common route.

Contributing factors
- Urolithiasis—renal and ureteric stones are very common.
- Vesico-ureteric reflux.
- Urinary stasis and acute pyelonephritis is more common in females—during childhood, at puberty, after coitus and during pregnancy.

Pathology
Suppurative necrosis of parenchyma which can progress to complications.

Complications
- Suppuration and parenchymal abscess in kidney
- Perinephric abscess
- Rupture of abscess into pelvis
- Pyonephrosis
- Septicemia.

Clinical Features
- Usually one side, uncommon to get bilateral.
- Symptoms may vary from a mild illness to a severe life threatening illness with renal failure and septic shock.
- Fever (temperature >38°C) with rigors.

Local symptoms: Flank pain, nausea and vomiting

Signs: Tenderness in costovertebral angle.

Note: Dysuria and frequency—indicate associated cystitis.

Differential Diagnosis

Pyonephrosis
Right Side
- Pericolic abscess
- Retrocecal appendicitis—appendix abscess
- Liver abscess pointing posteriorly.

Left Side
Pericolic abscess, retroperitoneal lymphangitis.

Pyelonephritis Complicating Pregnancy

- Commonly it is seen between 20 and 28 weeks of gestation.
- Malaise, fever, loin pain and rigors.
- Some may present with premature labor.
- More common on right side—due to greater dilatation of ureter on right side.

Investigations

- Urine—plenty of pus cells. Granular casts indicate renal damage.
- Urine and blood culture.
- Gram negative bacteria are common, e.g., *Escherichia coli* and *Klebsiella*.
- Urea splitters—*Proteus* or staphylococci—make urine alkaline.
- Renal function - blood urea and creatinine.
- Blood sugar and glycosylated hemoglobin
- WBC count and ESR.

Imaging Studies

Ultrasonography—entire urogenital tract.
To find or exclude:
- Obstruction of the collecting system by renal calculi, pyonephrosis, perirenal abscess.

Contrast Enhanced CT Scan

Shows decreased opacification of the affected parenchyma.

Treatment

- Best guess antibiotic initially and modified later as per the culture report.
  Generally—a quinolone or cephalosporin.
- Hydration and electrolyte balance—intravenous fluids are preferred in severe cases, presenting with vomiting.
- Symptomatic: Fever and pain—paracetamol (intravenous or oral tablets) is safe.
- Follow up scans to assess progress.
- Intensive care when the infection is very severe with threatening sepsis.
- Complications are dealt with accordingly.
- Interventions: Radiological and endoscopic.
  - Ureteric stenting for relief of obstruction.
  - Endoscopic lithotomy or lithotripsy.
  - Aspiration or pig tail drainage of renal abscess under image guidance.
- Surgery: For complications like perirenal abscess, pyonephrosis.

CHRONIC PYELONEPHRITIS

Causes

- Neglected acute pyelonephritis.
- Diabetes.
- Obstructive pathology in urinary tract.
- Diseased lower urinary tract like a neuropathic bladder.

Consequences

- Renal scarring and renal failure.
- All complications of acute pyelonephritis.

Treatment

- Treating the renal infection o its own merit.
- Treatment for the contributing cause.

Q. Short note on renal carbuncle.

Renal Carbuncle (Syn: Renal Cortical Abscess)

- Caused by *Staphylococcus aureus* in most of the cases, transmitted by hematogenous route.
- Diabetics are most prone for this condition.
- Patients with acquired immunodeficiency (HIV - AIDs), debilitating chronic illness and IV drug abusers also develop this.
- It is a life threatening infection.
- If diagnosed early—antibiotics and intervention to debride the necrotic renal part may be feasible; however, nephrectomy is more often performed as a life saving measure.

Corticomedullary Abscess and Perirenal Abscess

Renal Corticomedullary Abscess

- Secondary to ascending UTI and any underlying abnormality of urinary tract
- Obstructive uropathy
- Vesicoureteral reflux

Uropathogens: *E. coli* and other gram negative bacilli.

Pathology

- Abscesses—extending into parenchyma.
- Or/and perforating the capsule to cause perirenal abscess.

- The abscess may or may not communicate with pelvicalyceal system.

Clinical Features
- Fever high grade or mild.
- Pain—loin or back; abdominal pain.
- Fullness and tenderness over costovertebral tenderness.
- Urinary symptoms—only if the communicate with pelvicalyceal collecting system.

Diagnosis
- Ultrasonogaphy.
- CT scan—helps in accurate method to establish the diagnosis and location of a renal or perirenal abscess.

Treatment
- Antibiotics without drainage.
    - If small abscess or multiple micro abscesses are seen.
    - If the underlying urinary tract abnormality can be corrected (like ureteric obstruction).
- Antibioic and percutaneous drainage—most cases require this.
    - Two percutaneous drains.
    - First to drain the perirenal collection.
    - Second to decompress the obstructed collecting system of the kidney.
- **Open drainage of the abscess**
    - If pus is too thick to be drained by the percutaneous route.

> **Q. Short notes on emphysematous pyelonephritis.**

EMPHYSEMATOUS PYELONEPHRITIS
- A life-threatening condition.
- A fulminant, necrotizing variant of acute pyelonephritis caused by gas-forming organisms.
- *E. coli, Klebsiella pneumoniae, Pseudomonas aeruginosa* and *Proteus mirabilis.*
- About 90% of cases are seen in poorly controlled diabetic patients.
- Often seen with obstructive uropathy.

Clinical Features
- Symptoms are of severe pyelonephritis.
- May present with a loin mass—tender.
- Patients are severely toxic.

Investigations
- A plain X-ray - KUB shows gas around renal shadow.
- Ultrasound and CT scan also confirm diagnosis.

Treatment
- Intravenous broad-spectrum antibiotics
- Percutaneous catheter drainage
- Relief of obstruction of urinary tract—endoscopic D-J stenting of pelvi ureteric tract.
- Nephrectomy—in a very severe case with threat to life.

> **Q. Short note on xanthogranulomatous pyelonephritis.**

Xanthogranulomatous Pyelonephritis (XGP)
- A chronic severely destructive granulomatous inflammation of the renal parenchyma associated with obstruction and infection of the urinary tract.
- Middle-aged women mostly affected.

Symptoms—chronic flank pain, fever, malaise. irritative voiding symptoms (frequency, dysuria)

Signs—Flank tenderness, a palpable mass.

Differential diagnosis—renal carcinoma.

Investigations
- The urine culture—commonly shows *E. coli*, other gram-negative bacilli or *S. aureus*.
- CT—shows an enlarged, non-functioning kidney, with calculi and low-density masses (xanthomatous tissue) and evidence of peri renal extension inflammation.

Treatment

Nephrectomy is curative—but technically challenging as the kidney is adherent to adjacent structures.

> Q. Discuss pathogenesis, pathology, clinical diagnosis and management of renal tuberculosis.

GENITOURINARY TUBERCULOSIS (GUTB)

Tuberculosis (TB) of the Urinary Tract

Very common in India; accounts for about 20% of extrapulmonary tuberculosis.

Route of Infection

- Hematogenous: Hence it is always secondary tuberculosis.
- There is either reinfection or reactivation of old TB.

Pathogenesis of Genitourinry Tuberculosis

Refer **Table 29U-2**.

Complications of Tuberculosis of Upper Urinary Tract

Refer **Table 29U-3**.

Pathology of Renal Tuberculosis

Refer **Figure 29U-2**.

Clinical Diagnosis

Early diagnosis is difficult as most cases are asymptomatic. Others may have any or combination of the following:

Table 29U-2: Pathology of genitourinary tuberculosis.

Blood-borne bacilli reach juxtaglomerular site to evoke inflammatory reaction and activate macrophages →	
Granulomas are formed	
Bacterial growth continues	**Bacterial growth checked**
• Caseation necrosis • Extensive renal parenchymal destruction • Shedding of bacteria into collecting system • Tubeculous bacilluria • Disease extends to collecting system • Calyx is stenosed by fibrosis • Ureteric disease—granuloma, fibrosis, stricture • Vesico-ureteric junction—stricture • Ureteric orifice—bullous granulations and ulcers, fibrosis and shortening or ureter causing "golf hole" • TB cystitis— secondary to renal TB • Prostatitis • Seminal vesiculitis • Epididymis—retrograde or blood borne • Testis—secondary to epididymal TB	• Granulomas heal by fibrosis • Calcification follows fibrosis • Residual fibrosis at corticomedullary pyramids may result in hypertension.

Table 29U-3: Complications of tuberculosis of upper urinary tract

Kidney	**Calyces**
• Caseous necrosis—putty kidney • Renal cold abscesses • Perirenal/perinephric abscess • Dilatation, distortion, destruction • Fibrosis and shrinking of kidney • Amyloidosis • Xanthogranulomatous nephritis	• Papillary necrosis, fibrosis—caliectasis • Fibrosis calyces • Hydrocalycosis. **Pelvis** • Hydroureteronephrosis • Pyonephrosis **Ureter** • Stricture and obstruction

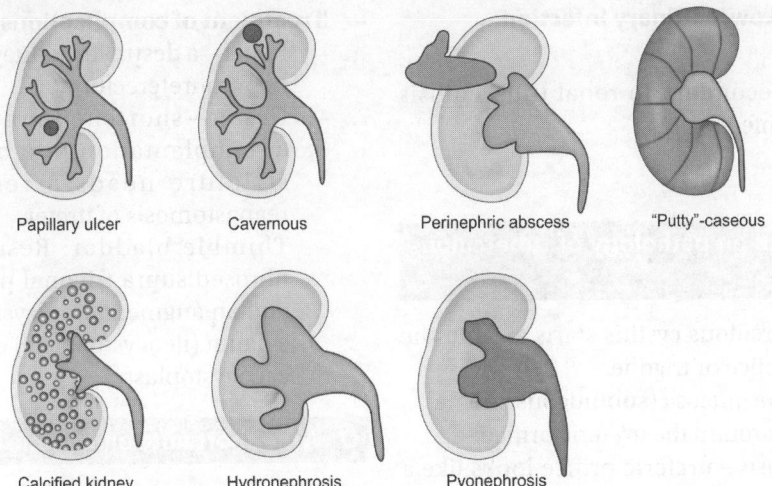

Fig. 29U-2: Pathology of renal tuberculosis

- Fever low grade or weight loss.
- Painless hematuria or microscopic hematuria or clot colic.
- Features of complications: Hydronephrosis, perinephric abscess.

Investigations

For diagnosis and assessment:
- Fluorescent microscopy or microscopy after Ziehl Neelsen staining of urine for acid fast bacilli (three consecutive early-morning whole specimens of urine).
- Urine culture for acid fast bacilli—readings taken at 3 weeks, 4 weeks, 6 weeks and 8 weeks.
- **Ultrasound**—to study renal parenchymal state and calyceal system; to study the distal genitourinary tract to detect obstructive uropathy and collections like pus.

CT scan—for identifying renal calcifications.

CT urography—identifies all manifestations of renal tuberculosis.

Early: Papillary necrosis (single or multiple) resulting in uneven caliectasis.
Progressive: Multifocal strictures—mainly ureters or calyx.
Generalised or focal hydronephrosis: Mural thickening and enhancement. Poorly enhancing renal parenchyma—(due to disease or hydronephrosis)
End-stage: Hydronephrosis with thinned out parenchyma—resemble multiple thin-walled cysts.

Dystrophic calcification of the full kidney—'putty kidney'.
Guided aspiration of fluid/pus is examined for AFB under microscope by RT- PCR- TB or GeneXpert- CB-NAAT for AFB.
Tissue biopsy from the lesions—kidney bladder, testis, epididymis - subjected to **histopathology** and **tissue culture** for a better yield of AFB.

Treatment

Tuberculosis is a notifiable disease by law and it is mandatory to notify to the authority.
Antituberculous treatment: (ATT) Currently 4 drug regimen is given in either 6 months or 8 months.
Drugs: Pyrazinamide, isoniazid and rifampicin and ethambutol.

Surgery

Surgery for GUTB—is always for complications
- Drainage of large collections/abscesses
  - Perinephric collection
  - Pyelostomy - for pyonephrosis
- Removal of diseased, dead or fibrosed tissue
  - Partial nephrectomy or nephrectomy, epididymectomy or orchiectomy
- Reconstructive surgery
  - Pyeloplasty for hydronephrosis
  - Ureteric reimplantation e.g. for ureteric strictures, mainly distal ureteric
  - Augmentation cystoplasty for thimble bladder

Tuberculous Lower Urinary Infection: Cystitis

Generally—secondary to renal tuberculosis (descending infection).

Pathology

> Q. Short note on pathology of tuberculous cystitis.

- Early tuberculous cystitis starts around the ureteric orifice or trigone.
- Pallor of the mucosa (submucous edema).
- Tubercles around the ureteric orifice.
- Later fibrosis—ureteric orifice looks like a Golf hole due to fibrosis and pulling up.
- Bladder shrinks—reducing the storage capacity (thimble bladder).

Diagnosis

Differentiated from carcinoma by cystoscopy.

Treatment

- **Antituberculous therapy**
  - Four drugs—rifampicin, pyrazinamide, Isoniazid and ethambutol for 2 months followed by
  - Three drugs (pyrazinamide withdrawn) for next 7 months (total 9 months)
  - Or officially recommended regimen.
  - Usually they respond well.

- **Treatment of complications**
  - Renal—a destroyed kidney—treated by a nephroureterectomy.
  - Ureter—shortened ureter—requires a reimplantation into bladder and a stricture needs a resection and reanastomosis of ureter.
  - Thimble bladder: Resection of the fibrosed supra trigonal part of bladder and an augmentation cystoplasty—with a ileum (ileocystoplasty) or cecum (ileal cecocystoplasty).

> Q. Write short note on thimble bladder.

THIMBLE BLADDER
Refer **Table 29U-4**.

> Q. Short note on vesicoureteric reflux.

VESICO-URETERIC REFLUX (VUR) (REFER TABLE 29U-5)

- Commonest cause of recurrent urinary infection in children.
- Affects male children in 1st year and the female children above 1 year of age.
- Also seen in adult life due to back pressure.

Etiopathogenesis of VU Reflux

- Urinary stasis due to VUR.
- Detrusor-sphincter dyssynergia.

Table 29U-4: Details of thimble bladder.

Thimble bladder: A shrunken bladder with severely reduced storage capacity.

Commonest cause	Complications
Tuberculous cystitis with severe fibrosis. Other causes: • Post irradiation • Long-standing in dwelling catheterization • Interstitial cystitis (Hunner's ulcer) • Schistosomiasis • Drug induced—intravesical caustics • Chemotherapeutic agents.	• Storage—causing frequency and urgency • High intravesical filling pressure causing back pressure and vesicoureteric reflux resulting in hydroureter or hydronephrosis and subsequent renal failure
Treatment	**Surgery**
• After treatment of the cause of shrinking. • Capacity of bladder is enhanced by surgery.	• The fibrosed supratrigonal bladder is removed and a bladder augmentation procedure is done. • Using an ileal segment—ileocystoplasty or Ileocecal segment—ilealcecocystoplasty.

Table 29U-5: Vesicoureteric reflux (VUR).

Grading of vesicoureteric reflux

Grade I	Reflux into the ureter
Grade II	Reflux into the ureter and renal pelvis
Grade III	Reflux is associated with mild/moderate dilatation on an IVU
Grade IV	Blunting of calyceal fornices
Grade V	Absent papillary impressions

- Poor bladder emptying habit.
- Outlet obstruction, stones.
- Neurological disorder causing stasis of urine (e.g., spina bifida).

Complications of UV Reflux
- Renal scarring due to renal parenchymal suppurative inflammation.
- Hypertension.
- **Chronic pyelonephritis (CPN) with renal failure.**

Diagnosis
- Ultrasonography—screening.
- CT—IV contrast enhanced CT or IVU—to demonstrate scarring.
- DMSA scan—Dimercaptosuccinic acid scan—to assess renal scarring.
- Diagnostic: MCU—micturating cystourethrography.

Treatment
General measures—antibiotic therapy to treat infection.

VUR grade I, II, III: Treatment of infection will lead to spontaneous resolution in the absence of any organic contributory pathology.

Surgery—indications:
- For VUR IV and V.
- Recurrent infections despite treatment.
- Renal scarring found.

Procedures
- Ureteric re-implantation with submucosal tunneling to prevent reflux.
- Periureteric injections of Teflon or collagen.
- Renal transplantation for a case with bilaterally scarred kidneys with renal failure.

LOWER URINARY TRACT INFECTION AND CYSTITIS

Isolated episode of infection—more in female.

Recurrent infection
- **Due to** bacterial resistance or an underlying predisposing cause.
- Postcoital infection.

Asymptomatic bacteriuria—clueless at investigation.

Infection in men—common:
- In male infants due to urinary tract anomalies and abnormalities.
- Infection in men—complicated or recurrent—requires prompt therapy and investigation.

Infection in pregnancy: Asymptomatic bacteriuria is common—more in pregnant.
- Antibiotics administered as per sensitivity—e.g., amoxicillin clavulenic acid, cephalosporin.
- Sonography to evaluate for underlying cause.

Predisposing Causes of Urinary Tract Infection

Incomplete Emptying of the Bladder
- Bladder outflow obstruction—BPH, bladder neck obstruction.
- A bladder diverticulum.
- A calculus, foreign body or neoplasm.
- Neurogenic bladder dysfunction or decompensation of the detrusor muscle.

Incomplete Emptying of the Upper Tract
- Dilated pelvicalyceal system—hydroureters—pregnancy, **vesicoureteric reflux**.
- Diabetes mellitus, immunosuppression.

Estrogen deficiency—can give rise to lowered local resistance.

Fecal colonisation (*Esch. Coli*) of the perineal skin.

In childhood, the mainstay of treatment of vesicoureteric reflux is antibiotic therapy; surgery is for recurrent infection despite antibiotics or severely dilated upper tract.

Investigations: Recurrent or complicated infection (hematuria, rigors) requires appropriate antimicrobial therapy and investigation to exclude a predisposing cause.
- Urine—microscopy and culture.
- Upper urinary tract imaging—sonography, CECT.
- Cystoscopy.
- Pyuria with a negative urine culture is suspicious of *Mycobacterium tuberculosis*
  - *Neisseria gonorrhoeae* or *Mycoplasma genitalium*.
- Cancer in situ (CIS) of bladder may present as Abacterial cystitis.

Routes of Infection

Ascending infection—most common
- Urethra—most common route.
- Vulval contamination by feces.
- Urethral instrumentation.
- Residual urine.

Descending infection—less common—from the kidney (tuberculosis).
- Hematogenous spread
- Lymphogenous spread
- Spread from adjoining structures —Fallopian tube, vagina or gut.

Pathological Consequences of UTI
- Pyelonephritis
- Cystitis
- Prostatitis
- Epididymitis

Bacteriology
- Bacterial virulence factors affect the ability of a pathogen to infect the host and cause.
- *E. coli* is the most common; *Proteus mirabilis*.
- *Staphylococcus epidermidis* and *Streptococcus faecalis* infection.

Mixed organisms found in patients with neurogenic bladder dysfunction or those with a longstanding urethral catheter - commonly *Pseudomonas* and *Klebsiella spp.*, *Staphylococcus aureus* and various streptococci. Tuberculous infection is also seen.

> **Q. Abacterial pyuria.**
>
> **Abacterial pyuria:** The presence of pus cells without organisms.
> **Differential diagnosis:**
>
> Infective causes:
> - Residual infection, recurrent infection
> - *Mycobacterium tuberculosis* and *Neisseria gonorrhoeae*
> - Abacterial cystitis due to Mycoplasma
>
> Non-infective causes:
> - CIS, renal papillary necrosis, stones.

Clinical Features
- Pain, hematuria and pyuria.
- Pyrexia and rigors and loin pain are a sign of upper tract infection or septicemia.
- Signs: Tenderness over the bladder.

Investigations

Midstream urine specimens—mid stream not intital stream—to avoid prostatic threads in initial stream (associated acute prostatitis)—subjected to microscopy and culture and sensitivity.

Treatment

Antibiotics

A best guess empirical antibiotic started immediately and modified after report is available. (Generally a quinolone—ciprofloxacin, norfloxacin).

Investigation to exclude predisposing factors
Allergies to drugs:
- Measurement of urinary flow rates and post-void residual urine.
- Ultrasound scan or IV contrast enhanced.
- CT scanning will usually be carried out together with cystoscopy.
- Difficult cases may require urodynamic investigation.

Special Forms of Lower Urinary Tract Infections

Acute Abacterial Cystitis (Acute Hemorrhagic Cystitis)

An acute attack of severe UTI with abacterial pyuria.

Cause: Mostly sexually acquired.
- Infection: Mycoplasma species, herpes simplex virus, tuberculosis
- Bladder cancer: Carcinoma *in situ*
- Drugs: Cyclophosphamide.

> **Q. Short note on Hunner's ulcer.**

Interstitial Cystitis (Hunner's Ulcer)
Almost always seen in women.

Pathology
- Chronic **pancystitis**—with granulation in submucosal layer.
- Involves trigone, ureter and the peritoneum of bladder too.
- Fibrosis of the detrusor muscle.
- Patchy areas of avascular atrophy of mucosa.
- **Mucosal ulceration in the fundus of the bladder** - linear bleeding ulcer.
- Late cases—shrunken bladder (capacity may be just 40–50 mL).

Clinical Features
- Frequency and pain, worse on full bladder (fundal ulceration), relieved by voiding.
- Hematuria—may be seen.

Treatment is difficult and unsatisfactory.
- Hydrostatic dilatation under anesthesia— gives temporary relief.

Drugs tried include —intravenous or intravesical - steroids and heparin.

PPS—Pentosal Polysulfate - oral or intravesical.

Intravesical chondroitin sulfate.

Immunosuppresants.

Role of surgery: Only in severe cases with severe fibrosis of bladder

Cystectomy along with the following options:
- With orthotopic transplantation of bladder.
- Urinary diversion:

Cystitis Cystica
Chronic inflammation of the mucosal epithelium which stimulates the extension of mucosal buds deeper down to cause cysts filled with fluid mostly near the trigone.

Symptoms—recurrent frequency and dysuria.

SCHISTOSOMIASIS (BILHARZIASIS) OF THE BLADDER

Geographical distribution:
Middle east countries, Egypt, Turkey, Lakes of China, far east countries.

Causative agent: Parasitic infestation by the trematode: *Schistosoma hematobium, S. japonicum, S. mansoni.*

Route of entry: Through the skin from the water inhabited by the parasite.

Life cycle: Definitive host—man; intermediate host—fresh water snail (*Bulinus truncatus*).

In man
- Entry of the Schistosoma embryos (cercariae) through skin into circulation to reach liver where they mature into adult.
- Adult worms enter portal vein.
- Pairing happens between the male and female worms.
- The pair moves through inferior mesenteric vein to reach the vesical venous plexus through the porta systemic anastomotic channels.
- The female worm enters submucous venule to lay eggs (about 20 ova in a chain).
- The ova are passed in urine to reach the water where they rupture (hatch) into a larva, the ciliated miracidium, which has to enter the snail, the intermediate host with in 36 hours of hatching.

In the snail:
The miracidium enlarges in the snail's liver and produces thousands of cercariae to complete the cycle.

Clinical Features
- Swimmer's itch—urticaria due to penetration of the ski by cercariae.
- Incubation period—4 to 12 weeks. Men affected more frequently than females (3:1).
- High evening temperature, sweating and asthma.
- Leukocytosis and eosinophilia.
- Or long asymptomatic of several months before the ova are released.

- Causing intermittent, painless, terminal hematuria.

Differential Diagnosis

Carcinoma bladder, tuberculous cystitis, chroinic cystitis.

Examination of the Urine

- Terminal specimen of morning urine—centrifuged and examined—shows ova but a negative result does not exclude bilharziasis.
- *Schistosoma mansoni* adult microsomal antigen (MAMA) antibody test by ELISA. The test is positive one month after infestation and specific for Schistosoma (both *S. mansoni* and *S. hematobium*.

Q. Cystoscopic findings in schistosomiasis.

Cystoscopy

Depending on the chronology of the disease, the findings are typically seen.
- **Bilharzial pseudotubercles**—are the earliest
- **Bilharzial nodules**—are caused by the **fusion of tubercles**
- '**Granulomas**—Bilharzial masses are caused by the **bunching of nodules**
- "**Sandy patches'**—result of calcified dead ova with degeneration of the overlying epithelium
- **Ulceration** is the result of **sloughing of the mucous** membrane containing dead ova
- **Fibrosis** is mainly the result of secondary infection
- **Papillomas** are more pedunculated
- **Carcinoma** is a common end-result in grossly infected bilharziasis, if neglected.

Treatment of urinary bilharziasis:
- **Treatment of the trematode:**
  - Praziquantel—60 mg/kg weight in three divided doses 4 hours apart, this kills the worm but dead ova are expelled over several months, repeat the course as needed
  - Metrifonate is also used
  - **Garlic** oil—anti-inflammatory effect of **garlic** helps reduce *Schistosoma infection*
    As a prophylaxis in areas where the **infection** is endemic

- **Endoscopy**—biopsy, fulguration for bleeding lesions
- **Treatment of complications**:
  - Urinary calculi—lithotomy or lithotripsy
  - Stricture of the ureters—ureteric reimplantation
  - Prostatoseminal vesiculitis—antibiotics.
  - Fibrosis of the bladder and bladder neck—TUIP (trans urethral Incision of prostate) or augmentation for thimble bladder
  - Bilharzial urethral strictures—dilatation or urethroplasty (if needed)
  - Squamous cell carcinoma bladder—radical cystectomy.

SU29.4: Describe the clinical features, investigations and principles of management of hydronephrosis.

Obstruction of the Urinary Tract

Definitions
- **Obstructive uropathy:** Obstruction to normal flow of urine caused by structural or functional changes in the urinary outflow tract from pyramidal level upto external urinary meatus.
- **Obstructive nephropathy:** Renal disease due to obstruction to flow of urine or tubular fluid.
- **Hydronephrosis:** Aseptic dilatation of pelvicalyceal system secondary to obstruction to outflow of urine.
- **Hydroureter:** Aseptic dilatation of ureter due to distal obstruction.

Q. Discuss hydronephrosis.

HYDRONEPHROSIS

Definition: Aseptic dilatation of pelvicalyceal system.

It may be congenital or acquired; unilateral or bilateral.

Congenital or Acquired.

Unilateral or bilateral

Anatomical types: Depending on the relationship of pelvis to the parenchyma.

- **Intrarenal hydronephrosis**: Intrarenal pelvis—early damage and pressure related parenchymal destruction.
- **Extra renal hydronephrosis**: Extrarenal pelvis—late damage to parenchyma.

Etiology

Obstruction of the lower urinary urinary tract—generally causes bilateral hydronephrosis (Refer **Table 29U-6**). Obstruction of upper urinary tract causes unilateral or bilateral hydronephrosis (Refer **Table 29U-7**).

Pathogenesis of Obstruction of Urinary Tract

Back pressure—on proximal structures (Refer **Figure 29U-3**).

- Urethra—bladder—ureter—pelvis—calyces—renal parenchyma.
- Renal parenchymal thinning to less than 2 mm signifies irretrievable loss of renal function.

Clinical Features

Unilateral Hydronephrosis

- Idiopathic PUJ obstruction—most common cause; calculus is next most common cause.
- Sex—more common in women.
- Side—more often on right side.

Symptoms and Signs

- Loin Pain: Mild or dull aching—worsened by excessive fluid intake.

Table 29U-6: Etiology of lower urinary tract obstruction.

Structural causes	*Functional causes*
Urethral causes • Posterior urethral valves • Urethral strictures—trauma, iatrogenic infection or TB • Stones, blood clots • Phimosis, paraphimosis, meatal stenosis **Prostate:** BPH, carcinoma **Bladder** • Bladder trauma, pelvic fracture • Bladder calculi • Tuberculous cystitis, schistosomiasis • Bladder cancer.	**Urethral causes** • Anticholinergic drugs • Antidepressants, levodopa **Bladder** Neurogenic bladder: • Spinal cord defects or trauma • Diabetes • Cerebrovascular accidents • Multiple sclerosis, Parkinson's disease

Table 29U-7: Causes of upper urinary tract obstruction—unilateral or bilateral hydronephrosis.

Intraluminal causes	**Extraluminal**

• Intra tubular deposition of crystals
• Uric acid and drugs
• Calculi, clots
 	
Intramural (within the wall)
• **Functional**: Dysfunction of
  – Pelviureteric junction (PUJ)
  – Vesicoureteral junction (VUJ)
• **Structural**
  – Infections, granulomas
  – Strictures
  – Tumors (benign or malignant
	• **Genital system**
	Prostate—carcinoma
	Uterus and adnexa:
	  – Pregnancy, endometriosis
	  – Pelvic inflammatory disease
	Tumors—fibroid, ovarian cysts, cancer—cervix, ovaries
	• **Vascular system**
	  – **Aberrant arteries—pelviureteral junction**
	  – Aneurysms—aorta, iliac vessels
	  – Venous—**retrocaval ureter**, ovarian veins
	• **Gastrointestinal tract**: Crohn's disease, diverticulitis, tumors
	  – **Retroperitoneal pathology**:
	     Hematomas, fibrosis: idiopathic, drugs
	     Lymph nodes, tumors—primary or metastatic
	  – **Radiation therapy**
	  – **Iatrogenic:** Surgical injury or inadvertant ureteral ligation

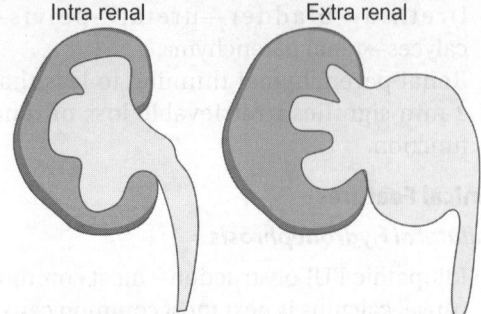

Fig. 29U-3: Types of hydronephrosis

- The kidney becomes palpable, retroperitoneal mass, ballotable with a fluid thrill.

Q. Short note on Dietl's crisis.

Intermittent hydronephrosis (Dietl's crisis). (Typical of the idiopathic PUJ obstruction).

Loin swelling associated with acute renal pain—disappears completely after the patient passes a large quantity urine; pain also subsides.

Bilateral Hydronephrosis

- From lower urinary obstruction—symptoms of bladder outlet obstruction seen.
- From bilateral upper urinary tract obstruction—idiopathic PUJ obstruction and idiopathic retroperitoneal fibrosis affects both ureters.

Hydronephrosis from pregnancy: Effected by the high levels of progesterone.

- Occurs from up to the 20th week and reverts to normalcy after parturition (12 weeks).
- Has a higher propensity for infection.

Complications

Pyonephrosis, perinephric abscess. Renal failure in bilateral cases.

Differential Diagnosis

- Loin pain—renal colic.
- Loin pain and fever—pyelonephritis, liver abscess.
- Mass: Cystic mass in flank—retroperitoneal cyst. Cystic tumor, ovarian tumor.

Q. Short note on CT/IVU findings in hydronephrosis and DTPA scan.

Investigations in hydronephrosis

Urine—culture and sensitivity and for AFB culture.

Renal function—blood urea and creatinine

Diagnostic—imaging

Ultrasonography: The best modality to diagnose hydronephrosis to diagnose PUJ obstruction. Helps assess the renal parenchyma thickness and degree of calyceal dilatation.

CT scan—intravenous contrast enhanced CT (CECT) has replaced intravenous urography (IVU).

Findings at CECT:

- Dilatation of the extrarenal pelvis.
- Loss of cupping and flattening of the calyces.
- Clubbing of calyces (later).
- Failure to opacify the renal shadow even after 36 hours of dye injection in extremes.

Isotope renography—best test to confirm obstructive dilatation of the collecting system.

DTPA scan—technetium -99 m—labeled DTPA (diethylene triamine pentaacetic acid).

- Injection of the dye and detection of accumulated dye in the obstructed collecting system with help of a gamma camera.

Whitaker test—monitoring of intrapelvic pressure after fluid is infused into the kidney, punctured percutaneously for access.

An abnormal rise in pressure confirms obstruction.

Retrograde pyelography to confirm the site of obstruction before surgery.

Treatment of Hydronephrosis

Aim: To prevent/reverse complications of obstructive uropathy and renal failure.

Goals:

- Treat complications
- Relief of pressure on collecting system and thereby on renal parenchyma.
- Treatment of the cause of obstruction.
- Restoring the drainage mechanism of the pelviureteric complex.

Indications for Surgery

Recurrent pain
- Enlarging hydronephrosis with calyceal dilatation.
- Progressive renal parenchyma damage.
- Compromised renal functional parameters.
- Risk of infection.

Obvious correctable lesion causing hydronephosis.
- Like stone, stricture, tumor renal pain, increasing.

Surgical Procedures

Q. Explain principles of pyeloplasties for hydronephrosis.

Aim at removal of obstruction and restoration of free drainage of urine into distal tract.
- **Pyeloplasty: For idiopathic pelviureteric obstruction**—unilateral or bilateral.
    - **Non-dismembered pyeloplasty** (Refer **Figure 29U-4**)
      Pelviuretic junction is not divided, but reconstruction is done to restore free drainage, e.g., **intubated pyelotomy**.
        ◆ A pyelotomy is done across the occluded segment and a tube is kept to drain.
    - **Foley's Y-V plasty (Figure 29U-4):** The Y incision over the occluded segment and advancement to make it a V-shaped anastomosis to ensure a free drainage.
    - **Dismembered pyeloplasties:**
        ◆ Anderson-Hynes pyeloplasty
        ◆ Culp pyeloplasty, scardino pyeloplasty—involve flaps of the redundant pelvis.

Anderson Hyne's pyeloplasty (Refer **Figure 29U-5**)
Performed by—
Open, laparoscopic or Robotic technique.

Principles of the Operation
- The PU junction is divided, the narrowed segment at PUJ is resected.
- The dilated pelvis is trimmed and reconstructed.
- Dependent urinary drainage is restored by reanastmosis of the ureter to the most dependent part of the trimmed pelvis to facilitate drainage.

Bilateral Hydronephrosis
- Bilateral hydronephrosis—the side with the better functioning kidey is repaired first.

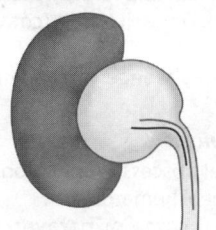
Intubated pyelotomy

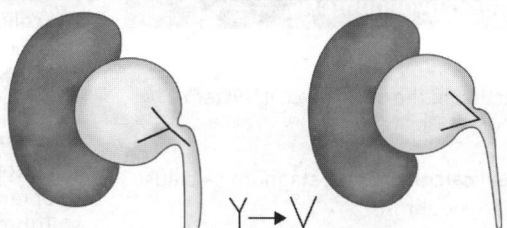
Foley's Y-V pyeloplasty

Fig. 29U-4: Non-dismembered pyeloplasty

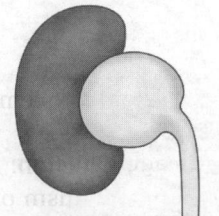
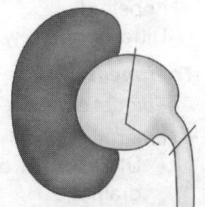
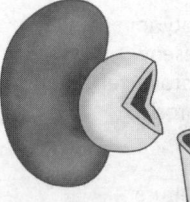
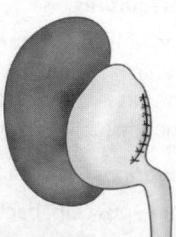

Fig. 29U-5: Anderson Hynes pyeloplasty

- Bilateral hydronephrosis with renal failure—bilateral tube nephrostomy or pyelostomy is done
- Renal function is allowed to improve and after that pyeloplasty is done.
- Bilateral disease with renal failure—bilateral nephrectomy with renal transplantation.

Nephrectomy—reserved only for a near defunct kidney with less than 10% residual function seen at DTPA scan.

- **Correction of causative pathology**:
  - Pelviureteric obstruction:
    - Aberrant vessel (artery or vein) divided and reanastomosis.
    - Stricture—resected.
    - Stone—lithotripsy (PCNL or ureteroscopic lithotripsy).
  - Re-implantation of ureter—for ureterocele, ureteric stricture.
  - Ureteric obstruction—resection (stricture or tumor) or release of narrowed segment of ureter (retroperitoneal fibrosis).

Procedures for lower urinary obstruction
- TURP, prostatectomy
- Urethral stricturoplasty
- Transurethral endoscopic fulguration of PUV.

Q. Short note on pyonephrosis.

Pyonephrosis
Purulent collection in the pelvicalyceaL system.

Etiology
- **Pelvicalyceal calculi** or Renal staghorn calculus
- Infected hydro nephrosis
- **Tuberculosis**
- Tumors obstructing pelvis or ureter
- Ascending lowet UTI—associated withV U reflux.

Clinical features
- Fever with chills/rigors, toxicity, loin pain
- Dysuria or pyuria may be present
- Loin mass—tender, full costovertebral angles, immobile (unlike hydronephrosis).

Investigations
- Urine—pus cells; bacterial culture
- Ultrasound study
- CT scan If renal function is not compromised.

Treatment
- Antibiotics
- Emergency—drainage of pyonephrosis: Percutaneous tube pyelostomy or nephrostomy or open Surgical pyelostomy
- Elective pyeloplasty.
- Subcapsular nephrectomy: When the kidney is destroyed and sepsis threatens life.

Q. Discuss perinephric abscess and what is Mathe's sign?

Perinephric abscess
A perinephric abscess is a collection of suppurative material in the perinephric space.

Causes
- Infection of a perinephric hematoma
- Rupture of renal cortical abscess or renal carbuncle into perinephric space
- Rupture of pyonephrosis
- Tuberculous perinephric abscess
- Periureteral lymphatic spread.

Extrarenal sepsis
- Hematogenous spread
- Extension of appendicular abscess
- Pericolic abscess—diverticulitis or growth
- Diabetes or immunosuppression may contribute.

Clinical features
- High fever
- Fullness in the loin
- Tenderness and rigidity
- Diffuse mass in loin and lumbar triangle
- Scoliosis to the opposite side (convexity to the opposite side)
- **Mathe's sign**—absence of movement during respiration.

Differential diagnosis
- Retroperitoneal abscess due t colonic pathology or retroperitoneal hematoma
- Tuberculosis of spine or paravertebral lymph nodes.

Investigations
- WBC counts: Elevated, renal function—may be impaired
- Ultrasonography, CT scan.

Treatment
Antibiotics coverage
- Emergency drainage
  - Ultrasound or CT—image guided pig tail drainage
  - Surgical drainage—with a tube drain.
- Followed by definitive treatment for the underlying cause.

SU29.5-SU29.6: Renal Calculi and Renal Tumors

> **SU29.5:** Describe the clinical features, investigations and principles of management of renal calculi.

UROLITHIASIS

> Q. Name the types of urinary stones, describe etiology of urolithiasis.

Calculi form in any part of urinay tract—the kidneys, pelvis, ureter, bladder or urethra. (Refer **Table 29U-8**).

Primary urinary calculi—form in sterile urine. Due to a metabolic o\abnormality.

Secondary urinary calculi—form in infected urine or owing to an underlying pathology.

Types of Urinary Stones (Biochemical Varieties)

Table 29U-8: Types of urinary stones.

Oxalate (75%)	Xanthine
Uric acid (5–7%)	Phosphate (12–15%)
Cystine (2%)	Rare types—indigo and struvite

- **Oxalate stones (75%):** (Syn: mulberry stone)—made of calcium oxalate with envelope shaped crystals. They are brownish in colour with sharp projections.
- **Uric acid stones (5%)**—hard, yellowish, smooth, multiple and radiolucent.
  - Associated with abnormal purine metabolism—with hyperuricemia and gout.
  - Urate stones—calcium urate—hard and opaque due to calcium.
- **Cystine stones (2%)**—are soft, and large, yellow in color, multiple and radioopaque (due to the sulfur content), formed only in acidic urine and commonly affects young girls.
  - An autosomal recessive trait with defective absorption of cystine ornithine, lysine and arginine from the renal tubules. It is seen in young girls.
- **Xanthine stones** are rare, smooth, brick red in color.
  - They are due to deficiency of the enzyme xanthine oxidase.
- **Indigo stones**—very rare, blue in color.
- **Struvite stone:** made of magnesium and ammonium phosphate mixed with carbonate.
  - It is formed in infections due to urea splitters, e.g., proteus.
- **Phosphate stones (10–15%): Secondary stone**
  - Composition—calcium phosphate
  - Triple phosphate stone—calcium, magnesium, ammonium phosphate
  - Formed in an infected urine more rapidly in an alkaline pH.
  - It is pale white and smooth surfaced can be very large and is radiopaque.
  - It fills the renal pelvis and calyces taking their shape and forming the Staghorn calculus or a very large bladder calculus.

Etiology of Urolithiasis

- **Idiopathic calcium urolithiasis—70% of all stone formers have this.**
  - Unexplained hypercalciuria with normal serum calcium (unlike hyperparathyroidism).
  - Renal or absorptive defect.
  - Associated with mild hyperoxaluria and hyperuricosuria and incomplete renal tubular acidosis.
- **Hypercalcemic disorders:**
  - Prolonged immobilisation causes resorption of bones resulting in hypercalcemia and hypercalciuria leading to stone formation.
  - Hyperparathyroidism causes hypercalciuria causing multiple bilateral stones or bilateral nephrocalcinosis (5%).
- **Milk-alkali syndrome:** Dietary excess of containing calcium (milk), vitamin D and alkali, soft-tissue calcification (nephrocalcinosis) and nephrolithiasis occur due to hypercalcemia.

- **Uric acid calculi:**
  - Excessive urinary uric acid or acidic urine (<pH 5.5) when uric acid is insoluble.
  - Excessive dietary purine and protein.
  - Overproduction of uric acid: Myeloproliferative disorder on chemotherapy with high cell turnover.
  - Due to low urine volumes inflammatory bowel disease and ileostomies.
- **Enzyme deficiency: Primary hyperoxaluria**
  - Autosomal recessive disorder of glyoxalate metabolism.
  - Type I—deficiency of alanine—glyoxalate aminotransferase.
  - Type II—a deficiency of D-glycerate dehydrogenase.
  Excess of endogenous oxalate production results in nephrocalcinosis and nephrolithiasis.
  - **Xanthinuria**—inherited deficiency of xanthine oxidase. Stones may form in them due to allopurinol, a xanthine oxidase inhibitor.
  - **2, 8-Dihydroadeninuria**—inherited deficiency of adenine phosphoribosyl transferase.
- **Renal tubular syndromes:** Renal tubular acidosis causes calcium phosphate stone.
  - Uric acid stones
  - Cystinuria.

Secondary Urolithiasis
- **Secondary hyperoxaluria**
  - Small bowel resection, inflammatory bowel disease, chronic pancreatitis or after jejunoileal bypass leads to increased oxalate absorption.
- **Dietary excess:** Spinach, tea, cocoa, chocolate and pepper commonly increase urinary oxalate.
- **Infection:** Urease-splitters (e.g. *Proteus, Pseudomonas* and *Staphylococcus*), break down urea to produce ammonia and CO_2. The alkaline urine, promotes formation of struvite calculi (magnesium ammonium phosphate) which can form a staghorn calculus.
- **Obstruction and stasis.**
- **Medullary sponge kidney**—about 20% of patients with calcium stones have this.
- **Urinary diversion:** These patients develop stones due to a combination of infection, acidosis and stasis.
- **Drugs**
  - Thiazide diuretics—uric acid stone. Allopurinol may cause xanthine stones.
  - Acetazolamide stimulates renal tubular acidosis.

Other Factors Include
- **Water intake**
- **Climatic conditions:**
  - Tropical and hot climate is conducive for urolithiasis.
  - Urinary colloids decrease and solutes increase causing chelation of solute with calcium.
  - Decrease in citrate level in urine (below 300-900 mg/24 hours) causes stone formation Urinary citrate maintains the calcium phosphate and carbonate in soluble state.
- **Occupation:** Sedentary jobs.
- **Diet:** Vitamin A deficiency—it causes desquamation of epithelium and forms a nidus for stone formation.

Epitaxy—a particular type of stone develops over a previously formed stone of different type (e.g., a phosphate stone over an oxalate or urate stone).

Pathology of Urinary Stones

> **Q. Describe the pathology and clinical features of urolithiasis.**

Stones cause problems through one or more of the following mechanisms:
- **Obstruction to urinary flow**—calyx, pelvis, ureter, bladder or urethra.
- Infection—renal cortical abscess, pyelonephritis, pyonephrosis, perinephric abscess, systemic sepsis.
- Epithelial erosion and hematuria—clot colic or severe hematuria.
- Malignancy—less often the urothelial metaplasia leads squamous carcinoma.

Obstruction due to Stone
- **Kidney:** Obstruction of pelvis and calyx—minor or major.

- **Ureter—any of the five sites**
  1. Ureteropelvic junction
  2. At the crossing of the common iliac artery
  3. Near the vas deferens or broad ligament
  4. At the entry into the bladder wall
  5. Ureteric orifice in the bladder.
- **Bladder**
  - Bladder outlet
  - Stone in a bladder diverticulum.
- **Urethra**
  - Prostatic urethra
  - Penile urethra and external meatus.

Clinical features: Features of both upper and lower tract calculi.

PAIN, HEMATURIA AND FEVER

Age: Common in patients aged between 25 and 40 years; but no age is exempt.

Pain: Depends on the level of stone and is due to the spasm of the smooth muscle in the wall of—the pelvis and ureter.

Renal and pelvic stone: Acute colic—felt in loin and renal angles associated with vomiting.

Acute ureteric colic—depends on level of stone:
- Upper and mid ureter—acute colicky pain—radiating from loin to groin.
- Lower ureter—pain felt in iliac fossa radiating along ilioinguinal nerve to the testicles.
- Terminal ureter (UV junction)—pain is referred to the tip of penis with strangury (due to irritation of trigone).
- Bladder stone: Suprapubic pain with dysuria and strangury.
- Urethral stone—burning and scalding pain.

Hematuria with pain.
- Hematuria with pain—visible or microscopic.
  - Initial—urethral
  - Midstream—upper urinary tract
  - Terminal—bladder and prostatic urethra.

Fever—only if accompanied by infection.

Differential diagnosis of renal and ureteric colic:
- Acute appendicitis
- Acute cholecystitis.
- Tuba-ovarian disease
- Mesenteric adenitis.

Investigations

Urine: pH-acid/alkaline, specific gravity
- Culture—for infection.
- Calcium, urate, cystine if suspected only.

Blood: ESR, serum calcium, phosphate, creatinine, blood, urea, uric acid, PTH level.

Plain X-ray, KUB: To see kidney shadow, stones (90% of stones are radio-opaque).

Ultrasound abdomen—the first noninvasive investigation—identifies all calculi and helps study parenchymal changes.

CECT scan: Helps detecting the small stones in ureter' assessing renal function and obstruction.

IVU—largely replaced by CECT

RGP (retrograde pyelography) to locate high upper ureteric obstruction.

Urine analysis and C/S to identify bacteria.

Treatment of Upper Urinary Tract Stones

The treatment may be for an emergency presentation or on elective basis.

Emergency treatment of urinary calculi—pain, hematuria or sepsis.

Diagnosis: USG or plain CT scan confirms the diagnosis, small stones (<5 mm).
- Stones less than 5 mm are observed and expected to pass spontaneously.
- Medical expulsive therapy.
  - A non-steroidal anti-inflammatory drug such as diclofenac for pain relief and observed for further episodes of pain.

Indications for early intervention: Repeated episodes of pain, signs of infection or a significant decline in renal function.

Signs of infection—temperature, pulse, blood pressure and white blood count. The estimated glomerular filtration rate (eGFR) shows the renal function.

Treatment Options for Urolithiasis of Upper Urinary Tract

- Extracorporeal shockwave lithotripsy (ESWL).
- Cystoscopy and insertion of a ureteric stent as a temporizing procedure.
- Primary ureteroscopic stone retrieval.
- Lasertripsy.

The treatment options for **sepsis secondary to an obstructing urinary tract calculus**:
- Percutaneous nephrostomy (PCN) under local anesthetic by an interventional radiologist.
- Cystoscopy and insertion of a ureteric stent after PCN.

Elective Treatment of Upper Urinary Tract Calculus

> Q. Write short note on extracorporeal shockwave lithotripsy (ESWL, ESL).

EXTRACORPOREAL SHOCKWAVE LITHOTRIPSY (ESWL, ESL)

Treating urinary tract stones by focusing shockwaves from outside the body, on the stones.

Methods of Generating Shock Waves
- Spark gap, piezoelectric, electromagnetic, and microexpulsive.
- Stones can be localized for treatment using either fluoroscopy or sonography.
- Stones up to approximately 1.5 cm in size are suitable for this form of treatment.
- More than one treatment session may be needed to fully treat the stone.
- Stone fragments left behind in the distal ureter after ESWL are called "Steinstrasse".
- Prophylactic antibiotics are used to prevent infection as stones are often colonised by bacteria. ESWL unsuitable for hard stones—cystine.

Complications: Infection, haematuria.
- Parenchymal hemorrhage and even perirenal hematoma.

Contraindications to ESWL
- Pregnancy
- Obesity
- Oral anticoagulant therapy.

Ureteroscopy
- Ureterorenoscopy can be used to access entire urinary tract and work.
- Ureteroscopes may be rigid, semi-rigid and flexible.
- Semi-rigid ureteroscopes are used for retrieval of ureteric calculi.

Stone retrieval
- Using wire retrieval baskets (Dormia basket) for distal ureteric calculi if <6 mm.
- Using lithotripsy—ultrasound or electrohydraulic (rarely) laser, electrokinetic.
- Lithoclast—mechanical breaking of stones.
- Cystoscopic ureteric meatotomy and extraction—vesicoureteric junction (VUJ) stone.

Complications of Ureteroscopy
- Injury to the ureteric mucosa or perforation.
- Tearing of ureteric wall and extravasation.
- Total avulsion of ureter.
- Ureteric stricture (late).

> Q. Short note on percutaneous nephrolithotomy (PCNL).

PERCUTANEOUS NEPHROLITHOTOMY (PCNL)

Used to treat larger stones in the renal pelvis, calyces and the proximal ureter.

Procedure: A tract is made into the renal collecting system using ultrasound or fluoroscopic guidance. The tract is dilated with dilators and a working sheath is inserted into the collecting system and the stone is visualised and fragmented (using ultrasound, laser or lithoclast). A nephrostomy is left behind after retrieval of fragments of stone for 2–3 days.

Indications for PCNL
- Larger stones—say 1.6 mm or more
- An obstruction: PUJ obstruction, calyceal diverticula or ureteric obstruction
- Obese patients
- Lower calyceal stones:
  - Stone composition: Struvite stones—nidus of infection and hence need total retrieval
  - Stones too hard for ESWL—cystine stones and calcium oxalate monohydrate.

Complications of PCNL include
- Injury to the spleen, pleura and colon.
- Hemorrhage from the renal parenchyma amd renal vessels.

- **Treatment**—for vessel bleed
  - Embolisation
  - Nephrectomy for severe uncontrollable bleed.
- Sepsis.
- Extravasation due to rupture of the collecting system.
- Retained stone fragments.

Surgery for stones: Done very infrequently these days.

Indications
- Pyelolithotomy.
- Ureterolithotomy.
- Nephrolithotomy with cooling of the kidney.
- **Total nephrectomy**—subcapsular nephrectomy due to the fibrous adhesions.
  - For a kidney destroyed and with poor function due to long-standing obstruction by a calculus (staghorn).
  - Xanthogranulomatous pyelonephritis (XGPN).

Medical Treatment of Stones
Aims
- Symptomatic relief of pain:
  - NSAID—diclofenac, mefenamic acid
  - Antispasmodic—hyoscine, dicyclomine, drotaverine
  - Alfa blockers—tamsulosin, alfuzosin, terazosin
- To prevent recurrent stone formation
- To halt growth of existing stones.

A High Fluid Intake
To avoid supersaturation of urine and ensure an daily output of at least 2500 mL.

Idiopathic Calcium Lithiasis
- High fluid intake.
- Correction of dietary excesses of calcium and oxalate.
- Thiazide diuretics may reduce urinary calcium excretion.
- Citrate mixtures—increase inhibitor activity in the urine.

Hypercalcemic Disorders
- Increased fluid—especially in immobilised patients.
- Oral orthophosphates—used to decrease urinary calcium excretion.
- Corticosteroids—in sarcoidosis reduce serum calcium.
  Thiazide diuretics are also given.

Renal Tubular Acidosis
Aim: Increase the urinary pH to 7.5-7.8 potassium citrate is given to increase renal citrate excretion. Sodium or bicarbonate is less preferred.

Cystinuria
6-mercaptopropionyl glycine (MPG). prevention and treatment of cystine stones.

Uric Acid Lithiasis
- Dissolved by increasing urinary pH to 6.5 using sodium bicarbonate or potassium citrate.
- Allopurinol, a xanthine oxidase inhibitor, to reduce uric acid excretion.

Primary Hyperoxaluria
- Pyridoxine reduces urinary oxalate excretion in half the patients.
- Orthophosphates—halt the growth of existing calculi.

Enteric hyperoxaluria: Restriction of dietary fat and oral calcium supplements.

Stones with Infection
- Antimicrobial prophylaxis—for 3 to 12 months after stone retrieval.
- Urinary acidification to prevent reformation of phosphate stones.

Q. Short note on Staghorn Calculus.

STAGHORN CALCULUS
- A calculus in the pelvis—with the shape congruent with that of the pelvi calyceal pouch.
- Typically a triple phosphate stone or ammonium, magnesium phosphate (pruvite).
- Forms in alkaline urine following infection by urea splitters.
- Large, smooth, pale white in color.

- It may be unilateral or bilateral.
- May be associated with hypercalcemic states, especially in those with prolonged recumbency.

Complications
- Pyelonephritis, pyonephrosis, perinephric abscess.
- Renal failure leading to end stage renal disease.

Clinical Features
- Pain in loin; fever; burning micturition; hematuria.
- Features of renal insufficiency.

Investigations
- Urine microscopy and urine culture and sensitivity.
- Blood urea and serum creatinine.
- Ultrasound abdomen; plain X-ray, KUB.
- Contrast enhanced CT urography or IVU to see the renal function.
- Isotope renogram-DTPA scan.

Treatment
Antibiotic—as per culture report.

Unilateral Staghorn
- PCNL—lasertripsy or lithoclastic
- Surgical nephro-pyelolithotomy.

Bilateral Staghorns
Kidney with the better function is operated upon first and the second after 3 months.

Bilateral Staghorn Calculi with Pyonephrosis
Bilateral nephrostomy - radiological image guided percutaneous nephrostomy or open pyelostomy followed by:
- PCNL or open pyelonephrolithotomy after kidney function improves- one side at a time, 3 months apart.

Non Functioning Infected Kidneys
Need nephrectomy and renal transplantation preceded by hemodialysis back up.

LOWER URINARY TRACT STONES

Bladder Stones

> Q. Classify bladder stones and enumerate types, describe the pathogenesis.

Types
- **Primary vesical calculus**—stone formed in sterile urine. Generally formed in kidney and pelvis and descends before enlarging in the bladder
  - Oxalate stone (Jack stone, mulberry)—single, sharp, hard and brownish black (blood pigment)
  - Uric acid and urate stones—single or multiple, radiolucent, smooth, pale yellow
    - Ulceration of mucosa causing hematuria
  - Cystine stones: Radiopaque (sulfur)—formed in acidic urine due cystinuria.
- **Secondary vesical calculus**. Formed in infected urine.
  - Triple phosphate or calcium phosphate stone—most common type
  - *E. coli* is the common organism.

Pathogenesis
Metabolic causes are same as in the case of upper tract lithiasis.

Local factors
- Stasis is the major factor
- Bladder outlet obstruction; BPH. Bladder neck hypertrophy
- Bladder diverticulum
- Indwelling catheter
- Recumbency
- Schistosomiasis.

Complications
- Hematuria
- Recurrent infection and asceding infection
- Renal failure
- Rupture of bladder diverticulum and extravasation of urine
- Metaplasia and carcinoma bladder.

Clinical Features

- Features of obstruction, infection, bleed, renal failure.
- Frequency, strangury.
- Hematuria—terminal.
- Pain—suprapubic or referred to tip of penis or labia, fever, hemturia.

Investigations

- Urine microscopy; crystals of oxalate (envelope) or cystine (hexagonal)
- Urine culture—for infection
- Renal function: Blood urea, serum creatinine
- Metabolic work up—serum calcium, magnesium, urinc acid, PTH assay
- Plain X-ray KUB (90% are radiopaque stones)
- Ultrasound abdomen is diagnostic
- IVU to see function of the kidney
- Cystoscopy to see radioluscent stone.

Treatment

- **Cystoscopic lilholapaxy:**
  - Mechanohydraulic lithotripsy; electro magnetic; pneumatic
  - LASER
- **Contraindications and limitations**
  - Children below 10 years of age
  - Stone characters—stone too large or too small, too soft or too hard and too many stones.
  - Bladder pathology: Stones associated with
    - Bladder diverticulum.
    - Bladder tumor
    - Thimble bladder (contracted)
    - Schistosomiasis.
- **Suprapubic percutaneous litholapaxy**
- **Suprapubic open cystolithotomy.**

Urethral Stones and Meatal Stones

- These may present with scalding and hematuria or with acute obstruction.
- Treatment is cystourethroscopic retrieval of stone
- A submeatal stenosis or urethral stricture need specific treatment—urethrotomy or meatoplasty.

> **SU29.6:** Describe the clinical features, investigations and principles of management of renal tumors.

> **Q.** Short note enumerate renal tumors.

RENAL TUMORS

Benign Tumors

- **Angiomyolipoma** (renal hamartoma)
  - May be associated with tuberous sclerosis—25%
  - Often bilateral and multiple
  - May turn malignant in 25%
  - May metastasize
  - CT—high fat content
- **Treatment**
  - Observe tumors of <4 cm
  - Angioembolization or partial nephrectomy.
- **Angioma**—may bleed and cause hematuria. Angiography and embolisation
- **Adenoma**—(metanephric adenoma) small cortical tumors—usually smaller than 3 cm.
  - Symptoms due to pressure when they grow large
- **Oncocytoma**—average 5 cm; affects more men than women can grow to large size
  - May show malignant elements
  - Radical nephrectomy is curative
- **Mesenchymal:** Leiomyoma, lipoma, fibroma

Malignant renal tumors

- Wilms' tumor (nephroblastoma)—children
- RCC—renal cell carcinoma (adenocarcinoma)
- TCC—transitional cell carcinoma—from renal pelvis
- SCC—squamous cell carcinoma
- Metastatic—from melanoma, adenocarcinoma

Renal Cell Carcinoma (RCC)

- A heterogeneous group of cancers from renal tubular epithelial cells. 2% of all cancers.
- Men are twice as often affected as the women.

Risk Factors for RCC include

- Age 60–70
- Sex—male
- Obesity
- Hypertension
- Cigarette smoking
- Occupational exposure—asbestos, cadmium.

Situations/Conditions Associated with RCC

- Chronic kidney disease, hemodialysis, kidney transplantation and acquired cystic disease of the kidney (ACDK).
- Genetic factors also contribute to RCC risk, familial RCC and at least eleven genetic mutations have been detected in association with VHL, the mutated gene—in von Hippel Lindau disease—with risk of a **ccRCC**.
- A family history of renal cancer doubles the risk of RCC.

Q. Classify renal cell carcinoma (histological and molecular basis).

Classification based on histopathology and molecular features

- **Clear cell RCC (ccRCC)**
  - Most common subtype and accounts for the majority of deaths from kidney cancer, 85% of all metastatic RCC is of clear cell type.
- **Non clear cell RCC - nccRCC**
  - Papillary RCC (pRCC) type I, pRCC type II
  - Chromophobe RCC (chRCC)

  Less common types of ncc RCC
  - Collecting duct RCC
  - Medullary RCC
  - Oncocytoma

Q. Describe pathology, staging and clinical features of renal cell carcinoma (RCC).

Pathology (Refer Table 29U-9 and Figure 29U-6)

Macroscopic appearance: Variegated appearance—golden yellow brown tumor with areas of hemorrhagic necrosis and cystic degeneration.

Spread

Direct spread: Into the perinephric space through the capsule and then through Gerota's fascia to the posterior abdominal wall.

Lymphatic spread: The renal hilar nodes and then through the para-aortic and mediastinal to the supra clavicular nodes.

Blood spread—early and extensive
- Lungs—75%, soft tissue—30%, bone (20%), liver (about 18%), CNS (8%) and skin (8%).

Microscopically

- ccRCC usually consists of tumor cells with clear cytoplasm (due to glycogen and lipids) arranged in nests or tubules surrounded by a rich vascular network.
- **Fuhrman grading system**: ccRCC—defines 4 nuclear grades (1-4) in order of increasing nuclear size, irregularity and nucleolar prominence.
- **Leibovich score following nephrectomy:** The Leibovich prognostic score runs from 0 to 11 and is based on the tumor size, stage, grade, state of lymph nodes and the presence of tumor necrosis at microscopy.
- RCC types also contain foci of high-grade malignant spindle cells (sarcomatoid differentiation).

Clinical Features

- Male: female ratio—2:1
- Age—most common group in 60-65
- Younger group (below 50) with a hereditary cancer syndrome is often seen (5% of all RCCs).

Presentation

- Asymptomatic—50%
- Hematuria seen in about 40-50%
- **Triad of RCC—pain, hematuria loin mass**. Seen in only 10%
- Weight loss
- Erythrocytosis
- Varicocele on left side due to renal vein occlusion.

Paraneoplastic Syndrome

- ACTH—led Cushing's syndrome
- Prolactin- Galactorrhea
- Hypercalcemia due to PTH like hormone secretion
- Hypertension is due to increased secretion of renin.

Atypical Presentations: 25%

Features due to secondaries:
- Pathological fractures
- Persistent cough and haemoptysis
- Fever of unknown origin (FUO)
- General symptoms—malaise, lethargy and severe anemia.

Differential Diagnosis
- Polycystic kidney disease
- Solitary cyst of kidney
- Xanthogranulomatous pyelonephritis
- Adrenal tumor
- Retroperitoneal sarcoma
- Lymphoma.
- Carcinoma colon.

Investigations for RCC
- Urine microscopy for RBCs
- Blood: Hemogram—for erythrocytosis and leukemoid picture
- Renal function test
- LFT—alkaline phosphatase
- Serum calcium and coagulation profile.

Ultrasound abdomen and Doppler study of renal vein and vena cava:
- To assess the lesions—the size, extent, lymph nodes, spread to renal vein and inferior vena cava node involvement, spread to the liver, hepatic metastases.

IVU: Spider leg—appearance—irregular and wider leg than cystic kidneys.
Mass lesion and irregular filling defect over the mass lesion.

CECT: Helps to study the tumor thrombus in renal vein and the vena cava.

MRI
- Best for evaluation of inferior vena cava and for caval tumor thrombus.
- Evaluate patients who can't receive intravenous contrast (allergy or renal impairment).

Bone scan—for metastases—h/o bone pain, tenderness over bones, high alkaline. Phosphatase, pathological fracture.

Bone scan and 18F-FDG PET scan—are not done routinely.

Q. Stage the renal cell carcinoma and summarise the treatment.

See **Table 29U-9**.

Staging of RCC
See **Fig. 29U-6**.

Treatment of Renal Cell Carcinoma
(Refer Tables 29U-10 and Table 29U-11)

Details for additional reading:

TNM staging of renal cell carcinoma—detailed—optional reading
Refer Table 29U-12.

Details
- **Radical nephrectomy is the gold standard** for all resectable tumors.
  - **Structures removed**: The kidney along with tumor, adrenal gland on the same side, perinephric fat, Gerota's fascia and proximal two thirds of the ureter. And lymph nodes from renal hilum and the nodes from crus of diaphragm to aortic bifurcation with renal hilar nodes
- **Nephron sparing nephrectomy** (partial nephrectomy)
  Indications
  - Tumors—T1 stage.
  - Solitary kidney with RCC
  - Bilateral RCC
  - Unilateral RCC with contra lateral diseased kidney—chronic nephritis, pyonephrosis or hydronephrosis, renal artery stenosis.

Table 29U-9: Staging of renal cell carcinoma.

Summary: Staging of RCC —must know	
Stage I	Tumor < 7 cm confined to kidney
Stage II	Tumor > 7 cm confined to kidney
Stage III: Extrarenal tumor extension	• Beyond capsule into perinephric fat—Gerota fascia intact. • Adrenal gland • Into a major vein or inferior vena cava
Stage IV: Metastases node	• Tumor spread beyond Gerota fascia • Any **lymph node** metastases stages N1, N2 - given up • Hematogenous metastases

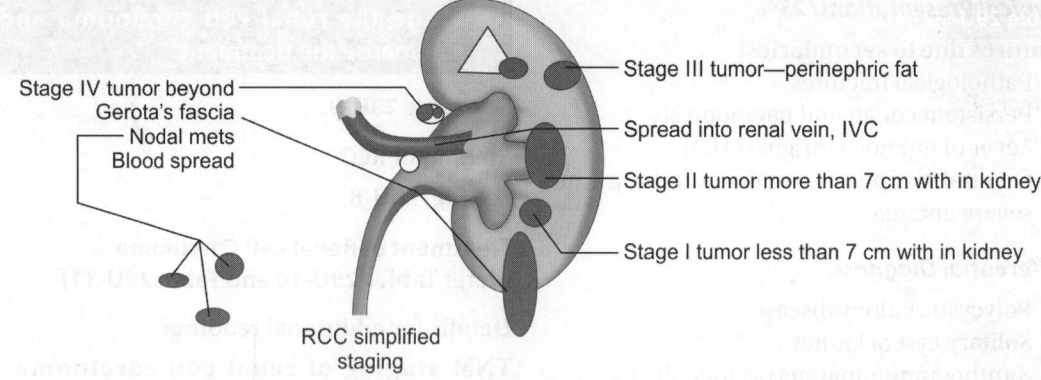

Fig. 29U-6: Staging of renal cell carcinoma

- **Palliative Nephrectomy**:
  - Principle—cytoreductive surgery
  - For advanced disease.
- **Nephrectomy and removal of IVC tumor thrombus**: Using cardiopulmonary bypass, for tumors extending above the diaphragm. (T3c)
- **Bench surgery and autotransplantation**: For larger tumors in a solitary kidney or bilateral tumors.

Nephrectomy is done, one kidney is preserved with cooling solution and dissected to remove the tumor off the normal part, which is re transplanted to the patient.

Other Local Ablative Treatment

- Radio frequency ablation (RFA)—for small tumors with metastases.
- Cryo ablation
  - Both can be done under ultrasound or CT image guidance through laparoscopy.

Radiotherapy: Generally Poor Result

- Limited role in advanced disease.
- As neoadjuvant to improve resectability of the tumor.

Table 29U-10: Nomenclature of renal surgeries in RCC.

Surgery is the sheet anchor: Nomenclature	For example,

• Laparoscopic - L
• Robotic assisted - RA
• Open - O
  – Radical nephrectomy—RN
  – Partial nephrectomy*
    (nephron sparing)—PN
  – Palliative (cytoreductive)
	LRN—laparoscopic radical nephrectomy
	RAPN—robotic assisted partial nephrectomy

Table 29U-11: Summary of treatment of renal cell carcinoma.

Summary of treatment of renal carcinoma				
RCC		CT	RT	immunotherapy/targeted therapy
Stage I, II	Radical nephrectomy	Post op	No	No
Stage III		Post op	Pre op	No
Stage IV	Palliative nephrectomy		Pre op	TKI/mTOR inhibitors
T1 tumors—low grade Bilateral RCC/single kidney	Partial nephrectomy/Bench surgery			
TCC	Nephroureterectomy			
SCC	Radical nephrectomy			

Table 29U-12: TNM staging of renel cell carcinoma.

Tumor - T		Stages			
		I	II	III	IV
T0/TX	Not assessed/No evidence				
T1	Confined to kidney < 7 cm	T1 N0			
T1a	<4 cm				
T1b	4 cm < 7 cm				
T2	Confined to kidney > 7 cm		T2 N0		
T3	Perinephric/adrenal or venous spread				
T3a	Spread to perinephric space, adrenal				
T3b	Extension to major vein or IVC			T3 N0	
T3c	Extends to IVC wall or Supradiaphragmatic IVC				
T4	Spread beyond Gerota's fascia				T4 Any N
Nodes Nx	Nodes not assessed				
N0	No nodal spread				
N1	Node positive - one or more				Any T N1
(N2 given up)					
Metastases-Mx	Mets—not assessed				
M0	No mets				
M1	Metastases present				Any T, N M1

- As adjuvant (postoperative RT, where local clearance is unsatisfactory with positive tumor margins or nonresectabillity.

Chemotherapy—chemoresistant tumor
- Used in advanced and metastatic disease, but with poor results.
- Combinations: Gemcitabine, 5 FU, carboplatin or cis platin.

Targeted therapies for metastatic RCC
- Tyrosine kinase inhibitors—anti VEGF (vascular endothelial growth factor), sorafenib, sunitinib, pazopanib, axitinib, lenvatinib and cabozantinib.
- The anti-VEGF monoclonal antibody-Bevacizumab; along with interferon- α.
- The mTOR inhibitors (**m**ammalian **T**arget **O**f **R**apamycin.inhibitors) - everolimus and temsirolimus.

Immunotherapy
- T cell-immune checkpoint inhibitors such as antibodies against programmed cell death protein 1 ligand 1 (PDL1), avelumab and tezolizumab.
- Antibodies against programmed cell death protein 1 (PD1) which include nivolumab and pembrolizumab.

UPPER TRACT TRANSITIONAL CELL CARCINOMA (UTTCC)

- Arising from pelvis, ureter and ureterovesical junction.
- Accounts for 5–10% of urothelial carcinomas
  - Frequently—multifocal and associated with carcinoma in situ (CIS) of bladder.

It may arise as a primary one or as a metachronous tumor after treatment for a bladder TCC.

Treatment
- Nephroureterectomy—kidney and entire ureter along with a cuff of bladder mucosa, around its entry into the bladder. Approach—open or laparoscopic assisted or robotic assisted.

- Regular endoscopic follow up of these patients is a must owing to a high incidence of metachronous TCC.
- Prophylactic intravesical instillation of mitomycin-C during treatment of TCC to reduce risk of recurrence.

Squamous Cell Carcinoma

Radical nephrectomy is the treatment of choice.

> **Q. Describe pathology, clinical features and management of Wilms' tumor.**

WILMS' TUMOR (NEPHROBLASTOMA) (REFER TABLE 29U-13)

Common Childhood Tumor

- This mixed tumor contains embryonic nephrogenic tissue.
- Nephroblastoma is usually discovered during the first five years of life, usually in one pole of one kidney. 5% are bilateral—pose a difficult problem.

Pathology

Gross

- A rapidly growing tumor.
- It is pinkish white, smooth, fleshy soft with hemorrhagic areas.

Microscopy: Primitive mesodermal elements (metanephric elements)—glomeruli and tubules along with epithelial elements.

Histological Types

Wilms' tumor classification depend on the dominance of epithelial or mesenchymal elements:

- Nephroblastoma
- Cystic nephroma.
- Mesoblastic nephroma.

Further Classified as per Histological Features Predictive of Prognosis

- Favorable histology (FH)—Wilms' has better differentiation (without anaplasia).
- Unfavorable histology (Un FH)—Wilms' has poorly differentiated or undifferentiated histological features.

Tumor Spread

- Local spread and blood spread early in the course, into the lungs, liver and rarely to bones.
- Lymphatic spread also is known.

Clinical Features

- Children: 2–5 years, more common in male
- A rapidly growing large abdominal mass
- Hypertension is seen often
- Hematuria signifies tumor spread into the renal pelvis.

Differential diagnosis: Neuroblastoma.

Investigations: Urinalysis—red blood cells.

Imaging: USG CT/MRI
- To find and assess
- The solid space-occupying lesion in the kidney or bilateral tumors.
- Assess the spread to veins, lungs and liver and
- Lymphatic spread is uncommon.

Treatment

- **Surgery—mainstay**—nephrectomy.
- Radiotherapy—RT

Table 29U-13: Staging and treatment of Wilms' tumor.

Wilms' tumor staging	Treatment
Stage I: Confined to kidney 40–45%	Resectable—nephrectomy + CT
Stage II: Perirenal spread 20–25%	Resectable—nephrectomy + CT
Stage III: Nonhematogenous spread -fixity to pelvic and abdominal structures + lymph nodes (uncommon)	Non resectable: Chemo- down stage and cytoreductive surgery and radiotherapy
Stage IV: Blood spread to lung/liver	CT+ palliative nephrectomy + RT
Stage V: Bilateral Wilms'	Nephrectomy on worse side, bench surgery nephrectomy on other side and retransplantation of kidney +RT +CT

- Chemotherapy CT—combination of actinomycin -D, vincristine, doxorubicin.

Treatment strategy depends on the stage of the tumor and histological type.

Wilms' tumnor - with favorable histology:
- Stage I and II: Nephrectomy and post op CT (vincristine + actinomycin + doxorubicin) + follow up.
- Stage III: Pre op RT followed by surgery post op CT.
- Stage IV: Chemotherapy + nephrectomy + RT.
- Stage V: Partial nephrectomy on better of the sides and total nephrectomy on worse affected kidney and CT+RT.

Unfavorable histology (anaplastic):
- St I, II and III—nephrectomy + CT + RT
- St IV—more aggressive CT + Nephrectomy and post op. irinotecan -+vincristine

Prognosis
- Eighty per cent survive long term with chemotherapy and surgery.
- The prognosis is worse in those with anaplastic features and metastases and in older children.

ADDITIONAL READING - GOOD TO KNOW
- Isotope renography
- DMSA/DTPA/MAG3
- TRUS-BIOPSY/TPTBP
- Narrow band imaging (NBI)
- Photodynamic diagnosis (PDD)—combined with cystoscopy
- PET CT SPECT CT
- Bone scan
- Renal cysts
- Renal trauma

INVESTIGATIONS IN SURGERY OF URINARY TRACT

Urine

Microscopy, culture and biochemical analysis.

Urinary Microscopy
- WBC—0-4 million cells per liter.
- Epithelial cells—0–55 million cells/liter.
- Blood and products.

Early morning urine samples—(3 days) for fluorescent microscopy or Ziel Nielsen staining for acid fast bacilli, followed by Culture for TB—reading taken at 4 weeks and 6 weeks.

Urinary cytology: For malignant cells—useful in TCC. But high false negative rates.

Cystoscopy and ureteroscopy:
- Visualization from urethra upto the renal pelvis

Diagnosis and therapy
- Innovation to improve the diagnostic accuracy of cystoscopy.

Narrow band imaging (NBI) and photodynamic diagnosis (PDD)—combined with cystoscopy.

NBI—a technique that filters the white light into two bandwidths—blue (415 nm) and green (540 nm) spectrum.

In the NBI mode, hemoglobin absorbs the light and light penetrates the tissue superficially helping in the identification of small capillaries and superficial structures. E.g., bladder tumors are vascular structures, appear in brown or green against a white background.

Photodynamic diagnosis (PDD): A fluorescent solution, with a preferential avidity to rapidly proliferating tissue (tumor or granuloma), is injected about 60 minutes before cystoscopy.

Cystoscopy is performed under blue light that excites the chemical accumulated in the tumor cells which stand out as pink cells against a blue bladder mucosa.

Bladder tumors and areas of CIS (carcinoma in situ) are diagnosed with greater accuracy and missed less often; they are easier to identify compared with white light cystoscopy.

CT SCAN—RENAL CYSTS

Bosniak classification of renal cystic masses:
1. Simple benign cysts
2. Benign cystic lesions
3. Complex cysts
4. Indeterminate masses
5. Malignant cystic mases.

TRUS Guided Prostatic Biopsy and Transperineal Template Biopsies of the Prostate (TPTBP) (Refer Table 29U-14)

Table 29U-14: Prostatic biopsy—TRUS guided and transperineal template.

TRUS - guided prostate biopsy	TPTBP
Local anesthesia	Generally Gen anesthesia
Limited number from PZ and TZ	Upto 36 samples -
First line biopsy	Used for negative TRUS
Anterior part of prostate nor accessible	Sampling from anterior part of prostate
Significant risk of sepsis	Less risk of sepsis

PET/CT and SPECT/CT

- Nuclear medicine imaging techniques help study the metabolic and functional status of cells. E.g., positron emission tomography (PET) and single photon emission computed tomography (SPECT) are combined with structural scans like CT and MRI to provide detailed anatomical and metabolic information.
- The most common radionuclide in clinical use is FDG (2-fluoro-2-deoxy-d-glucose). PET/CT - helps detect distant metastases in bladder cancer.
- Follow up of Seminoma Testis (11-C- Choline PET/CT) and prostatic cancer (18F Choline PET CT) after failed primary treatment.

Bone Scan

- Most frequently used in patients with urological cancers suspected of bone metastases present.
- In the routine staging of patients with high-risk prostate cancer.

Dimercaptosuccinic Acid (DMSA) Renogram

Tc-99m DMSA -is a technetium radiopharmaceutical; it binds to proximal convoluted tubules in the renal cortex with slow renal excretion causing in higher concentration on imaging.

- Used in renal imaging to assess renal structure, renal scarring and evaluation of the renal cortex.
- It also allows study of differential (split) renal function.

Diethylene-triamine-penta-acetate (DTPA) Renogram

Tc-99m DTPA—in patients suspected of having a ureteropelvic junction (UPJ)obstruction but it has largely been superseded by the **M**ercapto**a**cetyl**tri**glycine (MAG3) renogram.

MAG3 Renogram Tc-99m MAG3 is now the radiopharmaceutical of choice in the assessment of patients with suspected upper urinary tract obstruction.

The renogram curve (following subtraction of background activity) is dependent on uptake of MAG3 by the kidney from the circulation and its excretion from the kidney into the bladder.

Bladder Function Assessment

Flow Rate and Residual Urine Measurement - Indicated in

- Men with LUTS and females with recurrent UTIs or LUTS
- A peak flow rate- Q-max. < 10 mL/sec indicates BOO and >15 mL/sec rules out BOO.
- A very low flow rate with slow voiding suggests a urethral stricture.

Urodynamic Study (Refer Table 29U-15)

To evaluate bladder pressure and urine flow. (It is called pressure/flow study).

During urodynamics, fine per urethral catheters (or a dual-lumen catheter) are kept in bladder. Bladder is filled and intravesical pressure measured.

Indication: LUTS and incontinence.
- Suspected bladder neuropathy
- Selection of patients with BPH for TURP.

Two Phases of the Test

1. **Filling phase**—during which fluid is instilled into the bladder at a constant rate.
2. **Voiding phase**—the patient is asked to void.

Helps select patients for TURP—among BOO and exclude those with LUTS without BOO.

Also useful in assessing neuropathies.

Table 29U-15: Urodynamic study.

Bladder pressure		Flow rate	Interpretation
Filling phase	Voiding phase		
High	Urge to pass or nil		Overactive bladder
Normal	High	Reduced	BOO
Low	Low	Normal or low	Atonic bladder- DM or post APR
Normal	High	Low or normal	Detrusor sphincter dyssynergia Multiple sclerosis
Normal	High	Delay, low flow	Stricture urethra

RENAL TRAUMA

Seen in ten percent of all trauma cases.

It may be a blunt trauma due to fall or traffic mishap, or a penetrating one due to stabs, gun shots or industrial injuries.

Clinical Features
- Hematuria—50%.
- Shock with microscopic hematuria

Grading of Renal Injuries—American Association for the Surgery of Trauma (AAST)
Summary
- **Minor:** Confined to renal capsule and not communicating with collecting system.
- **Major:** Parenchymal tear extending to collecting system/vascular injuries/devascularisation.

Grade I: Renal contusion/subcapsular/perirenal hematoma.

Grade II: Superficial laceration <1 cm/no urinary extravasation.

Grade III: Laceration >1 cm, no urinary extravasation

Grade IV: laceration extending to pelvis or with extravasation ; or with injury to renal vein or artery.

Grade V: Shattered kidney, avulsion of renal hilum, ureteropelvic avulsion devitalised kidney/thrombus in renal artery/vein.

The indications for radiological assessment are:
- Penetrating injuries.
- Gross hematuria.
- Shock in combination with microscopic haematuria.
- Children—in whom the kidneys are much lower and less well protected.

Investigation: Immediate contrast enhanced CT scan.
- The extent of the injury, showing laceration, extravasation, surrounding hemorrhage and vessel injury.
- Helps classify pedicle injuries.
- Identifies associated non-renal trauma.

Management

Initial resuscitation as per ATLS protocols.
Penetrating injuries—require immediate surgical exploration.

Blunt Renal Trauma

Mostly managed by active observation and monitoring—GR I, II, III.

Surgery
- For Gr IV and V injuries—kidney is explored.
- If there is hemodynamic instability it reduces the risk of continued bleeding, sepsis and renal loss.

SU29.7-29.11: Lower Urinary Tract: Bladder, Prostate and Urethra

SU29.7: Describe the principles of management of acute and chronic retention of urine.

SU29.8: Describe the clinical features, investigations and principles of management of bladder cancer.

SU29.9: Describe the clinical features, investigations and principles of management of disorders of prostate.

SU29.10: Demonstrate a digital rectal examination of the prostate in a mannequin or equivalent.

SU29.11: Describe clinical features, investigations and management of urethral strictures.

SU29.7: Describe the principles of management of acute and chronic retention of urine.

SURGICAL ANATOMY OF THE BLADDER

Embryology

Bladder develops from hindgut (endoderm).
- Distal hindgut gets divided by the urorectal septum into an anterior bladder and posterior rectal component and both open into the primitive cloaca into which the genitalia also open.
- The upper part opens connects through the umbilicus as urachus, which disappears before birth.
- Adult bladder is lined by transitional epithelium overlying the lamina propria containing a plexus of vessels and lymphatic.
- The detrusor muscle is thick and trigone has only a thin area of muscle with an adherent epithelium without a submucosal layer, the urothelium extends as a sheath into proximal urethra distally and over the terminal ureters proximally.
- The internal sphincter around the male bladder neck is made of the smooth muscle and under adrenergic sympathetic control against retrograde ejaculation.
- The distal urethral sphincter is made of striated muscle anterior and on sides of post prostatic urethra(or the female urethra over its proximal two thirds), innervated by
  - Pudendal nerve- from S2-4 and
  - Somatic fibers through inferior hypogastric plexus (voluntary).

Fascial and Ligamentous Supports of the Bladder

- Pubo prostatic ligaments—lateral to dorsal vein from prostate to periosteum of pubic bone.
- At the posterolateral bladder neck, condensations of fascia pass forward medially and laterally to the ureter to join with the prostatic fascia; this fascia needs to be divided during cystectomy.
- Median and lateral umbilical ligaments: Respectively they are the urachus and obliterated hypogastric arteries, covered by folds of overlying peritoneum them.

Arterial Supply

- The superior and inferior vesical arteries—from the internal iliac artery.
- Also branches from the obturator, inferior gluteal arteries and the uterines in (female).

Venous Drainage

- The vesical plexus lateral and inferior surfaces of bladder drains into the internal iliac veins.
- The prostatic plexus and vaginal plexus are continuous with the vesical plexus in the male and females.

Lymphatic Drainage

The lymphatics accompany the veins to drain to nodes along the internal iliac vessels and then to the obturator and external iliac nodes and also into the hypogastric nodes.

Q. Nerve supply to urinary bladder.

Nerve supply to the bladder

- The parasympathetic "nerves of voiding"
  - The parasympathetic input—is from sacral segments S-2, 3 and 4.
  - The fibers pass through the pelvic splanchnic nerves to the inferior hypogastric plexus, which supply the bladder.
- The sympathetic "nerves of holding"
  - The sympathetic input—is from (T11 to L2) - eleventh thoracic to the second lumbar segments.
  - The fibers pass thorough pre sacral hypogastric nerve to the inferior hypogastric plexus.
- Somatic nerve supply: To the distal sphincter via the pudendal nerves and fibers passing through the inferior hypogastric plexus.

Afferent: Sympathetic nerves carry afferents from the fundus—arising from the mucosa, lamina and the detrusor and (they are sensitive to touch, pain and temperature and stretch of detrusor).

Stimuli are carried from the bladder to inferior hypogastric plexus; to the posterior roots of S2-4 and then to the pons which regulates coordinated detrusor contraction and inhibition of distal sphincter to effect the act of voiding. Any interruption of this connection with pons will result in a contraction of detrusor and no relaxation of distal sphincter (dyssynergia).

CONGENITAL DEFECTS OF THE BLADDER

Q. Ectopia vesicae.

Ectopia Vesicae (Exstrophy of Bladder)

- Males are four times more affected than females.
- Often associated with epispadias and abdominal wall defects, inguinal herniae.
- Congenital diastasis (separation of pubic bones and absence of symphysis)
- In males, the penis is broad and short, and bilateral inguinal herniae may be present. There is separation of the pubic bones. The penis is shot and broad and in female clitoris bifid.

Treatment

- First year of life:
  - Bladder is closed: The bladder is closed along with upper urinary diversion—ureterostomy or nephrostomy.
  - Along with bilateral iliac osteotomy lateral to sacroiliac joints.
- Later stage:
  - Reconstruction of the bladder neck and sphincters.
  - Augmentation cystoplasty—if needed with to increase bladder capacity.

Other Options

- One stage reconstruction of bladder and sphincter and abdominal wall.
- Urinary diversion onto bowel—uretero sigmoidostomy
  Or ileal or colonic conduit
  Risk of:
  - Anastomotic stricture and bilateral hydronephrosis and infection
  - Hyperchloremic acidosis
  - Twenty fold increased risk of tumor formation (adenoma and adenocarcinoma) at the site of a ureterocolic anastomosis.

RUPTURE OF BLADDER: TRAUMA

Q. Classify rupture of urinary bladder.

The bladder is invested by peritoneum, over the dome, anterior wall and upper part of posterior wall, and is without any peritoneal covering at the base and lower posterior wall.

Rupture of the bladder may be intraperitoneal (20%) or extraperitoneal (80%).

- Intraperitoneal rupture:
  Causes: An injury to a distended bladder
  - Such as a fall or blow
  - Iatrogenic—during surgery—inguinal or femoral herniotomy
  - Hysterectomy and excision of the rectum
- Extraperitoneal rupture—is caused
  - Blunt trauma or
  - Iatrogenic (surgical damage—TURP, cystoscopic procedures with diathermy or surgeries like laparoscopic hernia repair or hysterectomy).

Q. Clinical features of rupture of bladder.

Clinical Features

Intraperitoneal Rupture

- Sudden severe pain in the hypogastrium, hypotension, syncope.
- Abdominal distension: After the shock subsides and paralytic ileus sets in.
- There is no urge to pass urine. Abdominal rigidity is present.
- Peritonitis may set in later.

Extraperitoneal Rupture

- Similar to rupture of membranous urethra with urinary extravasation happening in retroperitoneum and extraperitoneal space.
- Gross hematuria is usually not seen.

Investigations

- Retrograde cystography will confirm the diagnosis
- Computed tomography (CT) is very useful—assessing bladder and associated injuries.
- Plain erect radiographs—a ground-glass appearance (fluid).
- Intravenous urography (IVU)—only if CT is not done—shows a leak.

Treatment of Intraperitoneal Rupture

- A lower midline laparotomy is performed; the bladder rent is sutured, after trimming its edges, (using 2/0 absorbable sutures—polyglactin or polydioxanone).
- A suprapubic and a urethral catheter are kept.
- A biopsy is taken if the rupture site is a bladder tumor.
- Laparoscopic exploration and suturing is also performed.

Injury to the Bladder During Operation

- If the injury is recognised, the bladder must be repaired and catheter.
- Drainage maintained for 7 days.
- If it is not recognised, treatment is similar to that of rupture of the bladder.

Extraperitoneal Rupture

- If it occurs during endoscopic resection, bladder is drained with a urethral catheter and antibiotic is administered.
- If a mass of extravasated fluid is present—a small drain through a stab incision.

Q. Etiology of retention of urine.

Retention of urine may be acute or chronic.

Causes of Acute Retention

Refer **Table 29L-1**.

Clinical Features

- History of inability to pass urine
- Severe pain

Table 29L-1: Causes of acute retention.

Causes of acute retention of urine	
Bladder • Bladder outlet obstruction (BOO) • Retroverted gravid uterus (female) • Bladder neck obstruction • Neurogenic bladder—spinal cord disease or injury. **Urethra** • Acute urethritis • Prostatitis • Urethral stricture • Urethral trauma with rupture urethra • Calculus stuck in urethra • Meatal stenosis • Phimosis	**Extrinsic** • Fecal impaction; tumor **Iatrogenic** – Postspinal anesthesia – Postoperative – Severe pain- hemorrhoidectomy – Drugs—atropine and other anticholinergics antihistamines, tricyclic antidepressants – Antihypertensives **Etiology: Chronic retention** Bladder atony • BOO with atony • Neurogenic bladder—post-trauma systemic disorders, diabetic neuropathy

- Distension of bladder—visible, painful, tender, palpable in hypogasrium.
- Neurogenic disorders—generally with perianal anesthesia and reduced lower limb reflexes.

Chronic Retention (Refer Table 29L-1)
- Usually they have high intravesical pressure and cause back pressure on upper urinary tract and uropathy including uremia.

Note: Chronic retention is painless.

Catheterization in Chronic Retention
Catheterisation drains urine but can precipitate post-obstructive diuresis and electrolyte loss. Hence they are monitored and resuscitated with replacement of fluid and sodium.

Hematuria—as the distended upper tract empties, there is risk of hematuria and obstruction of tract by blood clots. Renal recovery may take many days after catheterization.

"High pressure chronic retention"
High residual volume of urine and high filling bladder pressures.

Causes **back pressure**—to cause obstructive uropathy.
- Bilateral hydronephrosis—upper tract infection and renal failure.
- Overflow incontinence.
- Enuresis and renal insufficiency.

Diff diagnosis: Bladder dysfunction
- Impaired emptying—bladder decompensates
- Urinary infection and calculi.

Uroflowmetry—to confirm BOO and to differentiate between a dysfunctional bladder and high pressure BOO.

Retention with overflow
- The patient passes small quantities of urine involuntarily from a distended bladder.
- It is seen in an unrelieved retention.

Q. Treatment of acute retention of urine.

Treatment of acute retention
- A warm compress to lower abdomen may help in evacuation.
- A urethral catheter (14F – French gauge) is passed to relieve the pain and drain the urine.

Clinical evaluation along with ultrasonography will help in the diagnosis.
- Urethral catheter is passed under strict aseptic conditions.
- Failure to pass a catheter: Inadequate lubrication and local anesthesia, urethral trauma and false passage, urethral stricture, bladder neck stenosis and median lobe of prostate.

If catheterisation fails or is not advised:
- Suprapubic puncture—and catheter drainage under sonographic control
- Stab cystostomy
- Supra pubic cystostomy (less often done)

Further follow up—depends on the cause of retention
  - Sonography
  - Urodynamic study—evaluate a neuropathic bladder and bladder dysfunction.
  - Neurologic examination—reflexes.
  - Anal and bulbocavernosus reflex to rule out spinal cord damage.
- Treatment of chronic retention (refer above).

Q. Etiology of incontinence of urine and principles of treatment.

Incontinence of urine
Causes
- **Storage problems**
  - Small bladder capacity - "Thimble blader"—post fibrosis—tuberculosis, radiotherapy or interstitial cystitis.
  - Severe detrusor hyperactivity have a small functional capacity.
  - Infection
- **Impairment of emptying.**
  - Neurogenic bladder dysfunction—leads to small functional capacity of bladder.
- **Weak sphincter**
  - **Follows** surgical procedures such as radical prostatectomy in men
- **Problems of social control**
  - In dementia, the patients have uninhibited detrusor hyperreflexia and have incontinence.
- **Urinary tract fistulae:** Ectopic ureter—ureter joining the urethra rather than bladder.
  - Leakage from fistulae or upper tract duplication

- **Treatment of incontinence of urine**
  - Demented patients: Indwelling catheter.
  - Detrusor overactivity: Anticholinergics—Mirabegron.
  - Small bladder: Augmentation cystoplasty—ileal reinforcement of bladder.
  - Neuropathic patients with back pressure on upper tract.
    - Bladder substitution (near-total supratrigonal cystectomy with ileocecal segment bladder substitution) or
    - Augmentation with ileum (enterocystoplasty)
  - Overflow incontinence with impaired bladder emptying—prostatectomy
- **Weak sphincter**
  - Needs a gracilis sling operation to strengthen the sphincter
  - Or colpo suspension in females.
- **Appliances**
  - An indwelling catheter drained constantly into a leg urinal.
  - Penile clamps
- **Urinary diversions:**
- **Suprapubic cystostomy**

Q. Short note on residual urine in the bladder.

Importance of residual urine in the bladder
- It is the quantity of urine left in the bladder after voiding—post void residual urine (PVRU).
- Upto 30 mL of residual urine is accepted as normal, while 50 mL is considered significant.
- Residual urine may be due to outlet obstruction or failure of detrusor and sphincteric complex.

Causes
- BOO—residual PVRU exceeding 200 mL indicates need for surgery to relieve obstruction (TURP for BPH).
- Urethral strictures.
- Meatal stenosis.
- Neurogenic bladder—high volumes of PVRU may be seen.

Consequences
- Stasis and infection—ascending to the upper Urinary tract.
- Obstructive uropathy.

Evaluation
- Act of voiding is observed.
- Catheterization to assess volume of residual urine.
- Ultrasound study—evaluation of bladder and associated diseases.
- IVU and post void cystography.
- Flowmetry when possible.

BLADDER DIVERTICULA

Definition

The intravesical pressure, normally of 35–50 cm H_2O during voiding, shoots upto 150 cm of water in a hypertrophied bladder due to outflow obstruction.

This pressure forces the mucosa to project through hypertrophied muscle causing saccules between muscle fascicles and then turn into trabeculation. The complete projection through entire wall results in a diverticulum.

Classification

Congenital diverticula	Acquired diverticula
• Unobliterated vesical end of the urachus connecting the dome of the bladder	• Pulsion diverticula—high intravesical pressure • BOO, urethral stricture • Traction diverticula—herniation of bladder in a sliding hernia

Pathology
- Pulsion diverticulum: The mouth of the diverticulum is situated above and lateral to the ureteric orifice.
- Size variable—2 cm to 5 cm or larger.
- Structure—transitional epithelium and fibrous outer sheath (wall).
- Traction diverticulum—whole thickness of the bladder wall.

Complications
- Infection—diverticulitis, peridiverticulitis.
- Ureteric obstruction—by peridiverticulitis.
- Stone formation—due to stasis of urine.
- Squamous cell metaplasia and leukoplakia.
- Hydronephrosis and hydroureter—rare.
- Neoplasm: Uncommon. The prognosis is related to the tumor stage.

Clinical Features
- Mostly males above 50 years are affected
- Asymptomatic—if small and uninfected.
- Symptoms; due to infection, urinary tract obstruction and pyelonephritis.
- Hematuria—infecton or stone.
- Double micturition—back to back—after change of position.

Diagnosis

Diverticula are usually discovered incidentally on cystoscopy or ultrasonography.
- For treatment of complications, e.g., hematuria
- Treatment for the obstructing cause like BPH/stricture.
- Resection of large diverticula- (combined transvesical and extravesical diverticulectomy) is done for recurrent hematuria, risk of neoplasia, or ureteric obstruction.

> **SU29.8:** Describe the clinical features, investigations and principles of management of bladder cancer.

NEOPLASMS OF THE BLADDER

Primary bladder tumors
- Transitional epithelium—95%
- Connective tissue—angioma, myoma, fibroma and sarcoma
- Extra-adrenal pheochromocytomas.

Secondary metastatic tumors—common
- Local spread—from the prostate, the sigmoid and rectum, the uterus or the ovaries.
- Metastatic—although bronchial neoplasms may also spread to the bladder.

Pathology

Benign Papillary Tumors

The papilloma—is made of a single frond with a central vascular core with villi; the proliferative cells penetrate under normal mucosa so covered by smooth urothelium.

CARCINOMA OF THE BLADDER

One of the most common cancers in industrialized world.

> **Q.** What are the histological types of bladder carcinoma?

The World Health Organization (WHO) classification—for epithelial cancers of the bladder:

Four histologic types:
1. Urothelial carcinoma (90%)—transitional cell carcinoma (TCC)
2. Squamous cell carcinoma (7%)
3. Adenocarcinoma (2%)—due to glandular metaplasia
4. Other variants of urothelial carcinoma (<1%).

Mixed variety: Note—20% of urothelial carcinomas contain areas of squamous differentiation due to metaplasia in a TCC and 7% contain areas of adenomatous differentiation.

> **Q.** Briefly describe etiology, pathology and summary of urothelial cell carcinoma bladder.

Urothelial Cell Carcinoma

Etiology
- **Cigarette smoking**
- **Urothelial carcinogens**—aniline dye industry, benzidine
  - 2-naphthylamine, 4-aminobiphenyl; 4-chloro-o-toluidine; o-toluidine
  - Occupations associated with high risk of bladder cancer are the following:
  - Industries involving textile, chemicals, paints, dye, petroleum products, leather, cable, tyre and rubber, insecticides and anti rodent chemicals.
- **Genetic factors:**
  - **Activation of dominantly acting oncogenes—such as Ras and c-erbB-1 and -2,** and transcription factors such as E2F3
    Activation of factors dissolving basement membrane and metalloproteinases
    Factors and urinary plasminogenic factors—VEGF and EGF and their receptors
    Fibroblastic growth factor FGF and its receptor-3 (FGFR-3)
  - **Inactivation of tumor suppressor genes—p16, p53**
- Schistosomiasis—endemic countries—Schistosoma hematobium.

Pathology of urothelial cancer

Bladder is made of mucosa, lamina propria, muscularis propria, and serosa (in the dome).

Classification of Localized bladder cancer:
- **Non-muscle invasive bladder cancer, 70%**
  - limited to the mucosa and lamina propria
  - **Carcinoma in situ (CIS)**, an aggressive form of NMIBC, composed of flat, high-grade urothelial carcinoma limited to the mucosal layer.

- **Muscle invasive bladder cancer (MIBC), 30%**
  - Extends into the muscularis propria and beyond.
  - Extension through the basal layer of the mucosa, allows the tumor to invade blood vessels and lymphatics, and develop metastasis.

Grade: Low grade (well differentiated) and high grade (poorly differentiated)

Summary of bladder cancer stages: Stage I-IV must know

I Localized and non-muscle invasive
II Localized but muscle invasive
III Regional (locally advanced)—direct invasive disease
IV Extra-regional and metastatic—spread to pelvis/abdominal wall nodes and distant metastases

Tumor staging: Details for additional reading (Refer **Table 29L-2**)

Classification based on biological behavior of TCC bladder—WHO grading—system 2004—low grade (well differentiated) and high grade tumors (poorly differentiated).

The American Joint Committee on Cancer TNM staging systems

Clinical Features of Bladder Carcinoma

- Hematuria painless, intermittent—microscopic or gross—80%.
- Clot formation and clot urinary retention.
- Constant pain in the pelvis indicates extravesical spread.
- Irritative voiding symptoms (20%)—frequency and dysuria, strangury.
- Pyelonephritis—ureteric obstruction and hydronephrosis—due to obstructive uropathy—flank pain, edema of lower limbs.
- Neuropathic pain—suprapubic, perineal or anal and thighs—neuropathic.
- Anemia and weight loss.

Diagnosis—by thorough urologic evaluation consisting of a
- History, physical examination, urinalysis.
- Cystoscopic examination of the urinary bladder.
- Urine cytologic examination—cytology—positive in
  - 30% of patients with low-grade tumors.
  - 65% to 100% of patients with high-grade tumors or CIS.
- Flexible cystoscope
  - Papillary and sessile tumors are easily visualized through the cystoscope.
  - Carcinoma in Situ (CIS) is often missed as normal mucosa or as erythematous patch.
  - **Blue-light cystoscopy** with intravesical instillation of hexaminolevulinate—enhances detection rate of bladder cancer particularly CIS and helps **accurate staging of the tumor**.

Transurethral resection of the bladder tumor (TURBT) along with:

Table 29L-2: TNM staging systems for bladder cancer.

Tumor			Node		Metastases	
Tx/To	Not assessed/no evidenced of tumor		Nx		Mx	
Ta	Noninvasive papillary tumor		N0		M0- No metastases	
TIS	Noninvasive—flat (carcinoma in situ)		N1	Single pelvic node		
T1-invasive	subepithelial connective tissue: Lamina propria		N2	Multiple pelvic nodes		
T2	a	Muscle—superficial			M1 Metastases present	
	b	Muscle— deeper layers				
T3	a	Perivesical—micro	N3	Common iliac nodes		
	b	Perivesical—macro (mass)				
T4	a	Prostate, sem.vesicle, vagina, uterus				
	b	Pelvic or abdominal wall				

Stages	T	N	M
St 0 a	Ta		
St 0 is	Tis		
St I	T1	0	0
St II	T2a, T2b		
St III	T3a, T3b, T4a		
St IV	T4	Any T, Nl -3	Any T, Any N. M1

- Random biopsies of the bladder and prostatic urethra.
- To assess depth of invasion (T stage).
- The presence or absence of dysplasia or CIS.
- **Bimanual examination** should be performed at the time of resection to determine whether mass is present and, if so, whether it is fixed or mobile.

Metastatic work up
- CECT (intravenous Contrast-Enhanced CT scan) of the abdomen and pelvis.
  - CT scan detects fewer than 60% of bladder tumors;
- But useful for evaluation for -
  - Local extension into soft tissues, regional lymphadenopathy.
  - Other abnormalities in upper urinary tract (renal pelvis or ureteral tumors,
  - Associated hydronephrosis, etc.)
- MRI—plain or contrast enhanced—for evaluation of bladder wall and local extension as well as bone metastases.
- A chest radiograph
- Liver function tests,
- A bone scan (if the alkaline phosphatase is elevated).

Poor prognostic factors—predicting high risk for recurrence and progression
- Grade of tumor—high grade.
- Invasion of lamina propria (pT1).
- Tumors—3 cm or larger, multiple tumors.
- Concomitant Carcinoma in situ.
- Biological markers—expression of either epidermal growth factor.
  - Transforming growth factor-alpha.
- Mutations in *TP53*.

> **Summary**
> **Treatment of urothelial cancer of bladder (must know)**
> *Non-muscle invasive bladder cancer (NMIBC)*
> - TURBT with chemoprophylaxis—intravesical mitomycin-C within 6 hours
> - Follow up scopy—6 weeks—to check for recurrence in high grade tumors
> - Adjuvant intravesical chemotherapy—mitomycin/epirubicin/gemcitabine
> - BCG—alone or with alfa interferon 4-6 weeks after TURBT
> - Early radical cystectomy for high grade recurrence in 1 year.
>
> *Muscle invasive bladder cancer (MIBC)*
> - **Bladder sparing therapy**
>   - Re TURBT plus intravesical chemotherapy
>   - Partial cystectomy (solitary dome tumors) with a 2 cm margin and chemotherapy
>   - Multimodality— TURBT chemotherapy and radiotherapy (brachy or external).
> - **Radical cystectomy with pelvic lymphadenectomy and urinary diversion.**
>   **Also for**—SCC (associated with bilharziasis) and adenocarcinoma
> - **Urinary diversion and palliation for inoperable**

Urinary Diversion
Temporary: Tube cystostomy, pyelostomy, ureterostomy, nephrostomy.

Permanent: Internal diversions—uretero sigmoidostomy or colostomy.

External diversions
- Ileal conduits—with near spherical sphincter like designs.
- Suprapubic cystostomy—bilateral ureterostomy.

> **SU29.9:** Describe the clinical features, investigations and principles of management of disorders of prostate.
>
> **SU29.10:** Demonstrate a digital rectal examination of the prostate in a mannequin or equivalent.

DISORDERS OF PROSTATE

Applied Anatomy of Prostate

The prostate the male gland below the bladder, developing from the primitive urethra as a bud surrounded by the mesenchyme that forms the fibrous and muscular stroma. The female counterpart is the pair of Skene's glands. The bulbourethral glands (Cowper's glands) open into the prostatic urethra near the termination of the ejaculatory ducts.

> **Q. Explain anatomical zones/lobes of prostate.**

Zones (Lobes) of Prostate

Refer **Figure 29L-1**.
- Posterior or peripheral zone (PZ): Site of most carcinomas.
- Central zone (CZ): Posterior to urethral lumen above ejaculatory ducts which pass through the prostate before joining the urethra.
- Transitional zone (TZ): Mainly periurethral and more pronounced anteriorly harboring the "lateral lobes" seat of most of benign prostatic hyperplasia (BPH).

Sphincters

Smooth muscle is distributed in bladder neck and all over the prostate gland. Proximal sphincteric muscle (smooth muscle)—at the neck—to close during ejaculation helps a sexual function. The same has alfa adrenergic receptors which contract the bladder neck to prevent retrograde ejaculation (RE). Resection of bladder neck muscle or Alfa blockers allow allows RE.

The distal urethral sphincter (striated muscle) at the junction of prostate and the membranous urethra—horseshoe shaped.

Glands in the Prostate

- Peripheral zone: Glands lie in fibromuscular stroma. They are lined by columnar epithelium.
- The ducts branched, open into posterolateral grooves of verumontanum.
- Central and transition zone: Short ducts of glands open into common ejaculatory ducts, while the ducts of The prostatic utricle open into the prostatic urethra.

Benign Prostatic Hyperplasia (BPH)

Occurring in the periurethral transitional zone (TZ) compresses the outer peripheral zone (PZ), forming the false capsule while the prostatic true capsule is formed by tough fibrous capsule, separated by the intervening prostatic venous plexus from the periprostatic sheath made of endopelvic fascia.

> **Q. Prostatic specific antigen PSA.**
>
> **Prostate-specific antigen PSA**
> - PSA is a glycoprotein that is a serine protease. Its function is to facilitate liquefaction of semen. It is a marker for prostatic disease.

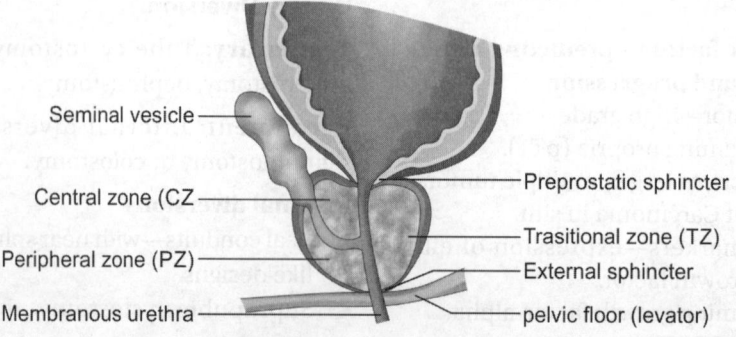

Fig. 29L-1: Prostatic zones

- There is no real normal upper limit of age. But the serum levels are elevated in elderly age, BPH, carcinoma, prostatitis. It is not specific of cancer. Serum levels below 3-4 ng/mL is considered as normal; but about 15-20% may have a cancer with these levels.
- It is good marker to monitor progress of cancer after diagnosis.
- Generally, PSA is a useful tumor marker in the post surgery setting, where a supersensitive assay, with sensitivity to 0.02 ng/mL, facilitates early detection of biochemical recurrence.

BENIGN PROSTATIC HYPERPLASIA (BPH)

- Half the men get BPH by 60 years of age.
- BPH is the most common cause of bladder outlet obstruction in men above 70 years.

> Q. Explain etiopathogeneis and pathology of benign prostatic hyperplasia.

Hormonal Physiology of Prostate and Pathophysiology of BPH

- LHRH from hypothalamus and LH from anterior pituitary stimulate Leydig cells in the testis to produce 90% of the body testosterone. Adrenal cortex produces 5-10%. The testosterone is converted into DHT (1, 5 -Dihydrotestosterone) by prostatic enzyme 5-alfa reductase II which is five times more potent than testosterone having trophic effect.
- The testosterone levels fall with age causing relative increase in estrogens, which suppress the hypothalamic LHRH level to effect low LH levels and low testosterone levels leading to atrophy of testicles.
- The estrogens stimulate the BPH through the locally acting growth factors—secreted by prostatic epithelium and mesenchymal stroma, viz., epidermal (EGF), insulin like IGF, fibroblastic GF and transforming GF).

Pathology of BPH

It affects the transition zone mainly—affecting lateral lobes and central zone at times, which projects median lobe into the bladder with in the line of internal sphincter at bladder neck. It affects the submucous group of glands in the transitional zone, forming a nodular enlargement.

Microscopy: Mixture of adenosis, epitheliosis and stromal proliferation.

Pathological Impact of BPH

Lengthening of urethra, detrusor hypertrophy—BOO, and venous congestion and LUTS.

- **Urethra**: The prostatic urethra is lengthened, but not narrowed or distorted in lateral lobe enlargement.
- **Bladder**: Hypertrophy of the bladder wall musculature if the BPH causes bladder outlet obstruction (BOO) and subsequently venous bleed from veins at bladder base.
- **Lower urinary tract symptoms (LUTS)**: The symptoms complex is a combination of various age related changes in bladder function, structure and neuromuscular activity. The following are often associated with each other.
  - BOO due to BPH
  - Idiopathic overactivity of detrusor
  - Neuropathic bladder—diabetes, centrally acting drugs, stroke, Alzheimer's disease, Parkinson's disease.

Lower Urinary Tract Symptoms (LUTS)

Related to voiding, storage, BOO-low flow.
- **Those related to act of emptying (voiding):**
  - Intermittent stream—stops and restarts
  - Poor flow—not improved by straining
  - Hesitancy worsened by a full bladder
  - Dribbling especially post void
  - Sensation of incomplete emptying
  - Episodes of near retention
- **Those related to urinary storage**: Irritative symptoms—mostly due to detrusor instability:
  - Frequency of urine
  - Urgency to void
  - Urge incontinence
  - Nocturia
  - Nocturnal incontinence (enuresis)
- **Bladder outflow obstruction (BOO)**
  - Low flow rates <10 mL/sec with high voiding pressures 80 cm of water
  - Pressure-flow studies to diagnose.

Q. Etiology of bladder outflow obstruction.

Etiology of BOO
- BPH
- Bladder neck hypertrophy
- Carcinoma of prostate
- Bladder neck stenosis
- Neuropathic causes—with functional obstruction functional obstruction
- Stricture of urethra.

Dynamics of BOO
- Low flow rate
- High voiding pressure

Effects of BOO on the Bladder
- May turn atonic due to detrusor decompensation and failure—retention v/s voiding.
- May become overactive due to irritation (diff diagnosis—neuropathic bladder or idiopathic) causing deficiency in filling capacity.

Complications of BOO

Acute Retention of Urine
- Precipitated—by illness, operations or excess of alcohol or postponement of micturition.
- May be the first prepreseting symptom.

Chronic Retention
- High residual volume of urine and high filling bladder pressures " **as high pressure chronic retention**".
- Causes **back pressure**—to cause obstructive uropathy.
- Bilateral hydronephrosis—upper tract infection and renal failure.
- Overflow incontinence.
- Enuresis and renal insufficiency.
- Bladder dysfunction: Impaired emptying—bladder decompensates.
- Urinary infection and calculi are prone to develop.
- Hematuria.

Uroflowmetry—to confirm the high pressure BOO and differentiate from a dysfunctional bladder cystoscopy to assess hematuria.

Table 29L-3: Clinical features of BPH—may vary presentation.

BPH	LUTS	Features of BOO
BPH	Nil	Nil
BPH	Nil	But only urodynamical features of BOO
BPH	Present—irritative symptoms	Nil
BPH	Present	Symptoms present
BPH	With complications	Acute retention, infection, stone formation or hematuria

Summary of Clinical Features of BPH (Refer Table 29 L-3)

Pain—a sign of complication of BOO not of BOO per se.

Pain is due to acute retention and differentiated from urinary infection, stones, carcinoma of the prostate and carcinoma of the bladder.

Digital Rectal Examination
- Prostate is smooth, convex and elastic surface of the posterior surface of the rectal mucosa moves freely over the prostate.
- Hard or nodular prostate is suspicious of malignancy and a palpable seminal vesicle indicates tuberculosis.

Investigations
- Urine culture
- Urine cytological examination
- Ultrasonography of full urinary tract with assessment of residual urine
- Serum creatinine and blood urea levels
- Urinary flow rate and residual volume assessed by uroflowmetry
- Prostate-specific antigen.

Q. Indication for surgery in benign prostatic hyperplasia.

Treatment of BPH

Prostatectomy is indicated for BPH with BOO.
- BPH with acute retention (25% of prostatectomies)
- Chronic retention and renal impairment
- Post void residual urine of more than 200 mL

- Elevation of blood urea or creatinine and sonographic evidence of obstructive uropathy (hydronephrosis or hydroureter) 15% of prostatectomies).
- Complications of bladder outflow obstruction: Formation of calculi, infection and diverticulum
- Hemorrhage: Occasionally, venous bleeding from a ruptured vein.
- Elective prostatectomy for severe symptoms.

Treatment of LUTS Secondary to BPH

- Mild LUTS—restriction of intake of water and caffeine.
- Alfa blockers: Relax bladder neck
  - Tamsulosin 0.4 mg per day. or,
  - Silodosin 8 mg or max 16 mg per day. - high incidence of retrograde ejaculation
  - Alfuzosin 5 mg (said to be causing less retrograde ejaculation)
- 5-alfa—reductase inhibitor (with alfa blocker) - dutasteride or finasteride block conversion of testosterone into DHT and cause shrinkage of a large prostate after about one year of therapy.

Surgery: TURP - trans urethral resection of prostate for large prostate with BOO_T-PAE (Transcatheter Prosatic Arterial Embolisation). Interventional radiology.

Prostatectomy

- **Trans urethral resection of prostate (TURP) is the gold standard**

Others:
- TULP—LASER vaporization—bloodless and less pain but histopathology can't be done.
- TUIP - Transurethral incision of prostate at bladder neck.
- Retropubic (Millin's) and transvesical (Freyer's) approach are rarely done now.
- Perineal (Young's) approach - given up.
- Robotic prostatectomy uncommon choice.

Complications of TURP

General

- Pulmonary atelectasis, pneumonia, myocardial infarction.
- Congestive cardiac failure and deep venous thrombosis.
- **Water intoxication**
- TURP syndrome—due to absorption of the water used for irrigation during TURP, into the circulation, can give rise to congestive cardiac failure, hyponatremia and hemolysis. Glycine is used instead of water to avoid this complication.

Local Complications

- Bleeding
- Infection
- Extravasation of urine due to perforation of prostatic urethra
- Incontinence
- Erectile dysfunction
- Retrograde ejaculation
- Stricture of bladder neck or urethra
- Worsening of LUTS.

Acute Retention in BPH

- Catheterization
- Evaluation for prostatic enlargement and excluding carcinoma
- Evaluate for other complications of BOO—renal failure in particular
- After sufficient time to allow subsiding of infection and bladder congestion
- TURP is preferred.

Chronic Retention in BPH

- Catheterization.
- Monitoring of water and electrolyte balance and sufficient hydration along with sodium replacement, against the diuresis and dehydration after decompression of retention, (resulting from failure of absorption of water and salt in distal tubules).

Bladder Neck Disorders Causing: Bladder Outflow Obstruction

- **Marion's disease**—"prostatism sans prostate"—congenital bladder neck hypertrophy
- Bladder neck sphincteric dyssynergy
- Bladder neck fibrosis
  - Post TURP
  - Post radical prostatectomy and worsened by external beam radiotherapy.

Diagnosis—along the lines of BPH

Treatment

- Alfa blockers—Alfuzosin 2.5 mg twice or thrice a day—upto 10 mg per day.
- Silodosin 16 mg per day.
- Tamsulosin 0.4 mg twice aday.

Surgery

- TUIP—transurethral incision of bladder neck.
- LASER—incision.

ACUTE PROSTATITIS

Etiology

Ascending infection:
- Iatrogenic—post instrumentation—cystoscopy.
- Long-term indwelling urinary catheter.

Descending infection—from upper urinary tract
- Blood spread—especially bedridden and immunocompromed persons.
- Common Bacteria: *Esch. coli, Klebsiella* species, *Proteus mirabilis; Staphylococcus; Streptococcus faecalis*; Gonococcus (now rare).

Predisposing Factors

- Diabetes mellitus
- Prolonged recumbency
- Immunocompromised state, debilitating illness
- BPH with BOO.

Complications

- Acute retention of urine
- Prostatic abscess.

Clinical Features

- Fever with chills and rigors
- Frequency
- Acute pain in perineum, heaviness, pain during defecation
- Retention of urine
- DRE: Acutely tender prostate. Tender prostate on per rectal examination.

Investigations

- Urine—culture and sensitivity
- Ultrasound abdomen and prostate.

Treatment

Long Course of Antibiotic

Initially a best bet broad spectrum antibiotic: Doxycycline 100 mg twice daily along with urinary alkalinizer (citrate) unless urinary pH is alkaline on preliminary examination (antibiotic changed as directed by the culture report); continued for at least 6 weeks to 2 months. Sexual abstinence for 6 to 8 weeks.

CHRONIC PROSTATITIS

Etiology

Microbiology: *E. coli, Chlamydia, Staphylococcus, Streptococcus, Trichomonas.*

Tuberculosis of prostate may also present with chronic prostatitis associated with genitourinary tuberculosis.

Associated conditions—posterior urethritis, epididymitis
- Fever—on and off, intermittent, low grade
- Continuous discomfort
- Pain in the perineum, rectum, low back pain, leg pain.
- Sexual dysfunction.

Digital Rectal Examination

- Prostate may be tender or mildly uneven or granular surface.
- Prostatic massage is done and fluid extracted—microscopy reveals pus cells.
- The fluid is tested for mycobacteria by Ziehl-Neelsen stain, culture for acid fast bacilli and cartridge based nucleic acid amplificationtest (CB-NAAT) for TB.

Treatment

- Antibiotics: Nitrofurantoin doxycycline and co-trimoxazole (trimethoprim - trimethoxazole), are useful.
- Tuberculosis should be treated with ATT.

PROSTATIC ABSCESS

- Suppuration and pus formation in the prostate.
- Preceded by prostatitis, common in diabetics and immunosuppressed.

Clinical Features

- Similar to those of prostatitis, which generally precedes the abscess.
- Ultrasonography helps accurate diagnosis.

Treatment

- Antibiotics.
- US guided aspiration—with wide bore needle in lithotomy position.
- Transperineal incision and drainage.
- Suprapubic trocar puncture and cystostomy—required in case of retention of urine.
- After drainage antibiotics are needed for longer period of 6 weeks to prevent recurrent infection.

CARCINOMA PROSTATE

- The most common malignant tumor in men over the age of 65 years.
- 15% have family history of the disease.
- Risk of a silent carcinoma focus in the prostate after the age of 60 is said to be equal to the age. Only a few are aggressive and symptomatic.

Pathology

- Originates in the PZ (peripheral zone) of the prostate.
- PSA as a screening tool: Those with PSA above 4 ng/L are screened and above 10 ng/L are subjected to prostatic biopsies. 30% of those with elevated PSA levels have cancer. 20% of the those with a confirmed cancer do not have an elevated level of PSA.

Spread of Prostatic Carcinoma

Local

- Proximally to the seminal vesicles, bladder neck and trigone; Distally to the distal sphincter mechanism.
- To ureter causing obstruction and anuria.
- The rectal invasion is unusual (due to the Denonvilliers' fascia) but a peri rectal spread causes stenosis of rectum.
- Also invasion of autonomic nerves supplying the sphincter occurs.

Lymphatic

- Periprostatic lymphatics to pelvic—obturator lymph nodes, then to internal iliac lymph nodes.
- Through seminal vesicles, into external iliac and retroperitoneal lymph nodes.
- Later stage—mediastinal, left supraclavicular lymph nodes.

Blood

- Spread to the bones mainly—pelvic bones, the lower lumbar vertebra, head of femur, ribs and the skull. The are mostly osteoblastic (unlike osteolytic deposits of other cancers).
- Paraplegia if spine is involved.

Pathological Fractures

> **Q. What is Gleason's scoring system for grading of prostatic cancer?**
>
> **Histopathology**: It is an adenocarcinoma—diagnosed and graded by Gleason's scoring.
>
> **Rationale of Gleason's scoring system**
>
> A layer of myoepithelial cells surround the prostatic glands, the seat of carcinoma.
>
> Carcinogenic changes: Loss of basement membrane followed by de-differentiation by sheets of cancer cells as the cancer grows.
>
> The degree of dedifferentiation and its relation to the prostatic stroma is the basis for the diagnosis and stratification of prostatic cancer, which also shows heterogeneity within the tissue.
>
> Hence, two areas of prostate are subjected to histological examination and each biopsy scored between 1 and 5 based on dedifferentiation of glandular cells and state of stroma and a total score of between 2 and 10 is arrived at to make a diagnosis and predict aggressiveness of the cancer as well as the tumor bulk.
>
> **Gleason's Histopathologic grade (G)**
> - GX: Can not be assessed
> - Gleason ≤6: Well differentiated (MILD anaplasia) 3 + 3
> - Gleason 7: Moderately differentiated 4 + 2 or 3 + 4
> - Gleason 8-10: Poorly differentiated (anaplastic) 4 + 3/5 + 2, any combination adding upto 8, 9, 10.

Q. Briefly mention the staging of prostatic carcinoma.

Staging of Carcinoma Prostate (TNM)

Summary

T1—found carcinoma found incidentally at histology after TURP or biopsies for high PSA
T2—nodule at digital rectal exam—but within capsule
T3—capsular spread, T3b—seminal vesicles
T4—spread to adjacent organs or beyond seminal vesicles

N0—no nodes
N1—regional nodes

M0—no metastases
M1—extraregional nodes (M1a), Bone (M1b), hematogenous metastases—liver, lung (M1c)

Q. Describe clinical features and investigation of carcinoma prostate.

Clinical Features of Carcinoma of Prostate

Early Disease

Asymptomatic—even some cases with advanced disease may be asymptomatic.

Symptoms of advanced disease include:
- Bladder outlet obstruction (BOO)
- Pelvic pain—sacroiliac
- Bone pain, 'arthritis'
- Generalized uneasy feeling, malaise
- Hematuria; frequency
- Anemia or pancytopenia; renal failure.

Digital rectal examination (DRE)
- Prostate feels hard gland, with nodule/s, irregular surface
- Obliterated median groove, if felt, is typical.

Prostatic biopsy: Transrectal ultrasound guided core needle biopsy (TRUCUT) is the gold standard to diagnose carcinoma prostate.

General blood tests
- Anemia in cases with metastases—leukoerythroblastic anemia due to invasion of marrow or anemia due to renal failure. Thrombocytopenia, DIC
- **Liver function tests**—elevation of alkaline phosphatase due to liver or bone metastases
- GGT is elevated in liver mets and also isoenzymes of ALP.

PSA
- PSA >10 ng/mL is suggestive of cancer and >35 ng/mL is diagnostic of advanced cancer.
- Prognostic value—post-treatment—tracking PSA value is a reliable index of recurrence.
- PSA falls to undetectable levels after radical prostatectomy.
- And any rise equal to 0.02 ng/mL is suspicious of recurrent or metastatic disease.

TRUS—high sensitivity to diagnose locally extensive disease (T2).

Triple assessment: DRE + PSA + TRUS
- Accuracy high only for advanced disease.
- Sensitivity to diagnose local early disease only 50%.

Magnetic resonance imaging (MRI)
MRI (1.5–3 Tesla) is the most accurate method of staging local disease.
- MRI—to assess pelvic lymph nodes and tumor stage.

Q. Outline treatment of carcinoma prostate.

Treatment of carcinoma of prostate

- Treatment options for prostate cancer depend on stage of disease, life expectancy of the patient and patient preference.
- Digital rectal examination (DRE) prostatic specific antigen, and biopsy—Gleason grade are used to predict pathological stage.

Localised cancer—treated by radical prostatectomy, radiation therapy and active monitoring.

Treatment of advanced disease is palliative, hormone ablation remains the first-line therapy.

Summary

Early disease
- Observant policy—T1, if Gleason score <6 - monitor with DRE - PSA and biopsy
- Radical prostatectomy: If Gleason score 7 and above, those tumors progressing on follow up, and in patients-life expectancy at least 10 years.
- External beam radiotherapy (EBRT)—for T1 and small T2 tumors, age >70 or patient's choice

- Brachytherapy (iridium needle or palladium or iodine 125)
  - Locally advanced: EBRT palliative.

Advanced disease: Hormonal ablation is the mainstay
- Orchidectomy—bilateral
- Medical castration
- Antiandrogens; Bicalutamide, flutamide, cyproterone acetate
- Luteinizing hormone-releasing hormone (LHRH) agonists—downregulate LH production and reduce testosterone output, e.g., Goserelin.
- GnRH receptor antagonist degarelix injections to block testosterone
- Chemotherapy—docetaxel and carbitaxel
- Abiroterone—testosterone precursor blockers (including adrenal cortex).

Treatment of carcinoma prostate: Optional advanced reading.

Early disease: Curative treatment
- Low grade Gleason score <6—surveillance with 6 monthly DRE + PSA and prostatic biopsy
- T1 T2, T 3- depends on age, and lifestyle.

Radical prostatectomy is for localised disease in men with a life expectancy of at least 10 years. Done for tumors - low grade T1 which progresses on follow up, and all T1 with high Gleason score, T2-T3.

Radical Radiotherapy for Early Prostate Cancer

External beam radiotherapy (EBRT)—is administered by focusing on the prostate, minimizing exposure of adjacent tissues.

Survival rates after EBRT:
- T1 and low-volume T2 disease—comparable to those of radical prostatectomy.

- (T3)—locally advanced disease may be treated by radiotherapy.
- On a daily basis for 4-6 weeks.

Brachytherapy: Iodine 125 or palladium-103 needles.
- Implantation of radioactive needles into prostate under TRUS (transrectal ultrasound) guidance.
- The patient is placed in the lithotomy position, under anesthesia and needles are placed transperineal puncture into prostate.

Advanced disease—The aim is to reduce testosterone levels.

Orchidectomy—for reducing testosterone effect.

Medical castration—androgen ablations:
- Stilbestrol was historically the first anti androgen drug tried.
- LHRH agonists stimulate hypothalamic LHRH receptors initially and later down regulate them, to effect stopping of pituitary LH production and decrease in testosterone production.
- Flutamide, bicalutamide or cyproterone acetate are the other antiandrogens.

Newer Agents
- GnRH Receptor antagonist—degarelix.
- Androgen receptor blocker enzalutamide.
- Abiraterone—blocks testosterone precursors—including the adrenal steroid production.

Chemotherapy

Docetaxel and carbitaxel have shown improvements in survival taxane chemotherapy to promote survival in metastatic prostate cancer.

Table 29L-4: Policy of treatment for carcinoma of prostate.

	Below 70 years	Above 70 years
Low risk	Surveillance or radical prostatectomy	Observe
Intermediate risk	RP/radical radiotherapy (if fit only)	TURP + Hormonal Ablation. (HA)
High risk	RP + hormonal ablation (HA)	Or HA only—if there is no BOO
Locally advanced (T3 disease)	Multimodal HA + RT + RP (RP= radical prostatectomy)	HA + (TURP FOR BOO) orchidectomy for HA
Metastatic	HA + Palliative RT + Abiraterone Systemic chemotherapy: Docetaxel	

> **SU29.10:** Demonstrate a digital rectal examination of the prostate in a mannequin or equivalent. DOAP session to be learnt in the ward.

Principles

- Explain to the patient
- Obtain consent
- Privacy to the patient
- Attendant—better a nurse
- Position—lateral or lithotomy (for better assessment of prostate)
- Lubricant jelly on the gloved finger
- Feel—prostate methodically—the surface, median sulcus or distorted
- Contour of prostate and relation to the seminal vesicles.
- Is the prostate pushed downwards by chronic retention?
- Above the prostate—free residual urine in the bladder feel seminal vesicles for any distention, nodularity or irregularity
- Lateral—nodes and masses
- Posterior - sacral hollow, sacroiliac joint
- Look at the finger tip for blood stain—upon withdrawal of finger.

> **SU29.11: Describe clinical features, investigations and management of urethral strictures.**

ANATOMY OF URETHRA

> **Q. Brief description of urethra and bladder neck.**

Female urethra is short—4 cm

Male urethra—4 parts
It extends from bladder neck to the external urinary meatus at the tip of the glans penis—4 parts.

1. **The prostatic urethra:** From the bladder neck to the verumontanum, is like a slit due to her side by the lateral lobes of the prostate.
2. **Membranous urethra:** Part just distal to the verumontanum, located at the level of urethral penetration of pelvic floor. It is most common site of rupture of urethra in a pelvic fracture. Surrounding musculature and external urethral sphincter make it the main site of continence, a crucial point in prostatic and urethral surgery.
3. **Bulbar urethra:** From the membranous urethra to the peno scrotal junction. Anteriorly located within the corpus spongiosum.
4. **Penile urethra:** Flattened anteroposteriorly but distends when filled with fluid. The urethral lining changes from transitional cell epithelium proximally to stratified squamous cell epithelium distally.

External urethral sphincter—made of circular striated muscle in its wall is innervated by pudendal nerve (S-2, 3, 4)

The bladder neck, innervated by T-10-12 is mainly a genital sphincter to prevent retrograde ejaculation, but contributes to urinary continence too.
It is mediated via alfa adrenergic receptors by release of noradrenaline. The alfa blockers are effective in relaxing the bladder neck spasm.

> **Q. Write short notes on posterior urethral valves (PUV).**

POSTERIOR URETHRAL VALVES

- Membranous slit like valves, distal to the verumontanum are seen in 1 in 5000–8000 male births. They are like flap valves and cause obstruction to the antegrade flow of urine.
- This causes obstructive uropathy and progressive renal failure
- The valves open cephalad direction and a catheter can be passed per urethrally.

Early diagnosis and treatment prevents renal damage and failure.

Diagnosis: Antenatal ultrasonography helps in detecting.

Neonatal sonography shows features of obstructive uropathy—bilateral hydroureteronephrosis. Later in life features of impaired renal function are seen.

Treatment

- Initial catheterization and decompression of the obstructed urinary tract will allow improvement of renal function.
- Endoscopic fulguration with diathermy or LASER correct the pathology.
- Follow up and continuing treatment of the dilated urinary tract, the recurrent urinary infections and the uremia.
- Adults with moribund failure with extreme destruction of renal parenchyma may be candidates for renal transplantation.

> **Q. Discuss hypospadias and write short note on types of hypospadias and its complications.**

HYPOSPADIAS

The most common congenital abnormality of the urethra (1 in 300 male births).
A condition where:

- External urinary meatus is on ventral side of penis from a point proximal to normal opening at the tip to anywhere upto the perineum.
- Chordee: A fibrous cord like thickening from glans to base of penis causing ventral bending of penis in an erect penis.
- Hood like prepuce: Ill developed ventral part of prepuce.

Classification of Hypospadias

Based on site of the ectopic meatus
- Glandular hypospadias meatus is proximal to normal on ventral side of glans penis, may be connected by a tunnel with the normal meatus.

- Coronal hypospadias. The meatus is in the coronal sulcus—junction of glans and shaft.
- Penile and penoscrotal hypospadias—meatus on the ventral side of penis.
- Perineal hypospadias—rarest, urethra opens between the two halves of a bifid scrotum.

Associated anomalies; testicular maldescent and micropenis.

Surgical Pathology

Absence of the urethra and distal corpus spongiosum, represented by a fibrous cord, the chordee, which causes ventral bending of the penis.

Treatment

Aim

- Top correct urinary stream
- To improve sexual function
- Cosmetic correction.

Surgical repair: Best done before the age of 18 months, complex and involves plastic reconstruction of the urethra and relocation of the meatus.

Involves

- Correction of chordee
- Relocation of external urinary meatus to the tip of the glans
- Urethral reconstruction.

Many Procedures are Practiced

- For the glandular and coronal hypospadias - the preferred procedure is the 'tubularized incised plate' urethroplasty,
- For penile and penoscrotal hypospadias, urethral reconstruction—utilizing the patient's prepucial skin is done.
- Circumcision should not be done before correction of hypospadias.

Epispadias

- The urethra opens on the dorsum of penis. penis may bend dorsally.
- It is generally associated with bladder exstrophy and defect or absence of pubic symphysis. Epispadias is very rare. Associated other developmental anomalies are common.

INJURIES TO THE MALE URETHRA

Causes

- Catheterization
- Urological Instrumentation—a cystoscope
- Accidental injuries—fall on perineum or blunt injuries associated with pelvic fractures.

Sites of Injuries

- At the point of bending of urethra—bulbous and membranous urethra
- At the site of narrowing of the urethra—submeatal urethra.

Pathogenesis

Injury causes bleeding and tear of urethra and this is followed by scarring leading to stricture. The commonest sites of such strictures are the submeatal area.

Rupture of the Bulbar Urethra

- Usually happens after a "fall astride injury" there is a history of a blow to the perineum.
- The bulbar urethra is crushed upwards between the pubis and the outer surface.
- For example, fall—gymnasium accidents astride the beam, cycling accidents, and loose manhole covers, workers falling on scaffolding.

Consequences: Extravasation of urine—in a space at mid perineal point—and collects in scrotum and under penile skin and also deep to the deep layer of superficial fascia of abdominal wall.

Clinical features: History of a fall or injury.
- Perineal bruises, hematoma
- Bleeding per urethra
- Retention of urine—full bladder.

Management

- Suspect or diagnose
  - History signs, emergency, ultrasound study
- Analgesia and antibiotic (best guess - like a ciprofloxacin or cephalosporin)
- Advise the patient not to attempt to pass urine nor strain at urine.
- Urinary diversion: Suprapubic puncture and catheterization—preferably under ultrasonic

guidance or trocar cystostomy or open cystostomy—reduces extravasation.
- Drainage of perineal of extravasated collection.

Investigations
- Contrast MRI study to evaluate urethra, bladder and pelvic muscles.
- Urethrography with water soluble contrast—to assess urethral injury and extravasation.
- Surgery for injured urethra: Delayed urethroplasty 8-12 weeks after injury when edema and infection have subsided. Excision of injured segment and anatomical repair and re anastomosis of urethra is ideal.
- Or else, secondary repairs involving reconstructive techniques for stricture urethra.

Rupture of the Membranous Urethra
- Usually it occurs in association with a fractured pelvis and may be complete or partial (less commonly). It may be associated with extraperitoneal rupture of bladder.
- The urethra also may be injured.
- Cause—road traffic accidents, falls and crush injuries.
- Associated injuries are common and need resuscitation along advanced trauma life support (ATLS) principles.

Clinical Features
- Urinary retention, blood at the urethral meatus.
- No bladder distension if there is rupture of bladder. Bruise over suprapubic area, scrotum and penis and tenderness over pubic area.
- Ultrasonography and MRI of bladder and pelvis are helpful in diagnosis.
- Urethrogram is performed with water-soluble contrast to confirm and document.

Treatment
- Emergency urinary diversion—if the bladder is distended.
An emergency suprapubic catheter should be inserted as soon as practicable (Seldinger technique) under ulrtasound guidance. Or else, a suprapubic cystostomy.
- Stabilization of the patient regarding poly trauma.
- No distended bladder indicates extraperitneal bladder rupture. It requires emergency exploration, repair of bladder and drainage of retropubic space.
- Delayed repair of urethra; injury site—3 to 6 months later—excision of scar tissue and re-anastomosis.

Complications of urethral injuries and treatment
- Hematoma between injured ends of urethra—large ones are explored and evacuated.
- Scarring and stricture—late urethroplasty.
- Incontinence of urine—difficult, permanent diversion may be needed
- Erectile dysfunction—oral sildenafil or intracavernosal prostaglandin injections.
  - Vacuum device or a penile implant.
- Extravasation of urine: Happen in the layers of the pelvic fascia.and retroperitoneum.
  - Treatment—suprapubic cystostomy—the extravasation persists—exploration of retropubic space and repair of urethral or prostatic or bladder injury and drainage is done.

URETHRAL STRICTURE

Q. Etiology and pathogenesis of urethral strictures.

Definition: Pathological narrowing of any part of the urethra.

Etiology (common causes): Causes of urethral stricture are:
- **Iatrogenic**
  - Secondary to urethral instrumentation including catheterization and transurethral prostatectomy
  - Secondary to radical prostatectomy for prostate cancer
- **Secondary to radiotherapy**
- **Post-traumatic**
  - Bulbar urethral injury
  - Pelvic fracture urethral disruption injury
- **Postinflammatory**
  - Secondary to urethritis
  - Secondary to balanitis xerotica obliterans (BXO)
- **Idiopathic**

Pathophysiology
- Iatrogenic strictures are due to a combination of trauma, infection and pressure necrosis; sensitivity to chemicals from a catheter may add to inflammatory reaction—may occur in any part of urethra (most commonly—sub meatal, bulbar and membranous urethra).
- Bladder neck stenosis—following TURP and radical prostatectomy (for prostate cancer).
- Post-traumatic strictures—refer section on urethral trauma- disruption or tear, hematoma formation and post inflammatory stricture.
- Postinflammatory strictures, e.g. gonorrhea—now uncommon.
- Generally—seen in the bulbar urethra because the persistence of infection in the periurethral glands causes fibrosis around ventral half of bulbar urethra causing crescentic stricture. Some strictures also occur in sub-meatal part.
- Balanitis xerotica obliterans (BXO)—meatal stenosis due to fibrosis of prepucial skin, extending to the glans and meatus and less commonly to the penile urethra. These strictures are long.

Clinical Features
History
- History of trauma, infection or instrumentation.
- Generally patient s are younger.
- Hesitancy.
- Urinary frequency—by day and night—stasis, cystitis and bladder overactivity.
- Straining to void and a narrow urinary stream with and low force.
- Progressive narrowing of stream.
- Prolongation of micturition and post-micturition dribbling from the pre-stricture dilatation of urethra.
- Acute retention—uncommon.

Investigations
- Urine—examination culture sensitivity.
- Ultrasonography—to assess bladder emptying and to detect any upper tract dilatation
- Uroflowmetry—plateau shaped, prolonged flow, low force.
- Urethroscopy—defines the stricture and
  - Detects false passages due to previous attempts to pass catheter.
- Urethrography—ascending or descending to depict and evaluate site and length of stricture.

Complications
- Urinary tract infections—often recurrent due to residual urine within the bladder.
- Complications of bladder outflow obstruction.
  - Bladder calculi and
  - Upper tract dilatation and renal failure.
- Retention of urine—rare.
- Urethral diverticulum—rare.
- Paraurethral abscess.

Treatment
- Endoscopic incision—internal urethrotomy.
  - For bladder neck stenosis and stricture including post- prostatectomy stricture. This can cause urinary incontinence.
- Reconstruction—urethroplasty.
- Urethral dilatation—indicated in short strictures in elderly patients. Complication includes false passage and bleeding.
- Intermittent self dilatation—recurrent strictures, patients unfit or unwilling for urethroplasty.
- Suprapubic cystostomy (trocar or open) is done for acute retention of urine or prior to definitive treatment.

Treatment Strategy
Stricture Newly Diagnosed
- Non-traumatic—internal urethrotomy.
  - Major urethroplasty procedures for recurrent strictures.
- Post-traumatic—stricture—short stricture—urethroplasty—cure rates in excess of 90%.
  - Excision of the stricture with end-to-end anastomosis.

Urethral dilatation not practiced as a first choice.

Endoscopic (internal) urethrotomy—performed under vision using the urethrotome.

Uncomplicated short stricture—single urethrotomy—50% cure rate.

Urethroplasty

- Anastomotic urethroplasty—excision of the stricture and reanastomosis.
  - For short stricture.
- Urethroplasty: For long strictures and complicated ones—using grafts.

  Free grafts of buccal mucosa, penile skin, lingual mucosa and bladder mucosa.

Technique of urethroplasty—depends upon the site, length and cause of the stricture.

> **Q. What is watering can perineum?**
>
> **Urethral fistula**
> - Cause of urethral fistula is a ruptured periurethral abscess or incision of an abscess
> - Fistula arises behind a tight stricture
> - Watering can perineum: Multiple abscesses burst open to cause fistulae
> - Post urethroplasty—due to necrosis of the flap or graft used to reconstruct the urethra
> - Tuberculosis is rarely a cause of urethral stricture
> - Treatment: Urethroplasty

Scrotum, Testis and the Penis

Chapter 30

SU30.1	Describe the clinical features, investigations and principles of management of phimosis, paraphimosis and carcinoma penis.
SU30.2	Describe the applied anatomy, clinical features, investigations and principles of management of undescended testis.
SU30.3	Describe the applied anatomy, clinical features, investigations and principles of management of epididymo-orchitis.
SU30.4	Describe the applied anatomy, clinical features, investigations and principles of management of varicocele.
SU30.5	Describe the applied anatomy, clinical features, investigations and principles of management of hydrocele.
SU30.6	Describe classification, clinical features, investigations and principles of management of tumors of testis.

SU30.1: Describe the clinical features, investigations and principles of management of phimosis, paraphimosis and carcinoma penis.

Q. Define phimosis.

PHIMOSIS

- It is inability to retract the prepuce.
- At birth the foreskin is adherent to glans penis; the adhesions begin to disappear after two years upto 6 years.
- True phimosis is due to narrowed preputial orifice.

Phimosis in Adults

Acquired phimosis
- Scarring of prepuce due to balanitis (glans).
- Posthitis (foreskin).

Q. Write a short note on Balanitis Xerotica Obliterans.

- **Lichen sclerosus et atrophicus (syn: balanitis xerotica obliterans) BXO.**
  - Affects—foreskin, glans penis and penile urethra.
  - Foreskin is thickened and whitish to form a constricting band (cicatrix)—that causes phimosis.
  - Glans penis—meatal stenosis.
  - Penile urethra—urethral stricture.
  - All these predispose to recurrent balanitis and synechiae between glans and prepuce.
  - Predisposes to carcinoma penis.

Treatment
- Young child with a non-retractile foreskin— observe for normal resolution of adhesions.

- Preputial cleaning to clear smegma and prevent infection.
- **Preputioplasty:** It involves division of tight preputial ring vertically and suturing horizontally to widen the sac and make the prepuce retractable.
- **Circumcision**—standard treatment.

BXO
- Preputial—circumcision is curative.
- Glans penis—steroid cream or ointment.
- Urethral meatal narrowing—meatotomy.

Dorsal Slit
- Division of prepuce vertically—to widen the preputial sac.
- To facilitate urethral catheterization in emergency.

> Q. Define circumcision, explain indications and complications of circumcision.

CIRCUMCISION
Indications
- Religious custom or social practice
- Medical indications:
  - Phimosis—infants and young children.
  - Recurrent attacks of balanoposthitis.
  - Recurrent urinary tract infections.
  - BXO—balanitis xerotica obliterans—in adults.
  - Tight frenum to facilitate coitus.
  - Recurrent balanitis—especially herpes simplex—to promote keratinization and thickening of skin to prevent infection.
  - Carcinoma—circumcision is curative for preputial carcinoma. It facilitates biopsy and radiotherapy for a subpreputial growth.

Technique of Circumcision
Infants
Guillotine method practiced earlier is not favored due to risk of amputating the glans.

Technique in Adolescents and Adults
The prepuce is pulled gently and divided upto about 10 mm from the corona to ensure that excess skin is not removed. The circumferential division of the skin 1.5 cm distal to the coronal sulcus and suturing the cut edges after ligating the dorsal vein and ventral renal artery.

> Q. Short note on paraphimosis.

PARAPHIMOSIS
- Inability to return a retracted prepuce.
- The retracted prepuce forms a tight ring around the glans causes edema.
- The venous and lymphatic return from the glans and distal foreskin is obstructed causing edema.

Treatment
- Reducton of paraphimosis followed by circumcision after the edema subsides.
- Methods for reduction: Ice bags, compresses with ether or gentle manual compression and retraction, local injection of hyaluronidase in normal saline.
- When reduction is not possible due to delayed presentation, division of constricting ring behind the corona is done under local anesthesia.

Circumcision is indicated as below:

Cicumcision is performed only after edema subsides or in cases where manual reduction is nor possible.

BALANOPOSTHITIS
- Balanitis, e.g, herpetic or posthitis—gonorrhea with urethritis or combination—common diabetics are more prone.
- 'Acute balanoposthitis—is seen more commonly in children.

Treatment
- Antibiotics—erythromycin or amoxicillin and ibuprofen syrup along with local hygiene.
- An phimosis or synechiae need release and circumcision.

Chronic Balanoposthitis
Adhesions develop between glans and prepuce and predisposes in the long run for carcinoma.

> Q. Classify penile malignancies, enumerate premalignant penile lesions and etiological factors in carcinoma of penis.

CARCINOMA PENIS

Penile Malignancies

- Squamous cell carcinoma—arising from skin of corona and glans—most common.
- Melanoma—less common.
- Adenocarcinoma—from glands of Tyson (tiny **glands** on either side of the frenulum—secrete smegma).
- Urothelial malignancy (transitional cell carcinoma)—from urethral lining.
- Sarcomas—form the mesenchymal supportive stroma—rare.

CARCINOMA OF PENIS

Etiology and Predisposing/Risk Factors

- Smegma: Inspissation of smegma in the coronal sulcus—leads to carcinogenic changes; circumcision at birth (not later) confers protection against carcinoma.
- HPV—human papilloma virus infection.
- BXO—balanitis xerotica obliterans.
- Chronic balanoposthitis and phimosis.
- Cigarette smoking.
- UV radiation.
- Immunosuppression.

PREMALIGNANT CONDITIONS

Each can be a short note question.
Penile Intraepithelia neoplasia (PeIN), erythroplasia of Queyrat, Bowen's disease, Leukoplakia of glans, HPV infections -HPV 6 and 11.

Penile Intraepithelial Neoplasia (PeIN)

Syn: Carcinoma in situ: PeIN—later turns invasive carcinoma.
Presents as a red patch on penile skin.

- **Erythroplasia of Queyrat:** PeIN over glans.
  - Elderly, white men—uncircumcised.
  - A solitary, bright-red eroded plaque—glistening, velvety, sharply defined and nontender—on the glans, in the coronal sulcus or inner layer of the prepuce.
- **Bowen's disease:** Elderly men, white race.
  - Solitary, dull-red plaque on shaft of penis—has areas of crusting and oozing.
  - Papillomatous or ulceration—growth suggests evolution to invasive SCC.

Pre-existing Dermatoses

Leukoplakia; HPV infections; penile lichen sclerosus, penile horn.

Leukoplakia of Glans Penis

Infiltrated, white, verrucous plaques on the glans or the prepuce due to squamous hyperplasia.

HPV Infections

Exophytic, fleshy, fibroepithelial proliferation.

PATHOLOGY OF CARCINOMA OF PENIS

> Q. Describe pathology and staging of penile carcinoma.

Macroscopy

Growth from coronal sulcus, glans, prepuce.
- Proliferative papillomatous.
- Ulcerative.
- Flat and infiltrating.

Direct Spread

To corpora cavernosa and less commonly to corpora spongiosa. Spread to urethra and meatus is late.

Lymphatic Spread

- From prepuce—inguinal nodes
- Glans and shaft—to the node at the root of penis; further spread to the external iliac.

Blood Spread

Less common—to lungs and rarely to skin.

Microscopy

- Carcinoma in situ
- Invasive—grades 1, 2, 3 and 4 depending on differentiation.

At times, it may be the first manifestation of diabetes.

STAGING (REFER TABLE 30.1)

TNM Staging of Carcinoma Penis

Special types: Penile verrucous carcinoma—associated with HPV.

> **Q. Short notes on Buschke–Löwenstein tumor.**

- The Buschke–Löwenstein tumor, an uncommon variant, resembles verrucous carcinoma in histologically.
- Locally invasive, destroys the tissue but does not spread to lymph nodes and does not spread through blood.

Treatment: Surgical excision.

Clinical Features of Penile Carcinoma

Presentation

Adults: Above 40 years make the most of the patients.

- Fleshy growth around corona gland is or under prepuce—gradually grows.
- History of recent phimosis in a non-diabetic is suspicious of a sub-preputial carcinoma.
- Foul smelling discharge from under the prepuce or bleeding from growth.
- Dysuria/hematuria if urethra is invaded. Induration is felt in the margin of the growth and penile shaft.

Inguinal and external iliac nodes may be palpably enlarged, hard and mobile or fixed.

Associated findings—previous papilloma, lichen planus, leukoplakia or BXO.

Differential Diagnosis

Papilloma, Buschke-Lowenstein tumor.

> **Q. Investigation and treatment of carcinoma of penis.**

Investigation

Wedge biopsy form the growth proves the diagnosis. Histopathology shows a squamous cell carcinoma.

- Immunohistochemistry (IHC) staining—for p53 and p16
- Ultrasound—groins and iliac nodes, other pelvic nodes
- Chest X-ray
- CT scan abdomen and chest—if metastases are suspected.
- **Assessment of primary growth:** MRI scan of penis and inguino-iliac nodes

Table 30.1: TNM staging of carcinoma of penis.

Tis PeIN: Syn: Ca in situ, Bowen's		Nx: Unassessed	Mx
Ta: Noninvasive (verrucous) Ca		N0: No nodes	M0
T-1: Glans and prepuce—sub-epithelial	T1a - Gr. 1-2, no LVI (lymphovascular invasion)	N1: Single superficial mobile unilateral inguinal node	M1a: Occult M1b: Single organ
	T1b - Gr. 3-4, LVI +		
T2: Corpora cavernosa/spongiosum		N2: Multiple unilateral or bilateral mobile inguinal nodes	M1c: Multiple mets in single organ
T3: Tumor invading the urethra		N3: Fixed inguinal nodes or involvement of pelvic nodes; unilateral or bilateral	M1d: Multiple organs
T4: Tumor invading other adjacent structures			
Clinical staging: Old classification		**TNM staging**	
Stage I: Confined to prepuce and glans Stage II: Spread to corpora cavernosa or spongiosum Stage III: Regional lymph nodes invaded Stage IV: Extra-regional/lymphatic metastases		T1a: N0 M0 T1b: T2 N0 M0 IIIa: T1- 3 N1, III b-T1-3 N2 IV: T4 any N, any TN3, M1	

- FNAC—groin lymph node under ultrasonic guidance for staging.
- SLNB—sentinel node biopsy in N0 tumor.

Q. Explain principles of treatment for carcinoma of penis.

Treatment of Carcinoma Penis

(Sum: Treatment for primary lesion, inguinal nodes and role of radiotherapy)

Modalities

- Surgery—for primary and secondary (refer below).
- Radiation therapy and chemotherapy.
- Local therapy—LASER.
- Immunotherapy—monoclonal Abs.

Primary Tumor: Treatment as per T Stage

- **Carcinoma in situ:** Local wide excision.
- **T1: (Glans)**—**balanectomy** (amputation of glans), with a proximal margin of at least 5 mm of normal penile tissue.
- **T2 and T3: (Corpora—cavernous or spongiosa)**
  - **Partial penectomy:** Partial amputation of penis with 1 cm of proximal margin if at least 2 cm of penile shaft can be retained for micturition clear of scrotal skin.
  - **Total penectomy**—(total amputation of penis) **with perineal urethrostomy:** Indicated for growth invading the proximal shaft or in a short penis where residual stump of 2 can not be obtained.
  - **Pierce Gould's Operation:** Total penectomy, perineal urethrostomy with bilateral orchiectomy with resection of scrotum:
    - This prevents scrotal dermatitis due to urinary soakage and claimed to reduce the sexual drive.
- **T4-salvage surgery**—post-neoadjuvant therapy and perineal urethrostomy.
  - Suprapubic cystostomy is performed where a perineal urethrostomy is not feasible or growth has involved proximal penile urethra.

Q. Role of circumcision in carcinoma penis.

Role of circumcision in penile carcinoma

- Diagnosis: Biopsy of a growth—sub-preputial or glandular with phimosis
- Therapeutic; curative effect for a growth confined to preputial inner layer.
- As an adjunct to: Radiotherapy
  - Carcinoma in situ,
  - T1 lesion of glans penis or
  - Well differentiated tumor in young individual, **circumcision and curative radiotherapy** to the penis—brachytherapy—radioactive tentalum wire or penile mould (6000 cGy in 7 days) or external beam radiation with linear accelerator.
- Preventive: Neonates and infants
  - In recurrent balanoposthitis to prevent the smegma from accumulating in coronal sulcus.

Surgery for Inguinal Nodes

Bilateral Ilioinguinal block dissection: Inguinal and external iliac nodes upto the common iliac division level are removed. Performed after a full course of antibiotics after a penectomy, to treat infection in the lymph nodes.

Indications for Bilateral Ilioinguinal Block Dissection

- **Therapeutic groin dissection:** For node positive disease—FNAC or SLNB positive.
- Elective (prophylactic) node dissection is indicated only in anaplastic (Gr 3 or 4) tumors, T3 and T4 tumor, tumors with lymphovascular invasion (LVI). Prophylactic dissection is usually not carried out as it can cause severe lymphorrhea.

Complications

- Severe lymphorrhea, lymphedema of lower limbs, ulcerations, infection and sepsis.
- Flap necrosis and hemorrhage.

Radiotherapy (RT)

RT to Primary

- **Curative:** For sub-preputial carcinoma or T1 well differentiated tumors (grade 1 and 2) along with circumcision.

- Postoperative therapy after penectomy—high grade T3 disease.
- **Palliative:** T4 disease.

RT to groin nodes: N2 and N3 disease.
Postoperative RT: To groin for N2.

Chemotherapy
- Combined with radiotherapy (chemoradiation (CTRT).
- **Chemotherapeutic regimens:** VBM—vincristine, bleomycin, methotrexate, or MBP—Methotrexate, bleomycin, cisplatin—5- fluorouracil (5-FU) added in some cases.

Immunotherapy - in advanced carcinomas - with Monoclonaol antibodies, e.g., ImiquimAb.
- Local therapy for carcinoma in situ—5 FU ointment after circumcision.
- Or Nd:YAG laser to the lesion.

> **SU30.2:** Describe the applied anatomy clinical features, investigations and principles of management of undescended testis.

UNDESCENDED TESTIS

The process is more properly called—**maldescent of testis**.

Applied Anatomy of Development of Testis

Each testis develops from the genital ridge of the mesoderm on respective side, supported by the primitive mesorchium below the developing kidneys.

During the 7th intrauterine week, the gubernaculum attaches the testis to the developing abdominal wall muscles and descends to scrotal bottom along with procesus vaginalis, an evagination of peritoneum that paves way to form inguinal canal. The testis descends to lie at internal inguinal ring at 3 months and into scrotum between 7th and 9th months. The scrotal descent to the base completes by birth over 4 weeks. Maternal chorionic gonadotrophin stimulates the growth and descent of the testis.

Pathology of Maldescent of Testis
Unilateral (80%) or bilateral (20%)
- More common on the right
- Secondary sexual features are developed.

The testis may be:
- Intra-abdominal—just deep to the internal inguinal ring lying extraperitoneally.
- Intracanalicular; ingunal canal.
- Extracanalicular at the root of scrotum.

Ectopic: An ectopic testis has taken a non-standard path.

Cryptorchidism denotes a hidden testis—usually intra-abdominal—it should be distinguished from agenesis.

Scrotal testis
- At root of scrotum.
- Funicular level—scrotum.

Deviated Testis and Ectopic Testis (Refer Table 30.2)

Theory of multiple split tails of the gubernaculum—pulling the descending testis to sites away from the scrotum.

Incidence
At birth: 4%; at 3 months—about 60% of the above descend; at 1 year only 1% remain.

Sites
- Superficial inguinal pouch—inferior and medial to the external inguinal ring.

Table 30.2: Retractile testis v/s undescended testis.

Retractile testis	Undescended testis
• The descent is complete	• Incomplete descent
• Testis can be milked to the bottom of scrotum	• Not possible to push testis to scrotal bottom
• Scrotum is normally developed	• Poorly developed scrotum
• The cord is normal	• Cord is not felt in scrotum

- Suprapubic—at the root of penis.
- Perineum and in the femoral triangle.

Microscopy: Degenerative changes in Leydig and Sertoli cell—starts by 1 year and spermatogenesis fails progressively.

Retractile testis: The cremasteric spasm pulls the testis proximally to the root of the scrotum.

Consequences and complications of incompletely descended testis—"TESTIS"
- Torsion
- Epididymo-orchitis
- Sterility (failure of spermatogenesis).
- Trauma—prone for trauma and tumor.
- Inguinal hernia (90% have a hernia—due to failure of the processus vaginalis to close).
- Seminoma—5-8 times higher risk in cryptorchids.

Investigations

Sonography: Shows the position of the testes and exclude agenesis of testis, and differentiate retractile from undescended testis.

Serum gonadotrophic hormone (FSH and LH levels): For any pituitatry failure in early infancy and childhood.

MRI—to search for a missing testis in cryptorchidism.

Treatment

Early orchidopexy by1st year—helps retaining function of testis. And prevents trauma and torsion. But surgery is not a protection against risk of infertility or tumor.

Principles

- Testis and spermatic cord are mobilised.
- The testis is repositioned in the scrotum.
- Associated inguinal hernia sac is ligated and divided (processus vaginalis).

In cases where there is shortening of testicular vessels, division of testicular artery and vein and **micro vascular anastomosis** with iliac artery and vein are performed.

Laparoscopic exploration for cryptorchism helps differentiating an abdominal testis from an absent testis.

Also it helps in mobilisation of testis in orchiopexy.

VANISHING TESTIS

A condition in which a testis develops but disappears before birth.

Cause: Most likely—a prenatal testicular torsion. Vas deferens is seen but without testis.

Diff. Diagnosis: True agenesis of the testis(even rarer).

Laparoscopy—helps to distinguish the clinically absent testis from intra-abdominal maldescent.

> **SU30.3:** Describe the applied anatomy, clinical features, investigations and principles of management of epididymo-orchitis.

ACUTE EPIDIDYMO-ORCHITIS

It may be epididymitis or epididymo-orchitis.

Route of Infection

- Retrograde—through tail of epididymis—in infections of urinary tract—bladder, prostate and seminal vesicles.
  - Urinary catheters, bladder outflow obstruction.
  - Sexually transmitted disease (in young)—*Chlamydia trachomatis, Neisseria gonorrhoeae.*
- Hematogenous—reaching head of epididymis—as in systemic sepsis.

Complications

- Abscess formation, sinus, spread to perineum and Fournier's gangrene.
- Testicular infarction, testicular atrophy.
- Chronic inflammation with fibrosis and infertility.

Clinical Features

Symptoms
- Pain in the groin and a fever.
- Dysuria, scalding micturition hematuria (in a urinary or a genital infection).

Signs
- Tender swelling of epididymis and testis.
- The scrotal wall—red, erythematous and later edematous gets adherent to epididymis.
- Scrotal rugosity is lost.

Investigations

- Urinalysis—shows leukocytes may shows formal urinary tract infection.
- A urine specimen or urethral swab is taken for culture and **nucleic acid amplification testing** (NAAT).
- NAAT is a sensitive way of identifying both gonococcal and chlamydial urethritis.
- Scrotal ultrasound—to assess epididymitis and abscess formation.

Differential Diagnosis

Torsion of testis.

Treatment

- **Young adults:** Immediate pharmacotherapy with quinolones (ciprofloxacin 500 mg twice daily or norfloxacin 400 mg twice daily.) or doxycycline (100–200 mg daily) for at least two weeks.
- Intravenous antibiotics—in presence of systemic sepsis.
- As per the urine culture report, appropriate antibiotic is administered for at least 2 weeks.
- **Supportive and symptomatic:** Analgesics—aceclofenac, ketorolac or paracetamol—scrotal support.
- **Drainage of abscess:** If suppuration occurs.

CHRONIC EPIDYMITIS

Non-tuberculous: After acute epididymitis, filarial epididymo-orchitis.

Tuberculous—epididymitis.

Tuberculous Epididymitis

Retrograde infection from seminal vesicles or bladder along the vas deferens—to affect the tail of epididymis. Blood borne—is rare.

Clinical Features

- General features of tuberculosis including weight loss and local features of hematuria.
- Epididymis—thickened, nodular and craggy.
- Vas deferens—beaded.
- The seminal vesicles—indurated and swollen.
- Tuberculous 'cold' abscess"—may form a discharging sinus.
- Usually bilateral.
- Renal tuberculosis—in two-thirds of cases.
- Previous disease—X-ray chest or residual disease in the abdomen = kidney.

Investigations

- Urine culture—for bacterial and for tuberculous (full night specimen in the morning to be collected on three successive days and incubated for AFB—reading after 4 and 6 weeks).
- CB NAAT—test/genexpert test for for TB.
- Biopsy—to confirm tuberculosis.

Treatment

- Antituberculous treatment—4 drugs, SHRZ (streptomycin, isoniazid, rifampicin, and pyrazinamide) regimen for 6-9 months.
- Epididymectomy done for residual disease. After 2 months of ATT.
- Cold abscess—and sinuses—scrotal exploration (after adequate ATT) and drainage/orchiectomy.

SU30.4: Describe the applied anatomy, clinical features, investigations and principles of management of varicocele.

Q. Discuss pathogenesis, clinical diagnosis and management of varicocele.

VARICOCELE

A varicocele is a varicose dilatation of the pampiniform plexus veins, draining the testis.

Surgical Anatomy

- The venous drainage from the testis and the epididymis is into the pampiniform plexus, through the cord and inguinal canal, and near the internal inguinal ring, the venous radicles join to form one or two testicular veins.
- The testicular veins pass upwards in the retroperitoneum. The left vein drains into the left renal and right into the inferior vena cava.
- The testicular veins are valved near their terminations. The alternative venous return from the testes is into the inferior epigastric veins through the cremasteric veins.

Etiology
- Varicoceles are seen in about 10–15% of adults and 80–90% are on left side.
- May be seen in late childhood and adolescents too.

Cause
- Absence or incompetence of valve in the testicular vein.
- Idiopathic—no cause detectable.
- Obstruction of the left testicular vein by a renal tumor or nephrectomy
- Iatrogenic—ligation or division of testicular vein during surgery on colon and retroperitoneum.

Clinical Features
- Most are asymptomatic and diagnosed during routine examination
- Symptoms seen in adolescence or young adults—dragging pain worse in the evening or prolonged standing.
- Findings in standing position—the scrotum hangs lower than normal.
- On palpation "a bag of worms" feeling of the varicosities.
- Varicosities empty by gravity—but emptying is not seen in varicocele due to venous obstruction, e.g., tumor infiltration.
- Testis may be smaller and softer.

Differential diagnosis—hernia, encysted hydrocele of cord.

Investigation
Ultrasonography with Doppler—to study the scrotum and in the diagnosis of varicoceles.

Grading of Varicocele
- Grade I: Diagnosed by ultrasound
- Grade II: Palpable
- Grade III: Visible

Ultrasonography of the kidneys to exclude renal tumor and to study gonadal vessels.
- Semen analysis.

Varicocele Affects Spermatogenesis
- Normal scrotal temperature is around 2.5°C below rectal temperature; varicocele will tend to 'warm' the testis and is believed to affect spermatogenesis.
- Oligospermia—oligospermia improves in 6–12 weeks (some reports disagree).

Treatment
Reassurance to the patient. And scrotal support while working. For an asymptomatic patient.

Non-surgical interventions—percutaneous embolization of gonadal veins is tried.

Indications for Surgery
- Significant oligospermia (if testicular and pituitary cause are excluded).
- For unbearable pain or discomfort. The patient needs to understand the limitations of unsure outcome.
- Recurrent varicocele.

Procedure: Surgical ligation of testicular veins is the appropriate treatment.

Approaches
- Inguinal approach: Inguinal canal is opened and veins ligated.
- Subinguinal approach: Incision at external inguinal ring—no muscle division.
- Paloma's operation: Suprainguinal extraperitoneal ligation of the testicular vein.
- Scrotal approach: For large varicoceles.
- Laparoscopic approach: Blamed for high recurrence rates by urologists.

Complications of Surgery
- Hemorrhage and scrotal hematoma—infection, pyocele
- Recurrence—10% approx.
- Injury to testicular artery, injury to ilioinguinal nerve and pain.

> **Q. Discuss etiology and differential diagnosis of acute scrotum.**

ACUTE SCROTUM
Any clinical condition with acute scrotal pain.

Etiology of Acute Scrotum
Torsion of testis—most common cause
- **Epididymitis**
- Torsion of appendix of testis

- Acute scrotal cellulitis
- Acute idiopathic scrotal edema
- **Fournier's gangrene**
- **Hernia—strangulation**
- Trauma—scrotal hematoma/acute hematocele/testicular laceration or rupture
- Tumor of testis—"acute hurricane tumor"
- Mumps—acute orchitis.

Acute Scrotum in Children and Adolescents
- Epididymitis accounts for 30 to 40%.
- But torsion of testis is still common and is misdiagnosed as epididymitis.
- Torsion—appendix of epididymis.

Differential Diagnosis of Acute Scrotum
Orchitis
- Especially viral—mumps
- Bacterial—less common
- Pain, fever
- Large testis, impalpable epididymis
- USG Doppler—to differentiate.

Other Acute Infective Conditions
- Acute scrotal cellulitis
- Acute scrotal abscess—abscess within scrotal layers
- Infected hydrocele—with in tunica vaginalis
- Infected hematocele
- Pyocele.

Acute Idiopathic Scrotal Edema
- Common in children
- Unknown infection is believed to trigger the onset of this condition
- Topical allergy/drugs
- Scrotal edema normal testis and epididymis
- Systemic and local symptoms
- Antibiotics may help.

Fournier's Gangrene
Refer next section on Fournier's Gangrene.

Testicular Trauma
- Generally blunt trauma—a blow, or compression of testis against bones.
- May be simple epididymitis/orchitis or severe causing hematoma, hematocele and pyocele.
- Testicular rupture.

Treatment
- Rupture needs exploration.
- Pyocele needs drainage.
- Other conditions are treated non-surgically.

> Q. Describe mechanism, clinical diagnosis and management of torsion of the testis.

TORSION OF THE TESTIS
Pathophysiology
- This is a surgical emergency wherein the testicle twists and its blood supply gets compromised and leading rapidly to infarction of the testis.
- Urgent surgery to untwist the testis is the only way to save the testis.

Acute torsion of testis. Early diagnosis is important
Testis is normally anchored to scrotal bottom by the gubernacular vestige and unable to rotate.

Predisposing Factors for the Torsion of the Testis
1. High investment of the tunica vaginalis causes the testis—"bell clapper testis" in a bell. This is the most common cause in adolescents and a bilateral abnormality.
2. Inversion of the testis—testis is rotated and it lies transversely or upside down.
3. Epididymo-testicular disjunction: Separation of the epididymis from the body of the testis.
4. With the factors 1, 2 and 3, testis rotates around the vertical axis following, any sudden muscle activity, due to the sudden contraction of cremaster.

Risk of testicular infarction depends on the extent of twist—(safer if <360 degree, worst if > 720 degree) and duration of the torsion.

Types of Testicular Torsion
Refer **Table 30.3** and **Figure 30.1**.

Complications of Torsion
- Testicular ischemia, infarction and gangrene.
- Infection abscess and sepsis.

- Torsion of opposite testis is common in over 50% due to bilaterality of predisposing cause.
- Breach of immunological blood testis barrier orchitis leads to formation of antisperm antibodies and infertility.

Clinical Features of Torsion Testis

- Commonly between 10 and 25 years of age.
- Sudden agonizing pain in the groin and hypogastrium, with vomiting.

Signs

- Usually normal body temperature.
- **Abnormally high testis**, swollen and tender but not warm.
- Transverse lie of testis (normally vertical) due to shortened cord "bell clapper deformity" the tender twisted cord can often be palpated.
- **Prehn's sign:** Elevation of testis—pain worsens in torsion (negative Prehn's sign) relieves pain in epididymitis **(positive sign)**.

- Note: Not very accurate.
- **Absence of cremasteric reflex—more reliable sign.**
- Epididymis is in front and opposite epididymitis is behind.
  - Except in bilateral congenital anteversion where both epididymis are in front.

Differential Diagnosis

- Epididymo-orchitis, acute orchitis.
- Torsion of a testicular appendage: Cyst of appendix of the testis—hydatid of morgagni.
- Recurrent intermittent torsion.

Investigation: Scrotal ultrasound with Doppler study—to check the position of testis and epididymis, state of the cord and state of the blood flow to testis.

Treatment of Torsion of Testis

Refer **Figures 30.2, 30.3** and **30.4** showing operative photographs.

- Immediate scrotal exploration, detorsion and fixation of testis—usually inversion of tunica vaginalis sac is done. If untwisted within 4-6 hours—most testicles survive.
- Delay beyond 4-6 hours of onset of pain—the risk of testicular gangrene are very; high.

Table 30.3: Types ot testicular torsion.		
Intravaginal	Extravaginal	Long mesorchium
Testis + epididymis	All contents	Only testis

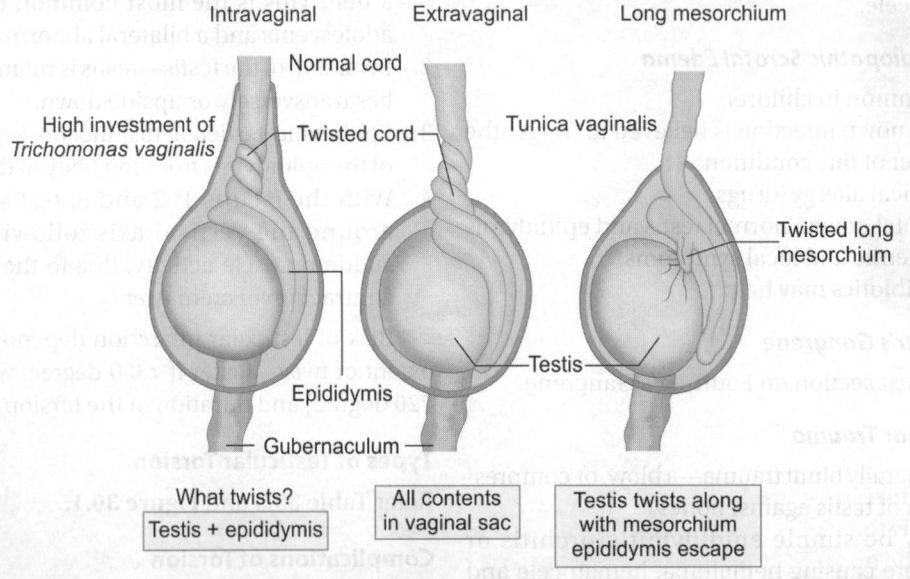

Fig. 30.1: Types ot testicular torsion.

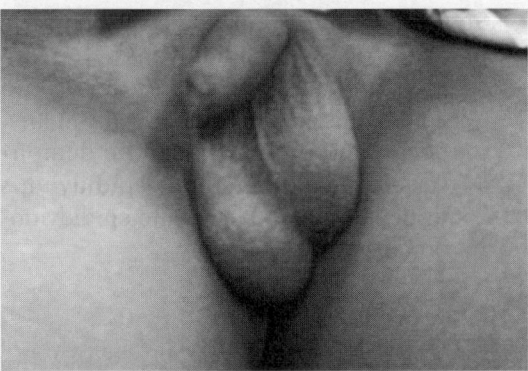

Fig. 30.2: Torsion left testis

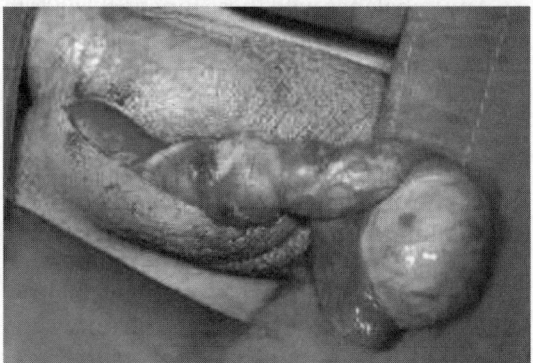

Fig. 30.3: Early torsion—detorsion done.
(For color version see Plate 4)

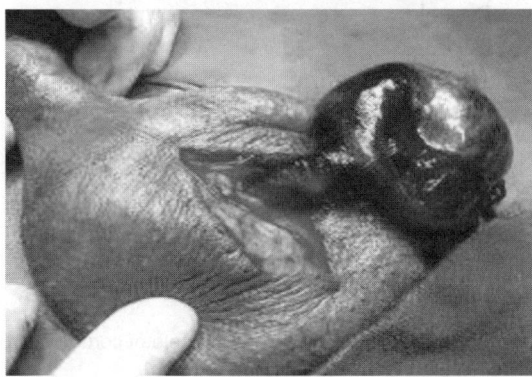

Fig. 30.4: Gangrenous torsion.
(For color version see Plate 4)

- **Explore opposite side and fix contralateral testis too.** Opinion is divided on the need to fix the opposite testis.
- Manual detorsion is generally recommended.
- **If gangrenous**—orchidectomy is performed.

Q. Short note on Fournier's gangrene.

FOURNIER'S GANGRENE

Syn: Idiopathic scrotal gangrene.

Pathogenesis

It is a polymicrobial infection causing arteriolar thrombosis and infective gangrene of skin and subcutaneous tissue of scrotum. Penis, perineum and perianal region— similar to a necrotizing fasciitis.

Infective Organisms

Mixed infection by aerobic and anaerobic organisms: Beta-hemolytic streptococci, anaerobic and microaerophilic streptococci, *Staphylococcus aureus* and *Cl. welchii, Bacteroides fragilis.*

Predisposing causes: Diabetes mellitus, malnourishment, immunocompromised state including steroid therapy, anticancer therapy and HIV, alcoholism.

Complications: Rapid local gangrene, systemic sepsis and high mortality.

Clinical Features

- Condition is common in old age.
- Sudden pain in the scrotum, fever, severe toxicity.
- Very fast spreading cellulitis of scrotal skin, extending to the groin, perineal skin and often to anterior abdominal wall leading to extensive gangrene of skin over large areas.

Treatment of a Case of Fournier's Gangrene is a Surgical Emergency

- Intravenous fluid resuscitation.
- Blood transfusion for severe anemia—pre and intraoperative.
- Aggressive treatment with broad spectrum intravenous antibiotics.
- **Emergency surgical necrosectomy**: Extensive debridement/excision of the dead and infected skin and subcutaneous tissue.
- Ancillary procedures—depending on the sites involved: Cystostomy to divert urine from perineum in a periurethral abscess.

Colostomy for a perineal wound. Urinary and supportive care is essential.
- Definitive suturing or reconstruction of raw areas once healing signs return.

> **SU30.5:** Describe the applied anatomy, clinical features, investigations and principles of management of hydrocele.

> **Q. Classify vaginal hydrocele. Describe pathophysiology and complications of hydrocele. Also discuss clinical diagnosis and management of vaginal hydrocele.**

VAGINAL HYDROCELE

A hydrocele is an abnormal collection of serous fluid any part of the processus vaginalis. Commonest type is the collection in tunica vaginalis.

Classification (Refer Figure 30.5)

Congenital hydrocele—patent processus vaginalis (essentially a hernia).
- Hydrocele of the cord.
- Infantile hydrocele (processus patent except at the internal ring).
- Vaginal hydrocele.

Acquired Hydrocele
- Primary—clinically unknown cause—large hydroceles, testis and epididymis not palpable, (e.g., filarial hydrocele).
- Secondary hydrocele—secondary to a pathology of testis or epididymis.
  - Lax and small hydroceles, testis and epididymis clearly palpable.
  - Secondary pathology can be demonstrated, e.g., tuberculous epididymitis testicular tumor, post-acute epididymo-orchitis.

Pathophysiology

Mechanisms of Hydrocele Formation

Tunica vaginalis has a secretory visceral layer and an absorptive parietal layer.

Any imbalance with these functions leads to collection of fluid the vaginal sac.
- Congenital—communication with peritoneal cavity (patent processus).
- Testicular or epididymal disease causing hyper secretion—tumor, epididymitis.
- Failure of parietal absorptive layer to absorb the fluid and interference with lymphatic drainage of scrotum, e.g., filarial hydrocele.

Complications of Hydrocele
- Hemorrhage into the sac and formation of hematocele.
- Infection of hydrocele.
- Chylocele.
- Pyocele.
- Rupture.
- Testicular atrophy.
- Hernia of hydrocele—the hydrocele sac herniates through scrotal layers to present

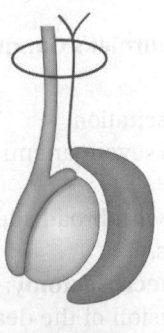 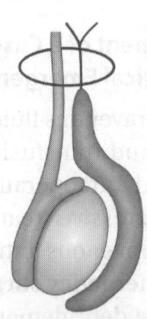 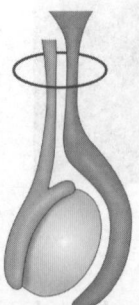 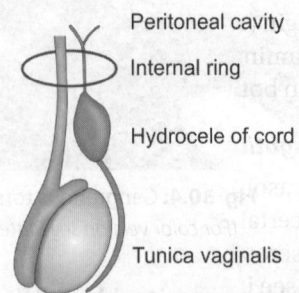

Vaginal hydrocele (most common)   Infantile hydrocele   Congenital hydrocele   Encysted hydrocele of cord

Fig. 30.5: Classification of hydrocele

under dartos as a subcutaneous cystic swelling.
- Elephantiasis of scrotum is a consequence of filarial lymphedema and fibroplasia resulting in hypertrophy and thickening of scrotal layers.

Clinical Features
- Scrotal swelling.
- Gradually enlarging.
- May appear following a trauma or infection or without any obvious cause.
- Pain is a feature of complication.

Examination
- Scrotal swelling soft and fluctuant.
- Mostly translucent, unless the sac is fibrotic and thickened.

Differential Diagnosis
Scrotal v/s Inguinal Swellings
- Possible to get above a scrotal swelling but not inguinal.
- The cord can be normally felt above and separate from a scrotal swelling.
- Hernia can be reduced and has an expansile impulse on coughing.
- Cystic swellings of the cord: "Drag test"—gentle traction on testis shows the swelling getting pulled down.

Scrotal Swelling
- Testicular v/s epididymal or both.
- Cord swelling.
- Tumor—lax and small hydrocele or recent origin (so called acute hydrocele).
Examination of a scrotal swelling should be done in both the upright and supine position.

Investigations
An ultrasound with Doppler
- Ascertain the nature of the swelling, and state of scrotal structures.
- To see if the testis itself is diseased.
- A hydrocele encloses the testis and epididymis.

Congenital hydrocele, the processus vaginalis is patent

- And connects with the peritoneal cavity with a tiny opening.
- Allows fluid to enter hydrocele.
- It can't be reduced but empties slowly in recumbent position due to "ink bottle effect".
- Associated ascites may be present.

Encysted hydrocele of the cord
- It is a smooth oval swelling above the testis near the spermatic cord.
- Drag test—swelling moves downwards on pulling the testis down and becomes less mobile.
- Differential diagnosis—inguinal hernia.

The hydrocele of the canal of nuck—cystic swelling in relation to the round ligament, partly or fully within the inguinal canal.

Treatment
Congenital hydrocele: Herniotomy and scrotal eversion of the processus sac.

Secondary hydrocele: Treatment of the cause and then reassess.
- Infections—antibiotics.
- Antituberculous treatment.
- Tumor—as per oncological protocol.

Primary hydrocele: Treated by surgery.

Injection of a sclerosant, such as tetracycline not favored due to risk of infection.

Aspiration: In patients unfit for surgery or
- To facilitate urology procedures like cystoscopy and TURP.
- Complications—bleeding into sac, infection and pyocele.
- Reaccumulation of fluid.

Surgery for Vaginal Hydrocele
Indications
- All primary hydroceles to remove the thick vaginal sac., and to prevent complications of hydrocele..

Principles
- Surgery aims to - empty the fluid from tunica vaginalis sac., and to prevent reaccumulation of fluid - by facilitating drainage of secretion in the vaginal sac scrotal wall lymphatics.

Lord's Plication: For small and thin hydrocele. But there is high risk of recurrence due to formation of loculi within the plicated folds of tunica.

Eversion—for thin and small sacs.

The sac is opened and the tunica vaginalis is everted behind the testis.

Partial excision and Eversion (Jabolay's procedure)—for moderately thick sacs.

Subtotal excision of the thickened and defunct parietal layer—for large and thick sacs. The tunica is divided about 1 cm away from its reflection onto the visceral layer.

Complications of Hydrocele Operation

- Hemorrhage—primary—on table or immediate postoperative.
- Reactionary bleeding.
- Scrotal hematoma.
- Infection.
- Septic epididymo-orchitis—requiring orchidectomy.

Filarial Hydroceles and Chyloceles

- Make most (90%) of the hydroceles in India and tropical countries.
- Follow repeated attacks of filarial epididymo-orchitis.
- Behave like primary hydroceles—by fibrosis ad occlusion of lymphatics.
- Contents of fluid—yellowish color, may contain cholesterol crystals due to rupture of a dilated (varicose) lymphatic vessel.
- Chyloceles: There are adhesions between scrotum and structures.
- Scrotal skin undegoes thickening and hypertrophy leads to elephantiasis of scrotum.

Treatment: As per treatment of primary hydrocele: Excision of the sac.
- Orchidectomy: If there is testicular atrophy and infection.
- Elephantiasis: Resection scrotal skin and reshaping of the scrotum.
- In severe cases: A liberal scrotectomy and reimplantation of testicles in thigh pouch on medial side of upper thigh is practiced.
- Antifilarial therapy: Diethyl carbamazine 100 mg tablets thrice daily for 3 weeks given yearly for 6 years.

> **Q. Short note on epididymal cyst.**

EPIDYMAL CYSTS

- They are due to cystic degeneration in epididymis, containing clear fluid.
- May be multiple varying in size or multi-locular.
- Age—middle age and young adults, and commonly bilateral.
- They lie posterior to testis.
- Transillumination test positive.

Investigation

Ultrasonography—to define them and to differentiate them from hydrocele.

Complications

- Hemorrhage into cyst and infection.
- Association with infertility due to degeneration of epididymal tubules.

Treatment

Reassurance and observation.
Surgery—for pain, infection or bleeding.
- Single cyst—excision.
- Multiple cysts—partial epididymectomy.

Complication of Surgery

Risk of infertility due to interference with sperm transportation path during surgery.

Spermatocele

- This is a unilocular retention cyst behind the upper pole of the testis.
- Formed by interference with sperm-conducting mechanism of the epididymis.

Clinical Features

- Scrotal swelling above testis.
- Lax, soft and transilluminating.
- Contents of the fluid—spermatozoa and turbid fluid.

Treatment

Excision is done for large and infected spermatoceles.

Hematocele

Collection of blood in tunica vaginalis
- Acute hematocele—testicular trauma, hemorrhage into a hydrocele sac. Iatrogenic—following aspiration of hydrocele or aspiration biopsy of testis.
- Chronic hematocele—long-standing hematocele.

Consequences and Complications
- Infection and pyocele formation.
- Organisation, calcification and pressure on testis leading to atrophy of testis.

Clinical Features
- **Acute** hematocele: Painful scrotal swelling, warm and tender to palpate, scrotal discoloration may be present.
- **Chronic hematocele**: Hard, heavy swelling resembling a tumor.

Ultrasound scrotum for both acute and chronic hematocele.

MRI of scrotum—may help differentiation from a tumor.

Treatment
- Acute hematocele.
- Analgesia and NSAIDs.
- Aspiration with wide bore needle for small swellings.
- Exploration of scrotum—evacuation of hematocele and hemostasis—depending upon the bleeding source—testicular vein (ligated) or rupture of testis (sutured) or orchidectomy when testis is badly shattered.
- Chronic hematocele—usually testis is atrophic and needs an orchidectomy.

PYOCELE

Collection of pus in the tunica vaginalis.

Etiology
- Infection in the tunica vaginalis—retrograde spread from urinary tract.
- Infection of hematocele or hydrocele or chylocele.

Post-traumatic
Iatrogenic
- Following aspiration of hydrocele.
- Postoperative.
- Diabetes, steroids and immunosuppression worsen the condition.

Complications
- Systemic spread—septicemia.
- Infective thrombosis of arterioles supplying testis and necrosis of testis.

Clinical Features
Fever, pain and swelling of scrotum, toxicity, tender swelling in the scrotum, with scrotal wall edema.

Differential diagnosis—torsion of testis.

Investigation
- Blood counts, culture, blood sugar.
- Urine culture.
- Ultrasonography and Doppler flow study—confirms diagnosis and differentiated from hydrocele.
- Also viability of testis is assessed by Doppler.

Treatment
- Scrotum is explored immediately and pus is evacuated.
- Viability of the testis is checked.
- Orchidectomy—for non-viable testis.

SU30.6: Describe classification, clinical features, investigations and principles of management of tumors of testis.

Q. Enumerate the etiology, pathology and staging of tumors of testis. Clnical diagnosis and management of tumors of testis.

TUMORS OF TESTIS

Etiological Factors and Risk Factors

For easy remembering
- *Ill developed testis:* Testicular hypoplasia.
- *Inheritance testis:* Klinefelter syndrome, Down's, testicular feminization syndrome.

- *In house testis:* Cryptorchidism—highest risk (400–800 percent higher risk).
- *Injured testis:* Recurrent testicular trauma.
- *Infertile testis:* Three times more likely.
- *Incinerated testis:* Regular and prolonged exposure to hot atmosphere and heat.
- *Inflamed testis :* Chronic/recurrent.
- *Indecent testis:* Maldescent of testis.
- *Insecure testis:* Ectopic testis.
- *Insulted testis:* Atrophic testis—post insult—trauma or inflammatory disease.
- *Irradiated testis:* Exposure to ionizing radiation.
- *Immunologic testis:* Diseases affecting testis.
- *Industrial testis:* Coal tar, cadmium, dye industries.
- *Other factors*—h/o contralateral tumor, tumors in family.

Pathogenesis: Cause not fully known

- Abnormal cell division of fetal gonocytes and postnatal invasive growth, stimulated by gonadotropin.
- Abnormality in germ cell development: Leading to overexpression of cyclin D2 gene (CCND2). This gene stimulates the failed cell causing ITGCN (intra tubular germ cell neoplasia).

Age Incidence: Two peaks—between 15 and 35 years and then after 60 years.

Seminomas—after 40 years and non seminomatous tumors below 35.

Seminoma is the most common tumor after 60 but rare in boys of age below 10 years.

Tumor Spread

Local—within the testis and through tunica albuginea, epididymis, along the cord.

Lymphatic—early spread to the para-aortic, mediastinal and supraclavicular.

Blood spread—to the lungs and then to other organs.

Q. Classify tumors of testis based on histopathology.

Refer **Table 30.4**.

WHO Histological Classification of Malignant Testicular Germ Cell Tumors

Germ Cell Tumors

- Intratubular germ cell neoplasia—unclassified—ITGCN or IGCN considered a precursor lesion for many GCTs.
- Pure germ cell tumor (a single cell type): Seminomatous or non seminomatous
- **Seminoma:**
  - Pure seminomas—50% of GCTs.
  - Mixed germ cell tumors (20% of GCTs)—
  - Spermatocytic seminoma—a less aggressive variant, rarely metastasize.
  - **Embryonal carcinoma** - rare in pure form but commonly seen in mixed GCT..

Teratoma (TD—Differentiated, TI—Intermediate, TA—Anaplastica, TT—Trophoblastica).

- Choriocarcinoma is the least common type of NSGCT, but are very aggressive.
  - Shows early blood metastases and less of lymphatics, high levels of beta HCG.
- Yolk sac tumor (syn: Endodermal sinus tumor), most common tumor in children,(40% of mixed GCTs). blood levels of AFP are high and those of beta-HCG low.
- **Mixed germ cell tumor** (showing more than one histologic germ cell pattern—with

Table 30.4: Tumors of testis .	
Germ cell tumors (GCT) (90%)	**Non-germ cell tumors (NGCT)**
Seminomatous—seminoma (SGCT) **Nonseminomatous** (NSGCT) Embryonal cell carcinoma, teratoma -TD TI TA and choriocarcinoma; yolk sac tumor **Mixed cell type**—more than 50%	**Interstitial tumors** (2%) Leydig cell tumor, Sertoli cell tumor **Lymphoma** (4–5%) **Other tumors** (1–2%) **Metastatic** (secondary)—rare—from gastric cancer, melanoma

combined patterns of seminoma, teratoma, embryonal carcinoma, yolk sac tumor or choriocarcinoma): These make about 35% of testicular cancer.
- **Polyembryoma:** A rare, very aggressive form of **germ cell tumor**. Features of both yolk sac tumor and undifferentiated teratoma/embryonal carcinoma.

Table 30.5: Staging of cancer testis—(abridged): TNMS.

I	Tumor confined to testis, N-0, S-0
II	Regional nodes or S1
III	Extra regional nodes or hematogenous mets
IIIa	M1a (extra regional nodes or lungs)/S1
IIIb	M1a, S2
IIIb	M1b (bone, liver) any S or any N/M S3

STAGING OF TESTICULAR TUMORS (REFER TABLE 30.5 AND FIGURE 30.6)

Always done after orchidectomy and by TNM-S staging (tumor, node, metastases and serum markers AFP, B-HCG, LDH).

> **Q. Clinical diagnosis and management of testicular tumors.**

Clinical Features (History and Findings)

Primary and Local Disease
- Painless swelling or nodule of one testicle—not felt separately from the testis.
- Dull ache or heavy sensation in the lower abdomen. Back pain in bulky retroperitoneal disease.
- A secondary hydrocele—lax, small with a palpable enlarged testis.

Metastatic disease: Depends on site of metastasis—lymphatic or hematogenous spread.

Lymphatic spread
- Neck mass in supraclavicular lymph node.
- Cough and stridor in mediastinal LN involvement
- Lymphedema of the lower limbs—in pelvic lymph node involvement.

Non lymphatic metastatic disease
- Lungs—cough, chest pain, hemoptysis and breathlessness.
- Central nervous system—(rare) they present as neurological symptoms.
- Bone pain in osseous metastasis.

Systemic manifestations
- Anorexia, nausea and other gastrointestinal symptom. Gynecomastia is seen in 5% of patients.
- Choriocarcinoma produces chorionic gonadotropin hyperthyroidism may be present.

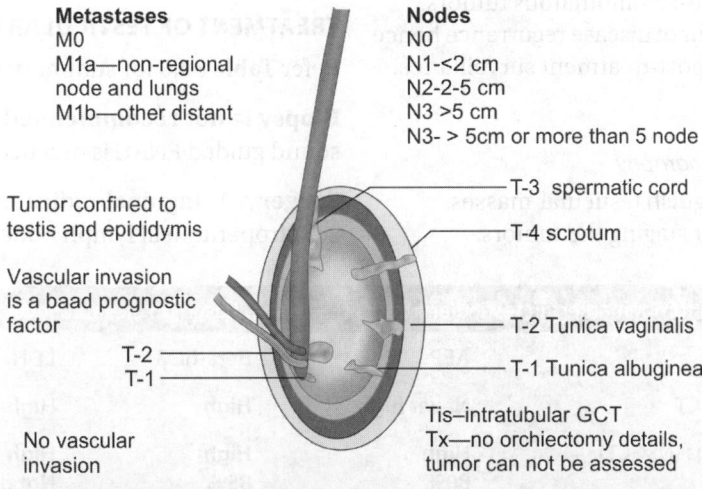

Fig. 30.6: TNM classification of testicular tumors (post-orchiectomy)

Physical Examination

- Examination of scrotum (normal testicles first) between thumb and fingers for any painless hard area, loss of testicular sensation and hydrocele, compression of epididymis or a thick cord.
- Examination of lower extremity: For edema—iliac or venacaval obstruction.
- Abdomen lymphadenopathy and hepatomegaly.
- Chest: Gynecomastia.
- Neck: Lymph nodes and distended veins.
- Bone: Tenderness in areas of pain.

Differential Diagnosis

- In patients with scrotal pain, chronic epididymitis, and epididymo-orchitis.
- In patients without pain hydrocele, hernia, hematocele-chronic, gumma of the testis.

Laboratory Studies

- Complete blood count
- Serum tumor markers (Refer **Table 30.6**).
Alpha fetoprotein (AFP), raised in non seminomas mainly (false positive in hepatitis, cirrhosis hepatoma). If in a pure seminoma AFP is raised, suspect non-seminomatous tumor.

Lactate dehydrogenase (LDH): Increased serum levels—reflect tumor burden, cellular proliferation rate.
- Elevated in 30% to 80% of pure seminoma and 60% of non-seminomatous tumors.
- Not an indicator of disease recurrence hence not useful for post-treatment surveillance.

Imaging Studies

Testicular Ultrasonography
- Used to distinguish testicular masses.
- Not reliable for staging the tumors.
- Seminoma—well defined homogenous and hypoechoic. Non-seminomatous tumors—non-homogenous, hyperechoic lesions with indistinct margins and calcification and cystc areas.

Other Radiographic Imaging

- Plain X-ray chest -routine.
- CT scan: High-resolution scan of the abdomen and pelvis.
- Chest CT is recommended if: 1. The chest X-ray is suspicious or 2. Thoracic metastatic disease is suspected clinically.
- MRI of the abdomen and pelvis or scrotum is not more informative than CT scan.
- MRI of the brain if metastases are suspected.
- Bone scan -Tc99 if metastases are suspected.
- PET scanning useful in the evaluation of post-therapy residual masses.

Staging-American Joint Committee on Cancer (AJCC)

- The AJCC stage groupings use both TNM staging and serum tumor marker levels.
- SX indicates that markers were unavailable or not performed; S0 indicates normal levels.

Risk Stratification of Testicular Tumors

Refer **Tables 30.7** and **30.8**.

TREATMENT OF TESTICULAR TUMOR

Refer **Table 30.9** for summary in next page.

Biopsy is not recommended (although ultrasound guided FNAC is practiced).

Surgery: 1. Inguinal radical orchiectomy and 2. Retroperitoneal lymph node dissection.

Table 30.6: Serum tumor markers in testicular tumors (" S" stage- based on elevated levels).

Tumor pathology	AFP	Beta-hCG	LDH
Seminomatous SGCT	Never high	High	High-poor prognostic
Non-seminomatous (NSGCT)	High 80%	High 85%	High Not diagnostic

Table 30.7: Markers of prognosis in testicular tumors.

Stage	LDH	HCG (mIU/mL)	AFP (ng/mL)
S1	< 1.5 times normal	< 5,000	< 1,000
S2	1.5–10 times normal	5,000–50,000	1,000–10,000
S3	>10 times normal	>50,000	>10,000

(LDH = lactate dehydrogenase; HCG = beta human chorionic gonadotropin, AFP = alpha-fetoprotein)

Table 30.8: Risk categories in testicular tumors.

Risk classification	Good-risk	Intermediate-risk	Poor-risk
Seminoma	S-GR	IR	PR
Non-seminoma	NS-GR	IR	PR

Inguinal Radical Orchiectomy (Syn: High Orchidectomy)

Inguinal approach, division of cord and deliver the testis through inguinal wound with all the fascial layers intact.

Scrotal incisions should not be used for Radical orchiectomy.

Retroperitoneal Lymph Node Dissection (RPLND)

The gold standard for finding nodal micrometastases and staging of the retroperitoneal disease.

Both the number and size of involved retroperitoneal lymph nodes have prognostic importance.

Surgical Approach for RPLND

- The transabdominal approach.
- Laparoscopic approach.
- Robotic approach is now gaining favor.

Medical Oncology in Cancer Testis

- Testicular cancers are often curable even in the presence of metastatic disease. If the cancer progresses or recurs despite initial chemotherapy, salvage therapy is indicated.
- Nonseminoma is more aggressive than seminoma: When the elements of both seminoma and nonseminoma are present or the AFP concentration is elevated, the tumor should be treated as a nonseminoma. The summary of treatment of testicular tumors is given in **Table 30.9**.

Fertility and Sperm Banking

Because 45% to 55% of testicular cancer patients have azoospermia or oligospermia from 2 years after therapy, they should be offered semen bank storing facility if they wish.

Second primary malignancies develop in survivors of testicular cancer and are the most common cause of death (sites—lung, bladder, kidney, colon, stomach, esophagus and pancreas and leukemia).

> **Q. Summarize the treatment of testicular tumors (Refer Table 30.9).**

Prognosis

The 5 year survival is as follows:
- **Seminomatous GCT—stage I:** 90-95%; advanced stage: 70%—if favorable prognostic factors.
- **NSGCT—stage I:** 90-95%.
- **Advanced stage—stage III:** 50-70%.

TUMORS OF SCROTUM

- Squamous cell carcinoma of scrotum—"chimney sweeper's cancer".

Table 30.9: Summary of treatment of testicular tumors.

Treatment strategy simplified

Seminomas

Stage 1, 2 and 3: Radical inguinal orchidectomy followed by:
- Stage 1:
  - Radiation therapy (RT) to para-aortic and ilioinguinal nodes.
  - Cisplatin single dose. If RT not possible (e.g., Horseshoe kidney or IBD)
- Stage 2: Radical inguinal orchidectomy followed by
  - RT to para-aortic and ilioinguinal nodes
  - If chemotherapy—etoposide, cisplatin 4 cycles.
- Stage 3: Radical inguinal orchidectomy followed by chemotherapy and No RT.
  If good risk—EP (etoposide, cisplatin) or BEP (bleomycin, etoposide cisplatin).

Residual retroperitoneal mass as detected by PET scan-biopsy
If positive-RPLND or salvage chemotherapy.

Non-seminomas

Stage 1 and 2: Radical inguinal **orchidectomy with RPLND**
- If node positive—chemotherapy EP/BEP
- If markers positive EP/BEP

Stage 3: Radical inguinal **orchidectomy. No RPLND but chemotherapy given**
- After chemotherapy, if node is positive at scanning
- Salvage RPLND or salvage chemo
- In both seminomas and non seminomas
- Salvage chemo is high dose chemo followed by stem cell transplantation

Favorable prognosis	*Unfavorable prognosis*
• Low tumor marker levels • Low-volume disease • Complete response to first-line chemo If they have an incomplete response or relapse, consider for high-dose chemotherapy with autologous stem cell transplantation	• High tumor marker levels • High-volume disease • Patients with an incomplete response to first-line chemotherapy • Extratesticular spread of primary

- Carcinoma of the scrotum is very rare in India and other Asian countries.

Etiology
- Occupational hazard—in workers coming in touch with oil and coal tar products due to the carcinogenicity of aromatic cyclic hydrocarbons.
- Other factors - unknown yet.

Clinical Features
Starts as a warty growth and may invade deeper including the testis.

Treatment
- Wide excision (with margin of healthy skin).
- The inguinal nodes—inguinal block dissection for early disease after a course of antibiotics.

Bibliography

1. AJCC Cancer Staging Manual, Version 8.
2. Anderson MD. Surgical Oncology Handbook, 6th edition.
3. Bailey and Love's, Short Practice Surgery, 27th and 28th edition.
4. Campbell, Walsh Urology.
5. Das K. Clinical Methods in Surgery.
6. Ellis' Clinical Anatomy for Medical Students.
7. Farquharson's Textbook of Operative Surgery.
8. Fisher et al. Mastery of Surgery, 6th edition.
9. Govt. of India Gazzette.
10. Illustrative Handbook of General Surgery, 2nd edition, Springer.
11. Lee McGregor's Surgical Anatomy.
12. Manipal Manual of Surgery, 4th and 5th editions.
13. Schwartz 's Principles of Surgery, 11th edition.
14. Smith & Tanagho's General Urology, 19th edition.
15. SRB Manual of Surgery, 6th and 7th editions.
16. Townsend et al. Sabiston Textbook of Surgery, 20th edition.
17. Washington Manual of Surgery, 8th edition.

Index

Page numbers followed by *f* refer to figure and *t* refer to table.

A

Abdomen 22, 351
  acute 499
  clinical examination of 451
  lower 487
  pit of 43
  ultrasonography of 227
  upper 117, 487
Abdominal wall
  hernia
    parts of 338
    sites of 337, 338*f*
    reconstruction 347
Abdominoperineal resection 526, 527*f*
Ablation, hormonal 597
Ablative techniques 95
ABO system 17
Abscess
  acute 262
  anorectal 529, 529*f*
  breast 260, 261
  chronic 261
  cold 49, 50
  complications of 49
  corticomedullary 554
  cryptoglandular 529
  drainage of 489
  formation, stage of 261
  intra-abdominal 355, 485
  intraperitoneal 355, 355*f*
  midpalmar 58
  open drainage of 555
  parotid 190
  pelvic 356
  perianal 530*f*
  pericolic 495
  perinephric 566
  perirenal 554
  peritoneal 355
  prostatic 594
  pyogenic 417
  renal corticomedullary 554
  space 59
  specific 529
  subdiaphragmatic 357
Accidents, surgical care of 72
Acetylcholine 389
Achalasia
  cardia 369, 370*f*
  clinical features of 369
  types of 369
Acid
  peptic attack 389*t*
    mechanism of 389

production
  inhibitors of 383
  three phases of 383
Acidity, hypersecretion of 396
Acidosis 12, 146
Acinic cell tumor 196
Acral lentiginous melanoma 162
Acropachy 208
Actinomyces 49
Actinomycosis 50
Acute appendicitis 484, 486
  clinical diagnosis of 484
  differential diagnosis of 486, 487*t*
  etiology of 484
  management of 484
  pathogenesis of 485*t*
  pathology of 484
Acute breast abscess 260
  complications of 261, 262
Acute cholecystitis 439, 439*f*
  complications of 439
  etiology of 439
  management of 439
  pathology of 439
Acute deep vein thrombosis
  clinical features of 322
  etiopathogenesis of 322
  management of 322
Acute intestinal obstruction 470
  cardinal features of 470*t*
  clinical features of 470
Acute intussusception 475
  clinical features of 475
  etiology of 475
  management of 475
  pathology of 475
Acute limb ischemia 305
  management of 309
  Rutherford's classification of 305, 305*t*
  treatment of 309
Acute liver failure 413
  treatment of 413
Acute lower gastrointestinal hemorrhage
  etiology of 501
  management of 501
Acute mastitis 260
  clinical diagnosis of 260
  etiology of 260
  management of 260
  pathology of 260
Acute pancreatitis 238, 239, 239*t*, 241, 434

classification of 239
clinical features of 239
complications of 238-240, 240*t*
differential diagnosis of 240, 240*t*
etiopathogenesis of 238
management of 241
pathology of 238, 239
pathophysiology of 238
phases of 238
Acute perforated peptic ulcer
  clinical diagnosis of 392
  management of 392
  pathology of 393*t*
Acute peritonitis 349, 355
  clinical features of 349
  complications of 355
  etiology of 349, 349*f*
  management of 349
  microbiology of 350
  treatment of 352
Acute pyelonephritis
  diagnosis of 553
  etiopathology of 553
  management of 553
Acute renal failure, postoperative 83
Acute respiratory distress syndrome 7, 148
Acute retention 593
  causes of 584*t*
  treatment of 585
Acute scrotum 612, 613
  differential diagnosis of 612, 613
  etiology of 612
Acute sialadenitis 190
  clinical features of 190
Acute trauma life support principles 35
Adamantinoma 174
Addison's disease 229
Addisonian crisis, acute 229
Adenitis, acute mesenteric 359
Adenocarcinoma 197, 248, 375, 522
  distal 398
  sequence 517
Adenoid cystic carcinoma 196
Adenolymphoma 193
Adenoma
  carcinoma sequence 517*t*, 518*t*
  hepatic 420
  monomorphic 193
  multi-step 518
  pleomorphic 193, 194
  sebaceum 161

Adnexa 165
 function of 155
Adrenal dysfunction, disorders of 227
Adrenal glands 225
 applied anatomy of 225
 disorders of 226
 disorders of 226, 226t
 function of 225
Adrenal insufficiency
 acute 11
 chronic 229
Adrenal medulla, tumors of 230
Adrenal tumors
 clinical features of 229
 management of 229
 staging of 230, 230t
Adrenalectomy 227, 232
Adrenocortical carcinoma 230
 management of 229
Adrenocortical insufficiency 229
Adrenogenital syndrome 228
Adson's maneuver 314
Adson's test 314
Advanced trauma life support 72
Aerobic gram-negative bacilli 48
Aganglionic zone 492
Air
 embolism 148
 filtration, inadequate 45
Airway 23, 134, 140
 maintenance of 89
 obstruction 86
 protection 27
 resuscitation of 13
 supraglottic 90
Alanine transaminase 75, 412
Albumin 106
Alcohols 116
Aldehydes 116
Alfa-fetoprotein 412
Alkaline
 gastritis 387
 phosphatase 75
Alloantibody 109
Alloantigen 109
Allograft 109
 dysfunction, causes of 111
Alpha-blockers 232
Alvarado score 486
Amebiasis
 extraintestinal 498
 intestinal 497
Amebic colitis, acute fulminant 498
Amebic liver abscess 415
 pathogenesis of 415
 pathology of 415
 treatment of 416
Amino acids 104
Aminoglycosides 49
Aminosalicylates 458

Amitriptyline 95
Amnesia
 post-traumatic 142
 retrograde 142
Amoxicillin 390, 393
Ampullary tumor 248f
Amputation 168, 310, 315, 608
 level of 315
 philosophy of 315
 principle steps of 316
 stump, types of 315
 types of 316
Amyand's hernia 341
Anal canal 505, 507f, 529
 anatomy of 505, 507f
 congenital anomalies of 451, 505
 development of 506f
 embryology of 505, 506f, 510
 lymphatic drainage of 508, 510f
 tumors of 515
 venous drainage of 508, 509f
Anal carcinoma 528
 treatment of 528
Anal crypts 505
Anal cushions 505, 537
Anal disease 459
Anal fissure
 distribution of 540t
 etiology of 540, 540t
 pathology of 540
 surgery for 541
 surgical procedures for 541f
 treatment of 540
Anal fistulae
 clinical features of 532
 complications of 532
Anal intraepithelial neoplasia 528
Anal sphincter 505, 508f
 dysfunction, internal 536
Analgesia 25, 97
 controlled 92, 93
 modes of 94
 nonopioid 94
 opioid 94
 oral opiate 95
 pre-emptive 94
 spinal 94
Anaphylaxis 10
Anderson Hynes pyeloplasty 565, 565f
Anemia, treatment of 19
Anesthesia 88, 91, 97, 125, 127
 epidural 9, 92, 94
 general 89, 91, 125, 489
 induction of 89, 100
 intravenous regional 92
 local 89, 91
 maintenance of 90
 preparation for 89
 regional 89, 91
 spinal 92
 total intravenous 90

Aneurysm 158
 etiology of 159
 intracranial 552
 mycotic 159
 saccular 159
 true 158
 types of 158f
Angina, mesenteric 482
Angiogenesis 33
Angiography 409
 coronary 286
 selective 405
Angioscopic laser atherectomy,
  percutaneous 310
Ankle-brachial pressure index 307
Annular carcinoma descending colon
 521f
Annular sigmoid carcinoma 521f
Anorectal abscesses 529, 529f
 anatomical classification of 529
 clinical features of 529
 etiology of 529, 529t
 pathogenesis of 529
 pathology of 529
 types of 529
Anorectal anomalies 510, 513t
 high 510, 512f, 513
 low 512, 513, 513f
Anorectal disease
 benign 536
 common 451, 505
Anorectal fistulae 530
 classification of 530
 etiology of 530, 531t
 Milligan Morgan classification of
  530, 531f, 531t
 Park's classification of 532f
Anorectal malformation, embryology
 for 512f
Anorectal myectomy 493
Anorectal surgery 505
Anorectal venous drainage 509f
Anthracycline 276
 regimens 276
Anti-beta lactamase 48
Antibioma 262
Antibiotic
 broad-spectrum 48
 coverage 50, 566
 selection of 48
 therapy 15, 52
Antibody
 antinuclear 75
 panel reactive 111
Anti-clostridial therapy 54
Anticonvulsants 95
Antifungal treatment 176
Antigen
 carcinoembryonic 243
 presenting cells 107

Index

Antimicrobial
 agents, topical 25
 intravenous 156
 prophylaxis 84
 therapy 48
Antineuropathic pain drugs 95
Antiproliferative agents 108
Anti-reflux barriers 364
Antisepsis 115
 beginning of 115
Antiseptic
 medicine, concept of 115
 prophylaxis 84
Antithyroid drugs 211, 212
Antitoxin 54
Antituberculous therapy 558
Antiviral agents 112
Aorta, coarctation of 290
Aortic aneurysms, traumatic 285
Aortic valve disease 287
Apoptosis 77
 failure of 77
Appendages 40
Appendicectomy 487
 complications of 487
 laparoscopic 488
Appendicitis 451, 485, 485f, 486
 acute 484, 486
 obstructive 484
 post-ileal 485f
 types of 484
Appendicular phlegmon 488
Appendix
 abscess 488
 anatomical positions of 483, 483f
 applied anatomy of 484
 carcinoid of 490
 epithelial tumors of 490
 gangrenous 484f
 mass 485, 488
  clinical course of 489t
  treatment of 488
 mucocele of 489
 perforation of 45, 484, 485f
Areola 256
Argon plasma coagulation 427
Aromatase inhibitors 277
Arrhythmias, cardiac 83, 151
Arterial disease 319
Arterial grafts 286
Arterial obstruction 469
 level of 307, 307t
Arterial occlusion
 causes of 304
 etiology of 305t
Arteriography 308
Arteriovenous fistula 159
 treatment of 160f
Arteritis 311
Artery 304
 aberrant 563
 forceps 119

Ascaris lumbricoides 461
Ascites
 management of 428
 pancreatic 242
Asepsis 115
 score system 47
Aspartate transaminase 75, 412
Aspiration 50
Aspirin 89, 95
Athelia 256
Atlanta classification, revised 239
Atresia
 biliary 435
 esophageal 370
 extrahepatic biliary 435
Atrial septal defects 290
Atrophic scar 39
Audit, types of 63
Auriculotemporal syndrome 191
Autoimmune disorder 188, 444
Autonomic nervous system 54
Autonomous toxic nodule 206, 209, 219
 treatment of 211
Axilla 271, 275
Axillary fascial tent 257
Axillary lymph 274
 management 277
 node 257f
  dissection 274
  metastases, surgery for 273
  surgical classification of 257
Axillary surgery, aim of 274
Axonal injury, diffuse 140
Azathioprine 302
Azithromycin 52

B

Bacillus fusiformis 185
Bacteria, translocation of 469
Bacteriology 51, 560
Bacteroides 36, 156
Balanectomy 608
Balanitis xerotica obliterans 601, 602, 604
Balanoposthitis 605
Ballance's sign 408
Balloon tamponade 427
Barbiturates 439
Bariatric surgery 124, 129, 130f, 131f
 types of 130
Barium swallow study 365
Barrett's esophagus 375
Barrett's ulcer 375
Bartholin duct 187
Basal cell carcinoma 165
 management of 165
Basal keratinocytes 155
Basic life support 133
Battle's para rectal incision 117

Beam radiotherapy, external 379, 597
Bench surgery 576
Benign prostatic hyperplasia
 clinical features of 592
 treatment of 592
Benzathine penicillin 52
Berry aneurysm 552
Beta-blockers 211, 232, 428
 propranolol 212
Beta-hemolytic *Streptococcus* 36
Bile ducts 235, 431, 433, 442
 cholangiocarcinoma of 444
 congenital abnormalities of 435
 tumors of 444
Bile peritonitis 353
Biliary colic 439, 445
Biliary dilatation, intrahepatic 447
Biliary disease 432
Biliary stones
 primary 442
 secondary 442
Biliary system, applied anatomy of 431
Biliary tract 431, 432
 evaluation, cornerstone of 432
Biliopancreatic diversion 131, 132t
Biochemical tests 75
Biological therapy 276
Biomedical waste 123t
 classification of 122t
 containers, label for 122
 disposal, steps of 121t
 management 122
  steps of 121, 122t
Biopsy 176, 259
 excision 76, 259
 laparoscopic 448
 multiple 404
 oropharyngeal 92
 prostatic 580t
 role of 448
 types of 76
Bisgaard's method 323
Bladder 547, 563, 548, 582, 583
 cancer
  clinical features of 547, 582
  investigation of 547, 582
  localized 587
  management of 547, 582
  TNM staging systems for 588t
 carcinoma
  clinical features of 588
  histological types of 587
 congenital defects of 583
 diverticula 586
 dysfunction 585
 exstrophy of 583
 fascial supports of 582
 function assessment 580
 incomplete emptying of 559
 ligamentous supports of 582

neck 599
   disorders 593
   stenosis 602
neoplasms of 587
outflow obstruction 591, 593
   etiology of 592
rupture of 583, 584
schistosomiasis of 561
sparing therapy 589
stones 572
surgical anatomy of 582
tumors, primary 587
urothelial cancer of 589
Blanching, signs of 157
Bleeding 126, 167
   control of 142
   internal 146
   nomenclature of 501
   peptic ulcer 393, 394
   signs of 146
   source of 146
   varices 427
      endotherapy for 427
Blind
   loop syndrome 463
   surgery 503
Blinding 67
   double 65, 67
Blisters 25
Blood 17, 106, 432
   autologous 18
   collection of 18, 139
   components 17
      shelf life of 18
   counts 457
   donation 17
      eligibility for 18
   escape of 43
   examination 75
   gas, arterial 83
   group 17
      matching 17
   loss, acute 19
   products 17
   spread 606
   substitutes 20
   tests 377
   transfusion 17, 84
      complications of 17-19
      indication for 19
      massive 19
      reactions 17
   use of 17
   vessels 43
Blue-light cystoscopy 588
Blunt 145
   dissection 85
   injuries 414
   renal trauma 581
   trauma 148

Boa's sign 440
Body
   fluid compartments 104
   nutrition, physiology of 101
Boerhaave's syndrome 366
Boil, fate of 50
Bone 34
   marrow 328
   scan 575
Borrmann's classification 398, 399*f*
Botulinum injection 370
Bowel
   congestion 469
   obstruction 471*f*, 471*t*
      chronic large 492, 481
Bowen's disease 166, 606
Boyd's classification 306
Brachytherapy 597
Bradycardia 138, 140, 142
Brain
   contusions 142
   damage 142
   death donation 111
   edema 138
   gut hormones 452
   injury 140, 142
   ischemia of 138
   metastases 279
   parts of 140
Brainstem hematoma 139
Branham's bradycardiac sign 159
Breast 98, 255, 271, 275
   abscess 260, 261
      acute 260
      clinical diagnosis of 260
      etiology of 260
      management of 260
      pathology of 260
      types of 261*f*
   anatomy of 255
   benign tumors of 264
   blood supply of 256
   cancer 280
      advanced 278
      early 275, 277, 278
      invasive 278
      non-invasive 269
      risk factors 258
      spread of 268
      treatment of 275
      triple negative 279
   carcinoma 267, 271, 272, 274
      AJCC staging of 270*t*
      TNM classification of 270
   congenital anomalies of 255
   conservation surgery 272, 277
   diseases 255, 257
      benign 259
      evacuation of 257, 258
   disorders 257*t*
   embryology of 255

   examination, self 258
   imaging report and data system 258*t*
   infections of 259
   inflammatory carcinoma of 279
   intra-ductal papilloma of 264
   invasive carcinoma of 277
   irradiation, accelerated partial 275
   lumps 264
   lymphatic
      deeper 257
      drainage of 256
   malignant tumors of 259
   recurrent carcinoma of 279
   surface, retraction of 256
   venous drainage of 256
Breathing 23, 134, 140
   resuscitation of 13
Broder's grading 166
Bronchi
   lungs, anatomy of 295
   lymphatic drainage zones of 296*t*
Bronchiectasis 293
Bronchodilators 84
Bronchoscopy 298
Bruising 43
Brush abrasion 43
Buccal sulcus 181
Budd-Chiari syndrome 426, 428, 430
Buerger's disease 311, 312*t*
Buerger's test 307
Bulbar urethra 599
   rupture of 600
Bupivacaine 92
Burkitt's lymphoma 328, 329
Burn 21, 23, 26
   acute 26
   circumferential 23
   classification of 21, 22
   depth of 21, 21*t*
   electrical 21, 23, 27
   eschar, early tangential excision of 26
   friction 43
   full thickness 22, 26
   inhalation 23
   injuries 21, 28, 29
   large 25
   management 29
   mechanism of 21
   partial thickness 22
   pathophysiology of 21, 22
   specific secondary survey 24
   surface area of 22
   surgical procedures of 26
   types of 22
   unit, management of 24
   victim 30
   wound care 25
Burst abdomen 36
Buschke-Löwenstein tumor 607

Index

C

Cadaveric donor 109
  transplantation 114
Calcineurin inhibitors 108
Calcium 105, 189
  channel blocker 370
  lithiasis, idiopathic 571
Calculus, removal of 189
Calot's triangle 431, 432*f*
  surgical anatomy of 431
Calyces 556
Campbell de Morgan spots 158
Cancer 401
  advanced stages of 95
  anal 528
  breast 280
  cardia 401
  cell 77
  colonic 528
  colorectal 516, 519
  development of 78
  early detection of 74, 78
  en cuirasse 271, 271*f*
  esophageal 379
  focused targeting of 79
  high-risk of 219
  localized 596
  management of 78
  nonsurgical treatment of 79
  oral 176, 177, 179
  oropharyngeal 175, 176
  pain 95
  pancreatic 251
  prostatic 595
  rectal 527
  risk of 375
  surgery, principles of 78
  syndromes 267
  testis 623
    staging of 621*t*
  therapy basis of 74
  treatment of 79
  urothelial 587
Cancrum oris 185
Candida albicans 57, 176
Candidiasis, chronic hyperplastic 176
Cantlie's line 411
Carbapenems 49
Carbimazole 212
Carbitaxel 597
Carbohydrate 102, 103
Carbon monoxide poisoning 27
Carbuncle 51
Carcinogens, urothelial 587
Carcinoid 297
  atypical 297
  syndrome 465, 491
    clinical features of 464, 465
    management of 464
    treatment of 465
  typical 297

Carcinoma 185, 206, 217, 256, 260, 558, 563
  adrenocortical 230
  anal 528
  anaplastic 197, 215, 218
  bladder 587
  breast 267, 271, 272, 274
    gene array based classification of 269*t*
    incidence of 271*f*
    pathology of 267
    treatment of 272, 276*t*
  cecum 491
  cheek 181
  colon 499
    differential diagnosis of 523
    surgery in 522
  colonic 522
  colorectal 517
  cylidromatous 196
  ductal 267
  embryonic antigen 522
  esophageal 376, 377*t*
  esophagus 375, 379
    clinical features of 376
  follicular 215, 216
  gallbladder 445
  head 251
  hepatocellular 421
  in situ 587, 608
  inflammatory 275, 279
  lip 181
  lobular 258, 267, 269
  metastatic 403
  mucoepidermoid 195, 196
  neuroendocrine 297
  non-functioning 230
  noninvasive 269, 277
  oropharyngeal 177
  pancreas 247, 250, 251
    stage of 249*t*
    treatment of 251
  pancreatic 247
  papillary 217
    follicular 215
  penis 606, 607, 607*t*, 608
    clinical features of 604
    investigation of 604
    management of 604
    TNM staging of 607
    treatment of 608
  periampullary 248, 251
  prostate 595, 597*t*
    clinical features of 596
    investigation of 596
    staging of 596
    treatment of 596, 597
  rectal 522, 525*f*, 526*t*
  rectum 524
    surgery for 524
    treatment of 526

  recurrent 279, 403
  salivary 195
    glands 195, 195*t*
  secondary 522
  sequence 518
  stomach 363, 380, 392, 394, 398, 400
    clinical features of 386
    etiology of 386
    investigation of 386
    management of 386
    staging of 399
    treatment of 401
  tail 251
  thyroid 216
  tongue 179
    distribution 179*f*
    treatment of 180
  transverse colon 523
Carcinomatosis peritonei 359
Cardiac arrest, acute 146
Cardiac function 285
Cardiac magnetic resonance imaging 286
Cardiogenic shock 10, 11
  causes of 11
Cardiological tests 83
Cardiology, interventional 290
Cardioplegia 284
Cardioplegic solutions 284
Cardiopulmonary bypass
  circuit 283*f*, 284
  complications of 284
  principles of 283
  steps of 283
Cardiothoracic surgery 283
Cardiovascular disease 74, 83, 130
Cardiovascular system 12, 13, 84, 159, 307
Caroli's disease 436
Caroli's syndrome 436
Carotid artery 183
Carotid ligation, external 184
Carotid sheath 215
Carr's classification 490
Causative pathology, correction of 566
Cavity
  abdominal 337
  peritoneal 349
Cecal volvulus 474
Cecostomy 496
Cecum, inflammation of 498
Ceftazidime 49
Cell 77
  neoplasms, immature 328
  origin 162, 267, 328
  surface erythroblastic oncogene B2 268
  types of 252, 302
Cellular stress responses 4, 5
Cellulitis 51, 156, 327

Cephalosporins 49
Cerebral perfusion pressure 141
Cervical rib 313
   syndrome 313
   types of 313
Cetrimide 116
Charcot's triad 442
Charle's procedure 327
Chemical
   burns 21, 23
   injury 27
   pleurodesis 150
   sterilization 116
   treatment 121
   waste 120, 122
Chemoembolization, transarterial 253
Chemokines 12
Chemoradiation 402, 528
Chemoradiotherapy 251
Chemotherapeutic regimens 609
Chemotherapy 169, 184, 232, 275, 293, 377, 379, 528, 597
   adjuvant 275, 299
   combination 276
   high dose 332
   hyperthermic intraperitoneal 403
   neoadjuvant 275, 402
   palliative 276
   regimens 276t, 278, 331, 528
   role of 275
Chest injuries
   classification of 145
   deadly dozen of 145, 145t
   management of 133, 147
   morbid physiology of 145
   pathophysiology of 133, 145
Chest wall 145, 275, 291
   mass 294t
   tumors of 293
Chest X-ray 146
Child-Turcotte-Pugh classification 413
Chlamydia trachomatis 610
Chlorhexidine 116
Chloroxylenol 116
Chlorpromazine 54
Cholangiography 434
   intravenous 432
   postoperative 434
Cholangitis, primary sclerosing 444
Cholecystectomy 441
   complications of 441
   emergency 441
   laparoscopic 441
Cholecystitis 445
   acalculous 433
   acute 439, 439f
   chronic 439
   diagnosis of 440
   glandularis proliferans 442

Cholecystography, oral 432
Cholecystohepatic duct, accessory 435
Cholecystostomy 441
Choledochal cysts 436
   types of 436
Choledocholithiasis 442
Choledochoscopy, operative 436
Cholelithiasis 436
Cholesterol stone 436, 437
Cholesterolosis 442
Chop wounds 44
Chorionic gonadotrophin stimulates 609
Chromosomal syndromes 266
Chronic constipation 499
   treatment of 500
Chronic ischemia 499
   Fontaine classification of 306
Chronic pain 94
   management of 93, 94
Chronic pancreatitis 236, 244
   clinical presentation of 244
   etiology of 244t
   pathogenesis of 244t
   surgery for 245, 246t
Chronic retention 585, 592, 593
   treatment of 585
Chronic wound 34, 37
   healing 34
Chyloceles 618
Ciprofloxacin 49
Circulation 140
Circulatory death 111
Circumcision
   complications of 605
   indications of 605
   role of 608
   technique of 605
Cirrhosis 414t
Cisplatin 402
Citrate phosphate dextrose solution 18
Clarithromycin 390
Cleft lip 170, 171, 172t
   classification of 171t
   repair 171
   surgery for 171
Cleft palate 170, 171, 172t
   classification of 171t
   repair 171
   surgery for 171
Clindamycin 52, 53
Clopidogrel 89
Clostridia 48, 156
   infections 48t
Clostridium 36
   difficile 49
   perfringens 45, 55, 439
   tetani 53
Cloxacillin 56, 262

Coagulopathy
   correction of 434
   indication for 19
   management of 19
Cock's peculiar tumor sebaceous horn 160
Codeine 95, 326
Colitis 495
   acute fulminant 496
   disintegrative 496
   ischemic 498
Collagen vascular disease 35
Collar
   button abscess 57
   stud abscess 50
Collis' gastroplasty 374
Colloid 105
   solutions 105
Colon
   angiodysplasia of 498
   lymphatic drainage of 453
   tumors of 515
   wall of 452
Colonic cancer 528
   non-surgical palliation of 524
Colonic carcinoma 522
   clinical diagnosis of 522, 523t
   complications of 522, 523, 523t
   surgery for 522
   treatment of 522, 523t
Colonic polyps
   microscopy of 515t
   types of 515
Colonic pseudo-obstruction 472
Colonoscopy 502
Color Doppler study 307
Colorectal adenomatous polyps 515
Colorectal cancers 516, 519
   distribution of 520f
   hereditary nonpolyposis 267
   staging of 518
Colorectal carcinoma 517
   macroscopic types of 519, 520f
   pathogenesis of 517
   pathology of 519
   spread of 518
   staging of 519f
   TNM staging of 518t
Colorectal malignancy, pathology of 519
Colostomy 472, 500, 514
   closure of 501
   complications of 500, 501, 501t
   double barrel 500
   indications 500
   permanent 500
   re-siting of 348
   types of 500, 500f
Commando operation 180, 184

Index

Common anorectal diseases
   clinical features of 451, 505
   investigation of 451, 505
   management of 451, 505
Common bile duct 431, 438, 442
   stone, surgery for 443
Compartment syndrome 36, 144
Complete blood counts 88
Compound volvulus 474
Congenital hypertrophic pyloric stenosis 386
   clinical features of 386
   etiology of 386
   investigation of 386
   management of 363, 380, 386
Connective tissue disorder 159
Constipation, chronic 499
Constrictions, esophageal 364
Contrecoup injury 138
Cord, encysted hydrocele of 617
Core biopsy 168
Coronary bypass surgery, indication for 286
Corticosteroid 95, 108
   therapy 229
Costoclavicular syndrome 313
Cough, chronic 37
Couinaud's liver segments 112, 112*f*, 411, 411*f*
Courvoisier's law 250, 443, 447
Cowden's syndrome 267, 398
Cowper's glands 590
Cranial nerves 54
Craniectomy 142
Craniotomy 142
Cremasteric reflex, absence of 614
Crepitus 156
Crisis, acute hypercalcemic 223
Crohn's disease 455-458, 546*t*
   colonic 497
   Montreal classification of 456*t*
   pathology of 455
   surgery for 458, 459*t*
Cryoprecipitate 18
Crypt abscesses 495
Crystalloids 105
Cullen's sign 239
Cushing's syndrome 228, 574
   medical therapy of 228
Cushing's triad 138, 142
Cutaneous melanoma 163*t*
   treatment of 164
Cyanoacrylate 320
Cyanosis 312
   local 312
   respiratory failure 149
Cyclophosphamide 276
Cyst 188
   choledochal 436
   chylolymphatic 359*f*
   dental 173
   dentigerous 173, 174
   deroofing of 552
   enterogenous 359*f*
   epidermal 160
   epidermoid 160
   epididymal 618
   hemorrhage 552
   infection 552
   renal 579
   sebaceous 160
   splenic 407
Cystadenoma 161
   lymphomatosum, papillary 193
Cystectomy, radical 589
Cystic duct 431
   absence of 435
   insertion 435
   low insertion of 435
Cystic kidney, types of 551
Cystic lump 265
Cystine stones 567
Cystinuria 571
Cystitis 559
   acute
      abacterial 560
      hemorrhagic 560
   cystica 561
   interstitial 561
   tuberculous 558
Cystolithotomy, suprapubic open 573
Cystoscopic lilholapaxy 573
Cystoscopy 558, 562, 579
Cytoarchitecture 103
Cytokines 12
   proinflammatory 6
   role of 12
Cytology 76

D

Dacarbazine 362
Damage control
   resuscitation 14, 136
   surgery 136, 415
Day care surgery 88, 96, 97
   principles of 96
   types of 96
De Quervain's goiter 210
De Quervain's thyroiditis 205, 212
Death 29
   causes of 379
   certificate 29
Deep vein thrombosis 52, 86, 322
   acute 322
   clinical signs of 319
   signs of 319
   treatment of 322
Delorme's procedure 544
Denervation 191

Dentate line, surgical importance of 505, 507*t*
Dermal grafts 40
Dermatoses, pre-existing 606
Dermis 155
Dermopathy 208
Dexamethasone 53
Dextrans 20
Diabetes mellitus 35, 83, 84, 129
Diabetic ulcers 37, 38
   management of 37
Diaphragm 145
   thoracoscopic repair of 151
Diazepam 54
Diethylene-triamine-penta-acetate renogram 580
Dietl's crisis 564
Dieulafoy's lesion 395
Digestive tract 337
Digital subtraction angiography 309
Dihydroadeninuria 568
Di-iodotyrosines 203
Dimercaptosuccinic acid renogram 580
Disability 23, 29, 30
Disasters activities 72
Disinfection 115
   beginning of 115
   methods of 115
Distributive justice theory 114
Diverticula
   acquired 586
   congenital 454, 586
   epiphrenic 368
   esophageal 368
   intestinal 454
Diverticulitis 494
Diverticulosis 494
   coli 493, 494
      complications of 493
      pathology of 493
   surgery for 494
Diverticulum, cricopharyngeal 368
Docetaxel 276, 597
Domestic violence 29
Donor
   group 17
   nephrectomy 112
   recipient matching 110
   types of 109
Doppler guided hemorrhoidal artery ligation 539
Dorothy-Reed-Sternberg cells 329
Down's syndrome 619
Dowry problem 29
Doxorubicin 362
Drainage, Hilton's method of 50
Dry gangrene 306
Dry mouth, causes of 188

Duct
  carcinoma in situ 269
  multiple 260
Ductal system 257f
Ductus arteriosus, constriction of 288
Ductus venosus, closure of 288
Duhamel operation, modified 493
Dumping syndrome 104, 391
Duodenal atresia 478
  types of 478, 479f
Duodenal switch gastric bypass 131, 132t
Duodenoduodenostomy 478
Duodenum 382
  investigation of 384
  part of 401
  secretes 383
  surgical physiology of 383
Duplex scan 307
Duplex ultrasound scan 320
  role of 320
Duplex ureters 553
Dysentery, amebic 498
Dyspepsia group 399
Dysphagia 365
  causes of 366
  etiology of 366, 366t
  evacuation of 366
Dysplasia 170, 397
  craniofacial 170

E

Ectopia vesicae 583
Eczema 326
Edema
  control 58
  peripheral 426
Edge biopsy 76
Electrolyte
  administration 106
  loss 469
  replacement of 101
Elevated jugular venous pulsations 82
Embryology 451, 582
Emergency medical services 134
Empathy 69
Emphysema, metastatic 338
Empyema 291, 293
  necessitans 292
  post-traumatic 151
  sites of 292
  surgery for 292
  thoracis 292
  typical 292
Endocrine 87, 233, 245, 246, 389
  deficiency 244
  secretions 234
  shock 10, 11
  system 12
  tumors 246, 252

Endoderm 582
Endomicroscopy 365
Endoscope 124
Endoscopic curative therapy 377
Endoscopic mucosal resection 378, 503
Endoscopic retrograde cholangiopancreatography 235, 245, 433
Endoscopic therapy 245
Endoscopy 365, 457
  biliary 434
  third space 366
Endosonography 365, 447
  transesophageal 377
Endotherapy 427
  methods of 394
Endotracheal intubation 27
Endovascular interventional revascularization procedures 310
Endovenous ablation 320, 321
Energy devices 86, 125
Enhanced recovery after surgery 8, 9, 104
Enucleation 194
Enzyme 234
  cardiac 75
  deficiency 568
Epidermis 40
Epididymitis
  chronic 611
  tuberculous 611
Epididymo-orchitis
  acute 610
  applied anatomy of 604, 610
  clinical features of 604, 610
  investigations of 604, 610
  management of 604, 610
Epispadias 600
Epitaxy 568
Epithelialization 33
Epithelioma 161
Epithelium 40
Epulides pleural 172
Epulis, types of 172, 173, 173t
Erysipelas 52, 156
Erythromycin 52
Erythroplakia 176
Escharotomy 26
Escherichia coli 36, 48, 156
Esomeprazole 390
Esophageal cancer 379
  distribution of 376t
Esophageal carcinoma
  staging of 376, 377t
  surgery for 378
  treatment of 377
Esophageal disease, clinical features of 365

Esophageal hiatus hernia 372
  types of 373f
Esophageal perforations 366
  treatment of 367t
Esophageal spasm 365
Esophageal sphincter, lower 364
Esophageal varices 394
  management of 426
Esophagectomy 370
Esophagogastrectomy 401
Esophagus 206, 363
  anatomical division of 363
  applied anatomy of 363
  behavior of 363
  cervical 363
  functional divisions of 364
  lower third of 378
  malignant disorders of 363
  middle third of 378
  physiology of 363
  spontaneous rupture of 366
  surgical anatomy of 364f
  thoracic 363
  upper third of 378
Estrogen 267
  receptors 268
Ethylene oxide gas 116
Eusol 116
Euthanasia, active 71
Ewings' tumor 294
Exocrine 233, 246
  deficiency 245
  function, pancreatic 235
  pancreatic
    deficiency 244
    tumors 247
  secretion 234
Extracorporeal shockwave lithotripsy 569, 570
Extraperitoneal drainage 489
Extremity, occlusive arterial disease of 304
Eye signs 209

F

Face
  development of 171f
  mask 24
Facial nerve 187
  weakness 192
Facies hippocratica 351
Fallot tetralogy 289
Fasciitis, typical necrotizing 36
Fasciotomy, emergency 36
Fat 103, 104, 256
  necrosis 266
    traumatic 266
Fatty liver disease, hepatic non-alcoholic 421

Index

Feeding
 artery, ligation of 394
 enteral 26
 timing of 103
Femoral canal 340
Femoral hernia 340, 342, 343
 diagnosis of 345
 surgery for 345
 surgical anatomy of 340
 treatment of 345
Femoral ring 340
Femoral vein 317
Fentanyl patch 94
Fertility 623
Fever 569
Fibers, partial tear of 143
Fibrinogen 19
Fibroadenoma 264
 intracanalicular 264
 pericanalicular 264
 types of 264
Fibroadenosis 263
 differential diagnosis of 263
 treatment of 263
Fibroblast migration 33
Fibrosis 562
 oral submucous 176
Fibula flap 41
Fine needle aspiration cytology 76, 207, 259
Finger invagination test 342
First aid 135
 principles of 133
 steps of 134
Fissure
 in ano 540
  clinical features of 541t
  pathology of 540, 541f
  treatment of 540
 portal 411
Fistula 204
 arteriovenous 159
 complications of 532
 enterocutaneous 463
 in Ano, treatment of 532
 intestinal 463
 low 533
 mammillary 262
 pancreatic 237
 salivary 190
Fistulography 76
Fitness, assessment of 98
Flail chest 148
 morbid respiratory physics of 148
 types 148
Flaps 40, 315
 classification of 40
 closure 315
 design of 41

Flexor
 pollicis longus, synovial sheath of 59
 synovial sheaths 59
 tendon sheath infection 58
 tenosynovitis
  acute suppurative 57
  etiology of 57
Fluctuation, signs of 50
Fluid 24
 administration 106
 collection 239t
  acute peripancreatic 242
 loss 469
 management
  intraoperative 106
  postoperative 106
 replacement of 101, 106
 requirement 105
 resuscitation 24, 156
 therapy 14
 supplemental 106
 therapy 101
Fluorodeoxyglucose 77
Foley's catheter, indwelling 25
Foley's Y-V plasty 565
Follicular thyroid carcinoma 217
Foramen ovale, closure of 288
Formaldehyde 116
Formalin solution 116
Fournier's gangrene 613, 615
 treatment of 615
Foxes' sign 239
Fractures, depressed 141
Fresh-frozen plasma 18
Frey's syndrome 191
Frostbite 28
Fruchaud's myopectineal orifice 341, 342f
Fundoplications, types of 374f
Fungal whitlow 57
Fusiform 158

G

Gabapentin 95
Galactocele 266
Galactorrhea 260
 drug induced 260
 physiologic 260
 spontaneous 260
Gallbladder 250, 431, 438
 congenital abnormalities of 435
 function of 432
 investigation of 432
 polyp 442
 porcelain 445
 radioisotope imaging of 433
Gallstone 436
 complications of 438
 disease, pre-existing 445

formation, pathogenesis of 437
 pathology of 438
 types of 436
Ganglioneuroma 230
Gangrene 306, 315
 causes of 306
 signs of 306
 types of 306, 315
Gangrenous torsion 615f
Gap analysis 64
Gas
 gangrene 55, 306
  management of 55
 insufflator 125
Gastrectomy 401f
 blind subtotal 394
 distal 394
 laparoscopic sleeve 130
 partial 272, 391, 392f
 radical 402
 subtotal 401
 total 401
Gastric
 acid secretion 383, 384
 antral venous ectasia 426
 band, laparoscopic adjustable 130
 cancer 397, 398, 401f, 403
  advanced 399f, 402
  early 398, 398f, 402
  histologic typing of 398t
  pathogenesis of 397
  pathology of 398
 carcinoma 402
  advanced 398
  classification of 398
  evacuation of 400
  treatment of 402
 dysmotility problems 385
 function study 384
 lumen 389
 lymph node stations 382f, 383, 383f
 lymphoma 404
 motility studies 385
 mucosa has 381
 mucosal barrier 384
 mucus 384
 resection, extent of 401
 surgery
  nomenclature of 401
  principles of 401
 ulcers 388, 389, 393
 volvulus 396
  types of 396
Gastrin 252, 385, 389
 level estimation 384
 stimulates acid production 385
Gastrinoma 254, 404
 treatment of 405
Gastritis 387
 autoimmune 387
 eosinophilic 388

erosive 387
granulomatous 388
lymphocytic 388
phlegmonous 388
types of 387t
Gastro-colic omentum 401
Gastroduodenal
  motility 384
  mucosa, microscopy of 381
  secretory functions 383
  stress ulcers 26
  ulcers, acute 394
Gastroesophageal reflux disease 371
  endoscopic treatment of 373
  Los Angeles classification of 372
  medical treatment of 373
  surgery for 373
  treatment of 373
Gastro-hepatic omentum 401
Gastrointestinal bleeding 501
  acute 503, 503t
  lower 501-503
  scintigraphy 503
  symptoms of 501
Gastrointestinal hemorrhage, acute
    lower 501
Gastrointestinal stromal tumors 395,
    403, 464, 465, 491
Gastrointestinal tract 563
Gastrojejunostomy 391, 391f
Gastroparesis 372
Gelatin 20
Gene
  array based classification 269, 269t
  therapy 311, 332
General anesthesia 89, 91, 125, 489
  induction of 89
Genetic
  mutations 162, 247
  pathways 517
  syndromes 162
Genital system 563
Genitourinary system
  clinical features of 547
  congenital anomalies of 547
  investigations of 547
Genitourinary tuberculosis 556
  pathogenesis of 556
  pathology of 556t
Germ cell tumor 302, 620
Germline mutations 397
Giant congenital pigmented nevus
    161
Giant hairy naevus 161
Glands 590
  bulbourethral 590
  sublingual 187
Glans
  amputation of 608
  penis, leukoplakia of 606

Glasgow coma scale score 140, 141,
    141t
Glasgow criteria 241, 241t
Gleason's histopathologic grade 595
Gleason's scoring system 595
  rationale of 595
Glomangioma 158
Glucagonoma 253
Glucose 104
Glutaraldehyde 116
Glycemic control 84
Glycopeptide antibiotics 49
Glycosaminoglycans 33
Goblet cells 495
Goiter 205
  classification of 205
  diffuse hyperplastic 206
  diffuse toxic 207
  hardness of 210
  hyperplastic 207
  inflammatory 205
  intrathoracic 210, 214f
  multinodular 207, 213
  nodular 205, 206
  pathogenesis of 206
  retrosternal 209
  simple 205
  toxic 205-207, 209
Goitrogenesis 205
Gompertzian growth, implications
    of 78
Goodsall's rule 531, 532f
Goodsall's suturing 543f
Graft
  disease 20, 110
  dysfunction 111, 112
    causes of 111
  full thickness 40
  multiple 112
  rejection
    mechanism of 109
    types of 110
  types of 109
  venous 286
Granuloma 562
  pyogenic 158
Grave's disease 207, 208, 211
  management of 208
Grave's ophthalmopathy 208
Gravel rash 43
Great saphenous vein 317, 321f
Grey Turner's sign 239
Groin hernia 339, 340
  classification of 340
  differential diagnosis of 343
  NYHUS' classification of 340
  repair 344
Guillotine amputation 315
Gums
  swellings of 170
  tumors of 170

Gut syndrome 466
Gynecomastia 266, 267

H

Hair follicle 161
  pits of 256
Halogen derivatives 116
Hamartoma tumor syndrome 398
Hand
  disease of 56
  infections 45, 56
    causes of 56
    diagnosis of 56
    treatment of 56
  rehabilitation 58
Hartmann's pouch 437
Hashimoto's disease 205
Hashimoto's thyroiditis 210, 212, 213
Head injury 138, 142
  classification of 138, 141
  clinical assessment of 140
  management of 133
  mechanism of 133, 138
  pathogenesis of 140
  pathophysiology of 138
  sequelae of 143
  treatment of 140, 141
Healing, abnormal 34
Heart
  disease
    acyanotic 289
    congenital 288
    cyanotic 289
    valvular 83, 552
  failure, congestive 83
  primary failure of 11
  walls, structure of 285
Heartburn 365
Helicobacter pylori 385, 398
Heller's cardiomyotomy 370, 370f
Helper T-cells 108
Hemangioma 157, 161, 420
  capillary 157
  cavernous 157
Hematemesis 393
  etiology of 393
Hematocele 619
Hematology 75
Hematolymphoid 172
Hematoma 414, 548, 552, 569
  acute extradural 139, 142
  acute subdural 139, 142, 143
  chronic subdural 139, 142
  epidural 93
  types of 139
Hematuria
  causes of 548f, 548t
  loin mass 574
  management of 547
  non-visible 548

Index

Hemifacial macrosomia, classification of 170, 170*t*
Hemiglossectomy 180
Hemimandibulectomy 180
Hemithyroidectomy 217
Hemocytopoiesis 407
Hemodynamic
   instability 16
   stabilization of 54
Hemolytic reaction, acute 17
Hemopericardium 146
Hemophilia 394
Hemoptysis 293
Hemorrhage 14
   acute subarachnoid 139
   intracranial 139
   intraparenchymal 139
   intraventricular 139
   surgical 97
Hemorrhagic shock 11, 146
   management of 14
Hemorrhoidectomy 538
   closed 539
Hemorrhoids 536, 537
   acute prolapsed 528*f*
   classification 536
   clinical features of 537, 538*t*
   differential diagnosis of 537, 538*t*
   etiopathogenesis of 536
   management of 537
   pathogenesis of 536
   primary 537*f*
   secondary causes for 537
   treatment of 538, 539, 539*t*
Hemostasis 33, 85, 427
Hemothorax 149, 150
Hepatectomy, terminology for 422
Hepatic disorders 82
Hepatic failure, signs of 413
Hepatic malignancy, primary 111
Hepatic resections 422*t*
   types of 423*f*
Hepatocellular carcinoma 421
   staging of 422*t*
   treatment of 422, 423
Hepatocellular function 414*t*
Hepatomegaly 250
Herceptin 268, 276
Hermann Taylor regimen 393
Hernia 337, 348, 613
   abdominal wall 338
   complications of 338
   diagnosis of 339
   epigastric 346
   etiology of 337
   external 337
   femoral 340, 342, 343
   gluteal 348
   groin 339, 340
   hiatus 372

incisional 337, 347
inguinal 340, 342, 343, 345, 345*f*
internal 337, 478
lumbar 348
obturator 348
parastomal 348
pathogenesis of 337, 338
perineal 348
reducible 338
repair, focus of 341
rolling 373
sciatic 348
sliding 342, 372
special types of 341
spigelian 348
strangulated groin 345
surgical repair of 347
treatment of 339
types of 337, 341
umbilical 346
uncomplicated 338
ventral 346
Herniogenesis 338
Herniology 337
Herpes simplex 57
Herpetic whitlow 57
Hiatus hernia
   clinical features of 372
   esophageal 372
Hidradenitis suppurativa 50, 156
Hidradenoma 161
High proliferation index 268
Hilar cholangiocarcinoma 444
Hinchey classification 494
Hirschsprung's disease 492
   classification of 492
   diagnosis of 492
   management of 492
   pathology of 492
Hodgkin's disease
   clinical features of 328, 329
   management of 328
Hodgkin's lymphoma 328-330, 330*t*
   treatment of 331
Hollander's insulin test 385
Homan's procedure 326
Homeostasis 3, 412
   concept of 3
Homeostatic control system 3
Hormonal therapy 275
Hormone
   binding of 203
   counter-regulatory 101
   receptors 268
   responsive tumors 278
   therapy 275
Horseshoe kidney 551
Hospital waste 120, 122
   disposal of 120, 121
Host disease 20, 110
Hot air oven 115

Hot nodules 207
House testis 620
Human albumin 18, 20
Human basic fibroblast growth factor 38
Human immune system 107
Human immunodeficiency virus gastritis 388
Human leukocyte antigen 109
Human major histocompatibility complexes 107
Human Organs and Tissues Rules, transplantation of 114
Human papilloma virus infections 606
Hunger, physiology of 129
Hunner's ulcer 561
Hurthle cell carcinoma 215
Hydatid
   cyst 293, 418, 419
   malignant 420
Hydrocele
   acquired 616
   applied anatomy of 604
   classification of 616*f*
   clinical features of 604
   complications of 616
   congenital 616, 617
   filarial 618
   formation, mechanism of 616
   investigations of 604
   management of 604
   pathophysiology of 616
Hydrochloric acid 384
Hydrocortisone 53
Hydrogen ions 384
Hydronephrosis 562, 564, 565
   bilateral 563*t*, 564, 565
   clinical features of 547, 562
   extra renal 563
   intermittent 564
   intrarenal 563
   investigations of 547, 562
   management of 547, 562
   treatment of 564
   types of 564*f*
   unilateral 563, 563*t*
Hydroureter 562
Hydroxyethyl starch 20
Hyperabduction
   maneuver 314
   syndrome 313
Hyperaldosteronism
   biochemistry of 228
   primary 227
Hyperamylasemia, causes of 234
Hyperbaric oxygen treatment 38
Hypercalcemia, differential diagnosis of 222
Hypercalcemic disorders 567, 571
Hypercarbia 127

Hyperemia 312
Hyperesthesia 305
Hypergastrinemia 385
  differential diagnosis of 405
Hyperglycemia 6
Hyperoxaluria
  enteric 571
  primary 568, 571
  secondary 568
Hyperparathyroidism 221
  primary 221
  secondary 221, 223
  tertiary 221
Hyperplasia, focal nodular 420
Hypertension 138, 140, 142, 552
  portal 413, 424, 425, 428
  venous 318
Hyperthyroid phase 212
Hyperthyroidism 10, 208
  control of 211
  signs of 209
Hypertonic saline solutions 105
Hypertrophic scar 39
Hypoparathyroidism 220
  clinical features of 221
Hypoperfusion 14
Hypoplasia, testicular 619
Hypoproteinemia 37
Hypospadias 599
  types of 599
Hypotension 140
Hypothermia 28
  signs of 28
Hypothesis 65
Hypothyroidism 11
  complications of 213
Hypotonic solutions 105
Hypoxemia 86
Hypoxia 12, 146

I

Iatrogenic strictures 602
Ifosfamide 362
Ileal gangrene 485f
Ileal strictures
  etiology of 462
  management of 462
Ileo-anal anastomosis 493
Ileocecal tuberculosis 491
  etiopathology of 459
Ileo-ileo colic intussusception,
    acute 477f
Ileostomy 458, 496
  care 458
Imatinib 168, 465
Imidazole 49
Iminodiacetic acid 433
Immune responses, adaptive 108
Immunization, passive 54
Immunohistochemistry 400
  staining 607

Immunosuppression 108, 109
  non-specific 109
  principles of 107
Immunosuppressive therapy 37, 108
Immunotherapy 80, 165, 169, 332, 609
In situ carcinoma 269
Incidentaloma 226
  treatment of 227
Incision
  abdominal 117
  biopsy 76, 259
  large 127f
  types of 37
Infarction, splenic 407
Infections 19, 109, 398, 568, 571
  anaerobic 55
  ascending 553, 560
  control of 39
  hematogenous 553
  hospital acquired 45, 47
  intra-abdominal 87
  pleural 291
  postoperative 45
  respiratory 87
  risk of 93
  route of 440, 459, 560, 610
  source of 15, 350
  spread of 45
  urogenital 87
Infectious diseases 18
Inferior vena cava 429
  filter 323
Inflammation, cardinal signs of 49
Inflammatory carcinoma 275, 279
  differential diagnosis of 261
Inguinal canal, anatomy of 339
Inguinal hernia 340, 342, 343, 345,
    345f
  clinical types of 342
  surgery, complications of 345
Inhalation burns 23
  injuries 27
Injury 42, 133
  arterial 144
  assessment of 414
  classification of 145
  cold 28
  corrosive 367
  diaphragmatic 151
  esophageal 151
  iatrogenic 514
  mechanism of 138
  mode of 133
  non-life-threatening 136
  potentially life threatening 145,
    150
  rectal 514
  reperfusion 311
  sites of 23, 600
  spinal 93
  thermal 21

tracheobronchial 151
  types of 145
  venous 144
Innate system 107
Insulinoma 253
Integrated day surgery centers 96
Intercostal drainage tube 150
Internal ring occlusion test 342
Intestinal disorders, large 492
Intestinal obstruction 468, 470, 478
  acute 470
  classification of 468, 468t
  clinical features of 470
  etiology of 468t
  pathophysiology of 468, 468t
  treatment of 471
Intestines 22, 451
  congenital disorders of 451
  large 492
  tuberculosis of 459
  volvulus of 472, 473t
Intracellular ice crystals, formation
    of 28
Intraductal papillary mucinous
    neoplasms 247
Intrahepatic ducts, congenital
    dilatation of 436
Intraoperative imaging techniques
    434
Intraperitoneal abscess 355, 355f
  clinical signs of 355
  post peritonitis, sites of 355f
Intraperitoneal rupture, treatment
    of 584
Intubation, complications of 90
Intussusception 475, 477, 491, 521f
  acute 475
  gangrenous 476
  parts of 476, 476f
  radiological signs of 476f
  target sign of 477f
  treatment of 476
  types of 476f
Invertogram 513
Iodide trapping 203
Iodine isotopes 207
Ionic calcium 75
Ipilimumab 165
Irradiation 275
  fractional dose of 79
Ischemia
  acute 305, 499
    mesenteric 481
  angle of 307
  chronic 499
    limb 310
    mesenteric 482
    progressive 499
  clinical features of 305
  non-occlusive mesenteric 481
  reperfusion syndrome 12

Ischiorectal abscess
  drainage of 530f
  investigations of 530
  treatment of 530
Isobaric bupivacaine 92
Isoniazid 439
Isotonic crystalloids 105
Isthmusectomy 213

J

Jabolay's procedure 618
Jaundice 244, 245, 249, 250
  extrahepatic obstructive 448
  mechanism of 446f
  obstructive 235, 445-449, 449f, 450t
  surgical 445, 449
Jaws
  swellings of 170, 172
  tumors of 170, 172
Jejunostomy, emergency 367
Jejunum 466
  anatomy of 451t
Jod Basedow thyrotoxicosis 208
Joffroy's sign 209
Joints
  extended interphalangeal 58
  interphalangeal 56
  movement of 40

K

Kanavel's cardinal signs 58
Kaposi's sarcoma 169
Kehr's sign 408
Keloid 26, 39
Keratosis, seborrheic 160
Kidney 547, 548, 556
  cystic diseases of 551
  ectopic 551
  enlarged 552
  injury, acute 87
  transplantation 112
Koch's peculiar tumor 160

L

Lactate dehydrogenase 622
Lamina propria 495
Laparoscope 124
Laparoscopy, diagnostic 126, 385
Laparotomy 147, 415, 477, 495
  staging of 331
Lapatinib ditosylate 276
Large intestine 492
  anatomy of 452
  applied anatomy of 451
  benign tumors of 515t
  blood supply of 452
  disorders of 451

function of 453
tumors of 515
Laryngeal mask airway 90
Laser ablation 176
Lauren's classification 398
Leg veins 317
Lentigo 161
  meligna maligna 162
Leprosy 50
Lesions, perianal 456
Letrozole 277
Leukocytosis 486
  polymorphonuclear 327
Leukoplakia
  proliferative verrucous 176
  speckled 175
  variants of 175
Levator ani, puborectalis sling of 510
Levobupivacaine 92
Leydig cell tumor 620
Lichen
  planus, oral 177
  sclerosus et atrophicus 604
Lichtenstein mesh onlay tension free repair 344
Lignocaine 92
Limb 37, 305, 315
  acute ischemic 305
  amputation of 36, 164
  ischemia of 305, 309
  lower 304
  morbid anatomy of 307
  perfusion, isolated 169
  reductive procedures 326
  sparing resection 168
  upper 304
Linea alba, fatty hernia of 346
Linezolid 56
Lingual thyroid 203
  resection of 204
Linitis plastica 399
Lipase 235
Lipoma 156, 229
  retroperitoneal 361
Liposomal bupivacaine 93
Lithium salts 211
Lithogenic bile 438
Litholapaxy, suprapubic percutaneous 573
Lithotomy position 85, 126
Littre's hernia 341
Live donor 109
Liver 411
  abscess, amebic 415
  actinomycosis of 420
  anatomy of 411
  cell failure 426
  cholangiocarcinoma of 423
  disease 412, 412t
    chronic 35, 37, 266, 413
    metabolic 111

enzymes 432
failure, acute 111, 413
function 412
  Child-Turcotte-Pugh classification of 413
  tests 75, 83, 412, 416, 596
hydatid cyst of 418
infectious conditions of 415
injuries 413, 414
metastases 465
pyogenic abscess of 417
segmental anatomy of 411
transplantation 111, 428, 449
  indications for 111
  steps of 112
trauma
  classification of 413, 414, 414t
  complications of 415
  etiology of 413
  management of 413, 414
  tumors of 420
Lobectomy 293
Local ablative therapy 423
Local anesthesia 89, 91
  complications of 92
Locoregional therapy 272
Loop
  colostomy 500
  ileostomy 458
Lord's plication 618
Lower gastrointestinal bleeding 501-503
  etiology of 501, 502t
Lower limb 304
  deep vein of 317
  superficial veins of 317
  venous system of 317
Lower urinary tract 582
  infection 559
    special forms of 560
  obstruction of 563
  stones 572
  symptoms 549, 591
L-thyroxine 203
Lucid interval 139, 142
Ludwig's angina 52
  complications of 52
Lumbar triangle
  inferior 348
  superior 348
Lumen, obstruction of 484
Luminal bile, composition of 436
Luminal toxins, intestinal 469
Lump 271
Lung
  abscess 293
    post-traumatic 151
  cancers 296
    clinical presentation of 297
    histological classification of 296, 297t

metastatic 299
staging of 297
surgical management of 298
treatment of 298
congestion 82
cysts 293
injury, acute 20
lymphatic drainage zones of 296t
resection, complications of 298
segments 295f
tumors 295
Lymph node 167, 210, 328, 376
dissection 164, 401
retroperitoneal 623
management of 164
metastases 180, 270, 575
Lymphadenectomy 378
pelvic 589
Lymphangioma 324
Lymphangiosarcoma 325
Lymphangitis 51, 52, 156
acute 51, 327
clinical features of 324
investigations of 324
management of 324
pathophysiology of 324
Lymphatic 304
drainage 202, 382
restoration of 326
rectal 524, 525f
spread 179, 249, 606
system 324
examination of 324, 332
Lymphedema 273, 319, 324
classification of 324, 325t
clinical features of 324
congenital primary 325
differential diagnosis of 326
grading of 324
investigations of 324
management of 324
pathogenesis of 324
pathology of 324t
pathophysiology of 324
primary 325
secondary 325
treatment of 326
Lymphoid tissue, gut-associated 46
Lymphoma 165, 193, 328, 464, 465, 620
Ann Arbor staging for 329, 330t
classification of 328, 328t
clinical features of 324, 329
investigations of 324
management of 324
pathophysiology of 324
treatment of 331
Lymphoscintigraphy 164
Lymphovascular units 453
Lynch syndrome 267, 516

M

Macroglossia 185
causes of 185t
Magnesium 105
sulphate infusion 55
Major injury, hypersecretion of 5
Malabsorptive procedures 130
Malignancy 109, 167, 196, 224
features of 192
incidence of 192
penile 606
risk of 227
Malignant disease 95
Malignant melanoma, management of 162
Mallory-Weiss syndrome 367, 394, 395
Malnutrition
assessment of 102
causes of 101, 102
consequences of 101, 102
Mammary duct ectasia 265
Mammary ridge 255f
Mammography 258
Manometry, esophageal 365
Margetuximab 276
Marjolin's ulcer 166
Mass
abdominal 250
adrenal 227
appendicular 491
casualties 135
management of 133, 135
closure 118
differential diagnosis of 491
epigastric 243
injuries 136
non-functional 227
Mastalgia 263
differential diagnosis of 263
treatment of 263
Mastectomy 280
radical 273
total 265, 273, 277
Mastitis
acute 260
bacterial 261
diffuse 260
carcinomatosa 279
cystic 263
granulomatous 262
stage of 261, 262
Mathe's sign 566
Maydl's hernia 341
McBurney's grid iron incision 487
McKeown's operation 378
McKeown's total esophagectomy 378
Meatal stones 573
Mechanical ventilation, indications for 91
Mechanochemical ablation 321

Meckel's diverticulum 394, 454
Meconium
ileus 480
peritonitis 353, 353f, 480
Mediastinal diseases 300
Mediastinal mass lesions, treatment of 301
Mediastinal pathology 302, 302t
Mediastinoscopy 302
Mediastinum
anatomy of 300, 300f
contents of 300t
inferior 300
middle 300
posterior 300
primary tumors of 301, 301t
superior 300
Medical therapy 223
Medical waste 120
classifications 120
types of 120
Medulla 225
Medullary sponge kidney 568
Medullary thyroid carcinoma 215
treatment of 218
Megacolon, congenital 492
Meige disease 325
Meissner's corpuscles 155
Melanocytes 155, 165
Melanocytic lesions 161
Melanoma 163, 163t, 522
amelanotic 162
clinical features of 162t, 163
cutaneous 163t
differential diagnosis of 163
nodular 162
staging of 163, 164, 164t
subungual 162
superficial spreading 162
Melena 393
etiology of 393
Membrane attack complex 107
Membranous urethra 599
rupture of 601
Menetrier's disease 388, 397
Menstrual irregularities 209
Merkel cells 155
Mesenchymal cells 33
Mesenteric artery
inferior 453, 524
superior 453, 524
Mesenteric cyst 358, 358f
clinical features of 359f
differentiation of 358t
Mesenteric vascular
insufficiency 481
ischemia, causes of 481
Mesenteric vein, superior 429
Mesentery, thrombosis of 485f
Mesh, types of 339

Mesoappendix 483
Mesonephric ducts 550
Metabolic stress response 3
Metaplasia, intestinal 397
Metastasectomy 299
   criteria for 299
Metastasis 164
   hematogenous 268
   number of 424
   removal of 78
Metastatic carcinoma 403
   breast, treatment of 279
Metastatic disease 621
Metastatic neck nodes, treatment of 183
Metastesectomy 528
Methimazole 211
Methotrexate 362
Methyldopa 439
Metoprolol 212
Metronidazole 49, 53, 55, 390
Metyrapone 232
Michon's stages 58t
Microbial flora 103
Microbial invasion 45
Microcarcinoma, papillary 215
Microscopy 165, 166, 455
Microvascular anastomosis 610
Midazolam 54
Mid-clavicular line 150
Midgut malrotation 479
   pathogenesis of 479
Midgut volvulus 479
Midpalmar space 58
   anatomy of 58
   infections of 59
Milan criteria 423
Milian's ear sign 52
Milk-alkali syndrome 567
Milligan Morgan classification 530, 531, 531f, 531t
Minimal access surgery 124
Minimal callus formation 34
Minimal incision 127f
Minimally invasive surgery 124, 127, 320
   advantages of 124, 127
   application of 126
   disadvantages of 124, 127
Minor salivary gland 187
   disorders of 188
   tumors 197
Mitogen activated protein kinase, dysregulation of 214
Mitotane 232
Mitral stenosis 287
Mitral valve disease, causes of 287
Mixed germ cell tumor 620
Modern digital technology, use of 79
Moebius' sign 209

Molecular therapy 80, 165
Mondor's disease 256
Monoclonal antibody 80, 108, 165, 301, 458
Monoiodotyrosines, coupling of 203
Monotherapy 48
Monro-Kellie doctrine 138, 139
Moral dilemmas 70
Morphine 95
   oral 95
Moses' sign 322
Motility disorders, esophageal 368
Motion exercises, range of 58
Motor response 141
Mucosa, vertical tear of 367
Mucoviscidosis 236
Mullerian duct 550
Multicystic disease 550
Multimodality pain management 93t
Multiple endocrine neoplasia 231
Multiple organ
   dysfunction syndrome 16
   system failure 351
Murphy's sign 440
Murphy's triad 485
Muscle 505, 522
   contusion of 144
   injuries 144
   invasive bladder cancer 588, 589
   lacerations 144
   necrosis, papillary 286
   relaxants 91
      non-depolarizing 91
Myasthenic crisis, management of 302
Mycobacterium 49
   marinum 57
Myeloma, multiple 294
Myocardial protection 284
Myopectineal orifice 341

N

Naffziger's sign 209
Nail, subungual abscess-excision of 56
Narath's hernia 341
Narrow band imaging 579
Nasogastric tube 25
Natural killer cells 107
Natural orifice transluminal endoscopic surgery 127
Nausea, postoperative 98
Neck 182
   dissection, elective 184
   extension 85
      restriction of 40
   lymph node 179, 184
      anatomy of 182
      clinical presentation of 183
      end stage 184
      groups 182t
      management of 182
      metastases, staging of 183t

Necrosis, pancreatic 242
Necrotic collection, acute 242
Necrotic tissue 34
   liberal surgical excision of 36
Necrotizing fasciitis 156
   treatment of 36, 39
Necrotizing soft-tissue infections
   management of 36
   types of 36
Needle
   biopsy 76
   decompression 134
   holder 119
Negative pressure wound closure therapy 38
Neisseria gonorrhoeae 610
Neonatal intestinal obstruction 478
   causes of 478
Nephrectomy 566, 576
   palliative 576
   partial 576
   radical 575, 576
   total 571
Nephroblastoma 578
Nephrolithiasis 552
Nephrolithotomy, percutaneous 570
Nephron sparing nephrectomy 575
Nephropathy, obstructive 562
Nerve 34
   blocks, complications of 92
   damage 93
   injuries 144
   supply 381
Nervous system, disease of 372
Neurectomy, tympanic 191
Neurilemmoma 157
Neuroblastoma 230, 231
Neuroendocrine reflex response 4
Neurofibroma 157
   types of 157
Neurofibromatosis 157, 231
Neuroma formation 34
Neuromuscular excitation 54
Neuropeptides 384
Neurotrauma 138
Neurovascular bundle, decompression of 314
Nevus
   atypical 161
   intradermal 161
   junctional 161
   sebaceous 161
Nifedipine 370
Nipple 256, 260t
   discharge 258, 263
      etiology of 260
      management of 260
      treatment of 260
   Paget's disease of 271
   retraction of 256
   sparing mastectomy 272

Nissen's fundoplacation 374f
Nitrogen
　balance 102
　equilibrium 8
Nitroglycerine 370
Nocturia 549
Nocturnal enuresis 549
Nodal metastases 270
Nodular goiter 205, 206
　clinical features of 209
　complications of 205
　management of 205
Nodule, bunching of 562
Non-anthracycline 276
　regimes 276
Non-breast disorders 259
Non-germ cell tumors 620
Non-Hodgkin's lymphoma 193, 328-330, 330t
　treatment of 332
Noninvasive breast cancer 269
　treatment of 277
Non-muscle invasive bladder cancer 587, 589
Non-seminomas 624
Non-small cell lung cancer 297
Non-surgical therapy
　application of 79
　intent of 79
Normothermia 84
Nuck canal 617
Nuclear medicine 77, 222
Nucleic acid amplification testing 611
Nutrition 26, 101
　enteral 103
　parenteral 103
Nutritional deficiency 37, 392
Nutritional support 101
　methods of 101, 103

O

Oat cell cancer 296
Obesity 129
　classification of 130t
　surgery 129, 130
　　complications of 131
　treatment of 129
Obstruction 469, 475, 568
　arterial 469
　closed loop 469, 470f
　extrahepatic biliary 445
　intestinal 468, 470, 478
　level of 425, 470
　neonatal 451
　non-malignant 492
　respiratory 206
　strangulated 469
Obstructive jaundice 235, 445–449, 449f, 450t

complications of 445
etiology of 445
pathology of 445
relief of 448
symptoms of 446
Ochsner-Sherren regimen 488, 489
Octreotide 405
Oddi's sphincter 433
Odynophagia 365
Off-pump coronary artery surgery 286
Ofloxacin 49
Olaparib 279
Omental torsion 360
Omeprazole 390
Open head injuries 138
Ophthalmopathy 208
Opiate drugs, epidural 95
Opioid 94
　analgesia 94
Oral cancer 176, 177, 179
　distribution of 177
　premalignant lesions of 177
Oral hypoglycemic agents 84
Orchidectomy 597, 623
Organ
　failure 239
　transplantation 108, 109, 111
Organisms, exogenous 45
Oropharyngeal cancer 175, 176
　staging of 177
Oropharyngeal carcinoma 177
　treatment of 177
Orthotopic liver transplantation 112, 423, 428
Osmolarity 105
Osteomyelitis 56
Oxalate stones 567
Oxygen 24
　humidified 24
Oxyphil cell 215

P

Pacemakers 84
Packed red cells 18
Paclitaxel 276
Paget's disease 271
Pain 365, 569, 574
　abdominal 390
　acute 25
　chest 365
　chronic 94
　control of 95
　ischemic 306
　neuropathic 94
　nociceptive 94
　postoperative neuropathic 95
　psychogenic 95
　recurrent 565
　relief of 25, 88
　severe 56
　treatment of 95, 245

Palate procedures, secondary 172
Palatoplasty 171
Palbociclib 279
Palliation 251, 280, 379, 403
Palliative therapy 80, 423
Pallor 312
Palmar spaces 59f
Pancreas 233
　anatomy of 233
　annular 236
　cystic neoplasms of 247
　divisum 236
　embryology of 233
　functions of 234
　neuroectodermal tumors 252
　pseudocyst of 243
　tumors of 246
Pancreatic cancer 251
　development of 248t
　staging of 249
Pancreatic carcinoma 247
　precursor lesions of 248
　TNM staging of 249t
Pancreatic disease 235
Pancreatic duct system 234f
Pancreatic function tests 235
Pancreatic intraepithelial neoplasia 248
Pancreatic neuroendocrine tumors 246, 252
　classification of 252
Pancreatic stone 246f
　retrieval 246f
Pancreaticoduodenectomy 405, 444
Pancreatitis 238
　acute 238, 239, 239t, 241, 434
　chronic 236, 244
　clinical features of 233
　etiology of 238
　management of 233
　prognosis of 233
Pantaprazole 390
Papillomas 562
Papillotomy 443
Para typhi 439
Paracetamol 93, 95, 326
Paraganglioma syndrome, familial 231
Paralytic ileus 469, 472, 472
Paramesonephric duct 550
Paraneoplastic syndrome 574
Paraphimosis 605
　clinical features of 604
　investigations of 604
　management of 604
Parathormone 75
Parathyroid 201, 220
　applied anatomy of 220
　carcinoma 224
　disorders 222
　glands 202

Park's classification 531, 532f
Parkland formula 24
Parona's space 58
Paronychia 56
    acute 56
    chronic 56
Parotid abscess 190
    diagnosis of 190
    management of 190
Parotid disorders 188
Parotid duct 187, 189
Parotidectomy
    complications of 194
    congestive 194
    extracapsular partial 194
    radical 194
    types of 194
Parotitis
    acute bacterial 190
    chronic 191
Pasteurella multocida 57
Patent ductus arteriosus 289
Peak acid output test 384
Peau d'orange 256
Pelvic abscess 356
    clinical features of 356
    etiopathology of 356
    management of 356
Pelvic floor 543
Pelvicalyceal calculi 566
Pelvicalyceal system 553
Pelvirectal fistula 533
Pelvis 487, 556
Pelviureteral junction 563
Pelviureteric obstruction, idiopathic 565
Pendulum movement 149
Penicillin 48
Penile carcinoma 608
    clinical features of 607
    pathology of 606
    staging of 606
Penile intraepithelial neoplasia 606
Penile lesions, premalignant 606
Penis 604
Pentagastrin test 384, 405
Peptic ulcer 388, 390, 391, 394
    acute perforation of 392
    benign 397
    chronic 394
    complications of 388, 392
    disease 363, 380
        clinical features of 386
        etiology of 386
        investigations of 386
        management of 386
    distribution of 389f
    medical treatment of 390
    pathology of 388
    surgical treatment 390
    treatment of 390

Peptides 384
Perforations, esophageal 366
Perforator ligation 322
Perianal abscess
    drainage of 530f
    investigations of 530
    treatment of 530
Pericarditis, constrictive 284
Peripheral nerve blocks 94
Peripheral vascular disease 83
Peristalsis
    primary 364
    secondary 364
Peritoneal abscess 355
    drainage of 356f
Peritoneal lavage, diagnostic 409
Peritoneum 337, 349
    functions of 349
Peritonitis 349-351, 351f, 352
    acute 349, 355
    chronic tuberculous 354
    clinical features 351
    generalized 351
    localization of 350
    postoperative 352
    primary 349, 350
    secondary 349
    special types of 352
    spontaneous bacterial 350
    tertiary 350
    tuberculous 354
Pertuzumab 268, 276
Petal flap 41f
Peutz-Jeghers syndrome 398, 464
Phalanx, prevent osteomyelitis of 56
Phantom limb 316
Pharyngoesophageal junction 368
Phenobarbitone 54
Phenols 116
Phenoxybenzamine 232
Pheochromocytoma 230, 231
    adrenal 232f
    hereditary 231
Phimosis 604
    clinical features of 606
    investigations of 606
    management of 606
Phlebectomy 321
Phlegmasia
    alba dolens 322
    cerulea dolens 322
Phosphate stones 567
Phrygian cap 435
Phyllodes
    benign 265
    tumor 265
Physiotherapy 148
Pierce Gould's operation 608
Pigment stones 436, 437, 438
Pilomatrixoma 161

Pilonidal sinus 533, 534, 534f
    Bascom procedure for 535f
Piperacillin tazobactam 27
Plasma
    half life 203
    levels 203t
    substitutes 20
    volume expanders 20
Plasmacytoma 294
Platelet 18
Pleura, mesothelioma of 293
Pleural abrasion 150
Pleural diseases 291
Pleural effusion 291
    malignant 291
Pleurectomy 150
Plummer's disease 208
Pneumatosis cystoides intestinalis 462
Pneumonitis 148
Pneumoperitoneum 124, 127
Pneumothorax 134, 149
Polycystic kidney disease
    adult 551
    autosomal dominant 551
Polycystic liver disease 552
Polymicrobial infection 156
Polypectomy, endoscopic 503
Polypeptide, pancreatic 252
Polypoid colonic carcinoma 521f
Polyposis
    familial adenomatous 516
    syndromes, hereditary 516
Polyps 515
    colorectal 515, 516
    hyperplastic 397, 515
    neoplastic 515
Popliteal vein 317
Porta caval shunts 428
Portal hypertension 413, 424, 425, 428
    etiology of 425, 425t
    etiopathogenesis of 425
    management of 426
    surgery for 428
    treatment of 426
Portal pressure, reduce 428
Portal vein 429
    embolization 422
Portosystemic disconnection,
    emergency 428
Portosystemic shunts 429t
    emergency 428
    types of 429f
Port-wine stain 158
Positive end expiratory pressure 91
Positron emission tomography 400
    scanning 77
Post-inflammatory destructive phase 33
Postoperative pain
    management 94
    treatment of 94

Post-orchiectomy 621f
Postsplenectomy infection, opportunistic 410
Post-thrombotic syndrome, prevention of 323
Potassium 105
　permanganate 116
　thiocyanate 211
Praecox 325
Pregabalin 95
Pre-gangrene 306
Pregnancy 554
Premalignant disease 388
Pressure
　arterial 318
　control ventilation 91
　intracranial 138
　sore
　　stages 38
　　treatment of 39
Prilocaine 92
Primary hemorrhoids 537f
　management of 536
　morphology of 537
Pringle maneuver 415
Proctitis 495
Proctocolectomy 493
Proctocolitis 495
Proctoscopy 510
Progesterone receptors 268
Prolapsed rectum
　clinical diagnosis of 542
　differential diagnosis of 542
　etiology of 542
　etiopathogenesis of 542
　investigations of 543
　management of 542
　morphology of 542f
　pathogenesis of 543
　treatment of 543
　types of 542
Prone Jackknife position 85
Propofol 89
Propranolol 232, 428
Prostate 547-549, 563, 582, 590
　applied anatomy of 590
　cancer 597
　digital rectal examination of 547, 582, 590, 598
　disorders of 547, 582, 590
　hormonal physiology of 591
　lobes of 590
　transperineal template biopsies of 580
　zones of 590
Prostatectomy 593
　radical 596
Prostatic carcinoma
　spread of 595
　staging of 596

Prostatic hyperplasia, benign 590, 591, 592
Prostatitis
　acute 594
　chronic 594
Prosthetic valve
　dysfunction 287
　types of 287
Protein 103
　acute phase 6
　metabolism 6
Proteoglycans 33
Proteolysis 7
Proteus 49
Prothrombin complex concentrate 19
Proton pump 384
　inhibitor 390
Protrusions, mucosal 515
Pseudoachalasia 369
Pseudoaneurysm 159
Pseudocyst 239, 243
　external drainage of 244
　sites of 243
Pseudohypoparathyroidism 221
Pseudomembranous colitis 48
Pseudomonas 36, 49, 51, 156
Pseudomyxoma peritonei 360, 490, 490f
Pseudo-obstruction 472
　intestinal 472
Psoas abscess 361
Psychological therapy 280
Pulmonary function test 83
Pulsation, arterial 306
Pulse
　oximetry 25
　rate 140, 209
Pulsion diverticula 368
Punch biopsy 76, 259
Pure cholesterol stone 437f
Purpura 394
Pus
　drainage of 50
　incision of 50
　release of 56
Pyelonephritis 554
　acute 553
　chronic 554, 559
　emphysematous 555
　xanthogranulomatous 555
Pyeloplasty 565
　non-dismembered 565f
　principles of 565
Pyelotomy, intubated 565
Pyemia, portal 418
Pylephlebitis 418
Pyloric stenosis 395
　physiological consequences of 395
Pyloroplasty 391, 391f, 394
Pyonephrosis 553, 566, 572

Pyrexia 486
Pyridostigmine 302
Pyuria, abacterial 560

Q

Quadrantectomy 272
Quinolones 49

R

Racial predisposition 328
Radiation 35, 116, 293
　burns 21, 28
　ionizing 116, 267
　therapy 298, 563
Radical mastectomy, modified 265, 273
Radical neck dissection 180, 183
　modified 179, 183
　types of 183
Radical orchiectomy, inguinal 623
Radical resections 401, 526
Radical surgery 78, 252, 293, 401
　indications for 377
Radio isotope 77
Radioactive iodine ablation 211
Radioactive medical waste, disposal of 122
Radiofrequency ablation 298, 321
Radiography
　contrast 76
　interventional 415
Radioiodine ablation therapy 217
Radioisotope 433
Radiology 412, 503
　role of 412
Radionuclide studies 286
Radiotherapy 79, 166, 178, 180, 184, 232, 274, 278, 377, 379, 601, 608
　curative 608
　palliative 95
　primary 180
　radical 597
Raised intracranial pressure 138
Ramstedt's pyloromyotomy 387
Randomized controlled trials 65, 67
Ranson's criteria 241t
Ranula 188
　simple 188
　types of 188
Rapid sequence induction 90
Raynaud's disease 312, 312t
　differential diagnosis of 312
　treatment of 312
Raynaud's phenomena 312
Raynaud's syndrome 312
Rectal biopsy, full thickness 493
Rectal cancer 527
　chemoradiation for 528

Rectal carcinoma 522, 525*f*, 526*t*
    clinical features of 525*t*
    complications of 525, 525*t*
    differential diagnosis of 525*t*
    treatment of 524
Rectal disease, symptoms of 508
Rectal examination 510*f*
Rectal injuries 514
    mechanism of 514
Rectal resections 526
    resection of 526
    restorative 527
Rectopexy 544
Rectum 505, 507*f*
    abdominoperineal resection of 527*f*
    anatomy of 505, 507*f*
    congenital anomalies of 451, 505
    development of 506*f*
    differentiation of 492, 510, 511*f*, 592, 596
    embryology of 505, 506*f*
    lymphatic drainage of 508, 510*f*, 524
    prolapse of 542, 542*t*
    surgical anatomy of 505
    tumors of 515
    venous
        anatomy of 536*f*
        drainage of 508, 509*f*
Refeeding syndrome 104
Reflux 365
    esophagitis 372
    gastritis 387
Regional chemotherapy, high dose 165
Regurgitation
    aortic 288
    mitral 287
Rehabilitation 143, 148, 280, 316, 365
Renal agenesis
    bilateral 550
    unilateral 550
Renal calculi 547
    clinical features of 547
    investigations of 547
    management of 547
Renal carbuncle 554
Renal cell carcinoma 573-575
    clinical features of 574
    staging of 574, 575*t*, 576*f*
    TNM staging of 577*t*
    treatment of 575, 576*t*
Renal cystic masses, Bosniak classification of 579
Renal disease 82, 83, 84
    end-stage 552
Renal failure 87, 559
Renal insufficiency 35
Renal parenchyma, acute suppurative inflammation of 553

Renal system 12
Renal transplantation 113*f*, 552
Renal trauma 581
Renal tuberculosis 611
    clinical diagnosis of 556
    management of 556
    pathogenesis of 556
    pathology of 556, 557*f*
Renal tubular
    acidosis 571
    syndromes 568
Renal tumors 547, 573
    clinical features of 547
    investigations of 547
    malignant 573
    management of 547
Renal vein, Doppler study of 575
Replacement fluid, types of 106
Respiration, irregular 138, 142
Respiratory system 12, 82
Resuscitation 13, 426
    cardiopulmonary 135
    emergency 414
    end points of 14
    monitoring of 25
    principles of 10
Retention, acute 593
Retromandibular vein 186
Retromolar pad 182
Retromolar trigone 182
Retroperitoneal pathology 361, 563
Retroperitoneum 337, 361, 487
    primary tumors of 361
Retrosternal nodule 213*f*
    signs of 210
Reynold pentad 447
Rhomboid flap reconstruction, steps of 534*f*
Rib fractures 148
Richter's hernia 341
Riedel's thyroiditis 210, 212, 213
Rifampicin 439
Risus sardonicus 54
Robotic laparoscopic surgery 127
Rocuronium 90
Root cause analyses 99
Ropivacaine 92
Roundworm, surgical complications of 461
Routine diagnostic testing 82
Roux-en-Y gastric bypass 131, 131*t*
Rovsing operation 552
Rovsing theory 438
Rutherford's classification 305, 305*t*
Rutherford's Morrison's pouch 118

S

Sac, coverings of 338
Sacral vertebrae, counting of 513
Sacrococcygeal teratoma 514

Sacrococcygeal, pilonidal sinus of 533, 534
Safe general surgery 88, 99
    principles of 99
Safe surgery saves lives 99
Saint's triad 438, 493
Saliva, secretion of 186
Salivary calculi 189
    submandibular 189
Salivary gland 186
    disorders of 187
    minor 187
    parotid 186
    primary malignancies of 195
    submandibular 187, 188
    surgical anatomy of 186
    tumors 192, 193*t*
        classification of 192
Salivary tumors
    benign 193, 229
    clinical features of 192
    excision of 195
    sublingual 193
    submandibular 193
Salmon patch 158
Salmonella typhi 439
Sandy patches 562
Saphenopopliteal junction ligation 321
Saphenous vein, short 317
Sarcomas 50, 246
    classification of 168
    retroperitoneal 168, 361
Savory-Miller classification 373
    reflux esophagitis 372
Scalenus anticus syndrome 313
Scar
    formation 33
    immature 39
    management 26
    mature 39
Schistosomiasis 561, 562
Sclerotherapy 538
    catheter directed 320, 321
    injection 539
Scratch test 395
Scrotal gangrene, idiopathic 615
Scrotum 604
    acute 612, 613
    tumors of 623
Scuff 43
Sebaceous horn 160
Secreto-motor function 381
Segmental grafts, types of 112
Selective neck dissection 184
    types of 184
Seminoma 620, 624
Sengstaken-Blackmore tube 427
Senile keratosis 160
Sentinel lymph node 273, 274
    biopsy 164, 259
    application of 274

Sepsis 22, 27
   cryptoglandular 529
   extrarenal 566
   pelvic 529
   severe 7
   syndrome 7
Septic shock 7, 10, 15
   treatment of 15
Septicemia 50
Sertoli cell tumor 620
Serum amylase 234
   elevation of 234
Serum gonadotrophic hormone 610
Sestamibi scan 222
Sheath 125
Shock 10, 10t, 12, 14, 15, 408
   cardiogenic 10, 11
   classification of 11
   clinical features of 10
   distributive 10, 11, 13
   end results of 13
   forms of 15
   hemorrhagic 11, 146
   hypovolemic 10, 11, 146
   inflammatory mediators of 12
   management of 13
   neurogenic 10
   obstructive 10, 11, 15
   pathophysiology of 10, 12
   prognosis of 10, 16
   septic 7, 10, 15
   severity of 12, 13, 13t
   treatment of 16
   types of 10, 12, 14
Short gut
   consequences of 466
   syndrome 451, 466, 466t
Short-stay surgery centers 96
Sialadenitis
   acute 190
      submandibular 190
   chronic submandibular 190
   granulomatous 192
   submandibular 189
Sialadenosis 192
Sialography 189
Sialorrhea, causes of 187
Sialosis 192
Sigmoid
   after resection, continuity of 474
   colon, volvulus of 473
   volvulus 473, 473f, 474f
Sigmoidectomy 544
Single incision laparoscopic surgery 127
Sinusography 76
Sistrunk's operation 204, 326
Sjögren's syndrome 192
Skene's glands 590

Skin 162, 166
   adnexa 155
   benign lesions of 160, 161
   defects 40
   erythema of 156
   function of 155
   grafts 40
      partial thickness 40
   infections of 155, 156
   malignant
      melanoma of 162
      tumors of 165
   nodules 456
   pigmented lesions of 161
   retraction of 256
   sparing mastectomy 273
      indications for 273
   tumors of 155
Sleeping pulse 209
Small bowel
   bleed 502
   enema 457
   malignant tumors of 464
Small cell lung cancer 296
Small intestinal
   pseudo-obstruction 472
   tumors 464
Small intestine
   anatomy of 451
   disorders of 451
   function of 452
Smear cytology 76
Soave's procedure 493
Sodium 105
Soft tissue
   injury 143, 144
      management of 144
      severity grades of 143
      treatment of 144
      types 143
   sarcomas 168
   total rupture of 143
   trauma 143
   tumors, malignant 167
Solid lump 265
Solid organ transplantation 108
Solitary nodule, differential diagnosis of 219
Solitary thyroid nodule 218t, 219
Somatostatinoma 253
Sonomammography 258
Southampton score 47
Speech 171
Spence axillary tail 256
Sperm banking 623
Spermatocele 618
Spermatogenesis 612
Sphincter 590
   esophageal 368, 369
   external 531

Sphincterotomy, endoscopic 443
Spider nevi 158
Spinal anesthesia 92
   complications of 92
Spine 487
Spirochaeta vincenti 185
Spironolactone 228
Spleen 328, 406
   applied anatomy of 406
   functions of 407
Splenectomy 410
   complications of 410
   emergency 410
   indications for 410t
Splenic anatomy 406f
Splenic rupture 408, 408t
   clinical features of 408
   complications of 408
   diagnosis of 408
   etiology of 408
   signs of 408
Splenic surgery, complications of 410
Splenic trauma 409
   classification of 409, 409t
   clinical diagnosis of 409
   management of 409
Splenic vein 429 429
Splenunculi 407
Sporadic gastrinoma, primary 405
Squamous cell carcinoma 166, 167, 167t, 179, 182, 197, 578
   management of 166
   oropharyngeal 178t
Stab wound 44, 71
Staghorn calculi, bilateral 572
Staghorn calculus 571
Staphylococcal whitlow 57
Staphylococcus 56, 156
   aureus 36, 51, 52, 56
   epidermidis 48
Stapled hemorrhoidopexy, principles of 539
Starch iodine test 191
Stasis 568
Stellwag's sign 209
Stelzner Corpus cavernosum recti 537
Stem cell
   therapy 311
   transplantation 332
Stenosis
   abnormal connections of 289
   aortic 287
   congenital 289
Stensen's duct, stricture of 189
Sterilization 115, 125
   methods of 115
   physical 115
Sternotomy 147
Steroid 35, 37, 458

Stomach 363, 380, 381
    acute dilatation of 397
    anatomy of 363, 380f
    applied anatomy of 380
    arterial supply of 380, 380f
    blood supply of 380f
    contents 383
    disorders of 380
    investigations of 384
    lymphatic drainage of 382
    nerve supply of 381f
    physiology of 363, 380
    structure of 381
    surgical physiology of 383
    tumors of 403
    venous drainage of 381
Stones 549, 571
    clinical features of 442
    management of 442
    medical treatment of 571
    pathology of 442
Strawberry
    gallbladder 442
    nevus 157
Streptococcus 56
    pyogenes 36, 51
    viridans 52
Stress 101
    echocardiography 286
    free peri-operative care 8
    gastritis 388
    incontinence 549
    test 286
    ulcers 395
Stroke 87
Stroma 522
    fibrous 256
Stylohyoid muscles 186
Subclavian artery 313
Subfascial endoscopic perforator surgery 126
Submucous lipoma 477f
Subphrenic abscesses 356, 357f, 358
    etiology of 357t
    treatment of 358
Subphrenic spaces 356, 356f
    anatomy of 357t
Sunitinib 168, 465
Suppurative flexor tenosynovitis 57, 58t
    complications of 58
    pathophysiology of 57
    treatment of 58
Supraclavicular node 399
Surgery 68, 144, 227, 293
    bariatric 124, 129, 130f, 131f
    basis of 129
    cytoreductive 403
    elective 495
    emergency 8, 69, 410, 414, 441

general 68
immediate 371
indications for 460
laparoscopic 126
open 284
palliative 251, 293, 378, 402, 527
preparation for 286
radical 78, 252, 293, 401
reconstructive 78
role of 78, 283, 288, 293
thoracoscopic 147, 150
types of 84
Surgical emergency, acute 156
Surgical infection 45, 48
    antimicrobial treatment of 48
    microbiology of 47
Surgical jaundice 445, 449
    etiology of 446f
    management of 445
    pre-treatment of 448
Surgical site infection 47, 84, 87
    classification of 47
    development of 46
    prophylaxis of 84
Surgical wounds 46
    classification of 46t
Suture material, types of 37
Suxamethonium 90
Swallowing 170, 172, 365
    physiology of 364
Sweat glands tumors, benign 161
Swellings
    inguinal 617
    scrotal 617
Swenson's operation 493
Swiss roll cake procedure 327
Sympathectomy 310
Synacthen test 229
Syncope, local 312
Syndrome of inappropriate antidiuretic hormone 142
Syphilis 185
Systemic inflammatory response syndrome 5, 7, 15
    pathogenesis of 5

T

Tachycardia 140
Tamoxifen 277
Tamponade 135
    pericanalicular 151
Tarda 325
Taxane 276
Tazobactam 53
T-cell
    cytotoxic 108
    receptor 108
Teicoplanin 49
Telescope 124
Tenesmus 508

Tenosynovitis 57
Tension
    free repair 344
    interfacial 438
    pneumothorax 133, 150
    repairs 344
Teratoma 620
Terminal ileum 452, 466
Terminal pulp space abscess 56
Testicular feminization syndrome 619
Testicular germ cell tumors, malignant 620
Testicular torsion, types of 613, 614f
Testicular tumors 622t, 623t
    clinical diagnosis of 621
    management of 621
    risk stratification of 622
    staging of 621
    TNM classification of 621f
    treatment of 622, 623, 624t
Testis 604, 610, 620
    acute torsion of 613
    descended 610
    development of 609
    ectopic 609
    incinerated 620
    indecent 620
    industrial 620
    infertile 620
    inflamed 620
    inheritance 619
    irradiated 620
    maldescent of 609
    retractile 609, 609t, 610
    scrotal 609
    torsion of 613, 614
    tumors of 604, 619, 620, 620t
    undescended 609, 609t
Testosterone, deficiency of 266
Tetanolysin 53
Tetanospasmin 53
Tetanus
    early 54
    immunoglobulin 54
    management of 54
    pathogenesis of 53t
    prophylaxis 25
    severe 54
    toxins 53
    toxoid 55
    treatment of 53
Tetany, differential diagnosis of 221
Therapeutic groin dissection 608
Thiazide diuretics 568
Thimble bladder 558, 558t
Thoracic aorta, disruption of 150
Thoracic aortic aneurysms 285
Thoracic outlet syndrome 312, 313f
Thoracic trauma 151
Thoracotomy 147
    emergency 147

Thromboangiitis obliterans 311
Thrombocytopenia 18
Thromboembolism, venous 26
Thrombophlebitis 86
Thrombotic complications 86
Thumb, long flexor of 59
Thymoma 301
　Masaoka staging system for 302
Thyroglobulin 203
Thyroglossal cyst 201, 204
　positions of 204f
　treatment of 204
Thyroid 201
　antibodies 207
　cancers
　　incidence of 214
　　treatment of 217
　carcinoma 216, 216t
　　papillary 214
　development of 201
　disorders 207
　　congenital 203
　　investigations of 206
　ectopic 201, 203
　embryology of 201, 201f
　function 75, 203, 206, 206t
　gland
　　enlargement of 205
　　physiology of 202
　hormones 203
　　half-life of 203t
　imaging recording and data system 207
　lobectomy 211, 213
　malignancies 214
　median ectopic 204
　neoplasms, classification of 214, 214t
　peroxidase 213
　　enzyme 203
　scintiscan 207
　stimulating antibodies 206
　storm 211
　swellings
　　diagnosis of 206
　　etiopathogenesis of 205
Thyroidectomy 213
　completion 214
　subtotal 207, 213
　total 207, 213
Thyroiditis 205, 210, 212
　acute granulomatous 212
　chronic lymphocytic 213
　subacute granulomatous 205
Thyrotoxic crisis 211
Thyrotoxic ophthalmopathy 209
Thyrotoxicosis 11, 208
　primary 208, 210, 210t, 211
　secondary 208, 210, 210t
　treatment of 211

Thyroxine 217
　replacement, lifelong 207
Tidy wound 35
Tissue
　elasticity of 43
　subcutaneous 160
　transfer, types of 40
　trauma 33
　types of 40
Toilet mastectomy 273
Tongue, large 185
Tonic muscle spasm, stage of 54
Torsion
　complications of 613
　testis, clinical features of 614
Total anomalous pulmonary venous
　　drainage 289
Total parenteral nutrition 26, 104
Total prolapse 542
　surgery for 543
　treatment of 543
Toxic adenoma 206, 208, 209, 219
Toxic goiter 205-207, 209
　causes of 207
　etiopathogenesis of 322
　exophthalmic 207
Toxic megacolon 496, 498
Toxic multinodular goiter 208
Toxic nodular goiter
　diagnosis of 208
　management of 208
　treatment of 211
Toxicity 49
　signs of 209
Toxins, bacterial 469
Trachea 206
Tracheal fixity 210
Tracheal obstruction, release of 213
Tracheoesophageal fistula 370
　types of 370, 371f
Tracheostomy, emergency 53
Traction diverticulum 368
Tramadol 95
Transabdominal restorative resections 526
Transanal endoscopic microsurgery 527
Transanal minimally invasive surgery 527
Transcatheter arterial embolization, emergency 394
Transcatheter interventional aortic
　　valve implantation 288
Transhepatic cholangiography,
　　percutaneous 434, 448
Trans-hiatal total esophagectomy 378
Transjugular intrahepatic
　　portosystemic shunt 428
Transluminal angioplasty,
　　percutaneous 310

Transperitoneal drainage 489
Transplantation
　ethics of 113
　heterotopic 112
　types of 109
Trastuzumab 268, 276, 277
Trauma 3, 133, 410, 583
　care 134
　chest 145, 148
　head 139
　impact of 7
　implications of 134t
　occurrence of 138
　primary 138
　repetitive 34
Trematode, treatment of 562
Trench mouth 185
Trendelenburg operation 320, 321
Trichilemmoma 161
Trichoepithelioma 161
Tricyclic antidepressants 95
Trocar 125
Trousseau' sign 250, 447
Truncal vagotomy 390
T-tube cholangiogram 444
Tube thoracostomy 146, 150
Tubercles, fusion of 562
Tuberculosis 37, 50, 293, 566
　abdominal 354
　general pathology of 354
　genitourinary 556
　hyperplastic 459
　ileocecal 491
　intestinal 459
　renal 611
　ulcerative 459
Tuberous sclerosis 161
Tubo-ovarian mass 491
Tuboembryonic cyst 204
Tumors 163, 395, 549
　accurate staging of 588
　aggressive 277
　behavior of 177
　benign 157, 420, 464, 515, 573
　　papillary 587
　carcinoid 464
　chemosensitive 362
　childhood 578
　debulking of 252
　deep lobe 194
　desmoid 168
　diagnosis 278
　distribution of 375
　extra-adrenal 232
　glomus 158
　growth, gompertzian curve of 77
　hyperfunctioning 230
　interstitial 620
　invasion, local 399
　larger 197

Index

malignant 192, 193, 197
markers 75, 250, 432
mesenchymal 246, 464
metastatic 193, 423
mixed 194
mucinous cystic 247
multiple 177
neuroendocrine 297
node metastasis stage 249
nonresectable 423
odontogenic 172
pancreatic 246
parotid 192
pathology 622
primary 270, 301, 301t, 361, 608
renal 547, 573
retroperitoneal 361
secondary 361
soft 157
spread of 248, 399, 620
stromal 193
superficial lobe 194
suppressor genes, inactivation of 587
Typhoid
  perforation 461
  surgical complications of 460
Tyrosine 203
  kinase inhibitor 80, 465

U

Ulcerative carcinoma cecum 521f
Ulcerative colitis 456, 456t, 495, 498
  extracolonic manifestations of 495
  investigations of 496
  pathology of 495
  severity of 496t
  treatment of 496
Ulcerogenic disorders 385
Ulcers 37
  acute 390
  chronic 37
  dental 185
  diabetic 37
  duodenal 388, 394, 395
  herpetic 185
  jejunal 388, 392
  oral 185
  painless 185
  peptic 388, 390, 391, 394
  tuberculous 185
Ulnar bursa 59
Ultrasonography 76, 206, 227, 432
  abdominal 447
  laparoscopic 434
  testicular 622
Ultrasound
  endoscopic 400, 447
  guided foam sclerotherapy 321
Umbilical nodule 399

Undescended testis 609, 609t
  applied anatomy of 604, 609
  clinical features of 604, 609
  investigations of 604, 609
  tumors of 604, 609
Upper abdominal surgery 126
Upper biliary obstruction 448
Upper gastrointestinal bleeding 427
  differential diagnosis of 394
  etiology of 427t
Upper urinary tract 512
  calculus, elective treatment of 570
  obstruction, causes of 563t
  stones, treatment of 569
  tuberculosis of 556, 556t
  urolithiasis of 569
Ureidopenicillins 49
Ureter 547, 548, 556, 569
  ectopic 553
  retrocaval 563
Ureterocoele 552
Ureteroscopy 570, 579
  complications of 570
Urethra 547, 548, 582, 591, 599, 601
  anatomy of 599
  bulbar 599
  female 599
  male 599, 600
  membranous 599
  penile 599
  prostatic 599
Urethral fistula 603
  causes of 603
Urethral injury, complications of 601
Urethral sphincter
  distal 590
  external 599
Urethral stones 573
Urethral strictures
  clinical features of 547, 582
  etiology of 601
  investigations of 547, 582
  pathogenesis of 601
  tumors of 547, 582
Urethral valves, posterior 599
Urethroplasty 603
  anastomotic 603
  technique of 603
Urethrostomy
  endoscopic 602
  perineal 608
Urge incontinence 549
Uric acid calculi 568
Uric acid
  lithiasis 571
  stones 567
Urinary bladder 583
  rupture of 583
Urinary calculi
  emergency treatment of 569
  primary 567
  secondary 567

Urinary cytology 579
Urinary diversion 568, 589
Urinary flow, obstruction of 568
Urinary microscopy 579
Urinary obstruction, lower 566
Urinary stones
  pathology of 568
  types of 567, 567t
Urinary stream, reduce 550
Urinary tract 550
  infection 552, 553
    causes of 559
    clinical features of 547
    investigations of 547
    lower 559
    pathological consequences of 560
    tumors of 547
  lower 582
  obstruction of 562, 563
  stones, lower 572
  surgery of 579
Urinary vanillylmandelic acid 75
Urine
  acute retention of 547, 582, 584, 585, 592
  analysis 75, 486
  chronic retention of 547, 582
  culture 75
  examination of 562
  incontinence of 585, 586
  output 25
  retention of 584
  tests 75
Urodynamic study 580, 581t
Urogenital system, embryology of 550
Urolithiasis
  clinical features of 568
  etiology of 567
  pathology of 568
  secondary 568
Uropathy, obstructive 562
Urothelial cell carcinoma 587
  bladder 587
    etiology of 587
    pathology of 587

V

VACTERL anomalies 512
Vaginal hydrocele 616
  clinical diagnosis of 616
  surgery for 617
  tumors of 616
Vagotomy 390
  selective 390, 391f
Vagus nerve 183, 363
Valentino's appendix 392
Valvular heart disease 83, 552
  surgery for 286
Vancomycin 49

Variceal bleed 428
 acute 426
 clinical features of 427
 surgery for 428
Varicocele 611, 612
 applied anatomy of 611, 604
 clinical features of 611, 604
 grading of 612
 investigations of 611, 604
 pathogenesis of 611
 tumors of 611, 604
Varicose veins 317, 321, 322
 complications of 320
 endothermal ablation of 320
 pathology of 318
 soft tissue complications of 318
 surgery for 321
Vascular injury 414
Vascular malformations 157
Vasoactive intestinal polypeptide 252
Vasodilatation, causes of 11
Vein 304, 431
 arterialization of 159
 compression of 469
 perforator 317
 wall 318
Vena cava 429
Venography, contrast 320
Venous disease
 differential diagnosis of 319
 evacuation of 320
Venous drainage 202, 508, 509f
Ventilation 91
 artificial 91
 inadequacy of 86
Ventricular septal defects 290
Veress' needle 125
Vermiform appendix 483
 diseases of 483
Verucous carcinoma, pathology of 166
Vesical calculus
 primary 572
 secondary 572
Vesicoureteric reflux 558, 559t
Vessels 249
 abnormal connections of 289
Video-assisted thoracoscopic surgery 298
Vincent's angina 185
Virchow's triad 322
Vitamin K antagonists 89
Vocational therapy 280
Volume control ventilation 91

Volvulus 474
 neonatorum 473
 primary 473
 secondary 473
Vomiting 244
 postoperative 98
Von Graefe's sign 209
Von Hippel-Lindau syndrome 231
von Recklinghausen's disease 157

W

Waldeyer's rings 175, 175f
Wallace's rule of 9 22, 22t
Walled off necrosis 242
War injury 136
Warm nodules 207
Warthin's tumor 193
Warts
 seborrheic 41f
 viral 161
Waste
 anatomical 121
 cytostatic 120
 cytotoxic 120
 general 120
 genotoxic 120
 hazardous 120
 hospital 120, 122
 infectious 120
 medical 120
 offensive 121
 pharmaceutical 120
 radioactive 120
 sharps 122
 treatment, types of 122
Water intoxication 593
WDHA syndrome 253
Webspace abscess 57
Wedge biopsy 76, 607
Weight loss 250, 466
Werner-Morrison syndrome 253
Wet gangrene 306
Wharton's duct 187
Whipple's operation 251
Whipple's procedure 444
Whipple's triad 253
Wide lump excision 259, 272
Willis circle 552
Wilms' tumor 578
 clinical features of 578
 staging 578
 treatment of 578t

Winslow's foramen 478
Wolf-Chaikoff effect 205
Wolffian ducts 550
Worms, bag of 612
Wound 32, 42
 care 32, 86, 224
  mainstay of 25
 chronic 34, 37
 classification of 42, 42t
 closure 37, 86
 contaminated 35
 contraction 33
 defence 43
 dehiscence 86
  abdominal 36
 diagnostic 44
 dressing 56
 evacuation of 35
 failure, acute 36
 healing 32, 34
  acute 32
  chronic 34
  classification of 34
  early 32
  intermediate 33
  late 33
  normal 32
  phases of 32t
 infections of 45
 management 55
 mechanical 43
 nature of 138
 repair, primary 35
 suicidal 43
 surgical 46
 therapeutic 44
 tumors of 35
 types of 35, 43, 46
Wuchereria bancrofti 325

X

Xanthine stones 567
Xanthinuria 568
Xenograft 109
Xerostomia 188
Xiphisternum 117

Z

Zenker's diverticulum 368
Zipper laparostomy 242
Zollinger-Ellison syndrome 404